The Effects of Drugs on the Fetus
and Nursing Infant

Rec'd 5-14-96
H 49.95

W9-CTE-465

THE EFFECTS OF DRUGS ON THE FETUS AND NURSING INFANT

A Handbook for Health Care Professionals

J. M. FRIEDMAN, M.D., PH.D.
Professor and Head, Department of Medical Genetics
University of British Columbia
Vancouver, British Columbia

and

JANINE E. POLIFKA, PH.D.
TERIS Project Coordinator, Department of Pediatrics
University of Washington
Seattle, Washington

THE JOHNS HOPKINS UNIVERSITY PRESS
Baltimore and London

© 1996 The Johns Hopkins University Press
All rights reserved. Published 1996
Printed in the United States of America on acid-free paper
05 04 03 02 01 00 99 98 97 96   5 4 3 2 1

The Johns Hopkins University Press
2715 North Charles Street, Baltimore, Maryland 21218-4319
The Johns Hopkins Press Ltd., London

Library of Congress Cataloging-in-Publication Data

Friedman, J. M. (Jan Marshall), 1947–
The effects of drugs on the fetus and nursing infant : a handbook for
health care professionals / J. M. Friedman and Janine E. Polifka.
p. cm.
Material in this book was extracted from the TERIS database and book.
ISBN 0-8018-5345-1 (pbk. : alk. paper)
1. Fetus — Effect of drugs on — Handbooks, manuals, etc.
2. Infants (Newborn) — Effect of drugs on — Handbooks, manuals, etc.
3. Teratogenic agents — Handbooks, manuals, etc.
4. Breast milk — Contamination — Handbooks, manuals, etc.
I. Polifka, Janine E.   II. Title.
[DNLM: 1. Abnormalities, Drug-Induced — handbooks.
2. Drugs — adverse effects — handbooks.
3. Genetic Counseling — handbooks. QS 629 F911e 1996]
RG627.6.D79F75 1996
618.3′2 — dc20
DNLM/DLC
for Library of Congress   95-46371

A catalog record for this book is available from the British Library.

CONTENTS

Acknowledgments   *vii*

Introduction   *ix*

The Effects of Drugs on the Fetus and Nursing Infant   1

Appendix 1: List of Agents Available in TERIS   635

Appendix 2: Resources for Information on Pregnancy
             Exposures   645

Acknowledgments

This book is partly derived from the TERIS database, a computerized database that was initially funded by the US Public Health Service Bureau of Maternal and Child Health.

We wish to thank members of the TERIS Advisory Board, Drs. Robert Brent, Jose Cordero, James Hanson, Richard Miller, and Tom Shepard for their expertise and dedication to TERIS. All of the teratology risk ratings included in this book were developed by consensus of this distinguished group of clinical teratologists, and we have depended heavily on their help in interpreting the teratology literature.

Special thanks to Dr. Beatrice Guyard-Boileau for her advice and friendship. Her expertise as an obstetrician and consultant for CARE Northwest, a teratogen information service located at the University of Washington, were invaluable in the development of the lactation component of the summaries included in this book. Her enthusiasm and encouragement will be greatly missed when she returns to France to continue her practice.

This book would not have been possible without the help of Barbara Brownfield, who unselfishly cancelled a trip to Ireland so that we could complete the book; Jenny Nakahara, who helped proof and put the book together; and Jennifer Johnston, who did much of the library work for the book. All three spent countless hours helping to prepare this book and we are grateful for their talent and commitment.

INTRODUCTION

PURPOSE AND ORGANIZATION OF THIS BOOK

This book is intended to provide a critical assessment of information that is available regarding the fetal and neonatal risks associated with maternal use of common medications during pregnancy or lactation. The book is **not** a guide for prescribing medications and should not be used in that way.

We have included information on the teratogenicity, transplacental carcinogenesis, embryonic or fetal death, and fetal and perinatal pharmacologic effects of the most commonly used medications. We also discuss effects that maternal use of such drugs during lactation may have on the nursing infant. Information on maternal and neonatal pharmacology is not included, but is available elsewhere (Windholz et al., 1989; Gilman et al., 1990; Briggs et al., 1994; USP DI, 1995). Other aspects of reproductive toxicology such as alterations of fertility and male-mediated effects have also been excluded.

The teratology information provided consists of a condensed version of selected summaries from TERIS, a computer-based teratology information system that is available on-line, on conventional and compact disks, and as a book (Friedman & Polifka, 1994). Appendix I includes a full list of current TERIS agent summaries.

Each agent summary is based on a thorough review of published data identified through MEDLINE, TOXLINE, and DART bibliographic searches. References provided in *Chemically Induced Birth Defects* (Schardein, 1993), *Drugs in Pregnancy and Lactation: A Reference Guide to Fetal and Neonatal Risks* (Briggs et al., 1994), and the *Catalog of Teratogenic Agents* (Shepard, 1995) are also used extensively. Statements regarding the absence of published studies are made on the basis of this literature review and are true to the best of our knowledge. Unpublished studies, such as those submitted by pharmaceutical companies to regulatory agencies, are not included because their unpublished state precludes conventional peer review and assessment.

This book contains information that is intended to help in teratogen risk assessment. Descriptions of each agent and its usual dosage are given to provide perspective on the exposure in a particular patient. We have not included information on the value (or lack of value) of treatment; such considerations are outside the scope of this book.

A risk rating is printed in italics at the beginning of the section entitled "Teratogenic Risk" in each agent summary. This rating is based on a consensus of opinion among the authors and five internationally recognized authorities in clinical teratology, Drs. Robert Brent, Jose Cordero, James Hanson, Richard Miller, and Thomas Shepard. The italicized risk rating has two parts:

♦ An estimate of the magnitude of teratogenic risk to a child born after maternal exposure to the drug during pregnancy, and

♦ An assessment of the quality and quantity of the data on which the teratogenic risk estimate is based.

The risk ratings apply only to *usual conditions of exposure*. The risk may be substantially higher with unusually large exposures.

The magnitude of the teratogenic risk is rated on a standard scale as *High, Moderate, Small, Minimal, None,* or *Unlikely*. Agents are assigned a risk of *Unlikely* if available evidence suggests that a substantial teratogenic risk is unlikely to occur with usual exposures but the data are insufficient to state that there is no risk. If the available data are insufficient to decide whether or not a teratogenic risk exists, the magnitude of risk is said to be *Undetermined*. Both the likelihood of a teratogenic effect and the severity of that effect contribute to the rating of the magnitude of the risk.

In some instances, the risk rating is amplified by a comment. For example, the magnitude of teratogenic risk for an agent may be *Undetermined,* but an accompanying statement may say "a small risk cannot be excluded, but there is no indication that the risk of congenital anomalies in the children of women treated with this agent during pregnancy is likely to be great." Such statements are based on general pharmacology, animal data, or analogy to a closely related agent that has been more thoroughly studied.

In general, risks that are *Minimal* or less ought not to alter decisions regarding the continuation or termination of an exposed pregnancy. *Moderate* or *High* risks may be considered important enough to influence such decisions, at least in some cases.

A standard scale is also used to indicate the quality and quantity of the data available to make each teratogenic risk assessment. The available data may be rated as *None, Very Poor, Poor, Fair, Good,* or *Excellent.* Risk assessments based on evidence that is *Poor* or *Fair* ought to be considered tentative and liable to change as more information becomes available. Even with *Good* data, only crude estimates of the magnitude of the risk are usually possible.

The narrative summary that follows the italicized risk assessment emphasizes information from human studies. Experimental animal data are briefly summarized in the content of their application (if any) to human pregnancy. The italicized teratogenic risk assessment should always be read in the context of the discussion that follows it.

Adverse effects other than teratogenesis (e.g., alterations of perinatal adaptation or transplacental carcinogenesis) are not considered in the teratogenic risk rating but are mentioned in the following narrative. The risk to nursing infants whose mothers are taking the agent is discussed under a separate heading, "Risk Related to Breast-feeding," and does not contribute to the teratogenic risk assessment.

A few references have been selected on the basis of their quality and accessibility for inclusion with each agent summary. These references are intended to help the clinician obtain a broader understanding of the agent's effects on the embryo, fetus, and nursing infant. Proprietary names are used only for purposes of identification, and such use does not imply any recommendation regarding the agent.

ASSESSMENT AND COUNSELING OF PATIENTS FOR TERATOGENIC RISK

A pregnant woman should not take any drug unless it is necessary for her own health or that of her fetus. Even though the use of a particular drug in pregnancy may be considered safe, such safety is *never* absolute. It is impossible to be certain that a drug never causes harm to a developing embryo or fetus. There is too much normal variability in human embryogenesis and pharmacokinetics: unexpected idiosyncratic effects may occur.

A teratogen may be defined as an agent that can produce a permanent abnormality of structure or function in an organism exposed during embryonic or fetal life. Concern about teratogenic effects arises in two circumstances--inadvertent exposure and intended exposure. Inadvertent exposure occurs when a woman takes a drug after conception but before her pregnancy is recognized. This often happens when a woman unexpectedly becomes pregnant while taking a medication. *It is essential, therefore, that the teratogenic potential of any medication prescribed for a woman who is capable of having children be considered and discussed with her at the time the prescription is given.*

Intended exposure occurs when a woman takes a drug while she knows that she is pregnant. A pregnant woman should not be given any medication unless its benefit is clearly greater than the risk to both her and her fetus. In practice, it may be difficult to determine whether the risk exceeds the benefit because, although the benefit is known, the risk to the fetus is uncertain.

The purpose of teratogen risk assessment is to determine the likelihood and nature of congenital anomalies in the child of a woman who has been exposed to a particular agent (or combination of agents) during pregnancy. Teratogen risk counseling seeks to provide a patient with accurate information about the teratogenic risk in an appropriate manner so that she can more effectively participate in decisions regarding further management of the pregnancy.

Teratogen risk assessment in an individual patient requires knowledge of her state of health, previous and current pregnancy history, and family history. Sometimes other factors increase the risk on a pregnancy as much as or more than exposure to a particular drug. This must be considered when providing counseling and considering options for management.

It is always necessary to determine as accurately as possible what the route and dose of a drug exposure was and whether there were concurrent exposures to other agents. Most drugs that exhibit teratogenic effects do so only when the dose exceeds a certain threshold value. A mother who has taken a drug in an amount or by a route that produces an absorbed dose below this critical threshold is usually *not* at increased risk of having a child with congenital anomalies. On the other hand, even a drug that is considered to have no teratogenic risk with usual exposures may produce substantial fetal damage in a pregnant woman who has had a toxic exposure to the agent. This may occur, for example, when the mother has taken a large overdose of medication in a suicide attempt.

Simultaneous exposure to more than one drug may modify the associated fetal risk. Depending on the particular combination of agents, the risk may be greater or less than that of exposure to the agents individually. In practice, the effect of a combination of agents is usually unknown. In such circumstances one must use the risks associated with the individual agents to estimate the overall risk but decrease the certainty of the assessment because of the combined exposure.

Accurate assessment of when the exposure occurred is critical. The greatest risk of teratogenesis exists during the period of embryonic organogenesis (i.e., between about 18 and 60 days after conception). Before this time, malformations are unlikely to be induced, but death of the embryo can be caused by drug exposures. Later in pregnancy, fetal damage is unlikely to produce malformations but can cause death, growth retardation, disruptions, or functional deficits.

One must consider all of the information available on the agent(s), dose, route of exposure, gestational timing, and other medical factors together in order to determine whether the risk of congenital anomalies in a particular pregnancy is similar to, greater than, or less than that usually associated with exposure to the agent under consideration. In other words, one must determine if the estimated magnitude of teratogenic risk as given in the agent summaries in this book applies to the patient under consideration. *The most frequent mistake made in teratogen risk counseling is failure to recognize that the circumstances in a particular pregnancy differ from those for which a risk has been established.*

Counseling provided as the result of this comprehensive risk assessment should be tailored to each patient's intellectual, educational, psychosocial, and cultural background. The risk associated with an exposure should be presented with reference to the 5% background risk of congenital anomalies or mental retardation apparent by one year of age that attends every pregnancy. Any teratogenic risk that is recognized must be explained in qualitative as well as quantitative terms. A high risk for dental staining, for example, may be much more acceptable than a small risk of severe mental handicap. Decisions regarding prenatal diagnosis and continuation or termination of pregnancy should be made by the patient in consultation with her physician, family, and other appropriate individuals.

Counseling a pregnant woman about possible effects of an environmental or drug exposure on her developing embryo or fetus is an important component of her medical care. Such counseling should be provided by physicians and other health professionals with competence in clinical teratology. Difficult or complex cases should be referred to appropriate specialists.

ASSESSMENT AND COUNSELING OF LACTATING MOTHERS

Breast-feeding for the first six months of life has many advantages over bottle-feeding. Breast-feeding is associated with decreased infant mortality rates, lower rates of respiratory illness, gastrointestinal diseases, and better immunological protection of the baby. Breast-feeding also has psychological benefits in facilitating maternal-infant bonding.

Exposures of the baby to drugs during lactation are intentional exposures in that the mother can usually choose between nursing or formula-feeding her infant while taking medication. Breast-feeding should always be avoided whenever drug therapy presents an unacceptable risk to the developing infant. Because of their low molecular weight and lipid solubility, most drugs are excreted into breast milk. As a result, the nursing infant will receive any medication that the mother is taking. Adverse pharmacological effects in breast-fed infants are usually "dose related" or the result of idiosyncratic reaction to the drug. The question is, how much drug in the breast milk is too much for the nursing infant and what factors determine whether or not drug exposure through breast milk will present an unacceptable risk to the infant?

Unfortunately, very little epidemiological data exist to assist the health care practitioner in assessing the risks of drug exposure to the nursing infant. The majority of relevant data in the published literature is in the form of case reports that involve measurements of milk and plasma levels from individual women. Although case reports may be useful in predicting possible adverse effects associated with a drug, it is difficult to know to what extent the finding can be generalized to all nursing infants. In addition, such case reports usually include no information on the presence or absence of adverse or pharmacological effects in the nursing infant.

In many of the published case reports, milk/plasma ratios are provided as an estimate of drug distribution in the breast milk. However, because this ratio does not take neonatal factors into consideration, such as age and reduced clearance and ability to bind proteins, it is only capable of providing information about the *availability* of drug to the infant and not how much active drug is actually present in the infant's circulation. Also, milk/plasma ratios measured at a single point in time may not accurately reflect the total transfer of drug from the mother to the nursing infant. Concentrations in milk and plasma differ as a function of time because of several factors: 1) variability in maternal plasma levels relative to when the drug was taken and the milk sampled, 2) equilibrium of the maternal plasma levels related to acute or chronic exposure and consequent changes in metabolism and excretion, and 3) variability in drug excretion in the milk related to volume of distribution, interval between feedings, and maturity of milk.

Infant plasma levels are usually not measured in published case reports. Instead the infant dose is often calculated from the concentrations of drug in maternal plasma and milk. Generally, less than 5% of the maternal dose is ingested by the nursing infant on a weight-adjusted basis. It must be remembered that these doses are usually only estimates and the effect of the ingested drug may be modified by the infant's age, medical condition, and ability to metabolize and excrete the drug.

Counseling a lactating woman with a condition that requires medication is an important component of her postpartum care. Because exposures during lactation are usually intentional, it is often possible to devise a plan for drug therapy that minimizes the risks to the infant and does not unnecessarily deprive the mother and infant of the benefits of breast-feeding. Breast-feeding women should refrain from taking any medication that is not absolutely necessary. If medication is indicated, then the possible risk of adverse effects in the nursing infant must be weighed against the benefits of continued breast-feeding for the period of treatment. If the duration of treatment is short, breast-feeding can usually be resumed after treatment is completed. If chronic treatment is required, the decision may be whether or not to continue nursing. If the decision to continue breast-feeding during treatment is made and more than one drug is available that has equivalent efficacy and safety for the mother, then the drug which is safest for the baby should be used. The therapeutic dose and duration of treatment should be kept to the minimum amount that will be effective. In some cases it may be possible to reduce the transfer of drug to the nursing infant by having the mother take the medication right after breast-feeding. All breast-fed infants whose mothers are on medication should be monitored for pharmacological effects such as irritability, rash, vomiting, and diarrhea.

ESTIMATION OF THE DOSE RECEIVED BY THE NURSING INFANT

To assist clinicians in assessing the risks associated with drug therapy while breast-feeding, the dose of the drug ingested by the infant has been estimated on the basis of the drug concentration measured in the breast milk using the following formula :

$$ID = DCM \times VM$$

where ID= estimated infant dose in mg/kg/d, DCM=drug concentration measured in breast milk in mcg/mL, and VM = volume of milk ingested by the infant per day on a weight-adjusted basis. The volume of milk ingested by the nursing infant usually ranges from 600-1000 mL per day, depending on the age and size of the infant. In calculating the amount of drug received by the nursing infant, we have used a volume of 150 mL/kg/d as a standard. The estimated infant dose is then expressed as a proportion of the lowest therapeutic dose for the drug in question. Therapeutic doses are obtained from standard reference sources such as the *USP DI* (1995), *Drugdex*® System of the MICROMEDEX drug information database (Gelman & Rumack, 1995),

Martindale: The Extra Pharmacopeia (Reynolds et al., 1993), and *AHFS Drug Information* (1989). The lowest therapeutic dose for infants is used whenever possible and adjusted for weight. An infant weight of 4 kg is used for the calculations. When infant or pediatric doses are not available, the lowest therapeutic dose for adults is used after adjusting for weight, assuming that the mother weighs 64 kg.

For example, if the adult dose of a drug is 320-640 mg/d and the concentration in the breast milk is about 0.01 mg/mL, the dose a nursing infant receives would be:

$$0.01 \text{ mg/mL} \times 150 \text{ mL/kg/d} = 1.5 \text{ mg/kg/d}$$

The dose equivalent to a therapeutic dose in the infant would be:

$$\frac{320 \text{ mg/d}}{64 \text{ kg}} = 5 \text{ mg/kg/d}$$

The dose ingested by the infant would therefore be:

$$\frac{1.5 \text{ mg/kg/d}}{5 \text{ mg/kg/d}} = 0.3 \text{ or } 30\% \text{ of the lowest therapeutic dose.}$$

REFERENCES

AHFS (American Hospital Formulary Service) Drug Information. Bethesda, Md.: Board of Directors of the American Society of Hospital Pharmacists, 1989.

Briggs GG, Freeman RK, Yaffe SJ: *Drugs in Pregnancy and Lactation: A Reference Guide to Fetal and Neonatal Risk*, 4th ed. Baltimore, Md.: Williams and Wilkins, 1994.

Friedman JM, Polifka JE: *Teratogenic Effects of Drugs: A Resource for Clinicians (TERIS)*. Baltimore, Md.: The Johns Hopkins University Press, 1994.

Gelman CR, Rumack BH (eds): *Drugdex*® Information System. MICROMEDEX, Englewood, Colo. (Edition expires [11/31/95]).

Gilman AG, Rall TW, Nies AS, Taylor P: *Goodman and Gilman's The Pharmacological Basis of Therapeutics*, 8th ed. New York: Macmillan Publishing Company, 1990.

Reynolds JEF, Parfitt K, Parsons AV, Sweetman SC (eds): *Martindale: The Extra Pharmacopoeia*, 30th ed. London: Pharmaceutical Press, 1993.

Schardein JL: *Chemically Induced Birth Defects*, 2nd ed. New York: Marcel Dekker, 1993.

Shepard TH: *Catalog of Teratogenic Agents*, 8th ed. Baltimore, Md.: The Johns Hopkins University Press, 1995.

USP DI: *USP DI (USP Dispensing Information), Volume 1. Drug Information for the Health Care Professional*, 15th ed. Rockville, Md.: The US Pharmacopeial Convention, 1995.

Windholz M, Budavari S, Blumetti RF, Otterbein ES (eds): *The Merck Index*, 11th ed. Rahway, NJ: Merck and Company, 1989.

The Effects of Drugs on the Fetus and Nursing Infant

ACCUTANE® *See* Isotretinoin

ACETAMINOPHEN
(Anacin-3®, Datril®, Tylenol®)

Acetaminophen is an oral analgesic and antipyretic agent. Doses range from 325-4000 mg/d.

Teratogenic Risk

Magnitude of teratogenic
risk to child born after
exposure during gestation: None

Quality and quantity of data
on which risk estimate is based: Good

The assessment given above is based on exposure to usual thera-peutic doses of acetaminophen.
The risks of fetal toxicity or death may be substantial when the mother takes a toxic overdose of acetaminophen during pregnancy (see below).

The frequency of congenital anomalies was no greater than expected among the children of 493 and 350 women who took acetaminophen during the first trimester of pregnancy in two cohorts of one large epidemiological study (Jick et al., 1981; Aselton et al., 1985). Similarly, there was no increase in the frequency of congenital anomalies among the infants of 226 women who took acetaminophen during the first four lunar months of pregnancy or of 781 women who took this drug anytime during gestation in another large study (Heinonen et al., 1977). No association with maternal use of acetaminophen during the first trimester of pregnancy was seen among 458 infants with various congenital anomalies (Nelson & Forfar, 1971) or 298 children with congenital heart disease (Zierler & Rothman, 1985). A marginal association with maternal acetaminophen use during the first trimester of pregnancy was seen among 76 infants with gastroschisis, but this equivocal finding requires independent confirmation (Werler et al., 1992).

1

Streissguth et al. (1987) found no association between maternal use of acetaminophen during the first half of pregnancy and IQ of 421 children at four years of age.

Among 51 women who were treated for acetaminophen overdose in pregnancy in one series, there were nine spontaneous abortions or fetal deaths; six of the spontaneous abortions occurred among the 11 patients with first-trimester overdoses (Riggs et al., 1989). Thirty-two liveborn infants were delivered in this series; the only one with a congenital anomaly was a child with positional deformity of the feet whose mother had taken an overdose of acetaminophen at 30 weeks gestation. All five infants born to mothers who had taken acetaminophen overdoses in the first trimester of pregnancy appeared normal at birth. In another series of 41 cases of acetaminophen overdose in pregnancy, there was one infant with cleft lip and palate (overdose at 28 weeks gestation), one with spina bifida occulta and strabismus (overdose at 26 weeks), and one who developed pyloric stenosis (overdose at 36 weeks) (McElhatton et al., 1990). Among 14 cases with first-trimester acetaminophen overdose in this series, there were two spontaneous abortions and 12 normal liveborn infants.

Hepatoxicity and nephrotoxicity occur as complications of acetaminophen overdosage in adults. Similar effects have been observed among infants born to women who took large therapeutic or toxic doses of acetaminophen late in pregnancy (Riggs et al., 1989; Kurzel, 1990). Fetal distress has been demonstrated in a pregnant woman who took a toxic overdose of acetaminophen in the third trimester (Rosevear & Hope, 1989).

The frequency of fetal death and eye anomalies was increased among the offspring of mice treated with 5-7.5 times the maximal human dose of acetaminophen in one investigation (Popp et al., 1979), but the clinical relevance of this observation is unknown.

Risk Related to Breast-feeding

Acetaminophen is excreted into breast milk in low concentrations. The amount of acetaminophen that the nursing infant would be expected to ingest is between 0.75-5.2% of the lowest infant therapeutic dose, based on data from seven lactating women (Blitzen et al., 1981; Notarianni et al., 1987).*

A case of skin rash was observed in one two-month-old nursing infant whose mother was taking 1 g acetaminophen for two days (Matheson et al., 1985). The rash disappeared following withdrawal of acetaminophen from the mother's system. The rash recurred when the mother again took 1 g acetaminophen two weeks later.

Both the American Academy of Pediatrics (Committee on Drugs, American Academy of Pediatrics, 1994) and the WHO Working Group on Drugs and Human Lactation (1988) consider it safe to use acetaminophen during breast-feeding.

Key References

Aselton PA, Jick H, Milunsky A, et al.: First-trimester drug use and congenital disorders. Obstet Gynecol 65:451-455, 1985.

Bitzen P-O, Gustafsson B, Jostell KG, et al.: Excretion of paracetamol in human breast milk. Eur J Clin Pharmacol 20:123-125, 1981.

Committee on Drugs, American Academy of Pediatrics: The transfer of drugs and other chemicals into human milk. Pediatrics 93(1):137-150, 1994.

Heinonen OP, Slone D, Shapiro S: *Birth Defects and Drugs in Pregnancy.* Littleton, Mass.: John Wright-PSG, 1977, pp 286-288, 434.

Jick H, Holmes LB, Hunter JR et al.: First-trimester drug use and congenital disorders. JAMA 246:343-346, 1981.

Kurzel RB: Can acetaminophen excess result in maternal and fetal toxicity? South Med J 83(8):953-955, 1990.

Matheson I, Lunde PKM, Notarianni LJ: Infant rash caused by paracetamol in breast milk? Pediatrics 76:651-652, 1985.

McElhatton PR, Sullivan FM, Volans GN, Fitzpatrick R: Paracetamol poisoning in pregnancy: An analysis of the outcomes of cases referred to the Teratology Information Service of the National Poisons Information Service. Hum Exp Toxicol 9:147-153, 1990.

*This calculation is based on the following assumptions: maternal dose of acetaminophen: 0.5-1 g; milk concentration of acetaminophen: 2-14 mcg/mL; milk intake by the nursing infant: 150 mL/kg/d; estimated dose of acetaminophen ingested by the nursing infant: 0.3-2.1 mg/kg/d; lowest infant therapeutic dose of acetaminophen: 40 mg/kg/d.

3

Nelson MM, Forfar JO: Associations between drugs administered during pregnancy and congenital abnormalities of the fetus. Br Med J 1:523-527, 1971.

Notarianni LJ, Oldham HG, Bennett PN: Passage of paracetamol into breast milk and its subsequent metabolism by the neonate. Br J Clin Pharmacol 24:63-67, 1987.

Popp RA, Sessions C, Owens S: Effect of acetaminophen in mice. Environ Mutagen 1:117, 1979.

Riggs BS, Bronstein AC, Kulig K, et al.: Acute acetaminophen overdose during pregnancy. Obstet Gynecol 74(2):247-253, 1989.

Rosevear SK, Hope PL: Favourable neonatal outcome following maternal paracetamol overdose and severe fetal distress. Case report. Br J Obstet Gynaecol 96:491-493, 1989.

Streissguth AP, Treder RP, Barr HM, et al.: Aspirin and acetaminophen use by pregnant women and subsequent child IQ and attention decrements. Teratology 35:211-219, 1987.

Werler MM, Mitchell AA, Shapiro S: First trimester maternal medication use in relation to gastroschisis. Teratology 45:361-367, 1992.

WHO Working Group on Drugs and Human Lactation. In: Bennet PN (ed). *Drugs and Human Lactation.* Amsterdam: Elsevier, 1988, pp 327-328.

Zierler S, Rothman KJ: Congenital heart disease in relation to maternal use of bendectin and other drugs in early pregnancy. N Engl J Med 313:347-352, 1985.

ACETAZOLAMIDE
(Ak-Zol®, Diamox®)

Acetazolamide is a carbonic anhydrase inhibitor used as a diuretic and in the treatment of glaucoma and certain kinds of epilepsy. Acetazolamide is also taken to prevent acute mountain sickness. The usual oral dose is 250-1000 mg/d. Oral doses up to 1500 mg/d or intravenous doses of 500-1500 mg/d are sometimes used to treat acute glaucoma.

Teratogenic Risk

*Magnitude of teratogenic
risk to child born after
exposure during gestation:*   Unlikely

Therapeutic doses of acetazolamide are unlikely to pose a sub-stantial teratogenic risk, but the data are insufficient to state that there is no risk.

Congenital anomalies were no more frequent than expected among the children of 1024 women treated with acetazolamide during pregnancy in one large epidemiological study, but only 12 of these mothers were treated during the first four lunar months of gestation (Heinonen et al., 1977). An increased frequency of malformations was observed among 28 children of women treated with acetazolamide during the first trimester of pregnancy in another study (Nakane et al., 1980), but the data presentation does not permit evaluation of the clinical significance of this association. It may have been due to factors other than the maternal acetazolamide therapy.

Acetazolamide produces an unusual and specific limb malformation when administered to rats, mice, or hamsters early in pregnancy in doses many times those used clinically (Layton & Hallesy, 1965; Layton, 1971; Scott et al., 1981; Biddle et al., 1993). These doses are often toxic to the mothers. Craniofacial and central nervous system malformations have also been reported, although less consistently, among the offspring of pregnant mice treated with acetazolamide in doses many times those used clinically (Scott et al., 1984). Fetal growth retardation, death, and axial skeletal malformations were observed with increased frequency among the offspring of pregnant rabbits treated with a few times the maximum human dose of acetazolamide (Nakatsuka et al., 1992). The relevance, if any, of these observations to the therapeutic use of acetazolamide in human pregnancy is unknown.

Risk Related to Breast-feeding

Acetazolamide is excreted into breast milk. The amount of acetazolamide that the nursing infant would be expected to ingest is approximately 5% of the lowest oral pediatric dose, based on data from a single patient (Soderman et al., 1984).* Serum concentrations meas-

---

*This calculation is based on the following assumptions: maternal dose of acetazolamide: 1g/d; milk concentration of acetazolamide: 1.3-2.1 mcg/mL; milk intake by the nursing infant: 150 mL/kg/d; estimated dose of acetazolamide by the nursing infant: 0.2-0.3 mg/kg/d; lowest oral pediatric dose of acetazolamide: 5 mg/kg/d.

ured in the infant were between 20-60% of the lowest adult therapeutic serum level.[†] No adverse effects were observed in the nursing infant at one week of age.

The American Academy of Pediatrics considers acetazolamide to be safe to use during breast-feeding (Committee on Drugs, American Academy of Pediatrics, 1994).

Key References

Biddle FG, Mulholland LR, Eales BA: Penetrance and expressivity of acetazolamide-ectrodactyly provide a method to define a right-left teratogenic gradient that differs between C57BL/6J and WB/ReJ mouse strains. Teratology 47:603-612, 1993.

Committee on Drugs, American Academy of Pediatrics: The transfer of drugs and other chemicals into human milk. Pediatrics 93:137-150, 1994.

Heinonen OP, Slone D, Shapiro S: *Birth Defects and Drugs in Pregnancy*. Littleton, Mass.: John Wright-PSG, 1977, p 495.

Layton WM Jr: Teratogenic action of acetazolamide in golden hamsters. Teratology 4:95-102, 1971.

Layton WM Jr, Hallesy DW: Deformity of forelimb in rats: Association with high doses of acetazolamide. Science 149:306-308, 1965.

Nakane Y, Okuma T, Takahashi R, et al.: Multi-institutional study on the teratogenicity and fetal toxicity of antiepileptic drugs: A report of a collaborative study group in Japan. Epilepsia 21:663-680, 1980.

Nakatsuka T, Komatsu T, Fujii T: Axial skeletal malformations induced by acetazolamide in rabbits. Teratology 45:629-636, 1992.

Scott WJ, Hirsch KS, DeSesso JM, Wilson JG: Comparative studies on acetazolamide teratogenesis in pregnant rats, rabbits, and rhesus monkeys. Teratology 24:37-42, 1981.

Scott WJ Jr, Lane PD, Randall JL, Schreiner CM: Malformations in nonlimb structures induced by acetazolamide and other inhibitors of carbonic anhydrase. Ann NY Acad Sci 429:447-456, 1984.

Soderman P, Hartvig P, Fagerlund C: Acetazolamide excretion into human breast milk. Br J Clin Pharmacol 17:599-600, 1984.

[†]Infant serum concentrations of acetazolamide: 0.2-0.6 mcg/mL; lowest adult therapeutic serum level of acetazolamide: 1 mcg/mL.

ACETISONE® *See* Cortisone

ACHROMYCIN V® *See* Tetracycline

ACITRETIN
(all-trans-etretin, Neotigasone®, Soriatane®)

Acitretin, a retinoid, is the active metabolite of etretinate. Acitretin is given orally in doses of 10-75 mg/d to treat psoriasis. Therapy with acitretin rather than etretinate is usually recommended for women of child-bearing age because the half-life for elimination of acitretin from the body is 50-60 hours while that of etretinate is 100-120 days (Pilkington & Brogden, 1992; Geiger et al., 1994).

Teratogenic Risk

Magnitude of teratogenic risk to child born after exposure during gestation:	*High*
Quality and quantity of data on which risk estimate is based:	*Poor to fair*

In eight cases reported to the manufacturer in which maternal treatment with acitretin occurred during pregnancy, there were four spontaneous abortions, one fetus with malformations typical of vitamin A embryopathy, one child with high-frequency hearing loss but no malformations, one normal child, and one induced abortion without information on the fetus (Geiger et al., 1994). The affected fetus had microtia and malformations of the face and extremities; these features resemble those seen in infants with retinoid embryopathy associated with maternal treatment with etretinate or isotretinoin during pregnancy (Happle et al., 1984; Rosa et al., 1986; Thomson & Cordero, 1989; Chen et al., 1990; Geiger et al., 1994). In 52 pregnancies in which conception occurred six weeks to 23 months after the mother had stopped taking acitretin and in which fetal outcome was known, there were no infants or fetuses with malformations typical of vitamin A embryopathy; nine miscarriages occurred (Geiger et al., 1994).

Acitretin is teratogenic in experimental animals at doses similar to or greater than those used in humans. Increased frequencies of craniofacial, limb, and other malformations have been observed among the offspring of pregnant mice, rats, or rabbits treated respectively with 2-

7

267, 10-33, or <1-1.3 times the maximum human dose of acitretin (Kistler & Hummler, 1985; Kochhar et al., 1989; Lofberg et al., 1990; Turton et al., 1992).

Risk Related to Breast-feeding

Acitretin is excreted in breast milk in low concentrations. The amount of acitretin that the nursing infant would be expected to ingest is between 0.1-1.5% of the minimum oral adult dose, based on data from a single patient (Rollman & Pihl-Lundin, 1990).* Vitamin A concentrations in maternal serum and milk did not vary significantly throughout the treatment period.

The American Academy of Pediatrics considers acitretin to be safe to take while breast-feeding (Committee on Drugs, American Academy of Pediatrics, 1994).

Key References

Chen DT, Jacobson MM, Kuntzman RG: Experience with the retinoids in human pregnancy. In: Volans GN (ed). *Basic Science in Toxicology*. London: Francis Taylor Publishing, 1990, pp 473-482.

Committee on Drugs, American Academy of Pediatrics: The transfer of drugs and other chemicals into human milk. Pediatrics 93(1):137-150, 1994.

Geiger J-M, Baudin M, Saurat J-H: Teratogenic risk with etretinate and acitretin treatment. Dermatology 189:109-116, 1994.

Happle R, Traupe H, Bounameaux Y, Fisch T: Teratogenic effects of etretinate in humans. Dtsch Med Wochenschr 109:1476-1480, 1984.

Kistler A, Hummler H: Teratogenesis and reproductive safety evaluation of the retinoid etretin (Ro 10-1670). Arch Toxicol 58:50-56, 1985.

Kochhar DM, Penner JD, Minutella LM: Biotransformation of etretinate and developmental toxicity of etretin and other aromatic retinoids in teratogenesis bioassays. Drug Metab Dispos 7:618-624, 1989.

Lofberg B, Chahoud I, Bochert G, Nau H: Teratogenicity of the 13-cis and all-trans-isomers of the aromatic retinoid etretin: Correla-

---

*This calculation is based on the following assumptions: maternal dose of acitretin: 40 mg/d for nine days; milk concentration of acitretin: 0.005-0.04 mcg/mL; milk intake by the nursing infant: 150 mL/kg/d; estimated dose of acitretin ingested by the nursing infant: 0.0007-0.006 mg/kg/d; lowest therapeutic dose of acitretin in adults: 0.39 mg/kg/d.

tion to transplacental pharmacokinetics in mice during organogenesis after a single oral dose. Teratology 41:707-716, 1990.

Pilkington T, Brogden RN: Acitretin. A review of its pharmacology and therapeutic use. Drugs 43(4):597-627, 1992.

Rollman O, Pihl-Lundin I: Acitretin excretion into human breast milk. Acta Derm Venereol (Stockh) 70:487-490, 1990.

Rosa FW, Wilk AL, Kelsey FO: Teratogen update: Vitamin A congeners. Teratology 33:355-364, 1986.

Thomson EJ, Cordero JF: The new teratogens: Accutane and other vitamin-A analogs. MCN 14:244-248, 1989.

Turton JA, Willars GB, Haselden JN, et al.: Comparative teratogenicity of nine retinoids in the rat. Int J Exp Pathol 73:551-563, 1992.

ACUTRIM® *See* Phenylpropanolamine

ACTIDERM® *See* Desoximetasone

ACYCLOVIR
(Avirax®, Zovirax®)

Acyclovir is a purine nucleoside analog that is used to treat infections due to herpes or varicella virus. The drug is used orally, parenterally, and topically. Systemic absorption of the topical preparation appears to be minimal through normal skin but may occur to a moderate degree through diseased skin. Oral doses are usually 400-4000 mg/d and intravenous doses range from 10-30 mg/kg/d.

Teratogenic Risk

*Magnitude of teratogenic
risk to child born after
exposure during gestation*
    Topical: *Undetermined*
    Systemic: *Unlikely*

*Quality and quantity of data
on which risk estimate is based*
    Topical: *Poor*
    Systemic: *Fair to good*

A small risk cannot be excluded, but a high risk of congenital anomalies is unlikely in the children of women in whom small areas of skin are treated topically with acyclovir during pregnancy.

Therapeutic doses of acyclovir given systemically are unlikely to pose a substantial teratogenic risk, but the data are insufficient to state that there is no risk.

Thirteen (4%) of 311 infants born to women treated with acyclovir systemically during the first trimester and followed prospectively to birth were found to have congenital anomalies in an international Acyclovir in Pregnancy Registry (Andrews et al., 1988, 1992). No recurrent pattern of anomalies was seen among these affected infants or among nine other infants with congenital anomalies born to women who took systemic acyclovir during the first trimester of pregnancy and reported to the registry after delivery. No congenital anomalies attributable to acyclovir were observed among the children of 73 women treated systemically with acyclovir in the second or third trimester of pregnancy and reported to the registry before delivery.

Maternal systemic treatment with acyclovir near term has been used to prevent recurrent genital herpes and perinatal transmission (Stray-Pedersen, 1990; Frenkel et al., 1991). No "short-term side-effects" of acyclovir were noted among the newborns in a controlled trial in which 92 women received such treatment (Stray-Pedersen, 1990).

The frequency of malformations was not increased among the offspring of pregnant marmosets, mice, rats, or rabbits treated with acyclovir in doses similar to those used in humans, but fetal death and craniofacial and skeletal malformations were seen in rat experiments when 5 or more times the human dose was used (Moore et al., 1983; Neubert et al., 1986; Chahoud et al., 1988; Stahlmann et al., 1988, 1992; Klug et al., 1992). The relevance of these observations to therapeutic use of acyclovir in women is unknown.

Risk Related to Breast-feeding

Acyclovir is excreted in breast milk and may be found in concentrations up to 4 times those found in maternal plasma (Lau et al., 1987; Meyer et al., 1988). The amount of acyclovir that the nursing infant would be expected to receive is <1% of the minimum weight-adjusted therapeutic dose, based on two mothers who took low doses of acyclovir

(Lau et al., 1987; Meyer et al., 1988).* In a third case where the mother took much larger doses of acyclovir, it is estimated that the nursing infant would be expected to receive between 2-3% of the minimum therapeutic dose of acyclovir on a weight-adjusted basis (Taddio et al., 1994).[†] Neonates have been treated with acyclovir at doses as high as 75 mg/kg/d for disseminated herpetic infections without evidence of toxicity (Lau et al., 1987).

The American Academy of Pediatrics regards acyclovir to be safe to use while breast-feeding (Committee on Drugs, American Academy of Pediatrics, 1994).

Key References

Andrews EB, Tilson HH, Hurn BAL, et al.: Acyclovir in Pregnancy Registry. An observational epidemiologic approach. Am J Med 85(Suppl 2A):123-128, 1988.

Andrews EB, Yankaskas BC, Cordero JF, et al.: Acyclovir in Pregnancy Registry: Six years' experience. Obstet Gynecol 79:7-13, 1992.

Chahoud I, Stahlmann R, Bochert G, et al.: Gross-structural defects in rats after acyclovir application on day 10 of gestation. Arch Toxicol 62:8-14, 1988.

Committee on Drugs, American Academy of Pediatrics: The transfer of drugs and other chemicals into human milk. Pediatrics 93(1):137-150, 1994.

Frenkel LM, Brown ZA, Bryson YJ, et al.: Pharmacokinetics of acyclovir in the term human pregnancy and neonate. Am J Obstet Gynecol 164(2):569-576, 1991.

Klug S, Stahlmann R, Golor G, et al.: Aciclovir in pregnant marmoset monkeys--oral treatment. Teratology 45(5):472, 1992.

Lau RJ, Emery MG, Galinsky RE: Unexpected accumulation of acyclovir in breast milk with estimation of infant exposure. Obstet Gynecol 69:468-471, 1987.

Meyer LJ, de Miranda P, Sheth N, et al.: Acyclovir in human breast milk. Am J Obstet Gynecol 158:586-568, 1988.

*This calculation is based on the following assumptions: maternal dose of acyclovir: 1 g/d; milk concentration of acyclovir: 0.75-1.3 mcg/mL; milk intake by the nursing infant: 150 mL/kg/d; estimated dose of acyclovir ingested by the nursing infant: 0.11-0.19 mg/kg/d; lowest oral pediatric dose of acyclovir: 30 mg/kg/d.

†This calculation is based on the following assumptions: maternal dose of acyclovir: 4 g; milk concentration of acyclovir: 4.2-5.8 mcg/mL; estimated dose of acyclovir ingested by the nursing infant: 0.62-0.87 mg/kg/d.

Moore HL Jr, Szczech GM, Rodwell DE, et al.: Preclinical toxicology studies with acyclovir: Teratologic, reproductive and neonatal tests. Fundam Appl Toxicol 3:560-568, 1983.

Neubert D, Blankenburg G, Chahoud I, et al.: Results of in vivo and in vitro studies for assessing prenatal toxicity. Environ Health Perspect 70:89-103, 1986.

Stahlmann R, Golor G, Klug S, et al.: Aciclovir in pregnant marmoset monkeys - intravenous treatment. Teratology 45(5):453, 1992.

Stahlmann R, Klug S, Lewandowski C, et al.: Prenatal toxicity of acyclovir in rats. Arch Toxicol 61:468-479, 1988.

Stray-Pedersen B: Acyclovir in late pregnancy to prevent neonatal herpes simplex. Lancet 336:756, 1990.

Taddio A, Klein J, Koren G: Acyclovir excretion into human breast milk. Ann Pharmacother 28:585-587, 1994.

ADALAT® *See* Nifedipine

ADAPIN® *See* Doxepin

ADVIL® *See* Ibuprofen

AEROLATE® *See* Theophylline

AEROLONE® *See* Isoproterenol

AEROSEB-DEX® *See* Dexamethasone

AEROSPORIN® *See* Polymyxin B

AFRINOL® *See* Pseudoephedrine

A-HYDROCORT® *See* Hydrocortisone

AKARPINE® *See* Pilocarpine

AK-TRACIN® *See* Bacitracin

AK-ZOL® *See* Acetazolamide

ALAZINE TABS® *See* Hydralazine

ALBUTEROL
(Proventil®, Ventolin®, Volmax®)

Albuterol is a β-sympathicomimetic agent used as a bronchodilator and to arrest premature labor. The daily dose varies substantially by route of administration, from 0.5-1.2 mg/d as an aerosol to 6-32 mg/d orally. The drug is also given parenterally in relatively small doses and by intermittent positive pressure breathing or nebulizer in relatively large doses.

Teratogenic Risk

Magnitude of teratogenic risk to child born after exposure during gestation:	*Undetermined*
Quality and quantity of data on which risk estimate is based:	*Poor*

No epidemiological studies of congenital anomalies among infants born to women treated with albuterol during pregnancy have been reported.

Pregnant rabbits given albuterol at thousands of times the usual human dose produced offspring with no increased frequency of malformations in one study (Szabo et al., 1975). In another study which has not been published, albuterol was said to have induced cranioschisis in the offspring of rabbits when administered in doses 78 times the maximum human oral dose (USP DI, 1995). An increased frequency of cleft palates was observed among the offspring of pregnant mice given albuterol parenterally in doses several times that used in humans (Szabo et al., 1975; USP DI, 1995). The relevance of these findings to the therapeutic use of albuterol in pregnant women is unknown.

Maternal albuterol treatment in late pregnancy produces fetal tachycardia, but this has not been associated with any important neonatal problems (Ryden, 1977; Hastwell et al., 1978).

Risk Related to Breast-feeding

No information regarding the distribution of albuterol in breast milk has been published.

Key References

Hastwell GB, Halloway CP, Taylor TLO: A study of 208 patients in premature labour treated with orally administered salbutamol. Med J Aust 1:465-469, 1978.

Ryden G: The effect of salbutamol and terbutaline in the management of premature labour. Acta Obstet Gynecol Scand 56:293-296, 1977.

Szabo KT, Difebbo ME, Kang YJ: Effects of several β-receptor agonists on fetal development in various species of laboratory animals: Preliminary report. Teratology 12:336-337, 1975.

USP DI: Albuterol. In: *USP DI (USP Dispensing Information), Volume 1. Drug Information for the Health Care Professional*, 15th ed. Rockville, Md.: The US Pharmacopeial Convention, 1995, pp 535-536.

ALCOHOL
(Ethanol)

Alcohol is a central nervous system depressant that is widely consumed in beverages for its intoxicating effect. Alcohol is frequently used in pharmaceuticals as a solvent and preservative; it is also employed as a surface disinfectant.

Teratogenic Risk

*Magnitude of teratogenic
risk to child born after
exposure during gestation
     Heavy drinking (more than six drinks,
     glasses of wine, or beers per day):*   *Moderate to high*

Moderate drinking (fewer than two
drinks, glasses of wine, or beers per day):   *None to minimal*

Quality and quantity of data
on which risk estimate is based
  Heavy drinking: *Good to excellent*
  Moderate drinking: *Fair to good*

Alcohol-related birth defects (ARBD) represent a continuum. *At any given amount of maternal alcohol intake during pregnancy, more childen will have ARBD that do not constitute full fetal alcohol syndrome (defined below) than will have the classical syndrome.* *The risk of ARBD of any severity decreases with decreasing alcohol use, but no safe amount of alcohol drinking during pregnancy has been determined.*

The risk associated with drinking alcohol in amounts that fall between those classified as heavy and moderate above is presumed to be intermediate.

The amounts given above for heavy and moderate drinking are approximate and vary somewhat from person to person. *Genetic differences are likely to be a factor in this variability (Streissguth & Dehaene, 1993).*

The risk associated with binge drinking is unclear, but available data suggest that even a single heavy binge at a critical time in pregnancy may cause fetal damage.

A pattern of congenital anomalies called the fetal alcohol syndrome occurs in infants born to women who suffer from chronic, severe alcoholism during pregnancy (Jones et al., 1973; Clarren & Smith, 1978; Ginsburg et al., 1991). Typical fetal alcohol syndrome is usually seen among the children of women who drink more (and often much more) than about six beers, six glasses of wine, or six mixed drinks a day. Fetal alcohol syndrome is defined by: (a) prenatal and/or postnatal growth retardation; (b) central nervous system dysfunction, including microcephaly, neurological impairment, developmental delay, and neurobehavioral deficits; and (c) characteristic facial anomalies such as short palpebral fissures, indistinct philtrum, thin upper lip vermillion, elongated face, and flat midface (Sokol & Clarren, 1989). Congenital heart disease and brain malformations are common, but other major malformations are less frequent. Although the characteristic physical features change somewhat as children with fetal alcohol syndrome grow, the neurobehavioral abnormalities persist

(Streissguth, 1992; Spohr et al., 1993; Day et al., 1994). Attention deficits, poor judgement, and impulsivity compound the intellectual limitations of adults with fetal alcohol syndrome.

Full fetal alcohol syndrome occurs in about 6% of children of women who drink heavily during pregnancy (Day & Richardson, 1991). The risk is probably higher for women with chronic severe alcoholism during pregnancy. Less severe manifestations of alcohol embryopathy occur in a larger proportion of these children, but the estimated frequency varies widely in different studies (Abel & Sokol, 1988; Day & Richardson, 1991). The risk of full fetal alcohol syndrome is much higher for alcoholic women who have already had an affected child (Abel, 1988). The effects appear to be less severe among the children of alcoholic women who stop drinking early in pregnancy (Coles et al., 1991; Autti-Ramo et al., 1992).

Lower levels of maternal alcohol consumption during pregnancy have been associated with a variety of less severe but persistent manifestations in children (Ouellette et al., 1977; Day & Richardson, 1991; Forrest & Florey, 1991; Euromac Project Group, 1992). Among the "normal" children of women who drink an average of more than two to four beers, glasses of wine, or mixed drinks a day, minor anomalies, growth deficiency, intellectual deficits, and behavioral abnormalities occur with increased frequency. Mild effects on growth have been observed among the children of women who drank as little as one to two drinks, glasses of wine, or beers per day during pregnancy (Euromac Project Group, 1992). The risks of maternal episodic ("binge") drinking have not been clearly defined, but may be substantial (Streissguth, 1992; see also animal data below). No safe level of maternal drinking during pregnancy has been established. Maternal alcohol use during pregnancy has also been associated with an increased risk of miscarriage and stillbirth (Ginsburg et al., 1991; Euromac Project Group, 1992).

Several animal models of fetal alcohol syndrome have been developed (West & Goodlett, 1990; Euromac Project Group, 1992). Species studied include rodents, rabbits, ferrets, guinea pigs, swine, dogs, and primates. Various physical and behavioral abnormalities similar to those seen in human fetal alcohol syndrome have been induced with administration of alcohol in dosages equivalent to those used by human chronic alcoholics. Exposure of rodents, ferrets, and primates to alcohol under conditions similar to "binge" drinking in humans produces increased frequencies of anomalies in the offspring (Goodlett & West, 1992).

At least a dozen children with fetal alcohol syndrome who also have malignant neoplasms of various kinds have been reported (Kiess et al., 1984). Such observations appear to be surprisingly frequent, raising the possibility that maternal alcohol abuse during pregnancy may increase the risk of malignancy in children. Epidemiological studies of children with primitive neuroectodermal brain tumors (Bunin et al., 1994) and of children with acute myeloid leukemia diagnosed before two years of age (Severson et al., 1993) support an association with maternal alcohol use during pregnancy. Transient withdrawal symptoms such as tremors, hypertonia, and irritability have been observed among infants born to women who chronically drank alcohol late in pregnancy (Coles et al., 1984; Beattie, 1986).

Risk Related to Breast-feeding

Alcohol is excreted in breast milk in amounts that approximate those found in maternal plasma (Keesaniemi, 1974; Flores-Huerta et al., 1992). Based on one study of 11 breast-feeding mothers who consumed the equivalent of one to three drinks of alcohol each day, the amount of alcohol ingested by the nursing infant would be between 4-11% of the amount consumed by the mother on a weight-adjusted basis (Flores-Huerta et al., 1992).*

Psychomotor development, as measured by the Psychomotor Development Index, was found to be significantly lower in nursing infants whose mothers consumed at least one alcoholic drink per day than those whose mothers consumed less (Little et al., 1989). This effect persisted even after prenatal exposure to alcohol was controlled for, and was enhanced when nursing infants supplemented with formula were excluded from the analysis. Further studies with larger, more heterogeneous samples of subjects are necessary to confirm these findings.

Despite equal amounts of time spent at the breast and more frequent sucking, nursing infants in one study consumed significantly less milk when their mothers ingested approximately one ounce of alcohol one to four hours prior to nursing than when their mothers ingested no alcohol prior to nursing (Mennella & Beauchamp, 1993).

*This calculation is based on the following assumptions: maternal dose of alcohol: 120-550 mg/kg/d; milk concentration of alcohol: 35-410 mcg/mL; milk intake by the nursing infant: 150 mL/kg/d; estimated dose of alcohol ingested by the nursing infant: 5.2-61.5 mg/kg/d.

Maternal ingestion of alcohol in amounts equivalent to five drinks or more may produce inhibition of the milk ejection reflex (Cobo, 1973).

The American Academy of Pediatrics regards alcohol to be safe to drink while breast-feeding, although they caution that large amounts of alcohol may have adverse effects on the nursing infant and a decrease in the milk ejection reflex (Committee on Drugs, American Academy of Pediatrics, 1994). Presumably this recommendation of breast-feeding compatibility refers only to drinking small amounts of alcohol since caution is advised regarding consumption of large amounts of alcohol while nursing.

Key References

Abel EL: Fetal alcohol syndrome in families. Neurotoxicol Teratol 10:1-2, 1988.

Abel EL, Sokol RJ: Alcohol use in pregnancy. In: Niebyl JR. *Drug Use in Pregnancy.* Philadelphia, Pa.: Lea & Febiger, 1988, pp 193-202.

Autti-Ramo I, Korkman M, Hilakivi-Clarke L, et al.: Mental development of 2-year-old children exposed to alcohol in utero. J Pediatr 120(5):740-746, 1992.

Beattie JO: Transplacental alcohol intoxication. Alcohol Alcohol 21:163-166, 1986.

Bunin GR, Buckley JD, Boesel CP, et al.: Risk factors for astrocytic glioma and primitive neuroectodermal tumor of the brain in young children: A report from the Children's Cancer Group. Cancer Epidemiol Biomarkers Prev 3:197-204, 1994.

Clarren SK, Smith DW: The fetal alcohol syndrome. N Engl J Med 298:1063-1067, 1978.

Cobo E: Effect of different doses of ethanol on the milk-ejecting reflex in lactating women. Am J Obstet Gynecol 115:817, 1973.

Coles CD, Brown RT, Smith IE, et al.: Effects of prenatal alcohol exposure at school age. I. Physical and cognitive development. Neurotoxicol Teratol 13:357-367, 1991.

Coles CD, Smith IE, Fernhoff PM, Falek A: Neonatal ethanol withdrawal: Characteristics in clinically normal, nondysmorphic neonates. J Pediatr 105:445-451, 1984.

Committee on Drugs, American Academy of Pediatrics: The transfer of drugs and other chemicals into human milk. Pediatrics 93(1):137-150, 1994.

Day NL, Richardson GA: Prenatal alcohol exposure: A continuum of effects. Semin Perinatol 15(4):271-279, 1991.

Day NL, Richardson GA, Geva D, Robles N: Alcohol, marijuana, and tobacco: Effects of prenatal exposure on offspring growth and morphology at age six. Alcohol Clin Exp Res 18(4):786-794, 1994.

Euromac Project Group: Euromac: A European concerted action: Maternal alcohol consumption and its relation to the outcome of pregnancy and child development at 18 months. Int J Epidemiol 21(Suppl 1):S1-S87, 1992.

Flores-Huerta S, Hernandez-Montes H, Argote RM, Villalpando S: Effects of ethanol Consumption during pregnancy and lactation on the outcome and postnatal growth of the offspring. Ann Nutr Metab 36:121-128, 1992.

Forrest F, Florey C du V: The relation between maternal alcohol consumption and child development: The epidemiological evidence. J Public Health Med 13(4):247-255, 1991.

Ginsburg KA, Blacker CM, Abel EL, Sokol RJ: Fetal alcohol exposure and adverse pregnancy outcomes. Contrib Gynecol Obstet 18:115-129, 1991.

Goodlett CR, West JR: Fetal alcohol effects: Rat model of alcohol exposure during the brain growth spurt. In: Zagon IS, Slotkin TA (eds). *Maternal Substance Abuse and the Developing Nervous System.* San Diego, Calif.: Academic Press, 1992, pp 45-75.

Jones KL, Smith DW, Ulleland CN, Streissguth AP: Pattern of malformation in offspring of chronic alcoholic mothers. Lancet 1:1267-1271, 1973.

Keesaniemi YA: Ethanol and acetaldehyde in the milk and peripheral blood of lactating women after ethanol administration. J Obstet Gynecol Br Commonw 81:84-86, 1974.

Kiess W, Linderkamp O, Hadorn H-B, Haas R: Fetal alcohol syndrome and malignant disease. Eur J Pediatr 143:160-161, 1984.

Little RE, Anderson KW, Ervin CH, et al.: Maternal alcohol use during breast-feeding and infant mental and motor development at one year. N Engl J Med 321:425-430, 1989.

Mennella JA, Beauchamp GK: Beer, breast feeding, and folklore. Dev Psychobiol 26(8):459-466, 1993.

Ouellette EM, Rosett HL, Rosman NP, Weiner L: Adverse effects on offspring of maternal alcohol abuse during pregnancy. N Engl J Med 297:528-530, 1977.

Severson RK, Buckley JD, Woods WG, et al.: Cigarette smoking and alcohol consumption by parents of children with acute myeloid leukemia: An analysis within morphological subgroups--A report from the Childrens Cancer Group. Cancer Epidemiol Biomarkers Prev 2:433-439, 1993.

Sokol RJ, Clarren SK: Guidelines for use of terminology describing the impact of prenatal alcohol on the offspring. Alcohol Clin Exp Res 13(4):597-598, 1989.

Spohr H-L, Willms J, Steinhausen H-C: Prenatal alcohol exposure and long-term developmental consequences. Lancet 341(8850):907-910, 1993.

Streissguth AP: Fetal alcohol syndrome and fetal alcohol effects: A clinical perspective of later developmental consequences. In: Zagon IS, Slotkin TA (eds). *Maternal Substance Abuse and the Developing Nervous System*. San Diego, Calif.: Academic Press, 1992, pp 5-25.

Streissguth AP, Dehaene P: Fetal alcohol syndrome in twins of alcoholic mothers: Concordance of diagnosis and IQ. Am J Med Genet 47:857-861, 1993.

West JR, Goodlett CR: Teratogenic effects of alcohol on brain development. Ann Med 22:319-325, 1990.

ALDACTONE® *See* Spironolactone

ALDOMET® *See* Methyldopa

ALKA-MINTS® *See* Calcium Salts

ALLERCHLOR® *See* Chlorpheniramine

ALLERGAN® *See* Diphenhydramine

ALLERGEFON® *See* Carbinoxamine

ALLOPURINOL
(Apo-Allopurinol, Purinol, Zyloprim®)

Allopurinol is a xanthine oxidase inhibitor. It is used in the treatment of chronic gout and hyperuricemia, which may result from leukemia, radiotherapy, or systemic antineoplastic therapy. Allopurinol is given orally in a dose of 100-800 mg/d.

Teratogenic Risk

*Magnitude of teratogenic
risk to child born after
exposure during gestation:*   *Undetermined*

*Quality and quantity of data
on which risk estimate is based:*   *Very poor*

No epidemiological studies of infants born to women who were treated with allopurinol during pregnancy have been published.

The frequency of malformations was not increased among the offspring of pregnant rats treated with a single injection of allopurinol at 4-63 times the usual human dose (Bragonier et al., 1964; Chaube & Murphy, 1968). The frequencies of fetal cleft palate, growth retardation, and death were increased when pregnant mice were treated with 5-10 times the usual human dose of allopurinol (Fujii & Nishimura, 1972). The relevance of this observation to the therapeutic use of allopurinol in human pregnancy is unknown.

Risk Related to Breast-feeding

Allopurinol and one of its active metabolites, oxypurinol, are excreted in the breast milk. The amount of allopurinol that the nursing infant would be expected to ingest is 8-13% of the lowest weight-adjusted therapeutic dose, based on data from a single patient (Kamilli & Gresser, 1993).* Although a large amount of oxypurinol was ingested by the infant,[†] no adverse effects were observed.

The level of oxypurinol in the infant's plasma was found to be 6.6 mcg/mL, which was 33% of the mother's plasma level. No detectable levels of allopurinol could be found in the infant's plasma.

The American Academy of Pediatrics regards allopurinol to be safe to take while breast-feeding (Committee on Drugs, American Academy of Pediatrics, 1994).

*This calculation is based on the following assumptions: maternal dose of allopurinol: 300 mg/d for four weeks; milk concentration of allopurinol: 0.9-1.4 mcg/mL; milk intake by the nursing infant: 150 mL/kg/d; estimated dose of allopurinol ingested by the nursing infant: 0.13-0.21 mg/kg/d; lowest oral adult dose of allopurinol: 1.56 mg/kg/d.

†This calculation is based on the following assumptions: milk concentration of oxypurinol: 48-53.7 mcg/mL; estimated dose of oxypurinol ingested by the nursing infant: 7.2-8 mg/kg/d.

21

Key References

Bragonier JR, Roesky N, Carver MJ: Teratogenesis: Effects of substituted purines and the influence of 4-hydroxyprazolopyrimidine in the rat. Proc Soc Exp Biol Med 116:685-688, 1964.
Chaube S, Murphy ML: The teratogenic effects of the recent drugs active in cancer chemotherapy. Adv Teratol 3:181-237, 1968.
Committee on Drugs, American Academy of Pediatrics: The transfer of drugs and other chemicals into human milk. Pediatrics 93(1):137-150, 1994.
Fujii T, Nishimura H: Comparison of teratogenic action of substances related to purine metabolism in mouse embryos. Jpn J Pharmacol 22:201-206, 1972.
Kamilli I, Gresser U: Allopurinol and oxypurinol in human breast milk. Clin Invest 71:161-164, 1993.

ALL-TRANS-ETRETIN *See* Acitretin

ALOPAM® *See* Oxazepam

ALPHATREX® *See* Beclomethasone

ALPRAZOLAM
(Xanax®)

Alprazolam is a benzodiazepine used for treatment of anxiety and panic attacks. It is given orally in a dose of 0.5-10 mg/d.

Teratogenic Risk

Magnitude of teratogenic risk to child born after exposure during gestation: Unlikely

Quality and quantity of data on which risk estimate is based: Fair

Therapeutic doses of alprazolam during pregnancy are unlikely to pose a substantial teratogenic risk, but the data are insufficient to state that there is no risk.

Transient neonatal withdrawal symptoms similar to those seen with other benzodiazepines have been observed among infants whose mothers took alprazolam throughout pregnancy (Barry & St. Clair, 1987; Anderson & McGuire, 1989).

The rate of congenital anomalies did not appear unusual in two series of infants born to women treated with alprazolam during the first trimester of pregnancy. One study included 276 liveborn infants of women reported to the manufacturer in the first trimester of pregnancy (St. Clair & Schirmer, 1992); 4.7% of the infants had congenital anomalies. Two additional exposed pregnancies were therapeutically aborted for prenatally diagnosed fetal anomalies. The other series included 128 liveborn infants of women who consulted a teratogen information service in the first trimester (Schick-Boschetto & Zuber, 1992); 3.9% of the infants had congenital anomalies. No recurrent pattern of anomalies was seen in either series.

The frequency of malformations was no greater than expected among the offspring of rats or rabbits treated with alprazolam at a dose 8 times that used in humans (Esaki et al., 1981a, b). At higher doses, increased frequencies of minor skeletal anomalies and fetal mortality were seen, but such doses also produced maternal toxicity in the rabbits (Esaki et al., 1981a, b). The relevance of this observation to the therapeutic use of alprazolam in human pregnancy is unknown.

Please see agent summary on diazepam for information on a closely related agent that has been more thoroughly studied.

Risk Related to Breast-feeding

Alprazolam was found to be excreted into the breast milk of six lactating women in one study (Oo et al., 1993). The average milk/serum ratio was found to be 0.4. However, breast milk concentrations and serum levels were not reported. Using the observed milk/serum ratio and the average adult serum level of alprazolam, the estimated amount of alprazolam that the nursing infant would be expected to ingest is 8% of the lowest weight-adjusted therapeutic dose.*

*This calculation is based on the following assumptions: maternal dose of alprazolam: 0.5 mg; milk concentration of alprazolam assuming an average adult plasma level of 10 ng/mL and an observed milk/serum ratio of 0.38: 3.8 ng/mL; milk intake by the nursing infant: 150 mL/kg/d; estimated dose of alprazolam ingested by the nursing infant: 0.6 mcg/kg/d; lowest therapeutic dose of alprazolam in adults: 7.8 mcg/kg/d.

Withdrawal symptoms characterized by restlessness, irritability, and sleep disturbance were observed in two nursing infants. The mother of one of the infants took alprazolam throughout pregnancy and for one week postpartum, while the other mother took alprazolam only during the postpartum period (Anderson & McGuire, 1989).

Because elimination of benzodiazepines is much slower in neonates and accumulation may occur, nursing infants should be monitored for signs of sedation or weight loss (USP DI, 1995).

Key References

Anderson PO, McGuire GG: Neonatal alprazolam withdrawal--possible effects of breast feeding. DICP Ann Pharmacother 23:614, 1989.

Barry WS, St. Clair SM: Exposure to benzodiazepines in utero. Lancet 1:1436-1437, 1987.

Esaki K, Oshio K, Yanagita T: [Effects of oral administration of alprazolam (TUS-1) on the rat fetus--Experiment on drug administration during the organogenesis period.] Jitchuken Zenrinsho Kenkyuho 7:65-77, 1981a.

Esaki K, Sakai Y, Yanagita T: [Effect of oral administration of alprazolam (TUS-1) on rabbit fetus.] Jitchuken Zenrinsho Kenkyuho 7:79-90, 1981b.

Oo CY, Stowe C, Kuhn R, McNamara PJ: Alprazolam transfer into human milk: In vivo evaluation of a diffusional model. Pharm Res 10(10 Suppl):S348, 1993.

Schick-Boschetto B, Zuber C: Alprazolam exposure during early human pregnancy. Teratology 45(5):460, 1992.

St. Clair SM, Schirmer RG: First-trimester exposure to alprazolam. Obstet Gynecol 80:843-846, 1992.

USP DI: Benzodiazepines. In: *USP DI (USP Dispensing Information), Volume 1. Drug Information for the Health Care Professional*, 15th ed. Rockville, Md.: The US Pharmacopeial Convention, 1995, p 460.

ALTERNAGEL® *See Aluminum Hydroxide*

ALU-CAP® *See Aluminum Hydroxide*

ALUMINUM HYDROXIDE
(AlternaGEL®, Alu-Cap®, Amphojel®)

Aluminum hydroxide is given orally as an antacid, often in combination with magnesium hydroxide, magnesium carbonate, calcium carbonate, and/or simethicone. Aluminum hydroxide is also used to prevent the absorption of phosphate in patients with renal failure. Small amounts of aluminum are absorbed when aluminum hydroxide is taken orally. The amount of aluminum hydroxide in various antacid preparations varies greatly, and doses as high as 12,000 mg/d may be taken in extreme cases. Single doses usually provide 200-1200 mg of aluminum hydroxide.

Teratogenic Risk

*Magnitude of teratogenic
risk to child born after
exposure during gestation:*   *Undetermined*

*Quality and quantity of data
on which risk estimate is based:*   *Poor*

A small risk cannot be excluded, but there is no indication that the risk of congenital anomalies in children of women treated with aluminum hydroxide during pregnancy is likely to be great.

No epidemiological studies of congenital anomalies among the children of women who took antacids containing aluminum hydroxide during pregnancy have been reported.

Studies in rats and mice suggest that treatment of pregnant women with aluminum hydroxide in usual therapeutic doses is unlikely to increase the children's risk of malformations greatly (Domingo et al., 1989; Gomez et al., 1990; Colomina et al., 1994). Decreased fetal weight occurs when pregnant mice or rats are treated with large doses of aluminum hydroxide under conditions that promote absorption of aluminum (Gomez et al., 1991; Colomina et al., 1992). Maternal toxicity is also seen in such circumstances.

Risk Related to Breast-feeding

Aluminum hydroxide is excreted into human breast milk in concentrations that are unlikely to produce an adverse effect on the nursing infant (USP DI, 1995).

Key References

Colomina MT, Gomez M, Domingo JL, et al.: Concurrent ingestion of lactate and aluminum can result in developmental toxicity in mice. Res Commun Chem Pathol Pharmacol 77(1):95-106, 1992.

Colomina MT, Gomez M, Domingo JL, Corbella J: Lack of maternal and developmental toxicity in mice given high doses of aluminium hydroxide and ascorbic acid during gestation. Pharmacol Toxicol 74:236-239, 1994.

Domingo JL, Gomez M, Bosque MA, Corbella J: Lack of teratogenicity of aluminum hydroxide in mice. Life Sci 45:243-247, 1989.

Gomez M, Bosque MA, Domingo JL, et al.: Evaluation of the maternal and developmental toxicity of aluminum from high doses of aluminum hydroxide in rats. Vet Hum Toxicol 32(6):545-548, 1990.

Gomez M, Domingo JL, Llobet JM: Developmental toxicity evaluation of oral aluminum in rats: Influence of citrate. Neurotoxicol Teratol 13(3):323-328, 1991.

USP DI: Antacids. In: *USP DI (USP Dispensing Information), Volume 1. Drug Information for the Health Care Professional*, 15th ed. Rockville, Md.: The US Pharmacopeial Convention, 1995, p 177.

ALZAPRAM® See Lorazepam

AMCILL® *See* Ampicillin

AMERICAINE® *See* Benzocaine

AMILORIDE
(Midamor®, Modamide®)

Amiloride is a potassium sparing diuretic that is administered orally in a dose of 5-20 mg/d.

Teratogenic Risk

*Magnitude of teratogenic
risk to child born after
exposure during gestation:*   Undetermined

*Quality and quantity of data
on which risk estimate is based:*   Poor

No epidemiological studies of malformations in the infants of women treated with amiloride during pregnancy have been published.

Studies in rats and mice suggest that treatment of pregnant women with amiloride in usual therapeutic doses is unlikely to increase the children's risk of malformations greatly (Nelson et al., 1989; Scott et al., 1990).

Risk Related to Breast-feeding

No information regarding the distribution of amiloride in breast milk has been published.

Key References

Nelson BK, Vorhees CV, Scott WJ Jr, Hastings L: Effects of 2-methoxyethanol on fetal development, postnatal behavior, and embryonic intracellular pH of rats. Neurotoxicol Teratol 11:273-284, 1989.

Scott WJ, Duggan CA, Schreiner CM, Collins MD: Reduction of embryonic intracellular pH: A potential mechanism of acetazolamide-induced limb malformations. Toxicol Appl Pharmacol 103:238-254, 1990.

AMINACRINE
(Monacrin®)

Aminacrine is an acridine derivative that is used as a topical disinfectant, often in combination with other agents, in the treatment of vaginal and eye infections.

Teratogenic Risk

Magnitude of teratogenic risk to child born after exposure during gestation:	*Unlikely*
Quality and quantity of data on which risk estimate is based:	*Poor to fair*

Topical use of aminacrine is unlikely to pose a substantial teratogenic risk, but the data are insufficient to state that there is no risk.

Prescriptions for aminacrine during the first trimester of pregnancy were not found to have been given more frequently than expected to mothers of 6564 infants with a variety of congenital anomalies or to 2326 women who had miscarriages in one epidemiological study (Rosa et al., 1987). The frequency of congenital anomalies was no greater than expected among the infants of 59 women treated with aminacrine during the first four lunar months of pregnancy in another study (Heinonen et al., 1977).

No experimental animal teratology studies of aminacrine have been published.

Risk Related to Breast-feeding

No information regarding the distribution of aminacrine in breast milk has been published.

Key References

Heinonen OP, Slone D and Shapiro S: *Birth Defects and Drugs in Pregnancy.* Littleton, Mass.: John Wright-PSG, 1977, pp 300-302.

Rosa FW, Baum C, Shaw M: Pregnancy outcomes after first-trimester vaginitis drug therapy. Obstet Gynecol 69:751-755, 1987.

AMINOSALICYLIC ACID
(Nemasol Sodium®, PAS, Therazid®)

Aminosalicylic acid and its salts are given orally in a dose of 10-20 g/d to treat tuberculosis. Aminosalicylic acid is usually administered in combination with other antitubercular drugs.

Teratogenic Risk

*Magnitude of teratogenic
risk to child born after exposure
during gestation:*   *Undetermined*

*Quality and quantity of data
on which risk estimate is based:*   *Very poor*

The frequency of congenital anomalies was not increased in the infants of 68 women who were treated with aminosalicylic acid during the first four months of pregnancy in one epidemiological study (Lowe, 1964). In another study, the frequency of congenital anomalies was somewhat higher than expected among the children of 43 women treated with aminosalicylic acid during the first four lunar months of pregnancy (Heinonen et al., 1977). No information is provided regarding the kinds of malformations that occurred or on the statistical significance of this observation. Studies such as this one that include multiple comparisons between maternal drug exposures and various birth defect outcomes are expected to show occasional associations purely by chance. A higher than expected frequency of congenital anomalies was seen among the children of 36 women who had been treated with aminosalicylic acid during the first trimester of pregnancy in a third study (Varpela, 1964). No consistent pattern of anomalies was apparent among the affected children. The associations observed may have been due to some other aspect of the treatment or to the illness in these patients.

No animal teratology studies of aminosalicylic acid have been published.

Risk Related to Breast-feeding

Aminosalicylic acid is excreted in breast milk in low concentrations. The amount of aminosalicylic acid that the nursing infant would be expected to ingest is <1% of the lowest pediatric dose, based on data from a single patient (Holdiness, 1984).*

Key References

Heinonen OP, Slone D, Shapiro S: *Birth Defects and Drugs in Pregnancy.* Littleton, Mass.: John Wright-PSG, 1977, pp 298-299, 302, 313.

Holdiness MR: Antituberculosis drugs and breast-feeding. Arch Intern Med 144:1888, 1984.

Lowe CR: Congenital defects among children born to women under supervision or treatment for pulmonary tuberculosis. Br J Prev Soc Med 18:14-16, 1964.

Varpela E: On the effect exerted by first-line tuberculosis medicines on the foetus. Acta Tuberc Scand 35:53-69, 1964.

*This calculation is based on the following assumptions: maternal dose of aminosalicylic acid: 4 g; milk concentration of aminosalicylic acid: 1.1 mcg/mL; milk intake by the nursing infant: 150 mL/kg/d; estimated dose of aminosalicylic acid ingested by the nursing infant: 0.15 mg/kg/d; lowest pediatric dose of aminosalicylic acid: 200 mg/kg/d.

AMITRIPTYLINE
(Elavil®)

Amitriptyline is a tricyclic antidepressant with marked anticholinergic and sedative properties. Amitriptyline is used to treat bulimia, neurogenic pain, and peptic ulcer disease, as well as depression. The drug is given orally in doses up to 150 mg/d to outpatients and up to 300 mg/d to inpatients. It may also be administered intramuscularly in doses of 80-120 mg/d.

Teratogenic Risk

Magnitude of teratogenic risk to child born after exposure during gestation: *Unlikely*

Quality and quantity of data
on which risk estimate is based: *Fair*

Therapeutic doses of amitriptyline are unlikely to pose a substantial teratogenic risk, but the data are insufficient to state that there is no risk.

Available epidemiologic data on malformations in the offspring of women treated with amitriptyline during the first trimester of pregnancy are sparse. None of 21 infants born to women who were treated with amitriptyline in the first four lunar months of pregnancy in one epidemiological study had malformations (Heinonen et al., 1977). Another study of 1370 infants with malformations found a statistically significant association with maternal use of amitriptyline in the first trimester of gestation, but this association was based on a very small number of exposed children with malformations (Bracken & Holford, 1981). Anecdotal case reports of limb reduction defects in the offspring of women who took amitriptyline early in pregnancy are unlikely to represent a causal relationship (Morrow, 1972).

The frequency of malformations was not increased among the offspring of pregnant rats treated with 1-4 times the usual human dose of amitriptyline, but central nervous system malformations were seen among the offspring of pregnant hamsters, mice, and rabbits treated with 10 or more times the human dose (Jelinek et al., 1967; Khan & Azam, 1969; Di Carlo et al., 1971; Jurand, 1980; Guram et al., 1982; Beyer et al., 1984; Henderson & McMillen, 1990). Behavioral alterations have been observed among the offspring of pregnant rats treated with 1-2 times the human therapeutic dose of amitriptyline (Bigl et al., 1982; Henderson & McMillen, 1990). The relevance of these observations to the clinical use of amitriptyline in human pregnancy is unknown.

Transient central nervous system depression has been observed in the infant of a woman treated with amitriptyline throughout pregnancy (Vree & Zwart, 1985). Serum amitriptyline levels were found to be in the moderately toxic range in the mother and in the severely toxic range in the child.

Risk Related to Breast-feeding

Amitriptyline and its active metabolite, nortriptyline are excreted in breast milk in concentrations higher than those found in maternal serum (Bader & Newman, 1980; Brixen-Rasmussen et al., 1982; Pittard & O'Neal, 1986). Based on data from these studies, the amount of amitriptyline and nortriptyline that the nursing infant would be expected to ingest is between 0.3-1.8% and <1%, respectively, of the lowest weight-adjusted therapeutic dose.* Neither amitriptyline nor nortriptyline could be detected in milk samples from six lactating women following administration of a single low dose of amitriptyline (Eschenhof & Rieder, 1969).

No detectable levels of amitriptyline or nortriptyline could be found in the serum of infants whose mothers were treated with amitriptyline (Erickson et al., 1979; Bader & Newman, 1980; Brixen-Rasmussen et al., 1982). No adverse effects were noted in any of the nursed infants.

The WHO Working Group on Drugs and Human Lactation (1988) regard amitriptyline to be "probably safe" to use during breast-feeding; however, the American Academy of Pediatrics regards amitriptyline to be a drug whose effect on the infant is unknown but may be of concern (Committee on Drugs, American Academy of Pediatrics, 1994).

Key References

Bader TF, Newman K: Amitriptyline in human breast milk and the nursing infant's serum. Am J Psychiatry 137:855-856, 1980.

Beyer BK, Guram MS, Geber WF: Incidence and potentiation of external and internal fetal anomalies resulting from chlordiazepoxide and amitriptyline alone and in combination. Teratology 30:39-45, 1984.

Bigl V, Dalitz E, Kunert E, et al.: The effect of d-amphetamine and amitriptyline administered to pregnant rats on the locomotor activity and neurotransmitters of the offspring. Psychopharmacology 77:371-375, 1982.

Bracken MB, Holford TR: Exposure to prescribed drugs in pregnancy and association with congenital malformations. Obstet Gynecol 58:336-344, 1981.

---

*This calculation is based on the following assumptions: maternal doses of amitriptyline: 75-150 mg/d; milk concentration of amitriptyline: 0.03-0.15 mcg/mL; milk concentration of nortriptyline: 0.03-0.08 mcg/mL; milk intake by the nursing infant: 150 mL/kg/d; estimated dose of amitriptyline and nortriptyline ingested by the nursing infant: 0.004-0.02 mg/kg/d and 0.004-0.01 mg/kg/d, respectively; lowest oral adult dose of amitriptyline and nortriptyline: 1.2 mg/kg/d.

Brixen-Rasmussen L, Halgrener J, Jorgensen A: Amitriptyline and nortriptyline excretion in human breast milk. Psychopharmacology 76:94-95, 1982.

Committee on Drugs, American Academy of Pediatrics: The transfer of drugs and other chemicals into human milk. Pediatrics 93(1):137-150, 1994.

Di Carlo R, Pagnini G, Pelagalli GV: Effect of amitriptyline and butriptyline on fetal development in rats. J Med 2:271-275, 1971.

Erickson SH, Smith GH, Heidrich F: Tricyclics and breast feeding. Am J Psychiatry 136:1483, 1979.

Eschenhof E, Rieder J: Antidepressivums amitriptylin in organisms untersvchungen uberdas schicksal des der ratte und des menscher. Arzneimittelforsch 19:957, 1969.

Guram MS, Gill TS, Geber WF: Comparative teratogenicity of chlordiazepoxide, amitriptyline, and a combination of the two compounds in the fetal hamster. Neurotoxicology 3:83-90, 1982.

Heinonen OP, Slone D, Shapiro S: *Birth Defects and Drugs in Pregnancy.* Littleton, Mass.: John Wright-PSG, 1977, pp 336-337.

Henderson MG, McMillen BA: Effects of prenatal exposure to cocaine or related drugs on rat developmental and neurological indices. Brain Res Bull 24:207-212, 1990.

Jelinek V, Zikmund E, Reichlova R: [The influence of some psychotropic medications on the development of the rat fetus.] Therapie 22:1429-1433, 1967.

Jurand A: Malformations of the central nervous system induced by neurotropic drugs in mouse embryos. Dev Growth Differ 22:61-78, 1980.

Khan I, Azam A: Study of teratogenic activity of trifluoperazine, amitriptyline, ethionamide and thalidomide in pregnant rabbits and mice. Excerpta Med Int Cong Ser 181:235-242, 1969.

Morrow AW: Limb deformities associated with iminodibenzyl hydrochloride. Med J Aust 1:658-659, 1972.

Pittard WB III, O'Neal W Jr: Amitriptyline excretion in human milk. J Clin Psychopharmacol 6(6):383-384, 1986.

Vree PH, Zwart P: [A newborn infant with amitryptyline poisoning.] Med Tijdschr Geneeskd 129:910-912, 1985.

WHO Working Group on Drugs and Human Lactation: In: Bennet PN (ed). *Drugs and Human Lactation.* Amsterdam: Elsevier, 1988, pp 391-392.

AMOBARBITAL
(Amytal®)

Amobarbital is a barbiturate that is given orally in single doses of 65-200 mg as a hypnotic and in divided doses of 50-300 mg/d as a sedative. It is also used parenterally in doses up to 1000 mg/d during labor and in the treatment of status epilepticus.

Teratogenic Risk

Magnitude of teratogenic risk to child born after exposure during gestation:	*None to minimal*
Quality and quantity of data on which risk estimate is based:	*Poor to fair*

This risk is for occasional therapeutic use of amobarbital during pregnancy. The risk for chronic use and for amobarbital overdose during pregnancy is unknown.

The frequencies of congenital anomalies in general, of major malformations, and of minor anomalies were not significantly increased among the children of 298 women treated with amobarbital during the first four lunar months of pregnancy in one epidemiological study (Heinonen et al., 1977). The frequencies of cardiovascular malformations and inguinal hernias did appear to be increased, however. Congenital anomalies were no more frequent than expected among the children of 867 women who were treated with amobarbital anytime during pregnancy in this study. A significant association with maternal use of amobarbital during the first trimester of pregnancy was found in an investigation of 175 infants with major congenital anomalies (Nelson & Forfar, 1971). Both of these studies include multiple comparisons between maternal drug exposures and various birth defect outcomes. In such circumstances, associations observed with nominal statistical significance often occur by chance alone.

In 20 cases in which the mother took an overdose (1300-12,500 mg) of amobarbital, usually in combination with other medications, there were two fetal deaths, but the frequency of congenital anomalies did not appear to be increased (Czeizel et al., 1984, 1988). There were four cases of mental retardation among 18 liveborn children, but in three of these cases there was also a mentally retarded brother. The overdose occurred in the first trimester of pregnancy in only three cases, and none of these children had malformations.

No animal teratology studies of amobarbital have been published.

Risk Related to Breast-feeding

No information regarding the distribution of amobarbital in breast milk has been published

Key References

Czeizel A, Szentesi I, Szekeres I, et al.: A study of adverse effects on the progeny after intoxication during pregnancy. Arch Toxicol 62:1-7, 1988.

Czeizel A, Szentesi I, Szekeres I, et al.: Pregnancy outcome and health conditions of offspring of self-poisoned pregnant women. Acta Paediatr Hung 25(3):209-236, 1984.

Heinonen OP, Slone D, Shapiro S: *Birth Defects and Drugs in Pregnancy.* Littleton, Mass.: John Wright-PSG, 1977, pp 336-344, 438, 476, 491.

Nelson MM, Forfar JO: Associations between drugs administered during pregnancy and congenital abnormalities of the fetus. Br Med J 1:523-527, 1971.

USP DI: Barbiturates. In: *USP DI (USP Dispensing Information), Volume 1. Drug Information for the Health Care Professional,* 15th ed. Rockville, Md.: The US Pharmacopeial Convention, 1995, p 428.

AMOXICILLIN
(Amoxil®, Polymox®, Wymox®)

Amoxicillin, a penicillin derivative, is a widely used antibiotic. It is given orally in doses of 750-6000 mg/d.

Teratogenic Risk

*Magnitude of teratogenic
risk to child born after
exposure during gestation:*   *Undetermined*

Quality and quantity of data
on which risk estimate is based: Very poor

A small risk cannot be excluded, but there is no indication that the
risk of congenital anomalies in the children of women treated with
amoxicillin during pregnancy is likely to be great.

No significant increase in the frequencies of major or minor congenital anomalies was observed among the children of 14 women treated during the first 14 weeks of gestation with amoxicillin and probenecid or among the children of 57 women so treated after the fourteenth week in a randomized controlled trial (Cavenee et al., 1993). No animal teratology studies of amoxicillin have been published.

Please see agent summaries on penicillin and ampicillin for information on related drugs that have been more thoroughly studied.

Risk Related to Breast-feeding

Amoxicillin is excreted in breast milk in low concentrations. The amount of amoxicillin that the nursing infant would be expected to ingest is <1% of the lowest neonatal dose, based on data obtained from six lactating mothers (Kafetzis et al., 1981).*

Both the American Academy of Pediatrics (Committee on Drugs, American Academy of Pediatrics, 1994) and the WHO Working Group on Drugs and Human Lactation (1988) regard amoxicillin to be safe to use while breast-feeding.

Key References

Cavenee MR, Farris JR, Spalding TR, et al.: Treatment of gonorrhea in pregnancy. Obstet Gynecol 81:33-38, 1993.

Committee on Drugs, American Academy of Pediatrics: The transfer of drugs and other chemicals into human milk. Pediatrics 93(1):137-150, 1994.

Kafetzis DA, Siafas CA, Georgakopoulos PA, Papadatos CJ: Passage of cephalosporins and amoxicillin into the breast milk. Acta Paediatr Scand 70:285-288, 1981.

*This calculation is based on the following assumptions: maternal dose of amoxicillin: 1 g; milk concentration of amoxicillin: 0.68-1.3 mcg/mL; milk intake by the nursing infant: 150 mL/kg/d; estimated dose of amoxicillin ingested by the nursing infant: 0.10-0.19 mg/kg/d; lowest neonatal dose of amoxicillin: 50 mg/kg/d.

WHO Working Group on Drugs and Human Lactation. In: Bennet PN (ed). *Drugs and Human Lactation.* Amsterdam: Elsevier, 1988, pp 213-214.

AMOXIL® *See* Amobarbital

AMPHOJEL® *See* Aluminum Hydroxide

AMPICILLIN
(Amcill®, Omnipen®, Polycillin®)

Ampicillin is a widely used antibiotic that is derived from penicillin. Ampicillin is given orally in doses of 1000-4000 mg/d. The parenteral dose in serious infections may be as great as 14,000 mg/d.

Teratogenic Risk

Magnitude of teratogenic risk to child born after exposure during gestation:	*None*
Quality and quantity of data on which risk estimate is based:	*Fair to good*

The frequency of congenital anomalies among the infants of 309 and 409 women treated with ampicillin during the first trimester of pregnancy was no greater than expected in two separate cohorts of one epidemiological study (Jick et al., 1981; Aselton et al., 1985). Rothman et al. (1979) observed an association with maternal ampicillin treatment "about the time pregnancy began" in a study of 390 infants with congenital heart disease. This finding was not confirmed in a follow-up study of similar design by the same investigators (Zierler & Rothman, 1985) or in an independent study of about the same size (Bracken, 1986). In two of these studies but not in the third, a significant association of maternal ampicillin use with one particular kind of heart malformation, transposition of the great arteries, was observed. Studies such as these that include multiple comparisons between maternal drug exposures and various birth defect outcomes are expected to show occasional associations with nominal statistical significance purely by chance.

37

Studies in rats suggest that treatment of pregnant women with ampicillin in usual therapeutic doses is unlikely to increase the children's risk of malformations greatly (Bachev et al., 1974; Korzhova et al., 1981).

Risk Related to Breast-feeding

Ampicillin is excreted in breast milk in low concentrations (Anderson, 1977; Matsuda, 1984; Branebjerg & Heisterberg, 1987; Matheson et al., 1988). The amount of ampicillin that the nursing infant would be expected to ingest is <1% of the lowest neonatal dose, based on data from more than 20 lactating women who had taken either ampicillin or pivampicillin, which is metabolized to ampicillin (Matsuda, 1984; Branebjerg & Heisterberg, 1987; Matheson et al., 1988).*

Diarrhea, candidiasis, and skin rash have been reported in two nursing infants whose mothers took ampicillin while breast-feeding (Williams, 1976; Taddio & Ito, 1994).

Key References

Anderson P: Drugs and breast feeding--a review. Drug Intell Clin Pharm 11:208-223, 1977.

Aselton P, Jick H, Milunsky A, et al.: First-trimester drug use and congenital disorders. Obstet Gynecol 65:451-455, 1985.

Bachev S, Petrova L, Voicheva V, et al.: [Experimental studies on the teratogenic effect, acute and chronic toxicity of ampicillin.] Savremenna Medicina 25:29-32, 1974.

Bracken MB: Drug use in pregnancy and congenital heart disease in offspring. N Engl J Med 314:1120, 1986.

Branebjerg PE, Heisterberg L: Blood and milk concentrations of ampicillin in mothers treated with pivampicillin and in their infants. J Perinat Med 15:555-558, 1987.

Jick H, Holmes LB, Hunter JR, et al.: First-trimester drug use and congenital disorders. JAMA 246:343-346, 1981.

Korzhova VV, Lisitsyna NT, Mikhailova EG: Effect of ampicillin and oxacillin on fetal and neonatal development. Bull Exp Biol Med 91:169-171, 1981.

*This calculation is based on the following assumptions: maternal dose of ampicillin or pivampicillin: 1-2 g/d; milk concentration of ampicillin: 0.03-1 mcg/mL; milk intake by the nursing infant: 150 mL/kg/d; estimated dose of ampicillin ingested by the nursing infant: 0.004-0.15 mg/kg/d; lowest neonatal dose: 50 mg/kg/d.

Matheson I, Samseth M, Sande HA: Ampicillin breast milk during puerperal infections. Eur J Clin Pharmacol 34:657-659, 1988.

Matsuda S: Transfer of antibiotics into maternal milk. Biol Res Pregnancy 5:57-60, 1984.

Rothman KJ, Fyler DC, Goldblatt A, Kreidberg MB: Exogenous hormones and other drug exposures of children with congenital heart disease. Am J Epidemiol 109:433-439, 1979.

Taddio A, Ito S: Drug use during lactation. In: Koren G (ed). *Maternal-Fetal Toxicology. A Clinician's Guide*, 2nd ed. New York: Marcel Dekker, 1994, pp 133-219.

Williams M: Excretion of drugs in milk. Pharm J (Sept 18):217-219, 1976.

Zierler S, Rothman KJ: Congenital heart disease in relation to maternal use of Bendectin and other drugs in early pregnancy. N Engl J Med 313:347-352, 1985.

AMYTAL® *See* Amobarbital

ANACIN-3® *See* Acetaminophen

ANACOBIN® *See* Cyanocobalamin

ANADROL® *See* Oxymetholone

ANAFRANIL® *See* Clomipramine

ANAPOLON® *See* Oxymetholone

ANAPROX® *See* Naproxen

ANASPAZ® *See* Hyoscyamine

ANGEL DUST *See* Phencyclidine

ANTI-SPAS® *See* Dicyclomine

ANTI-TUS® *See* Guaifenesin

ANTIVERT® *See* Meclizine

APO-ALLOPURINOL *See* Allopurinol

APO-CHLORPROPAMIDE
See Chlorpropamide

APO-CHLORTHALIDONE
See Chlorthalidone

APRANAX® *See* Naproxen

APRESOLINE® *See* Hydralazine

APROZIDE® *See* Hydrochlorothiazide

AQUASOL A® *See* Vitamin A

AQUASOL E® *See* Vitamin E

AQUATENSEN® *See* Methyclothiazide

ARGICILLINE® *See* Gramicidin

ARALEN® *See* Chloroquine

ARTHROCINE® *See* Sulindac

ASA *See* Aspirin

ASCABIOL® *See* Benzyl Benzoate

ASCORBIC ACID
(Cecon®, C-Span®,Vitamin C)

Ascorbic acid is vitamin C, an essential nutrient. The US recommended dietary allowance (RDA) of ascorbic acid during pregnancy is 70 mg/d (NRC, 1989). Ascorbic acid is given orally or parenterally as a nutritional supplement in doses of 50-1000 mg/d, although some people take larger doses for various purported health benefits.

Teratogenic Risk

Magnitude of teratogenic risk to child born after exposure during gestation:	*None*
Quality and quantity of data on which risk estimate is based:	*Poor*

The frequency of supplemental ascorbic acid use during the first trimester of pregnancy was no greater than expected among the mothers of 175 infants with major malformations or of 283 women with minor anomalies in one study (Nelson & Forfar, 1971). No epidemiological investigations of malformations in infants born to women who took exceptionally large doses of ascorbic acid during pregnancy have been reported.

Studies in rats and mice suggest that treatment of pregnant women with ascorbic acid in usual therapeutic doses is unlikely to increase the children's risk of malformations greatly (Kola et al., 1989; Vogel & Spielmann, 1989; Pillans et al., 1990; Colomina et al., 1994). Fetal deaths were increased in pregnant mice treated with 4800 times the human RDA in one study (Pillans et al., 1990). The relevance of this finding to use of ascorbic acid in conventional therapeutic doses in human pregnancy is unknown.

Increased ascorbic acid catabolism and consequently increased dietary requirements have been observed in newborn guinea pigs whose mothers were fed 100-200 times the guinea pig minimal daily requirement of ascorbic acid during pregnancy (Cochrane, 1965; Norkus & Rosso, 1975, 1981). A report of scurvy despite documented adequate ascorbic acid intake in two children born to women who took about 8 times the RDA of vitamin C during pregnancy raises the possibility that a similar effect may occur in humans (Cochrane, 1965). If this does occur in humans, however, it must rarely be of clinical significance.

Risk Related to Breast-feeding

Breast-milk concentrations of ascorbic acid do not correlate with maternal ascorbic acid intake when mothers are well-nourished (Thomas et al., 1979, 1980; Sneed et al., 1981; Byerley & Kirksey, 1985). No significant changes in the ascorbic acid content of breast milk, for example, were found between women supplemented with 90 mg of ascorbic acid per day and women not supplemented (Thomas et al., 1979). The women in both groups were already consuming over 100% of the RDA for ascorbic acid in their diets. The amount of ascorbic acid that the nursing infant would be expected to ingest is approximately 1.5 times the RDA for infants.*

In contrast, progressive supplementation for eight months with ascorbic acid at doses up to 200 mg/d in lactating women who had low dietary intakes of ascorbic acid (1.5 mg/d) steadily increased the ascorbic acid content of breast milk (Deodhar et al., 1964).

Key References

Byerley LO, Kirksey A: Effects of different levels of vitamin C intake on the vitamin C concentration in human milk and the vitamin C intakes of breast-fed infants. Am J Clin Nutr 41:665-671, 1985.

Cochrane WA: Overnutrition in prenatal and neonatal life: A problem? Can Med Assoc J 93:893-899, 1965.

Colomina MT, Gomez M, Domino GL, Corbella J: Lack of maternal and developmental toxicity in mice given high doses of aluminium hydroxide and ascorbic acid during gestation. Pharmacol Toxicol 74:236-239, 1994.

Deodhar AD, Rajalakshmi R, Ramakrishnan CV: Studies on human lactation. Part III. Effect of dietary vitamin supplementation on vitamin contents of breast milk. Acta Pediatr 53:42-48, 1964.

Kola I, Vogel R, Spielmann H: Co-administration of ascorbic acid with cyclophosphamide (CPA) to pregnant mice inhibits the clastogenic activity of CPA in preimplantation murine blastocysts. Mutagenesis 4(4):297-301, 1989.

*The RDA of ascorbic acid for infants up to one year of age: 35 mg.

Nelson MM, Forfar JO: Associations between drugs administered during pregnancy and congenital abnormalities of the fetus. Br Med J 1:523-527, 1971.

Norkus EP, Rosso P: Changes in ascorbic acid metabolism of the offspring following high maternal intake of this vitamin in the pregnant guinea pig. Ann NY Acad Sci 258:401-409, 1975.

Norkus EP, Rosso P: Effects of maternal intake of ascorbic acid on the postnatal metabolism of this vitamin in the guinea pig. J Nutr 111:624-630, 1981.

NRC (National Research Council): *Recommended Dietary Allowances, 10th ed. Report of the Subcommittee on the Tenth Edition of the RDAs, Food and Nutrition Board, Commission on Life Sciences.* Washington, DC: National Academy Press, 1989, p 262.

Pillans PI, Ponzi SF, Parker MI: Effects of ascorbic acid on the mouse embryo and on cyclophosphamide-induced cephalic DNA strand breaks in vivo. Arch Toxicol 64:423-425, 1990.

Sneed SM, Zane C, Thomas MR: The effects of ascorbic acid, vitamin B_6, vitamin B_{12}, and folic acid supplementation on the breast milk and maternal nutritional status of low socioeconomic lactating women. Am J Clin Nutr 34:1338-1346, 1981.

Thomas MR, Kawamoto J, Sneed SM, Eakin R: The effects of vitamin C, vitamin B_6, and vitamin B_{12} supplementation on the breast milk and maternal status of well-nourished women. Am J Clin Nutr 32:1679-1685, 1979.

Thomas MR, Sneed SM, Wei C, et al.: The effects of vitamin C, vitamin B_6, vitamin B_{12}, folic acid, riboflavin, and thiamin on the breast milk and maternal status of well-nourished women at 6 months postpartum. Am J Clin Nutr 33:2151-2156, 1980.

Vogel R, Spielmann H: Beneficial effects of ascorbic acid on preimplantation mouse embryos after exposure to cyclophosphamide in vivo. Teratogenesis Carcinog Mutagen 9:51-59, 1989.

ASPARTAME
(Equal®, Nutrasweet®)

Aspartame is a low-calorie sweetening agent that is widely used in beverages and foods. It is a dipeptide ester composed of phenylalanine and aspartic acid. The allowable daily intake of aspartame set by the US Food and Drug Administration is 50 mg/kg/d, the equivalent of about 17 12-ounce cans of soft drink sweetened with aspartame (Sturtevant, 1985; Anonymous, 1993).

Teratogenic Risk

*Magnitude of teratogenic
risk to child born after
exposure during gestation:*   *Unlikely*

*Quality and quantity of data
on which risk estimate is based:*   *Poor*

> *Use of aspartame in small or moderate amounts is unlikely to pose a substantial teratogenic risk, but the data are insufficient to state that there is no risk.*

No epidemiological studies of congenital anomalies in infants born to women who used aspartame during pregnancy have been reported.

No teratogenic effect was observed among the offspring of rats fed diets containing 1% aspartame during pregnancy (Lederer et al., 1985). Treatment of pregnant rabbits with aspartame in doses 40 times greater than the human allowable daily intake did not affect fetal weight or litter size in one study (Ranney et al., 1975). Behavioral alterations have been observed among the offspring of guinea pigs or mice treated respectively with 10 or 20-80 times the human allowable daily intake of aspartame during pregnancy (Mahalik & Gautieri, 1985; Dow-Edwards et al., 1989). The clinical relevance of these findings is unknown.

It has been suggested on theoretical grounds that use of aspartame by pregnant women who are heterozygous carriers of phenylketonuria may increase the risk of mental retardation in their offspring (Bhagavan, 1975), but this risk is unlikely to be of clinical significance (Sturtevant, 1985; Caballero et al., 1986; Trefz et al., 1994).

Risk Related to Breast-feeding

Aspartame is metabolized to phenylalanine and aspartate, both of which are naturally present in breast milk. Although a single very large dose of aspartame (50 mg/kg) was found to produce a slight increase in breast milk levels of aspartate and phenylalanine in one study, the amount of these amino acids that the nursing infant would ingest in addition to that normally received in the breast milk is insignificant (Stegink et al., 1979). The maternal dose of aspartame used in this study was substantially greater than that which would be ingested in a single day when used as a sweetener.

The American Academy of Pediatrics regards aspartame to be safe to use while breast-feeding although they recommend that caution be used if either the mother or infant has phenylketonuria (Committee on Drugs, American Academy of Pediatrics, 1994).

Key References

Anonymous: Position of The American Dietetic Association: Use of nutritive and nonnutritive sweeteners. J Am Diet Assoc 93:816-821, 1993.

Bhagavan NV: Hazards in indiscriminate use of sweeteners containing phenylalanine. N Engl J Med 292:52-53, 1975.

Caballero B, Mahon BE, Rohr FJ, et al.: Plasma amino acid levels after single-dose aspartame consumption in phenylketonuria, mild hyperphenylalaninemia, and heterozygous state for phenylketonuria. J Pediatr 109:668-671, 1986.

Committee on Drugs, American Academy of Pediatrics: The transfer of drugs and other chemicals into human milk. Pediatrics 93(1):137-150, 1994.

Dow-Edwards DL, Scribani LA, Riley EP: Impaired performance on odor-aversion testing following prenatal aspartame exposure in the guinea pig. Neurotoxicol Teratol 11:413-416, 1989.

Lederer J, Bodin J, Colson A: [Aspartame and its effect on gestation in rats.] J Toxicol Clin Exp 5:7-14, 1985.

Mahalik MP, Gautieri RF: Reflex responsiveness of CF-1 mouse neonates following maternal aspartame exposure. Res Commun Psychol Psychiatr Behav 9:385-403, 1985.

Ranney RE, Mares SE, Schroeder RE, et al.: The phenylalanine and tyrosine content of maternal and fetal body fluids from rabbits fed aspartame. Toxicol Appl Pharmacol 32:339-346, 1975.

Steginik LD, Filer LJ Jr, Baker GL: Plasma, erythrocyte and human milk levels of free amino acids in lactating women administered aspartame or lactose. J Nutr 109:2173-2181, 1979.

Sturtevant FM: Use of aspartame in pregnancy. Int J Fertil 30:85-87, 1985.

Trefz F, de Sonneville L, Matthis P, et al.: Neuropsychological and biochemical investigations in heterozygotes for phenylketonuria during ingestion of high dose aspartame (a sweetener containing phenylalanine). Hum Genet 93:369-374, 1994.

ASPIRIN
(ASA, Ecotrin®, Salicylates)

Aspirin is a frequently used oral analgesic and antipyretic agent. Common occasional usage of aspirin for treatment of headache, muscle ache, fever, etc., is generally in "low" doses of 325-1300 mg/d. Administration of aspirin to prevent thrombosis generally involves lower doses (325-1000 mg/d), and much lower doses (50-150 mg/d) are used to prevent the development of pregnancy-induced hypertension and other complications of pregnancy. Much higher doses of aspirin (as much as 6000-8000 mg/d) are used to treat rheumatic disease.

Teratogenic Risk

*Magnitude of teratogenic
risk to child born after
exposure during gestation:*   *Unlikely*

*Quality and quantity of data
on which risk estimate is based:*   *Fair to good*

This rating is based on maternal use of occasional low doses of aspirin. The risks associated with chronic high doses (such as those used to treat rheumatic diseases) and with toxic overdoses of aspirin are unknown.

Occasional low doses of aspirin are unlikely to pose a substantial teratogenic risk, but the data are insufficient to state that there is no risk.

Maternal aspirin use just prior to delivery may be associated with intracranial hemorrhage in premature infants (see discussion below).

The extensive epidemiological data available regarding the risk of congenital anomalies among women who took aspirin during pregnancy is inconsistent, but overall this risk does not appear to be substantially increased among pregnant women who took occasional low doses of aspirin (Slone et al., 1976; Corby, 1978; Rudolph, 1981; Hertz-Picciotto et al., 1990). Various malformations have been associated with maternal aspirin use early in gestation in some studies (Nelson & Forfar, 1971; Richards 1972; Saxen, 1975; Rothman et al., 1979; Zierler & Rothman, 1985; Correy et al., 1991), but the types of anomalies associated with maternal aspirin use have varied among the studies and the findings have not been consistently reproducible (Turner & Collins, 1975; Slone et al., 1976; Jick et al., 1981; Winship et al., 1984; Aselton et al., 1985; Werler et al., 1989; Hertz-Picciotto et al., 1990; Tikkanen & Heinonen, 1991, 1992).

One infant with malformations was observed among 31 born to women who had taken overdoses of aspirin at various times during pregnancy in one series (McElhatton et al., 1991).

Maternal aspirin use during the first half of pregnancy was associated with slightly lower IQ scores in 421 four-year-old children in one study (Streissguth et al., 1987), but no such effect was seen in another similar study of the children of more than 19,000 women (Klebanoff & Berendes, 1988).

Aspirin in doses similar to or greater than those used to treat rheumatic disease in humans is teratogenic in rats, mice, dogs, cats, and monkeys (Wilson et al., 1977; Klein et al., 1981; Khera, 1984; Hamed et al., 1994). A variety of anomalies may be produced, including neural tube defects, skeletal malformations, and facial clefts. Behavioral alterations have been found among the offspring of rats treated during pregnancy with aspirin in doses several times those used to treat rheumatic disease in humans (Vorhees et al., 1982).

Aspirin is an inhibitor of prostaglandin synthesis. More potent prostaglandin synthesis inhibitors are used therapeutically to produce closure of the ductus arteriosus and consequent changes in cardiovascular and pulmonary function in newborns with patent ductus arteriosus. There is anecdotal evidence of an association between maternal high-dose aspirin use and premature closure of the fetal ductus arteriosus (Levin et al., 1978), but a causal relationship is uncertain. If maternal high-dose aspirin use does cause premature closure of the fetal ductus arteriosus, it must do so infrequently.

The onset of labor may be delayed and its duration prolonged in women who take high-dose aspirin chronically in late pregnancy (Lewis & Schulman, 1973). Some studies suggest that babies born to such women have lower birth weights than expected (Turner & Collins, 1975), but other studies do not support this conclusion (Shapiro et al., 1976).

Maternal aspirin use within a week of delivery causes abnormalities of hemostasis in human newborns as well as their mothers (Stuart et al., 1982). These hemostatic defects usually produce very little, if any, clinical manifestation in term infants but may be associated with an increased risk of intracranial hemorrhage in premature and low birth weight infants (Rumack et al., 1981).

Aspirin is metabolized more slowly and is less completely bound to serum proteins in neonates than in adults (Levy & Garrettson, 1974; Levy et al., 1975). Thus, the serum concentration of aspirin in the fetus or immediate newborn is often higher than that in a mother who has taken the drug. Salicylate intoxication in the infant of a mother who took large doses of aspirin during pregnancy (Lynd et al., 1976) and fetal death associated with maternal toxic salicylism have been reported (Rejent & Baik, 1985).

Maternal treatment with very low doses of aspirin during the second and third trimesters of pregnancy has been used for the prevention of fetal growth retardation, pregnancy-induced hypertension, and stillbirth in high-risk pregnancies (Benigni et al., 1989; Schiff et al., 1989; Hertz-Picciotto et al., 1990; Imperiale et al., 1991; Uzan et al., 1991; Anonymous, 1993, 1994; Dekker & Sibai, 1993; Sibai et al., 1993). Studies of this treatment have involved thousands of pregnant women and have not found any adverse effect on the children (Dekker & Sibai, 1993; Valcamonico et al., 1993). There were no significant differences in health or development among 427 18-month-old children born to women who had been treated with low-dose aspirin during pregnancy in one trial (Parazzini et al., 1994).

Risk Related to Breast-feeding

Aspirin is excreted in the breast milk. Based on data obtained from two lactating women, the amount of aspirin that the nursing infant would receive is <1% of the lowest neonatal dose (Findlay et al., 1981).*

A serum concentration three times the lowest therapeutic serum level in adults was measured in the infant of a woman who took a large dose of aspirin (2.4 g/d) for seven weeks postpartum (Unsworth et al., 1987).† No adverse effects were observed in the infant. No detectable levels of aspirin could be detected in the infant's serum or the breast milk of a mother who took very large doses of aspirin (4 g/d) while breast-feeding (Erickson & Oppenheim, 1979). No adverse effects of aspirin on the nursing infant were reported. However, metabolic acidosis was observed in the infant of a breast-feeding mother who took similar amounts of aspirin (Clark & Wilson, 1981). The infant's serum level of aspirin was 240 mcg/mL, which is 10 times the lowest therapeutic serum level in adults. Because of this case, the American

*This calculation is based on the following assumptions: maternal dose of aspirin: 454 mg; milk concentration of aspirin: 0.9-3.3 mcg/mL; milk intake by the nursing infant: 150 mL/kg/d; estimated dose of aspirin ingested by the nursing infant: 0.13-0.49 mg/kg/d; lowest neonatal dose of aspirin: 65 mg/kg/d.

†This calculation is based on the following assumptions: infant serum level of aspirin: 80 mcg/mL; lowest therapeutic serum level of aspirin in adults: 25 mcg/mL.

Academy of Pediatrics recommends that aspirin be taken by nursing mothers with caution (Committee on Drugs, American Academy of Pediatrics, 1994).

Rashes have been observed in nursing infants whose mothers ingested aspirin (Chaplin et al., 1982). Although use of high doses of aspirin have the potential of causing abnormal platelet function in nursing infants, no such effects have been reported.

Key References

Anonymous: CLASP: A randomised trial of low-dose aspirin for the prevention and treatment of pre-eclampsia among 9364 pregnant women. Lancet 343:619-629, 1994.

Anonymous: Low-dose aspirin in prevention and treatment of intrauterine growth retardation and pregnancy-induced hypertension. Lancet 341:396-400, 1993.

Aselton P, Jick H, Milunsky A, et al.: First-trimester drug use and congenital disorders. Obstet Gynecol 65:451-455, 1985.

Benigni A, Gregorini G, Frusca T, et al.: Effect of low-dose aspirin on fetal and maternal generation of thromboxane by platelets in women at risk for pregnancy-induced hypertension. N Engl J Med 321:357-362, 1989.

Chaplin S, Sanders GL, Smith JM: Drug excretion in human breast milk. Adv Drug React Ac Pois Rev 1:255-287, 1982.

Clark JH, Wilson WG: A 16-day-old breast-fed infant with metabolic acidosis caused by salicylate. Clin Pediatr 20:53-54, 1981.

Committee on Drugs, American Academy of Pediatrics: The transfer of drugs and other chemicals into human milk. Pediatrics 93(1):137-150, 1994.

Corby DG: Aspirin in pregnancy: Maternal and fetal effects. Pediatrics 62(Suppl):930-937, 1978.

Correy JF, Newman NM, Collins JA, et al.: Use of prescription drugs in the first trimester and congenital malformations. Aust NZ J Obstet Gynaecol 31(4):340-344, 1991.

Dekker GA, Sibai BM: Low-dose aspirin in the prevention of preeclampsia and fetal growth retardation: Rationale, mechanisms, and clinical trials. Am J Obstet Gynecol 168:214-227, 1993.

Erickson SH, Oppenheim GL: Aspirin in breast milk. J Fam Pract 8(1):189-190, 1979.

Findlay JWA, DeAngelis RL, Kearney MF, et al.: Analgesic drugs in breast milk and plasma. Clin Pharmacol Ther 29:625-633, 1981.

Hamed MR, Al-Assy YS, Ezzeldin E: Influence of protein malnutrition on teratogenicity of acetylsalicylic acid in rats. Hum Exp Toxicol 113:83-88, 1994.

Hertz-Picciotto I, Hopenhayn-Rich C, Golub M, Hooper K: The risks and benefits of taking aspirin during pregnancy. Epidemiol Rev 12:108-148, 1990.

Imperiale TF, Petrulis AS: A meta-analysis of low-dose aspirin for the prevention of pregnancy-induced hypertensive disease. JAMA 266:261-265, 1991.

Jick H, Holmes LB, Hunter JR, et al.: First-trimester drug use and congenital disorders. JAMA 246:343-346, 1981.

Khera KS: Adverse effects in humans and animals of prenatal exposure to selected therapeutic drugs and estimation of embryo-fetal sensitivity of animals for human risk assessment. Issues Rev Teratol 2:399-507, 1984.

Klebanoff MA, Berendes HW: Aspirin exposure during the first 20 weeks of gestation and IQ at four years of age. Teratology 37:249-255, 1988.

Klein KL, Scott WJ, Wilson JG: Aspirin-induced teratogenesis: A unique pattern of cell death and subsequent polydactyly in the rat. J Exp Zool 216:107-112, 1981.

Levin DL, Fixler DE, Morriss FC, Tyson J: Morphologic analysis of the pulmonary vascular bed in infants exposed in utero to prostaglandin synthetase inhibitors. J Pediatr 92:478-483, 1978.

Levy G, Garrettson LK: Kinetics of salicylate elimination by newborn infants of mothers who ingested aspirin before delivery. Pediatrics 53:201-210, 1974.

Levy G, Procknal JA, Garrettson LK: Distribution of salicylate between neonatal and maternal serum at diffusion equilibrium. Clin Pharmacol Ther 18:210-214, 1975.

Lewis RB, Schulman JD: Influence of acetylsalicylic acid, an inhibitor of prostaglandin synthesis, on the duration of human gestation and labor. Lancet 2:1159-1161, 1973.

Lynd PA, Andreasen AC, Wyatt RJ: Intrauterine salicylate intoxication in a newborn. Clin Pediatr 15:912-913, 1976.

McElhatton PR, Sullivan FM, Walton L: Analgesic overdose during pregnancy. Teratology 44:(3)17A, 1991.

Nelson MM, Forfar JO: Associations between drugs administered during pregnancy and congenital abnormalities of the fetus. Br Med J 1:523-527, 1971.

Parazzini F, Bortolus R, Chatenoud L, et al.: Follow-up of children in the Italian Study of Aspirin in Pregnancy. Lancet 343:1235, 1994.

Rejent TA, Baik S-O: Fatal in utero salicylism. J Forensic Sci 30:942-944, 1985.

Richards IDG: A retrospective enquiry into possible teratogenic effects of drugs in pregnancy. Adv Exp Med Biol 27:441-455, 1972.

Rothman KJ, Fyler DC, Goldblatt A, Kreidberg MB: Exogenous hormones and other drug exposures of children with congenital heart disease. Am J Epidemiol 109:433-439, 1979.

Rudolph AM: Effects of aspirin and acetaminophen in pregnancy and in the newborn. Arch Intern Med 141:358-363, 1981.

Rumack CM, Guggenheim MA, Rumack BH, et al.: Neonatal intracranial hemorrhage and maternal use of aspirin. Obstet Gynecol 58:52S-56S, 1981.

Saxen I: Associations between oral clefts and drugs taken during pregnancy. Int J Epidemiol 4:37-44, 1975.

Schiff E, Peleg E, Goldenberg M, et al.: The use of aspirin to prevent pregnancy-induced hypertension and lower the ratio of thromboxane A_2 to prostacyclin in relatively high risk pregnancies. N Engl J Med 321:351-356, 1989.

Shapiro S, Siskind V, Monson RR, et al.: Perinatal mortality and birth-weight in relation to aspirin taken during pregnancy. Lancet 1:1375-1376, 1976.

Sibai BM, Caritis SN, Thom E, et al.: Prevention of preeclampsia with low-dose aspirin in healthy nulliparous pregnant women. N Engl J Med 329:1213-1218, 1993.

Slone D, Siskind V, Heinonen OP, et al.: Aspirin and congenital malformations. Lancet 1:1373-1375, 1976.

Streissguth AP, Treder RP, Barr HM, et al.: Aspirin and acetaminophen use by pregnant women and subsequent child IQ and attention decrements. Teratology 35:211-219, 1987.

Stuart MJ, Gross SJ, Elrad H, Graeber JE: Effects of acetylsalicylic-acid ingestion on maternal and neonatal hemostasis. N Engl J Med 307:909-912, 1982.

Tikkanen J, Heinonen OP: Congenital heart disease in the offspring and maternal habits and home exposures during pregnancy. Teratology 46:447-454, 1992.

Tikkanen J, Heinonen OP: Maternal hyperthermia during pregnancy and cardiovascular malformations in the offspring. Eur J Epidemiol 7(6):628-635, 1991.

Turner G, Collins E: Fetal effects of regular salicylate ingestion in pregnancy. Lancet 2:338-339, 1975.

Unsworth J, d'Assis-Fonseca A, Beswick DT, Blake DR: Serum salicylate levels in a breast fed infant. Ann Rheum Dis 46:638-639, 1987.

Uzan S, Beaufils M, Breart G, et al.: Prevention of fetal growth retardation with low-dose aspirin: Findings of the EPREDA trial. Lancet 337:1427-1431, 1991.

Valcamonico A, Foschini M, Soregaroli M, et al.: Low dose aspirin in pregnancy: A clinical and biochemical study of effects on the newborn. J Perinat Med 21:235-240, 1993.

Vorhees CV, Klein KL, Scott WJ: Aspirin-induced psychoteratogenesis in rats as a function of embryonic age. Teratogenesis Carcinog Mutagen 2:77-84, 1982.

Werler MM, Mitchell AA, Shapiro S: The relation of aspirin use during the first trimester of pregnancy to congenital cardiac defects. N Engl J Med 321:1639-1642, 1989.

Wilson JG, Ritter EJ, Scott WJ, Fradkin R: Comparative distribution and embryotoxicity of acetylsalicylic acid in pregnant rats and rhesus monkeys. Toxicol Appl Pharmacol 41:67-78, 1977.

Winship KA, Cahal DA, Weber JCP, Griffin JP: Maternal drug histories and central nervous system anomalies. Arch Dis Child 59:1052-1060, 1984.

Zierler S, Rothman KJ: Congenital heart disease in relation to maternal use of Bendectin and other drugs in early pregnancy. N Engl J Med 313:347-352, 1985.

ATARAX® *See* Hydroxyzine

ATENOLOL
(Tenormin®)

Atenolol is a cardioselective β-adrenergic receptor blocking agent. It is used orally to treat hypertension and angina pectoris, the usual dose being 50-100 mg/d. Doses as large as 200 mg/d are sometimes used. Atenolol may also be given intravenously to patients with myocardial infarction; the usual dose is 10 mg.

Teratogenic Risk

*Magnitude of teratogenic
risk to child born after
exposure during gestation:*   *Undetermined*

Quality and quantity of data
on which risk estimate is based: *Poor*

A small risk cannot be excluded, but there is no indication that the risk of congenital anomalies in children of women treated with atenolol during pregnancy is likely to be great.

There are no published epidemiological studies of congenital anomalies among the children of women treated with atenolol during early pregnancy.

Studies in rats and rabbits suggest that treatment of pregnant women with atenolol in usual therapeutic doses is unlikely to increase the children's risk of malformations greatly (Esaki, 1980; Esaki & Imai, 1980).

Fetal growth retardation and neonatal bradycardia have been associated with second- and third-trimester atenolol therapy of hypertensive pregnant women in controlled therapeutic trials (Rubin et al., 1983; Butters et al., 1990; Marlettini et al., 1990). Similar effects have been observed in infants born to women treated with other, chemically-related β-blockers during pregnancy *(please see agent summary on propranolol).* No abnormalities were found on follow-up physical and developmental examinations to one year of age in 55 children of women who had been treated with atenolol for hypertension during pregnancy (Reynolds et al., 1984).

Risk Related to Breast-feeding

Atenolol is excreted in breast milk in concentrations up to seven times higher than those found in maternal serum (Liedholm et al., 1981; White et al., 1984). The amount of atenolol that the nursing infant would be expected to ingest is between 5-37% of the lowest weight-adjusted therapeutic dose, based on data obtained from 11 lactating women (Liedholm et al., 1981; Kulas et al., 1984).* Serum levels in five infants were between <2-30% of the average adult serum level (Liedholm et al., 1981; Kulas et al., 1984).[†] No abnormalities

*This calculation is based on the following assumptions: maternal dose of atenolol: 0.8-1.6 mg/kg/d; milk concentration of atenolol: 0.25-2.1 mcg/mL; milk intake by the nursing infant: 150 mL/kg/d; estimated dose of atenolol ingested by the nursing infant: 0.04-0.31 mg/kg/d; lowest adult therapeutic dose: 0.8 mg/kg/d.

†This calculation is based on the following assumption: infant serum levels of atenolol: <0.01-0.12 mcg/mL; average adult serum level of atenolol: 0.4 mcg/mL.

were observed in any of the infants. In another study, serum levels of atenolol in one nursing infant were below the detection level of 0.01 mcg/mL (White et al., 1984).

Symptoms characteristic of β-adrenergic blockade (bradycardia, cyanosis, jaundice, fever, and hypothermia) were reported in an infant whose mother was taking 100 mg of atenolol per day while breast-feeding (Schmimmel et al., 1989). Levels of atenolol five times the average adult serum level were measured in the infant's serum (0.14-2 mcg/mL). The symptoms resolved upon discontinuance of the drug.

The American Academy of Pediatrics (Committee on Drugs, American Academy of Pediatrics, 1994) considers atenolol to be safe to use during breast-feeding. Nursing infants exposed to atenolol via the breast milk should be monitored for signs of β-blockade.

Key References

Butters L, Kennedy S, Rubin PC: Atenolol in essential hypertension during pregnancy. BMJ 301:587-589, 1990.

Committee on Drugs, American Academy of Pediatrics: The transfer of drugs and other chemicals into human milk. Pediatrics 93:137-150, 1994.

Esaki K: Effects of oral administration of atenolol on the rabbit fetus. Preclin Rep Cent Inst Exper Anim 6:259-264, 1980.

Esaki K, Imai K: Effects of oral administration of atenolol on reproduction in rats. II. Experiments on drug administration during the organogenesis period. Preclin Rep Cent Inst Exper Anim 6:247-252, 1980.

Kulas J, Lunell NO, Rosing U, et al.: Atenolol and metoprolol. A comparison of their excretion into human breast milk. Acta Obstet Gynecol Scand 118(Suppl):65-69, 1984.

Liedholm H, Melander A, Bitzen P-O, et al.: Accumulation of atenolol and metoprolol in human breast milk. Eur J Clin Pharmacol 20:229-231, 1981.

Marlettini MG, Crippa S, Morselli-Labate AM, et al.: Randomized comparison of calcium antagonists and β-blockers in the treatment of pregnancy-induced hypertension. Curr Ther Res 48(4):684-694, 1990.

Reynolds B, Butters L, Evans J, et al.: First year of life after the use of atenolol in pregnancy associated with hypertension. Arch Dis Child 59:1061-1063, 1984.

Rubin PC, Clark DM, Sumner DJ, et al.: Placebo-controlled trial of atenolol in treatment of pregnancy-associated hypertension. Lancet 1:431-434, 1983.

Schmimmel MS, Eidelman AJ, Wilschanski MA, et al.: Toxic effects of atenolol consumed during breast-feeding. J Pediatr 114:476-478, 1989.

White WB, Andreoli JW, Wong SH, Cohn RD: Atenolol in human plasma and breast milk. Obstet Gynecol 63:42S-44S, 1984.

ATIVAN® *See* Lorazepam

ATROPINE
(Atropin Minims®)

Atropine is an anticholinergic alkaloid that is often used as a preanesthetic medication to reduce airway secretions. It is also employed in the treatment of gastrointestinal disorders, bronchial asthma, bradycardia, Parkinsonism, and organophosphorous insecticide poisoning. Atropine is given orally, parenterally, or as an inhalant in doses ranging from 1.2-7.2 mg/d. Atropine is also used in ophthalmic preparations as a mydriatic; systemic absorption of the drug may occur after ophthalmic administration.

Teratogenic Risk

*Magnitude of teratogenic
risk to child born after
exposure during gestation:*   *Unlikely*

*Quality and quantity of data
on which risk estimate is based:*   *Fair*

Therapeutic doses of atropine are unlikely to pose a substantial teratogenic risk, but the data are insufficient to state that there is no risk.

The frequency of congenital anomalies was no greater than expected among the children of 401 women treated with atropine during the first four lunar months of pregnancy or the children of 1198 women treated with this drug anytime during pregnancy in one epidemiological study (Heinonen et al., 1977). Similarly, congenital anomalies were observed no more often than expected among the infants of more than 50 women who took atropine during the first trimester of pregnancy in another study (Jick et al., 1981).

The frequency of skeletal variations, but not of brain or visceral malformations, was increased among the offspring of mice treated once during pregnancy with atropine in doses about 1500 times those used clinically (Arcuri & Gautieri, 1973). Behavioral alterations have been observed among the offspring of rats treated during pregnancy with about 4 times the usual human dose of atropine (Watanabe et al., 1985). The relevance, if any, of these observations to the risks associated with therapeutic use of atropine in human pregnancy is unclear.

Risk Related to Breast-feeding

Atropine is excreted in breast milk, although this has not been quantitated in published reports (USP DI, 1995).

The American Academy of Pediatrics regards atropine to be safe to use while breast-feeding (Committee on Drugs, American Academy of Pediatrics, 1994.

Key References

Arcuri PA, Gautieri RF: Morphine-induced fetal malformations. III: Possible mechanisms of action. J Pharm Sci 62:1626-1634, 1973.

Committee on Drugs, American Academy of Pediatrics: The transfer of drugs and other chemicals into human milk. Pediatrics 93(1):137-150, 1994.

Heinonen OP, Slone D, Shapiro S: *Birth Defects and Drugs in Pregnancy.* Littleton, Mass.: John Wright-PSG, 1977, pp 346, 439.

Jick H, Holmes LB, Hunter JR, et al.: First-trimester drug use and congenital disorders. JAMA 246:343-346, 1981.

USP DI: Anticholinergics/Antispasmodics. In: *USP DI (USP Dispensing Information), Volume 1. Drug Information for the Health Care Professional,* 15th ed. Rockville, Md.: The US Pharmacopeial Convention, 1995, p 211.

Watanabe T, Matsuhashi K, Takayama S: Study on the postnatal neurobehavioral development in rats treated prenatally with drugs acting on the autonomic nervous systems. Folia Pharmacol Jpn 85:79-90, 1985.

ATROPIN-MINIMS® *See* Atropine

ATTENUVAX® *See* Measles Vaccine, Live

AUREOMYCIN® *See* Chlortetracycline

AVENTYL® *See* Nortriptyline

AVIRAX® *See* Acyclovir

AYERCILLIN® *See* Penicillin

AZALINE® *See* Sulfasalazine

AZATADINE
(Optimine®, Trinalin Repetabs®)

Azatadine is an antihistamine used to treat allergic disorders. It is given orally in a dose of 2-6 mg/d.

Teratogenic Risk

Magnitude of teratogenic risk to child born after exposure during gestation:	*Undetermined*
Quality and quantity of data on which risk estimate is based:	*None*

No epidemiological studies of congenital anomalies in children born to women who took azatadine during pregnancy have been reported.

No animal teratology studies of azatadine have been published.

Risk Related to Breast-feeding

No information regarding the distribution of azatadine in breast milk has been published.

Key References

None available.

AZATHIOPRINE
(Imuran®)

Azathioprine is a purine antimetabolite. It is used as an immunosuppressant in treatment of autoimmune diseases and in prevention of transplant rejection. Azathioprine is given orally or parenterally in a dose of 1-5 mg/kg of body weight per day. This would amount to 50-250 mg/d for a 110 pound woman.

Teratogenic Risk

Magnitude of teratogenic risk to child born after exposure during gestation:	*Minimal to small*
Quality and quantity of data on which risk estimate is based:	*Poor to fair*

Serious and even fatal neonatal anemia, thrombocytopenia, and lymphopenia have been observed among the children of women treated with azathioprine during pregnancy (see below).

No controlled epidemiological studies of congenital anomalies in infants born to women treated with azathioprine during pregnancy have been reported. In two series of infants born to renal transplant recipients who had been treated with azathioprine and prednisone throughout pregnancy, the frequency of congenital anomalies was 4/44 (9%) and 7/110 (6.4%), respectively (Penn et al., 1980; Registration Committee of the European Dialysis and Transplant Association, 1980). No specificity was seen in the kinds of anomalies that occurred. It is difficult to know whether or not this rate of congenital anomalies is higher than expected because these mothers took other drugs besides azathioprine and often had azotemia. In more recent series of renal transplant recipients who were treated with azathioprine during pregnancy, none of 23 liveborn children in one group and none of 24 liveborn children in another had congenital anomalies (Brown et al., 1991). No congenital anomalies occurred among 20 infants born to women who had previously received cardiac transplantation and were treated with azathioprine during pregnancy or among 14 infants of women treated with azathioprine during the first trimester of pregnancy for inflammatory bowel disease (Alstead et al., 1990; Wagoner et al., 1994).

The frequencies of prematurity and fetal growth retardation appear to be increased in pregnancies of renal transplant recipients treated with azathioprine, especially if the woman has reduced renal function, previous rejection, or requires high-dose immunosuppressive therapy (Brown et al., 1991; Sturgiss & Davison, 1991; Cararach et al., 1993).

Increased frequencies of limb malformations, ocular anomalies, and cleft palate were observed among the offspring of rabbits treated with azathioprine in doses 1-2 times those used in humans (Tuchmann-Duplessis & Mercier-Parot, 1964). Similar anomalies were observed among the offspring of mice treated with azathioprine at 4-6 times the human therapeutic dose in one study (Rosenkrantz et al., 1967). The rate of malformations was not increased among the offspring of mice or rats treated during pregnancy with azathioprine in doses within the human therapeutic range or twice as great, but increased frequencies of fetal loss and growth retardation were regularly seen (Tuchmann-Duplessis & Mercier-Parot, 1964; Rosenkrantz et al., 1967; Scott, 1977; Fein et al., 1983).

Fatal neonatal anemia, thrombocytopenia, and lymphopenia have been reported in an infant born to a renal transplant recipient treated with azathioprine and prednisone during pregnancy (DeWitte et al., 1984). Neonatal lymphopenia and thrombocytopenia have been observed in several other children born to women who received similar therapy (Lower et al., 1971; Price et al., 1976; Rudolph et al., 1979; Penn, 1980; Davison et al., 1985). It seems likely that these hematologic abnormalities resulted from a toxic effect of azathioprine on the fetus similar to that which occasionally occurs with the drug in adults.

Increased frequencies of acquired chromosomal breaks and rearrangements have been observed in blood cells of renal transplant recipients receiving azathioprine therapy and, transiently, in the infants of women who were given such treatment during pregnancy (Sharon et al., 1974; Price et al., 1976). One case has also been reported of a child with two separate de novo constitutional chromosomal anomalies who was born to a woman treated before and during pregnancy with azathioprine and prednisone (Ostrer et al., 1984). These observations raise the possibility, but do not prove, that parental azathioprine treatment during gametogenesis may predispose to constitutional cytogenetic abnormalities in subsequently conceived children. If this does occur, it must be infrequent (Penn et al., 1980; Registration Committee of the European Dialysis and Transplant Association, 1980; Pirson et al., 1985).

Risk Related to Breast-feeding

The active metabolite of azathioprine, 6-mercaptopurine, has been found to be excreted in very low concentrations in breast milk (Coulam et al., 1982). The amount of 6-mercaptopurine that the nursing infant would be expected to ingest is <1% of the lowest weight-adjusted therapeutic dose of azathioprine, based on data from two breast-feeding patients (Coulam et al., 1982).* In this study, IgA concentrations in the breast milk of both mothers were similar to IgA concentrations measured in the breast milk of women not taking azathioprine. Only one of the mothers chose to breast-feed her infant and this infant was reported to have normal blood cell counts, no increase in infections, and an above-average growth rate. Although azathioprine and IgA breast milk levels were not measured in another case report, no abnormalities were observed in two infants whose breast-feeding mothers were treated with azathioprine (Grekas et al., 1984).

Because of the potential risk of bone marrow depression, susceptibility to infection, and hepatitis to the nursing infant, the WHO Working Group on Drugs and Human Lactation (1988) does not recommend breast-feeding in mothers taking azathioprine.

Key References

Alstead EM, Ritchie JK, Lennard-Jones JE, et al.: Safety of azathioprine in pregnancy in inflammatory bowel disease. Gastroenterology 99:443-446, 1990.

Brown JH, Maxwell AP, McGeown MG: Outcome of pregnancy following renal transplantation. Ir J Med Sci 160(8):255-256, 1991.

Cararach V, Carmona F, Monleon FJ, Andreu J: Pregnancy after renal transplantation: 25 years experience in Spain. Br J Obstet Gynaecol 100:122-125, 1993.

*This calculation is based on the following assumptions: maternal dose of azathioprine: 0.4-1.2 mg/kg/d; milk concentration of 6-mercaptopurine: 0.003-0.02 mcg/mL; milk intake by the nursing infant: 150 mL/kg/d; estimated dose of 6-mercaptopurine ingested by the nursing infant, assuming similar bioavailability, activity, and molecular weights: 0.0004-0.003 mg/kg/d; lowest adult therapeutic dose of azathioprine: 1 mg/kg/d.

Coulam CB, Moyer TP, Jiang N-S, Zincke H: Breast-feeding after renal transplantation. Transplant Proc 14:605-609, 1982.

Davison JM, Dellagrammatikas H, Parkin JM: Maternal azathioprine therapy and depressed haemopoiesis in the babies of renal allograft patients. Br J Obstet Gynaecol 92:233-239, 1985.

DeWitte DB, Buick MK, Cyran SE, Maisels MJ: Neonatal pancytopenia and severe combined immunodeficiency associated with antenatal administration of azathioprine and prednisone. J Pediatr 105:625-628, 1984.

Fein A, Gross A, Serr DM, Nebel L: Effect of Imuran® on placental and fetal development in rats. Isr J Med Sci 19:73-75, 1983.

Grekas DM, Vasiliou SS, Lazarides AN: Immunosuppressive therapy and breast-feeding after renal transplantation. Nephron 37:68, 1984.

Lower GD, Stevens LE, Najarian JS, Reemtsma K: Problems from immunosuppressives during pregnancy. Am J Obstet Gynecol 111:1120-1121, 1971.

Ostrer H, Stamberg J, Perinchief P: Two chromosome aberrations in the child of a woman with systemic lupus erythematosus treated with azathioprine and prednisone. Am J Med Genet 17:627-632, 1984.

Penn I, Makowski EL, Harris P: Parenthood following renal transplantation. Kidney Int 18:221-233, 1980.

Pirson Y, Van Lierde M, Ghysen J, et al.: Retardation of fetal growth in patients receiving immunosuppressive therapy. N Engl J Med 313:328, 1985.

Price HV, Salaman JR, Laurence KM, Langmaid H: Immunosuppressive drugs and the foetus. Transplantation 21:294-298, 1976.

Registration Committee of the European Dialysis and Transplant Association: Successful pregnancies in women treated by dialysis and kidney transplantation. Br J Obstet Gynaecol 87:839-845, 1980.

Rosenkrantz JG, Githens JH, Cox SM, Kellum DL: Azathioprine (Imuran®) and pregnancy. Am J Obstet Gynecol 97:387-394, 1967.

Rudolph JE, Schweizer RT, Bartus SA: Pregnancy in renal transplant patients. Transplantation 27:26-29, 1979.

Scott JR: Fetal growth retardation associated with maternal administration of immunosuppressive drugs. Am J Obstet Gynecol 128:668-676, 1977.

Sharon E, Jones J, Diamond H, Kaplan D: Pregnancy and azathioprine in systemic lupus erythematosus. Am J Obstet Gynecol 118:25-28, 1974.

Sturgiss SN, Davison JM: Perinatal outcome in renal allograft recipients: Prognostic significance of hypertension and renal function before and during pregnancy. Obstet Gynecol 78:573-577, 1991.

Tuchmann-Duplessis H, Mercier-Parot L: [Teratogenic tests. Difference of reaction of three animal species to an antitumoral agent.] C R Soc Biol 158:1984-1990, 1964.

Wagoner LE, Taylor DO, Olsen SL, et al.: Immunosuppressive therapy, management, and outcome of heart transplant recipients during pregnancy. J Heart Lung Transplant 13:993-1000, 1994.

WHO Working Group on Drugs and Human Lactation. In: Bennet PN (ed). *Drugs and Human Lactation*. Amsterdam: Elsevier, 1988, pp 286-287.

AZT *See* Zidovudine

AZULFIDINE® *See* Sulfasalazine

AZUREN® *See* Bromperidol

BACIGUENT® *See* Bacitracin

BACITRACIN
(Ak-tracin®, Baciguent®)

Bacitracin is a polypeptide antibiotic produced by the bacterium *Bacillus subtilis*. Bacitracin is used topically on skin or in the eye to treat susceptible infections. Systemic absorption of bacitracin after topical administration is minimal.

Teratogenic Risk

Magnitude of teratogenic risk to child born after exposure during gestation: *Undetermined*

Quality and quantity of data on which risk estimate is based: *None*

A small risk cannot be excluded, but there is no indication that the risk of congenital anomalies in children of women treated topically with bacitracin during pregnancy is likely to be great.

No epidemiological studies of infants born after maternal treatment with topical bacitracin during pregnancy have been reported.
No animal teratology studies of bacitracin have been published.

Risk Related to Breast-feeding

No information regarding the distribution of bacitracin in breast milk has been published.

Key References

None available.

BARBITAL® *See* Phenobarbital

BARIDIUM® *See* Phenazopyridine

BECLOMETHASONE
(Alphatrex®, Betamethasone®, Vancerase®)

Beclomethasone is a synthetic glucocorticoid used to treat skin disorders and in the prevention and therapy of asthma. Systemic absorption occurs after administration topically or by inhalation. The usual dose by inhalation is 0.25-0.8 mg/d up to 2 mg/d.

Teratogenic Risk

Magnitude of teratogenic risk to child born after exposure during gestation:	*Unlikely*
Quality and quantity of data on which risk estimate is based:	*Poor to fair*

Therapeutic doses of beclomethasone are unlikely to pose a substantial teratogenic risk, but the data are insufficient to state that there is no risk.

The frequency of malformations was not obviously increased in a series of 42 children born to women who used beclomethasone throughout pregnancy or beginning in the first trimester for treatment of asthma (Greenberger & Patterson, 1983).

Beclomethasone, when administered to pregnant mice in doses 7 or more times greater than those used in humans, produces an increased frequency of cleft palate in the offspring (Nomura et al., 1977; Tamagawa et al., 1982). No such effect was seen with lower doses (Esaki et al., 1976; Furuhashi et al., 1977). Similar results have been observed in rabbits (Furuhashi et al., 1977). No malformations were observed among the offspring of seven rhesus monkeys treated with 4-17 times the usual human dose of beclomethasone during pregnancy, although severe growth retardation was seen in one animal and fetal demise in another (Tanioka, 1976). The relevance of these findings to the therapeutic use of beclomethasone in human pregnancy is unknown.

Risk Related to Breast-feeding

No information regarding the distribution of beclomethasone in breast milk has been published.

Key References

Esaki K, Izumiyama K, Yasuda Y: [Effects of the inhalant administration of beclomethasone dipropionate on reproduction in mice. 2. Administration during the fetal organogenesis stage.] Jitchuken Zenrinsho Kenkyuho 2:213-222, 1976.

Furuhashi T, Nomura A, Hasegawa T, Nakazawa M: [Teratological studies on beclomethasone dipropionate. 1. Teratogenicity in rabbits by oral administration.] Oyo Yakuri (Pharmacometrics) 13:71-77, 1977.

Greenberger PA, Patterson R: Beclomethasone diproprionate for severe asthma during pregnancy. Ann Intern Med 98:478-480, 1983.

Nomura A, Furuhashi T, Nakazawa M: [Teratological studies on beclomethasone dipropionate. 4. Teratogenicity in mice by inhalation.] Oyo Yakuri (Pharmacometrics) 13:195-204, 1977.

Tamagawa M, Hatori M, Ooi A, et al.: [Comparative teratological study of flunisolide in mice.] Oyo Yakuri (Pharmacometrics) 24:741-750, 1982.

Tanioka Y: [Teratogenicity test on beclomethasone dipropionate by inhalation in rhesus monkeys.] Jitchuken Zenrinsho Kenkyuho 2:155-164, 1976.

BEDOZ® *See* Cyanocobalamin

BEESIX® *See* Pyridoxine

BENADRYL® *See* Diphenhydramine

BENTYL® *See* Dicyclomine

BENYLIN E® *See* Guaifenesin

BENZEMUL® *See* Benzyl Benzoate

BENZOCAINE
(Americaine®, Orajel®)

Benzocaine is a topical anesthetic of the PABA-derivative ester class. The drug is minimally absorbed after topical administration.

Teratogenic Risk

Magnitude of teratogenic
risk to child born after
exposure during gestation: *Unlikely*

Quality and quantity of data
on which risk estimate is based: *Poor*

Topical administration of benzocaine is unlikely to pose a substantial teratogenic risk, but the data are insufficient to state that there is no risk.

The frequency of congenital anomalies was not significantly greater than expected among the children of 47 women treated with benzocaine during the first four lunar months of pregnancy or among the children of 238 women treated anytime during pregnancy in one epidemiological study (Heinonen et al., 1977).

No animal teratology studies of benzocaine have been published.

Please see agent summary on lidocaine for information on a related agent that has been more thoroughly studied.

Risk Related to Breast-feeding

No information regarding the distribution of benzocaine in breast milk has been published.

Key References

Heinonen OP, Slone D, Shapiro S: *Birth Defects and Drugs in Pregnancy*. Littleton, Mass.: John Wright-PSG, 1977, pp 358, 360, 440.

BENZONATATE
(Tessalon®)

Benzonatate is used as a cough suppressant. It is taken orally in doses of 300-600 mg/d.

Teratogenic Risk

Magnitude of teratogenic risk to child born after exposure during gestation:	Undetermined
Quality and quantity of data on which risk estimate is based:	None

No epidemiological studies of congenital anomalies in infants born to women who took benzonatate during pregnancy have been reported.

No animal teratology studies of benzonatate have been published.

Risk Related to Breast-feeding

No information on the distribution of benzonatate in breast milk has been published.

Key References

None available.

BENZYL BENZOATE
(Ascabiol®, Benzemul®)

Benzyl benzoate is used topically as an insect repellent and as an insecticide to treat mite and lice infestations. Benzyl benzoate is also used as a solubilizing agent in foods and injectable medications.

Teratogenic Risk

*Magnitude of teratogenic
risk to child born after
exposure during gestation:*   *Undetermined*

*Quality and quantity of data
on which risk estimate is based:*   *Very poor*

A small risk cannot be excluded, but there is no indication that the risk of congenital anomalies in the children of women treated with benzyl benzoate during pregnancy is likely to be great.

No epidemiological studies of congenital anomalies in infants whose mothers were exposed to benzyl benzoate during pregnancy have been reported.

No teratogenic effect was observed in the offspring of pregnant rats or mice that had been given 5-130 or 60 times the World Health Organization acceptable daily intake of benzyl benzoate for humans (Morita et al., 1981; Eibs et al., 1982).

Risk Related to Breast-feeding

No information regarding the distribution of benzyl benzoate in breast milk has been published. Topical application directly to the breasts should be avoided.

Key References

Eibs HG, Spielmann H, Hagele M: Teratogenic effects of cyproterone acetate and medroxyprogesterone treatment during the pre- and postimplantation period of mouse embryos. I. Teratology 25:27-36, 1982.

Morita S, Yamada A, Ohgaki S, et al.: Safety evaluation of chemicals for use in household products. (II) Teratological studies on benzyl benzoate and 2-(Morpholinothio)-benzothiazole in rats. Annu Rep Osaka City Inst Publ Health Environ Sci 43:90-97, 1981.

BETA-CAROTENE
(Max-Caro®, Provatene®, Solatene®)

Beta-carotene, a carotenoid that occurs naturally in foods such as carrots and dark green leafy vegetables, can be converted in the body to vitamin A (retinol), a fat-soluble nutrient essential for normal vision. One international unit (IU) of vitamin A (retinol) is equivalent to 0.0006 mg of beta-carotene. The current US recommended dietary allowance (RDA) for vitamin A in pregnant women is the equivalent of 4.8 mg (8000 IU) of beta-carotene per day. Beta-carotene has a long biological half-life and accumulates in the body. The conversion of beta-carotene to vitamin A (retinol) decreases substantially when large amounts of beta-carotene are ingested (USP DI, 1995). Consequently, intake of high doses of beta-carotene does not lead to toxicity or abnormally high serum concentrations of vitamin A (Bendich, 1988).

Beta-carotene is given orally in doses of 6-60 mg (10,000-100,000 IU) per day to treat vitamin A deficiency states. Doses as large as 150 mg (250,000 IU) per day are used to treat certain skin diseases. Beta-carotene has been taken in very large doses for various other purported health benefits, but this use is not generally accepted.

Teratogenic Risk

Magnitude of teratogenic
risk to child born after
exposure during gestation
  Low dose (<10,000 IU):   None
  High dose (>25,000 IU):   Undetermined

Quality and quantity of data
on which risk estimate is based
  Low dose (<10,000 IU):   Poor
  High dose (>25,000 IU):   Poor

The risks related to treatment with high-dose retinol are substantially greater than those associated with high-dose beta-carotene treatment. It is essential to distinguish between beta-carotene and retinol when evaluating a pregnant woman who has taken vitamin A in high doses.

No epidemiological studies of congenital anomalies in children born to women who took large amounts of beta-carotene during pregnancy have been reported. A few cases have been described in which normal infants were born to women whose diets contained unusually large amounts of beta-carotene (Mathews-Roth, 1988; Fonda Allen & Rosenbaum, 1992).

The frequency of malformations was not increased among the offspring of rats or rabbits treated during pregnancy with beta-carotene in doses, respectively, 2600-18,750 or 1040-4170 times the human RDA (Komatsu, 1971; Heywood et al., 1985; Mathews-Roth, 1988). In contrast, the frequencies of fetal death, growth retardation, and malformations were increased among the offspring of pregnant rats which were given 1-3 mL palm oil, a rich source of beta-carotene (Singh, 1980). It is not possible to attribute the teratogenic effects observed in this experiment to beta-carotene, however, because the fetal damage may have been produced by other constituents of the palm oil.

Please see agent summary on retinol for information on vitamin A itself. The teratogenic risks related to ingestion of large doses of retinol during pregnancy are much greater than those associated with ingestion of equivalent doses of beta-carotene.

Risk Related to Breast-feeding

Beta-carotene is a normal constituent of breast milk (Ostrea et al., 1986; Giuliano et al., 1992). Colostrum contains three times the amount of beta-carotene than that found in mature milk (Ostrea et al., 1986). Although serum levels of beta-carotene in newborns are substantially lower than maternal levels, the serum levels of nursing infants progressively increase, reaching comparable maternal levels (>40 mcg/dL) in some infants within four to six days of breast-feeding (Ostrea et al., 1986).

Carotenemia has been observed at two months of age in two nursing infants of women who ingested excessive amounts of carrots (0.5-1 pounds per day) throughout their pregnancies and during breast-feeding, and who themselves were carotenemic (Almond & Logan, 1942; Thomson, 1943). Serum levels of beta-carotene were not measured in either the infants or the mothers. The infants were otherwise healthy and carotenemia disappeared following termination of breast-feeding.

Key References

Almond S, Logan RFL: Carotinaemia. Br Med J 2:239-241, 1942.

Bendich A: The safety of beta-carotene. Nutr Cancer 11:207-214, 1988.

Fonda Allen JF, Rosenbaum KN: Counseling after exposure to excessive amounts of beta-carotene in the first trimester: A case report. Teratology 45(5):459-460, 1992.

Giuliano AR, Neilson EM, Kelly BE, Canfield LM: Simultaneous quantitation and separation of carotenoids and retinol in human milk by high-performance liquid chromatography. Methods Enzymol 213:391-399, 1992.

Heywood R, Palmer AK, Gregson RL, Hummler H: The toxicity of beta-carotene. Toxicology 36:91-100, 1985.

Komatsu S: Teratogenic effects of vitamin A. 1. Effects of beta-carotene. Shika Gakuho 71:2067-2074, 1971.

Mathews-Roth MM: Lack of genotoxicity with beta-carotene. Toxicol Lett 41:185-191, 1988.

Ostrea EM Jr, Balun JE, Winkler R, Porter T: Influence of breast-feeding on the restoration of the low serum concentration of vitamin E and beta-carotene in the newborn infant. Am J Obstet Gynecol 154:1014-1017, 1986.

Singh JD: Palm oil induced congenital anomalies in rats. Senten Ijo 20:139-142, 1980.

Thomson ML: Carotinaemia in a suckling. Arch Dis Child 18:112, 1943.

USP DI: Beta-carotene. In: *USP DI (USP Dispensing Information) Volume 1. Drug Information for the Health Care Professional*, 15th ed. Rockville, Md.: The US Pharmacopeial Convention, 1995, pp 512.

BETAMETHASONE
(Betnesol®, BSP®, Prelestone®)

Betamethasone is a synthetic glucocorticoid used to treat inflammatory and allergic disorders. Betamethasone is given orally, rectally, intramuscularly, by injection into joints or other inflamed structures, and topically to the eye, ear canal, or skin. Usual oral doses range from 0.6-7.2 mg/d. Systemic parenteral doses may be up to 9 mg/d and intra-articular injections may be as great as 12 mg.

Teratogenic Risk

Magnitude of teratogenic risk to child born after exposure during gestation:	*Undetermined*
Quality and quantity of data on which risk estimate is based:	*Poor*

No epidemiological studies of congenital anomalies among infants born to women treated with betamethasone during pregnancy have been reported.

Short-term betamethasone therapy has been used to accelerate fetal pulmonary development in women with premature labor (Cosmi & Di Renzo, 1989; Roberts & Morrison, 1991; Kattner et al., 1992). No consistent abnormalities of growth or intellectual function have been observed among children born after such treatment and followed through childhood (MacArthur et al., 1982; Schmand et al., 1990; Smolders-de Haas et al., 1990;).

Constriction of the ductus arteriosus can sometimes be demonstrated by echocardiography in fetuses after maternal betamethasone therapy to promote lung maturation, but this effect does not appear to be of clinical significance (Wasserstrum et al., 1989). Leukemoid reactions and milder transient leukocytosis have been observed in premature infants whose mothers were treated with betamethasone prior to delivery (Barak et al., 1992; Cohen et al., 1993). The effect resembles that observed after steroid treatment in adults.

Clinical features of Cushing syndrome with suppression of the hypothalamic-pituitary-adrenal axis were observed in an infant born after seven courses of antenatal betamethasone therapy (Bradley et al., 1994).

The frequency of cleft palate is substantially increased in the offspring of pregnant rats, mice, and rabbits treated during pregnancy with betamethasone in doses similar to or greater than those used in humans (Walker, 1971; Ishimura et al., 1975; Yamada et al., 1981; Mosier et al., 1982). An increased frequency of omphalocele or umbilical hernia was also seen in the offspring of exposed rats (Yamada et al., 1981; Mosier et al., 1982). Similar results have been observed with other corticosteroids in experimental animal studies, but not in humans. The clinical relevance of these observations with respect to betamethasone treatment in human pregnancy is uncertain.

Decreased fetal body and organ weights and increased rates of fetal death were observed in the offspring of rabbits and rats treated with betamethasone during pregnancy in doses <1-3 or more times those employed in humans (Saijo et al., 1990; Takeshima et al., 1990; Tabor et al., 1991; Sun et al., 1993). Similar effects were observed in rhesus monkeys after treatment for two days in the last third of pregnancy (Epstein et al., 1977; Johnson et al., 1979, 1981).

Please see agent summary on prednisone/prednisolone for information on a related agent that has been more thoroughly studied.

Risk Related to Breast-feeding

No information regarding the distribution of betamethasone in breast milk has been published.

Key References

Barak M, Cohen A, Herschkowitz S: Total leukocyte and neutrophil count changes associated with antenatal betamethasone administration in premature infants. Acta Paediatr 81:760-763, 1992.

Bradley BS, Kumar SP, Mehta ON, Ezhuthachan SG: Neonatal cushingoid syndrome resulting from serial courses of antenatal betamethasone. Obstet Gynecol 83:869-872, 1994.

Cohen A, Barak M, Herschkowitz S, Zecca S: Leukemoid reaction induced by prenatal administration of betamethasone. Acta Paediatr Jpn 35:534-536, 1993.

Cosmi EV, Di Renzo GC: Prevention and treatment of fetal lung immaturity. Fetal Ther 4(Suppl 1):52-62, 1989.

Epstein MF, Farrell PM, Sparks JW, et al.: Maternal betamethasone and fetal growth and development in the monkey. Am J Obstet Gynecol 127:261-263, 1977.

Ishimura K, Honda Y, Neda K, et al.: Teratological studies on betamethasone 17-Benzoate (MS-1112). II. Teratogenicity test in rabbits. Oyo Yakuri 10:685-694, 1975.

Johnson JWC, Mitzner W, Beck JC, et al.: Long-term effects of betamethasone on fetal development. AM J Obstet Gynecol 141:1053-1064, 1981.

Johnson JWC, Mitzner W, London WT, et al.: Betamethasone and the rhesus fetus: Multisytemic effects. AM J Obstet Gynecol 133:677-684, 1979.

Kattner E, Metze B, Waiss E, Obladen M: Accelerated lung maturation, following maternal steroid treatment in infants born before 30 weeks gestation. J Perinat Med 20:449-457, 1992.

MacArthur BA, Howie RN, Dezoete JA, Elkins J: School progress and cognitive development of 6-year-old children whose mothers were treated antenatally with betamethasone. Pediatrics 70:99-105, 1982.

Mosier HD Jr, Dearden LC, Jansons RA, et al.: Disproportionate growth of organs and body weight following glucocorticoid treatment of the rat fetus. Dev Pharmacol Ther 4:89-105, 1982.

Roberts WE, Morrison JC: Pharmacologic induction of fetal lung maturity. Clin Obstet Gynecol 34(2):319-327, 1991.

Saijo T, Fujita T, Sadanaga O, Deguchi T: Betamethasone butyrate propionate (BBP). Kiso To Rinsho 24(11):127-135, 1990.

Schmand B, Neuvel J, Smolders-de Haas H, et al.: Psychological development of children who were treated antenatally with corticosteroids to prevent respiratory distress syndrome. Pediatrics 86(1):58-64, 1990.

Smolders-de Haas H, Neuvel J, Schmand B, et al.: Physical development and medical history of children who were treated antenatally with corticosteroids to prevent respiratory distress syndrome: A 10- to 12-year follow-up. Pediatrics 85:65-70, 1990.

Sun B, Jobe A, Rider E, Ikegami M: Single dose versus two doses of betamethasone for lung maturation in preterm rabbits. Pediatr Res 33(3):256-260, 1993.

Tabor BL, Rider ED, Ikegami M, et al.: Dose effects of antenatal corticosteroids for induction of lung maturation in preterm rabbits. Am J Obstet Gynecol 164:675-681, 1991.

Takeshima T, Tauchi K, Imai S: Betamethasone butyrate propionate (BBP). Kiso To Rinsho 24(11):95-111, 1990.

Walker BE: Induction of cleft palate in rats with anti-inflammatory drugs. Teratology 4:39-42, 1971.

Wasserstrum N, Huhta JC, Mari G, et al.: Betamethasone and the human fetal ductus arteriosus. Obstet Gynecol 74:897-900, 1989.

Yamada T, Nakano M, Ichihashi T, et al.: Fetal concentration after topical application of betamethasone 17, 21-dipropionate (S-3440) ointment and teratogenesis in mice and rabbits. Oyo Yakuri (Pharmacometrics) 21:645-655, 1981.

BETAPEN-VK® *See* Penicillin

BETAXIN® *See* Thiamine

BETNESOL® *See* Betamethasone

BIAMINE® *See* Thiamine

BISMUTH
(Pepto-Bismol®)

Bismuth is a heavy metal that is toxic to humans. As a salt or metal it was formerly given by injection to treat syphillis and yaws. Insoluble preparations have been used topically as protective agents and orally as antacids and to treat diarrhea in doses of 500-1200 mg/d.

Teratogenic Risk

Magnitude of teratogenic risk to child born after exposure during gestation: *Undetermined*

Quality and quantity of data on which risk estimate is based: *Poor*

The frequency of congenital anomalies was no greater than expected among the children of 144 women treated with bismuth subgallate (an insoluble salt) anytime during pregnancy in one epidemiological study (Heinonen et al., 1977). Only 13 of these women used bismuth during the first four lunar months of gestation.

In a study in which four ewes were given bismuth tartrate during pregnancy in doses similar to those used in humans, one of the lambs had multiple congenital anomalies, one was spontaneously aborted, and two were normal (James et al., 1966). Bismuth was not detectable in either maternal or fetal tissues at parturition. The relevance of this observation to the risks associated with bismuth exposure in human pregnancy is unknown.

Risk Related to Breast-feeding

No information regarding the distribution of bismuth subsalicylate in breast milk has been published.

Key References

Heinonen OP, Slone D, Shapiro S: *Birth Defects and Drugs in Pregnancy.* Littleton, Mass.: John Wright-PSG, 1977, pp 385, 497.

James LF, Lazar VA, Binns W: Effects of sublethal doses of certain minerals on pregnant ewes and fetal development. Am J Vet Res 27:132-135, 1966.

USP DI: Bismuth Subsalicylate. In: *USP DI (USP Dispensing Information), Volume 1. Drug Information for the Health Care Professional,* 15th ed. Rockville, Md. The US Pharmacopeial Convention, 1995, p 518.

BLACK TAR *See* Heroin

BLEPH-10® *See* Sulfacetamide

BLOCADREN® *See* Timolol

BLOW *See* Cocaine

BONAMINE® *See* Meclizine

BRETHAIRE® *See* Terbutaline

BRETHINE® *See* Terbutaline

BRICANYL® *See* Terbutaline

BROMOCRIPTINE
(Parlodel®)

Bromocriptine, an ergot derivative, is a dopamine D_2 receptor agonist. It is given orally to suppress prolactin secretion in the treatment of infertility and galactorrhea. It is also used in the symptomatic treatment of pituitary tumors and Parkinson's disease. The usual dosage is 1.25-7.5 mg/d for treatment of infertility, but much higher doses are used for other indications: up to 100 mg/d for pituitary prolactinomas, up to 100 mg/d for acromegaly, and up to 300 mg/d for parkinsonism.

Teratogenic Risk

*Magnitude of teratogenic
risk to child born after
exposure during gestation:*   *Unlikely*

*Quality and quantity of data
on which risk estimate is based:*   *Fair to good*

Women who conceive while taking bromocriptine for infertility have twins and other multifetal gestations with increased frequency (see below). This risk rating does not include deformations that are associated with multifetal pregnancies.

This rating is for bromocriptine treatment for infertility around the time of conception. Use of bromocriptine in this manner is unlikely to pose a substantial teratogenic risk, but the data are insufficient to state that there is no risk. The risk related to treatment with bromocriptine in larger doses is unknown.

In a series of 1406 pregnancies in women treated with bromocriptine for a variety of indications during the first few weeks after conception and reported to the manufacturer, the rates of major congenital anomalies (1%), minor anomalies (2.5%), and spontaneous abortions (11.1%) were lower than those expected in the general population (Turkalj et al., 1982). Similar rates of congenital anomalies were found in subsequent series of 687 and 448 prospectively-identified infants born to women who had been treated with bromocriptine during pregnancy (Krupp & Monka, 1987). Most of these women were treated for amenorrhea and most received bromocriptine for only a few weeks after conception. Postnatal growth and development of these children followed from four months to nine years of age was generally normal (Krupp & Monka, 1987). Similar results were reported in several smaller series of children born to women treated with bromocriptine during pregnancy (Randall et al., 1982; Raymond et al., 1985; Weil, 1986a, b).

No chromosome abnormalities and no evidence of mosaicism for aneuploid cell lines were found in 31 children of women who had been treated with bromocriptine around the time of conception (Czeizel et al., 1989).

Multifetal gestation, usually twinning, occurs in 1.2-2.5% of pregnancies in women treated with bromocriptine at the time of conception (Scialli, 1986; Krupp & Monka, 1987). The rate of multifetal gestation appears to be higher with concomitant clomiphene or human menopausal gonadotropin treatment.

Failure of implantation was observed in rats treated in the first few days after conception with about 2-13 times the dose of bromocriptine used to treat infertility in humans (Narburgh et al., 1990; Cummings et al., 1991; Vijayan & Jayashree, 1993), and miscarriage occurred in two of four dogs treated later in pregnancy with a dose of bromocriptine similar to that used for infertility in humans (Wichtel et al., 1990). In contrast, studies in rats and rabbits suggest that treatment of women during embryonic organogenesis with bromocriptine in doses used for infertility is unlikely to increase the children's risk of malformations greatly (Elton & Langrall, 1979; Weinstein et al., 1982; Narburgh et al., 1990).

Risk Related to Breast-feeding

Bromocriptine is contraindicated during breast-feeding because of its ability to suppress lactation (Committee on Drugs, American Academy of Pediatrics, 1994; USP DI, 1995). However, no adverse effects of bromocriptine on the nursing infant have been reported.

Key References

Committee on Drugs, American Academy of Pediatrics: The transfer of drugs and other chemicals into human milk. Pediatrics 93(1):137-150, 1994.

Cummings AM, Perreault SD, Harris ST: Use of bromoergocryptine in the validation of protocols for the assessment of mechanisms of early pregnancy loss in the rat. Fundam Appl Toxicol 17:563-574, 1991.

Czeizel A, Kiss R, Racz K, et al.: Case-control cytogenetic study in offspring of mothers treated with bromocriptine during early pregnancy. Mutat Res 210(1):23-27, 1989.

Elton RL, Langrall HM: Is bromocriptine teratogenic? Ann Intern Med 91:791, 1979.

Krupp P, Monka C: Bromocriptine in pregnancy: Safety aspects. Klin Wochenschr 65:823-827, 1987.

Narburgh LJ, Turner J, Freeman SJ: Evaluation of the teratogenic potential of the dopamine agonist bromocryptine in rats. Toxicol Lett 50:189-194, 1990.

Randall S, Laing I, Chapman AJ, et al.: Pregnancies in women with hyperprolactinaemia: Obstetric and endocrinological management of 50 pregnancies in 37 women. Br J Obstet Gynaecol 89:20-23, 1982.

Raymond JP, Goldstein E, Konopka P, et al.: Follow-up of children born of bromocriptine-treated mothers. Horm Res 22:239-246, 1985.

Scialli AR: The reproductive toxicity of ovulation induction. Fertil Steril 45(3):315-323, 1986.

Turkalj I, Braun P, Krupp P: Surveillance of bromocriptine in pregnancy. JAMA 247:1589-1591, 1982.

USP DI: Bromocriptine. In: *USP DI (USP Dispensing Information), Volume 1. Drug Information for the Health Care Professional*, 15th ed. Rockville, Md.: The US Pharmacopeial Convention, 1995, p 530.

Vijayan E, Jayashree J: Prolactin suppression during pre and post-implantation periods on rat uterine glucosamine synthase activity. Indian J Exp Biol 31(4):386-388, 1993.

Weil C: The safety of bromocriptine in hyperprolactinaemic female infertility: A literature review. Curr Med Res Opin 10:172-195, 1986b.

Weil C: The safety of bromocriptine in long-term use: A review of the literature. Curr Med Res Opin 10:25-51, 1986a.

Weinstein D, Ben-Amitay D, Schenker JG, et al.: Teratogenicity of bromocryptine in pregnant rats. Arch Gynecol 233:31-35, 1982.

Wichtel JJ, Whitacre MD, Yates DJ, Van Camp SD: Comparison of the effects of $PGF_{2\alpha}$ and bromocryptine in pregnant beagle bitches. Theriogenology 33(4):829-836, 1990.

BROMPERIDOL
(Azuren®, Tesoprel®)

Bromperidol is a butyrophenone neuroleptic agent used in treating psychoses. Bromperidol is given orally, usually in a dose of 1-15 mg/d, although doses as high as 50 mg/d are sometimes employed.

Teratogenic Risk

Magnitude of teratogenic risk to child born after exposure during gestation:	*Undetermined*
Quality and quantity of data on which risk estimate is based:	*Very poor*

No epidemiological studies of congenital anomalies in infants born to women treated with bromperidol during pregnancy have been been reported.

Studies in rats suggest that treatment of pregnant women with bromperidol in usual therapeutic doses is unlikely to increase the children's risk of malformations greatly (Imai et al., 1984).

Please see agent summary on haloperidol for information on a closely related drug that has been more thoroughly studied.

Risk Related to Breast-feeding

Bromperidol is excreted in the breast milk (Henke & Henke, 1995); however, no adverse effects on the nursing infant have been reported.

Key References

    Henke D, Henke W: Bromperidol--Drug Evaluation Monographs. In: Gelman CR, Rumack BH (eds). *Drugdex®* Information System. Englewood, Co.: *Micromedex* [edition expires 08/31/95].
    Imai S, Tauchi K, Huang KJ, Takeshima T, et al.: Teratogenicity study on bromperidol in rats. J Toxicol Sci 9:109-126, 1984.

BRONKAID MIST® *See* Epinephrine

BRONKODYL® *See* Theophylline

BSP® *See* Betamethasone

BUPIVACAINE
(Marcain®)

    Bupivacaine is a long-acting anesthetic of the amide class. It is administered by injection locally, epidurally, and regionally, and is completely absorbed systemically from these sites. The dose varies but may be as great as 175 mg in a single dose or 400 mg/d.

Teratogenic Risk

Magnitude of teratogenic risk to child born after exposure during gestation:	*Undetermined*
Quality and quantity of data on which risk estimate is based:	*None*

    No epidemiological studies of congenital anomalies in children born to women exposed to bupivacaine during pregnancy have been reported.
    No animal teratology studies of bupivacaine have been published.
    Transient fetal bradycardia and increased fetal heart rate variability have been observed in some studies of women who had epidural or regional anesthesia with bupivacaine during labor (Stavrou et al., 1990; Eddleston et al., 1992). The neurobehavioral status of infants born of such pregnancies is usually normal (Lieberman et al., 1979; Merkow et

al., 1980; Abboud et al., 1982; Harrison & Cullen, 1986; Thorp et al., 1993), although alterations of neonatal behavior are sometimes observed (Rosenblatt et al., 1981; Morikawa et al., 1990; Sepkoski et al., 1992).

Please see agent summary on lidocaine for information on a related agent that has been more thoroughly studied.

Risk Related to Breast-feeding

Bupivacaine is excreted in breast milk. Based on data from a single breast-feeding patient, the amount of bupivacaine that the nursing infant would be expected to receive is approximately 14% of the lowest dental dose of bupivacaine (Baker & Schroeder, 1989).* No detectable levels of bupivacaine could be measured in the serum of the nursing infant. No bupivacaine could be detected in the breast milk of a woman who had given epidural anesthesia containing bupivacaine during labor (Naulty et al., 1983).

Key References

Abboud TK, Khoo SS, Miller F, et al.: Maternal, fetal, and neonatal responses after epidural anesthesia with bupivacaine, 2-chloroprocaine, or lidocaine. Anesth Analg 61:638-644, 1982.

Baker PA, Schroeder D: Interpleural bupivacaine for postoperative pain during lactation. Anesth Analg 69:400-402, 1989.

Eddleston JM, Maresh M, Horsman EL, et al.: Comparison of the maternal and fetal effects associated with intermittent or continuous infusion of extradural analgesia. Br J Anaesth 69:154-158, 1992.

Harrison RF, Cullen R: A comparative study of the behaviour of the neonate following various forms of maternal intrapartum analgesia and anaesthesia. Ir J Med Sci 155:12-18, 1986.

Lieberman BA, Rosenblatt DB, Belsey E, et al.: The effects of maternally administered pethidine or epidural bupivacaine on the fetus and newborn. Br J Obstet Gynaecol 86:598-606, 1979.

Merkow AJ, McGuinness GA, Erenberg A, Kennedy RL: The neonatal neurobehavioral effects of bupivacaine, mepivacaine, and 2-

---

*This calculation is based on the following assumptions: maternal dose of bupivacaine: 9.4 mg/kg/d; milk concentration of bupivacaine: 0.45 mcg/mL; milk intake by the nursing infant: 150 mL/kg/d; estimated dose of bupivacaine ingested by the nursing infant (assuming only 35% of bupivacaine is absorbed): 0.02 mg/kg/d; lowest dental dose of bupivacaine: 0.14 mg/kg/d.

chloroprocaine used for pudendal block. Anesthesiology 52:309-312, 1980.

Morikawa S, Ishikawa J, Kamatsuki H, et al.: Neurobehavior and mental development of newborn infants delivered under epidural analgesia with bupivacaine. Nippon Sanka Fujinka Gakkai Zasshi 42(11):1495-1502, 1990.

Naulty JS, Ostheimer G, Datta S, Weiss JB: Bupivacaine in breast milk following epidural anesthesia for vaginal delivery. Reg Anesth 8:44-45, 1983.

Rosenblatt DB, Belsey EM, Lieberman BA, et al.: The influence of maternal analgesia on neonatal behaviour: II. Epidural bupivacaine. Br J Obstet Gynaecol 88:407-413, 1981.

Sepkoski CM, Lester BM, Ostheimer GW, Brazelton TB: The effects of maternal epidural anesthesia on neonatal behavior during the first month. Dev Med Child Neurol 34:1072-1080, 1992.

Stavrou C, Hofmeyr GJ, Boezaart AP: Prolonged fetal bradycardia during epidural analgesia. Incidence, timing and significance. S Afr Med J 77:66-68, 1990.

Thorp JA, Hu DH, Albin RM, et al.: The effect of intrapartum epidural analgesia on nulliparous labor. A randomized, controlled, prospective trial. Am J Obstet Gynecol 169:851-858, 1993.

BUTALBITAL

Butalbital is a short-acting barbiturate that is administered orally. Single doses of up to 100 mg are used as a hypnotic; up to 120 mg/d in divided doses may be given as a sedative.

Teratogenic Risk

*Magnitude of teratogenic
risk to child born after
exposure during gestation:*   *Unlikely*

*Quality and quantity of data
on which risk estimate is based:*   *Fair*

Therapeutic doses of butalbital are unlikely to pose a substantial teratogenic risk, but the data are insufficient to state that there is no risk.

The frequency of malformations was no greater than expected among the children of 112 women who were treated with butalbital during the first four lunar months of pregnancy in one epidemiological study (Heinonen et al., 1977).

No animal teratology studies of butalbital have been published.

Transient neonatal withdrawal symptoms similar to those which occur with phenobarbital have been reported after chronic maternal use of butalbital in therapeutic doses late in pregnancy (Ostrea, 1982).

Risk Related to Breast-feeding

No information regarding the distribution of butalbital in breast milk has been published.

Key References

Heinonen OP, Slone D, Shapiro S: *Birth Defects and Drugs in Pregnancy*. Littleton, Mass.: John Wright-PSG, 1977, p 336.

Ostrea EM: Neonatal withdrawal from intrauterine exposure to butalbital. Am J Obstet Gynecol 143:597-599, 1982.

CAFFEDRINE® *See* Caffeine

CAFFEINE
(Caffedrine®, NoDoz®, Vivarin®)

Caffeine is a methylated xanthine that acts as a central nervous system stimulant. Caffeine is contained in many commonly used beverages including coffee, tea, and colas. Many over-the-counter and prescription medicines include caffeine, usually in combination with other agents. A 5-ounce cup of coffee averages about 100 mg of caffeine in the US, but this can vary more than two-fold in either direction (Sobotka, 1989; Dlugosz & Bracken, 1992). The maximum recommended dose of caffeine as oral tablets is 1000 mg/d.

Teratogenic Risk

Magnitude of teratogenic
risk to child born after
exposure during gestation
    Malformations: *None*
    Spontaneous abortion: *None to minimal*

Quality and quantity of data
on which risk estimate is based
    Malformations: *Good*
    Spontaneous abortion: *Fair to good*

This risk assessment is for usual caffeine intake as occurs with moderate drinking of coffee, tea, or colas.
The available data are inadequate to determine the risk related to very high intake of caffeine.

The frequency of congenital anomalies was not increased among the children of 595 women who drank four or more cups of coffee per day during the first trimester of pregnancy in a well-controlled epidemiological study (Linn et al., 1982). Similarly, the frequency of congenital anomalies was no greater than expected among the infants of 5378 women who took medicines containing caffeine during the first four lunar months of pregnancy or among the infants of 12,696 women who took such medicines anytime during pregnancy in another study (Heinonen et al., 1977). The frequency of heavy maternal consumption of caffeinated beverages or maternal use of caffeine-containing medications during pregnancy was no more frequent than expected in studies involving 458, 2030, and 706, children with a variety of congenital anomalies (Nelson & Forfar, 1971; Rosenberg et al., 1982; Kurppa et al., 1983;). In two other studies, significant associations were observed with consumption of caffeinated beverages during pregnancy among mothers of 464 anencephalic infants and 190 children with various malformations (Fedrick, 1974; Borlee et al., 1978). The association was weak in both instances, however, and both studies have serious methodological limitations (James & Paull, 1985; Pieters, 1985;).

Associations between maternal coffee drinking during pregnancy and miscarriage or poor fetal growth have been repeatedly observed in epidemiological studies (Wilcox et al., 1990; Fenster et al., 1991a, b; Kline et al., 1991; Narod et al., 1991; Peacock et al., 1991; Fortier et al., 1993; Infante-Rivard et al., 1993; Larroque et al., 1993; Leviton,

1993), but in many instances these associations are attributable to confounding effects of maternal cigarette smoking or other factors. Some of these studies have very serious methodological limitations (Dlugosz & Bracken, 1992; Leviton, 1993; Mills et al., 1993; Shiono & Klebanoff, 1993). If maternal consumption of caffeine-containing beverages in conventional amounts during pregnancy does adversely influence the rate of miscarriage or fetal growth retardation, the effect is small.

Fetal and neonatal cardiac arrhythmias have been reported among the infants of women who drank large amounts of caffeine-containing beverages during pregnancy; these arrhythmias resolved after elimination of the caffeine intake (Oei et al., 1989; Hadeed & Siegel, 1993).

Stillbirths and miscarriages were observed with increased frequency among the offspring of macaque monkeys treated during pregnancy with caffeine in a dose equivalent to five to seven or 12-17 cups of coffee per day (Gilbert et al., 1988). The cause for the stillbirths was not apparent on necropsy; no malformations were seen. Body weight of the male but not the female infants of treated monkeys was reduced (Gilbert & Rice, 1991). An increased frequency of malformations, especially of the limbs and palate, has been observed among the offspring of rats or mice treated with caffeine during pregnancy in doses equivalent to human consumption of 40 or more cups of coffee daily (Smith et al., 1987; Muther, 1988; Nolen, 1989; Purves & Sullivan, 1993). Fetal death, growth retardation, and skeletal variations are often seen in these animal experiments after maternal treatment with very high doses of caffeine during pregnancy.

In one study an increased frequency of cleft palate was observed among the offspring of rats given caffeine in doses equivalent to five to 19 cups of coffee a day during pregnancy (Palm et al., 1978). An increased rate of cardiac defects was observed among the offspring of rats treated during pregnancy with caffeine in amounts equivalent to 15 or more cups of coffee per day in another study (Matsuoka et al., 1987). Most investigations do not show an increased frequency of malformations among the offspring of rodents treated during pregnancy with caffeine in similar or somewhat greater doses (Collins et al., 1987; Smith et al., 1987; Nolen, 1989; Purves & Sullivan, 1993). Doses and methods of caffeine administration that are teratogenic in animal studies generally cause maternal toxicity or death as well, and equivalent human doses would also be highly toxic or lethal (Nolen, 1989; Purves & Sullivan, 1993). Thus, the relevance of these observations to the risks in infants born to women who drink large amounts of caffeinated beverages during pregnancy is unknown.

Persistent behavioral alterations have been observed among the offspring of rats and mice treated during pregnancy with caffeine in doses equivalent to ten to 60 cups of coffee a day (Hughes & Beveridge, 1986, 1990; Nolen, 1989; Sobotka, 1989;). Behavioral alterations have also been observed among the offspring of monkeys born to mothers treated with an unspecified dose of caffeine during pregnancy (Rice & Gilbert, 1990). No effect of maternal caffeine use during pregnancy was observed on the development of about 500 children who were evaluated at four and seven years of age (Barr & Streissguth, 1991).

Risk Related to Breast-feeding

Caffeine is distributed in breast milk in low concentrations. Infants of women who consume 36-598 mg of caffeine (the equivalent of <1-6 cups of typical American coffee) per day would be expected to ingest between 3-43% of the minimal dose of caffeine used to treat neonatal apnea (Dorfman & Jarvik, 1970; Tyrala & Dodson, 1979; Berlin et al., 1984; Sagraves et al., 1984; Ryu, 1985b; Blanchard et al., 1992).* In another study, the estimated dose ingested through breast-feeding by infants of women who took 750 mg of caffeine (the equivalent of about 7.5 typical American cups of coffee) per day ranged from 0-170% of the minimal dose used to treat neonatal apnea (Ryu, 1985a).[†]

No evidence of alteration of heart rate or sleep time was observed in 11 nursing infants whose mothers were given 500 mg of caffeine per day (Ryu, 1985b).

The American Academy of Pediatrics regards maternal caffeine use to be safe while breast-feeding (Committee on Drugs, American Academy of Pediatrics, 1994). Presumably this recommendation refers to moderate maternal use of caffeine.

Key References

Barr HM, Streissguth AP: Caffeine use during pregnancy and child outcome: A 7-year prospective study. Neurotoxicol Teratol 13(4):441-448, 1991.

*This calculation is based on the following assumptions: milk concentration of caffeine: 0.54-7.17 mcg/mL; milk intake by the nursing infant: 150 mL/kg/d; estimated dose of caffeine ingested by the nursing infant: 0.10-1.01 mg/kg; lowest neonatal dose to treat apnea: 2.5 mg/kg/d.

†This calculation is based on the following assumptions: milk concentration of caffeine: 0-28.6 mcg/mL; estimated dose of caffeine ingested by the nursing infant: 0-4.3 mg/kg/d.

Berlin CM Jr, Denson HM, Daniel CH, Ward RM: Disposition of dietary caffeine in milk, saliva, and plasma of lactating women. Pediatrics 73(1):59-63, 1984.

Blanchard J, Weber CW, Shearer L-E: Methylxanthine levels in breast milk of lactating women of different ethnic and socioeconomic classes. Biopharm Drug Dispos 13:187-196, 1992.

Borlee I, Lechat MF, Bouckaert A, Misson C: Le cafe, facteur de risque pendant la grossesse? Louvain Med 97:279-284, 1978.

Collins TFX, Welsh JJ, Black TN, et al.: Potential reversibility of skeletal effects in rats exposed in utero to caffeine. Food Chem Toxicol 25(9):647-662, 1987.

Committee on Drugs, American Academy of Pediatrics: The transfer of drugs and other chemicals into human milk. Pediatrics 93(1):137-150, 1994.

Dlugosz L, Bracken MB: Reproductive effects of caffeine: A review and theoretical analysis. Epidemiol Rev 14:83-100, 1992.

Dorfman LJ, Jarvik ME: Comparative stimulant and diuretic actions of caffeine and theobromine in man. Clin Pharmacol 11:869-872, 1970.

Fedrick J: Anencephalus and maternal tea drinking: Evidence for a possible association. Proc R Soc Med 67:356-360, 1974.

Fenster L, Eskenazi B, Windham GC, Swan SH: Caffeine consumption during pregnancy and fetal growth. Am J Public Health 81:458-461, 1991a.

Fenster L, Eskenazi B, Windham GC, Swan SH: Caffeine consumption during pregnancy and spontaneous abortion. Epidemiology 2:168-174, 1991b.

Fortier I, Marcoux S, Beaulac-Baillargeon L: Relation of caffeine intake during pregnancy to intrauterine growth retardation and preterm birth. Am J Epidemiol 137(9):931-940, 1993.

Gilbert SG, Rice DC: Somatic development of the infant monkey following in utero exposure to caffeine. Fundam Appl Toxicol 17:454-465, 1991.

Gilbert SG, Rice DC, Reuhl KR, Stavric B: Adverse pregnancy outcome in the monkey (*Macaca fascicularis*) after chronic caffeine exposure. J Pharmacol Exp Ther 245(3):1048-1053, 1988.

Hadeed A, Siegel S: Newborn cardiac arrhythmias associated with maternal caffeine use during pregnancy. Clin Pediatr 32(1):45-47, 1993.

Heinonen OP, Slone D, Shapiro S: *Birth Defects and Drugs in Pregnancy.* Littleton, Mass.: John Wright-PSG, 1977, pp 11, 366-370, 436, 440, 477, 493.

Heller J: What do we know about the risks of caffeine consumption in pregnancy? Br J Addict 82:885-889, 1987.

Hughes RN, Beveridge IJ: Behavioral effects of prenatal exposure to caffeine in rats. Life Sci 38:861-868, 1986.

Hughes RN, Beveridge IJ: Sex-and age-dependent effects of prenatal exposure to caffeine on open-field behavior, emergence latency and adrenal weights in rats. Life Sci 47:2075-2088, 1990.

Infante-Rivard C, Fernandez A, Gauthier R, et al.: Fetal loss associated with caffeine intake before and during pregnancy. JAMA 270:2940-2943, 1993.

James JE, Paull I: Caffeine and human reproduction. Rev Environ Health 5:151-167, 1985.

Kline J, Levin B, Silverman J, et al.: Caffeine and spontaneous abortion of known karyotype. Epidemiology 2:409-417, 1991.

Kurppa K, Holmberg PC, Kuosma E, Saxen L: Coffee consumption during pregnancy and selected congenital malformations: A nationwide case-control study. Am J Public Health 73:1397-1399, 1983.

Larroque B, Kaminski M, Lelong N, et al.: Effects on birth weight of alcohol and caffeine consumption during pregnancy. Am J Epidemiol 137:941-950, 1993.

Leviton A: Coffee, caffeine, and reproductive hazards in humans. In: Garattini S (ed). *Monographs of the Mario Negri Institute for Pharmacological Research, Milan: Caffeine, Coffee and Health.* New York: Raven Press, 1993, pp 343-358.

Linn S, Schoenbaum SC, Monson RR, et al.: No association between coffee consumption and adverse outcomes of pregnancy. N Engl J Med 306:141-145, 1982.

Matsuoka R, Uno H, Tanaka H, et al.: Caffeine induces cardiac and other malformations in the rat. Am J Med Genet (Suppl 3):433-443, 1987.

Mills JL, Holmes LB, Aarons JH, et al.: Moderate caffeine use and the risk of spontaneous abortion and intrauterine growth retardation. JAMA 269(5):593-597, 1993.

Muther TF: Caffeine and reduction of fetal ossification in the rat: Fact or artifact? Teratology 37:239-247, 1988.

Narod SA, de Sanjose S, Victora C: Coffee during pregnancy: A reproductive hazard? Am J Obstet Gynecol 164:1109-1114, 1991.

Nelson MM, Forfar JO: Associations between drugs administered during pregnancy and congenital abnormalities of the fetus. Br Med J 1:523-527, 1971.

Nolen GA: The developmental toxicology of caffeine. Issues Rev Teratol 4:305-350, 1989.

Oei SG, Vosters RPL, van der Hagen NLJ: Fetal arrhythmia caused by excessive intake of caffeine by pregnant women. BMJ 298:568, 1989.

Palm PE, Arnold EP, Rachwall PC, et al.: Evaluation of the teratogenic potential of fresh-brewed coffee and caffeine in the rat. Toxicol Appl Pharmacol 44:1-16, 1978.

Peacock JL, Bland JM, Anderson HR: Effects on birthweight of alcohol and caffeine consumption in smoking women. J Epidemiol Community Health 45(2):159-163, 1991.

Pieters JJL: Nutritional teratogens: A survey of epidemiological literature. Prog Clin Biol Res 163B:419-429, 1985.

Purves D, Sullivan FM: Reproductive effects of caffeine: Experimental studies in animals. In: Garattini S (ed). *Monographs of the Mario Negri Institute for Pharmacological Research, Milan: Caffeine, Coffee and Health.* New York: Raven Press, 1993, pp 317-342.

Rice DC, Gilbert SG: Automated behavioral procedures for infant monkeys. Neurotoxicol Teratol 12:429-439, 1990.

Rosenberg L, Mitchell AA, Shapiro S, Slone D: Selected birth defects in relation to caffeine-containing beverages. JAMA 247:1429-1432, 1982.

Ryu JE: Caffeine in human milk and in serum of breast-fed infants. Dev Pharmacol Ther 8:329-337, 1985a.

Ryu JE: Effect of maternal caffeine consumption on heart rate and sleep time of breast-fed infants. Dev Pharmacol Ther 8:355-363, 1985b.

Sagraves R, Bradley JM, Delgado MJM, et al.: Pharmacokinetics of caffeine in human breast milk after a single oral dose of caffeine. Drug Intell Clin Pharm 18:507, 1984.

Shiono PH, Klebanoff MA: Invited commentary: Caffeine and birth outcomes. Am J Epidemiol 137(9):951-954, 1993.

Smith SE, McElhatton PR, Sullivan FM: Effects of administering caffeine to pregnant rats either as a single daily dose or as divided doses four times a day. Food Chem Toxicol 25(2):125-133, 1987.

Sobotka TJ: Neurobehavioral effects of prenatal caffeine. Ann NY Acad Sci 562:327-339, 1989.

Tyrala EE, Dodson WE: Caffeine secretion into breast milk. Arch Dis Child 54:787-789, 1979.

Wilcox AJ, Weinberg CR, Baird DD: Risk factors for early pregnancy loss. Epidemiology 1:382-385, 1990.

CALAN® *See* Verapamil

CALCIFEDIOL® *See* Vitamin D

CALCILEAN® *See* Heparin

CALCIUM SALTS
(Alka-mints®, Citracal®, Tums®)

Calcium is an essential electrolyte; its concentration in the blood is regulated within narrow limits. Calcium ions are required for normal cardiac, muscle, nerve, and hemostatic function. The US RDA of calcium for pregnant women is 1200 mg/d (NRC, 1989; NIH, 1994). Additional calcium (most often in a dose of 1000-1500 mg/d) is administered as a dietary supplement and to prevent the development of hypertension in pregnancy (Seely & Graves, 1993; Carroli et al., 1994; Prentice, 1994a).

Teratogenic Risk

*Magnitude of teratogenic
risk to child born after
exposure during gestation:*   *Unlikely*

*Quality and quantity of data
on which risk estimate is based:*   *Fair*

Supplemental doses of calcium salts are unlikely to pose a substantial teratogenic risk, but the data are insufficient to state that there is no risk.

The frequencies of malformations in general, of major malformations, and of minor anomalies were no greater than expected among the children of 1007 women who took calcium supplements during the first four lunar months of pregnancy in one epidemiological study (Heinonen et al., 1977). The frequencies of most major classes of congenital anomalies were also no greater than expected among the children of these women, but the frequency of central nervous system malformations were slightly, but significantly, increased. No specific anomaly accounted for this association, and it may well be due to chance. Studies such as this one that include multiple comparisons between maternal drug exposures and various birth defect outcomes are expected to show occasional associations with nominal statistical significance purely by chance. Congenital anomalies were not found more often than expected among the infants of 3739 women who took calcium salts anytime during pregnancy in this study. No adverse treatment-related effects have been observed among the infants of women given supplemental calcium in the second half of pregnancy in controlled clinical trials (Ito et al., 1994; Sanchez-Ramos et al., 1994).

Most studies in mice, rats, and rabbits suggest that treatment of pregnant women with calcium salts in usual therapeutic doses is unlikely to increase the children's risk of malformations greatly (Anonymous, 1974; McCormack et al., 1979; Hayasaka et al., 1990; Shackelford et al., 1993).

Risk Related to Breast-feeding

Approximately 200-300 mg of calcium per day is excreted into breast milk, but this amount varies greatly depending on the volume of breast milk produced and stage of lactation (Prentice, 1994b). Although calcium requirements are increased during pregnancy and lactation, it is not certain if breast milk levels of calcium are affected by maternal intake of calcium (Prentice, 1994b). Breast milk concentrations were found to be independent of maternal dietary calcium intake or use of calcium supplements in some studies (Walker et al., 1954; Kirksey et al., 1979; Vaughan et al al., 1979; Specker, 1994), but not in others (Prentice & Barclay, 1991; Dagnelie et al., 1992).

No information regarding the distribution of calcium chloride or calcium gluconate in breast milk has been published. Adverse effects of maternal supplementation with calcium on the nursing infant have not been reported.

Key References

Anonymous: Teratologic evaluation of FDA 71-86 (calcium sulfate) in mice, rats and rabbits. NTIS (National Technical Information Service) Report/PB-234 873, 1974.

Carroli G, Duley L, Belizan JM, Villar J: Calcium supplementation during pregnancy: A systematic review of randomised controlled trials. Br J Obstet Gynaecol 101:753-758, 1994.

Dagnelie PC, van Staveren WA, Roos AH, et al.: Nutrients and contaminants in human milk from mothers on macrobiotic and omnivorous diets. Eur J Clin Nutr 46:355-366, 1992.

Hayasaka I, Murakami K, Kato Z, et al.: Preventive effects of maternal electrolyte supplementation on azosemide-induced skeletal malformations in rats. Environ Med 34:61-67, 1990.

Heinonen OP, Slone D, Shapiro S: *Birth Defects and Drugs in Pregnancy.* Littleton, Mass.: John Wright-PSG, 1977, pp 444, 479, 498.

Ito M, Koyama H, Ohshige A et al.: Prevention of preeclampsia with calcium supplementation and vitamin D_3 in antenatal protocol. Int J Gynaecol Obstet 47:115-120, 1994.

Kirksey A, Ernst JA, Roepke JL, Tsai T-L: Influence of mineral intake and use of oral contraceptives before pregnancy on the mineral content of human colostrum and of more mature milk. Am J Clin Nutr 32:30-39, 1979.

McCormack KM, Ottosen LD, Sanger VL, et al.: Effect of prenatal administration of aluminum and parathyroid hormone on fetal development in the rat. Proc Soc Exp Biol Med 161:74-77, 1979.

NIH (National Institutes of Health): Optimal calcium intake. JAMA 272(24):142-148, 1994.

NRC (National Research Council): *Recommended Dietary Allowances, 10th ed. Report of the Subcommittee on the Tenth Edition of the RDAs, Food and Nutrition Board, Commission on Life Sciences.* Washington, DC: National Academy Press, 1989, pp 284.

Prentice A: Calcium requirements in pregnancy and lactation in rural Africa. S Afr Med J (Suppl):19-20, 1994b.

Prentice A: Maternal calcium requirements during pregnancy and lactation. Am J Clin Nutr 59(Suppl):477S-483S, 1994a.

Prentice A, Barclay DV: Breast-milk calcium and phosphorous concentrations of mothers in rural Zaire. Eur J Clin Nutr 45:611-617, 1991.

Sanchez-Ramos L, Briones DK, Kaunitz AM, et al.: Prevention of pregnancy-induced hypertension by calcium supplementation in angiotensin II-sensitive patients. Obstet Gynecol 84:349-353, 1994.

Seely EW, Graves SW: Calcium homeostasis in normotensive and hypertensive pregnancy. Compr Ther 19(3):124-128, 1993.

Shackelford ME, Collins TFX, Welsh JJ, et al.: Foetal development in rats fed AIN-76A diets supplemented with excess calcium. Food Chem Toxicol 31(12):953-961, 1993.

Specker BL: Nutritional concerns of lactating women consuming vegetarian diets. Am J Clin Nutr 59(Suppl):1182S-1186S, 1994.

Vaughan LA, Weber CW, Kemberling SR: Longitudinal changes in the mineral content of human milk. Am J Clin Nutr 32:2301-2306, 1979.

Walker ARP, Arvidsson UB, Draper WL: The composition of breast milk of South African Bantu mothers. Trans R Soc Trop Med Hyg 48:395-399, 1954.

CAPOTEN® *See* Captopril

CAPTOPRIL
(Capoten®)

Captopril is an inhibitor of angiotensin converting enzyme (ACE). It is given orally in a dose of 18-75 mg/d to treat hypertension. Doses as large as 450 mg/d are sometimes used in the treatment of congestive heart failure.

Teratogenic Risk

*Magnitude of teratogenic
risk to child born after
exposure during gestation*
    First trimester use: *Undetermined*
    Use later in pregnancy: *Moderate*

*Quality and quantity of data
on which risk estimate is based*
    First trimester use: *Poor*
    Use later in pregnancy: *Fair to good*

A small risk cannot be excluded, but a high risk of congenital anomalies in the children of women treated with captopril during the first trimester is unlikely.

There is a substantial risk of oligohydramnios and fetal distress or death in hypertensive women treated with captopril in the latter part of pregnancy. The effect may be related to the pharmacological action of this drug on the fetus (see below).

The risk associated with maternal use of captopril during the second or third trimester of pregnancy increases with the duration of treatment.

In one clinical series, no malformations were observed among 14 infants born to women who were treated with captopril during the first trimester of pregnancy (Kreft-Jais et al., 1988). In another series of 12 infants born to women given captopril or another ACE inhibitor during the first trimester of pregnancy, one malformed infant was observed (Piper et al., 1992). This child had an occipital encephalocele.

Three cases have been reported in which hypocalvaria, an unusual underdevelopment of the skull bones, and other skeletal anomalies occurred in the infant or fetus of a woman treated with captopril throughout pregnancy (Duminy & Berger, 1981; Rothberg & Lorenz, 1984; Barr & Cohen, 1991; Pryde et al., 1993). Four infants with similar unusual skull defects have been observed after maternal treatment throughout pregnancy with other ACE inhibitors (Mehta & Modi, 1989; Cunniff et al., 1990; Barr & Cohen, 1991; Bhatt-Mehta & Deluga, 1993; Pryde et al., 1993).

Oligohydramnios, fetal growth retardation and neonatal renal failure, hypotension, pulmonary hypoplasia, joint contractures, and death have been repeatedly observed after maternal treatment with captopril or related drugs during pregnancy (Hanssens et al., 1991; Bhatt-Mehta & Deluga, 1993; Pryde et al., 1993; Shotan et al., 1994). One infant among 15 who were born to women treated with captopril or other ACE inhibitors during the second or third trimester of pregnancy in one series had oligohydramnios and neonatal hypotension and anuria (Piper et al., 1992). It is important to note that these effects do not appear to reflect abnormal embryogenesis but rather a pharmacologic response of the fetus to captopril during the second half of gestation (Beckman & Brent, 1990; Brent & Beckman, 1991).

No increase in malformations but increased frequencies of fetal growth retardation and death were observed among the offspring of rats treated during pregnancy with 1.5-5 times the human therapeutic dose of captopril (Al-Shabanah et al., 1991). Decreased ossification of the skull and other bones was observed at the higher dose. Pregnant rabbits and sheep given captopril late in gestation in doses similar to those used in humans had an unexpectedly high frequency of fetal deaths (Broughton Pipkin et al., 1982; Keith et al., 1982; Ferris & Weir, 1983). Fetal hypotension and anuria have been demonstrated in sheep after such treatment (Broughton Pipkin et al., 1982; Robillard et al., 1983Lumbers et al., 1992, 1993;).

Please see agent summary on enalapril for information on a related agent.

Risk Related to Breast-feeding

Captopril is excreted in breast milk in low concentrations. The amount of captopril that the nursing infant would be expected to ingest is approximtely 3% of the lowest neonatal dose, based on data obtained from 12 lactating mothers (Devlin & Fleiss, 1981).* No adverse effects were observed in any of the nursed infants.

Both the American Academy of Pediatrics (Committee on Drugs, American Academy of Pediatrics, 1994) and the WHO Working Group on Drugs and Human Lactation (1988) regard captopril to be safe to use while breast-feeding.

Key References

Al-Shabanah OA, Al-Harbi MM, AlGharably NMA, Islam MW: The effect of maternal administration of captopril on fetal development in rat. Res Commun Chem Pathol Pharmacol 73:221-230, 1991.

Barr M Jr, Cohen MM Jr: ACE inhibitor fetopathy and hypocalvaria: The kidney-skull connection. Teratology 44:485-495, 1991.

Beckman DA, Brent RL: Teratogenesis: Alcohol, angiotensin-converting-enzyme inhibitors, and cocaine. Curr Opin Obstet Gynecol 2:236-245, 1990.

Bhatt-Mehta V, Deluga KS: Fetal exposure to lisinopril: Neonatal manifestations and management. Pharmacotherapy 13(5):515-518, 1993.

Brent RL, Beckman DA: Angiotensin-converting enzyme inhibitors, and embryopathic class of drugs with unique properties: Information for clinical teratology counselors. Teratology 43:543-546, 1991.

Broughton Pipkin F, Symonds EM, Turner SR: The effect of captopril (SQ14,225) upon mother and fetus in the chronically cannulated ewe and in the pregnant rabbit. J Physiol 323:415-422, 1982.

*This calculation is based on the following assumptions: maternal dose of captopril: 4.7 mg/kg/d; milk concentration of captopril: 0.005 mcg/mL; milk intake by the nursing infant: 150 mL/kg/d; estimated dose of captopril ingested by the nursing infant: 0.0007 mg/k/d; lowest neonatal dose of captopril: 0.02 mg/kg/d.

Committee on Drugs, American Academy of Pediatrics: The transfer of drugs and other chemicals into human milk. Pediatrics 93(1):137-150, 1994.

Cunniff C, Jones KL, Phillipson J, et al.: Oligohydramnios sequence and renal tubular malformation associated with maternal enalapril use. Am J Obstet Gynecol 162:187-189, 1990.

Devlin RG, Fleiss PM: Captopril in human blood and breast milk. J Clin Pharmacol 21:110-113, 1981.

Duminy PC, Burger P du T: Fetal abnormality associated with the use of captopril during pregnancy. S Afr Med J 60:805, 1981.

Ferris TF, Weir EK: Effect of captopril on uterine blood flow and prostaglandin E synthesis in the pregnant rabbit. J Clin Invest 71:809-815, 1983.

Hanssens M, Keirse MJNC, Vankelecom F, Van Assche FA: Fetal and neonatal effects of treatment with angiotensin-converting enzyme inhibitors in pregnancy. Obstet Gynecol 78(1):128-135, 1991.

Keith IM, Will JA, Weir EK: Captopril: Association with fetal death and pulmonary vascular changes in the rabbit. Proc Soc Exp Biol Med 170:378-383, 1982.

Kreft-Jais C, Plouin P-F, Tchobroutsky C, Boutroy M-J: Angiotensin-converting enzyme inhibitors during pregnancy: A survey of 22 patients given captopril and nine given enalapril. Br J Obstet Gynaecol 95:420-422, 1988.

Lumbers ER, Burrell JH, Menzies RI, Stevens AD: The effects of a converting enzyme inhibitor (captopril) and angiotensin II on fetal renal function. Br J Pharmacol 110:821-827, 1993.

Lumbers ER, Kingsford NM, Menzies RI, Stevens AD: Acute effects of captopril, an angiotensin-converting enzyme inhibitor, on the pregnant ewe and fetus. Am J Physiol 262(5 PT 2):R754-R760, 1992.

Mehta N, Modi N: ACE inhibitors in pregnancy. Lancet 2:96-97, 1989.

Piper JM, Ray WA, Rosa FW: Pregnancy outcome following exposure to angiotensin-converting enzyme inhibitors. Obstet Gynecol 80:429-432, 1992.

Pryde PG, Sedman AB, Nugent CE, Barr M Jr: Angiotensin-converting enzyme inhibitor fetopathy. J Am Soc Nephrol 3:1575-1582, 1993.

Robillard JE, Weismann DN, Gomez RA, et al.: Renal and adrenal responses to converting-enzyme inhibition in fetal and newborn life. Am J Physiol 244:R249-R256, 1983.

Rothberg AD, Lorenz R: Can captopril cause fetal and neonatal renal failure? Pediatr Pharmacol 4:189-192, 1984.

Shotan A, Widerhorn J, Hurst A, Elkayam U: Risks of angiotensin-converting enzyme inhibition during pregnancy: Experimental and clinical evidence, potential mechanisms, and recommendations for use. Am J Med 96:451-456, 1994.

WHO Working Group on Drugs and Human Lactation. In: Bennet PN (ed). *Drugs and Human Lactation.* Amsterdam: Elsevier, 1988, pp 125-126.

CARAMIPHEN

Caramiphen is an anticholinergic agent that is used in cough medicines. In such preparations, caramiphen is given orally in doses of 20-80 mg/d in combination with other ingredients.

Teratogenic Risk

Magnitude of teratogenic risk to child born after exposure during gestation:	*Unlikely*
Quality and quantity of data on which risk estimate is based:	*Poor to fair*

Therapeutic doses of caramiphen do not pose a substantial teratogenic risk, but the data are insufficient to state that there is no risk.

The frequency of congenital anomalies was no greater than expected among 38 infants whose mothers took caramiphen during the first four lunar months of pregnancy or among 236 infants whose mothers who took the drug anytime during pregnancy in one epidemiological study (Heinonen et al., 1977).

No animal teratology studies of caramiphen have been published.

Risk Related to Breast-feeding

No information regarding the distribution of caramiphen in breast milk has been published.

Key References

Heinonen OP, Slone D, Shapiro S: *Birth Defects and Drugs in Pregnancy.* Littleton, Mass.: John Wright-PSG, 1977, pp 378, 442.

CARBAMAZEPINE
(Epitol®, Mazepine®, Tegretol®)

Carbamazepine is an anticonvulsant agent used to prevent grand mal, psychomotor, and partial seizures. It is also used to treat depression and certain kinds of cranial nerve pain. Carbamazepine is given orally in doses of 200-1200 mg/d. Doses as great as 1600 mg/d are sometimes used to treat pyschosis. Therapeutic plasma levels for carbamazepine as an anticonvulsant are considered to be in the range of 6-12 mcg/mL.

Teratogenic Risk

Magnitude of teratogenic risk to child born after exposure during gestation:	*Small to Moderate*
Quality and quantity of data on which risk estimate is based:	*Fair to Good*

Teratogenic risks associated with polydrug therapy that includes carbamazepine are greater than those associated with carbamazepine monotherapy.

Folate supplementation is generally recommended for women who are taking carbamazepine and who are or may become pregnant to reduce the risk of neural tube defects among future children (Delgado-Escueta & Janz, 1992; Lindhout & Omtzigt, 1994; Oakeshott, 1994; Yerby & Devinsky, 1994).

Prenatal diagnosis by high-resolution ultrasound examination and α-fetoprotein measurement can detect most fetal neural tube defects and should be offered to women treated with carbamazepine during pregnancy (Delgado-Escueta & Janz, 1992; Lindhout & Omtzigt, 1994; Yerby & Devinsky, 1994).

Epidemiological studies of malformations in infants born to women who took carbamazepine during pregnancy are difficult to interpret because almost all of the women studied were taking carbamazepine for epilepsy. Assessment of the effects of anticonvulsant drug exposure is confounded in such cases by many other factors including the facts that most women with seizures are treated with some anticonvulsant drug, that many women are treated with more than one anticonvulsant at a time, and that women who are not treated or are treated with a single agent probably have milder seizure disorders (Dansky & Finnell, 1991).

In several epidemiological studies, each of which involved fewer than 100 epileptic women treated with carbamazepine during the first trimester of pregnancy, the frequency of malformations in the infants was 2-3 times as great as that generally seen among normal populations but similar to that in children born to epileptic women who had been treated with other anticonvulsants (Starreveld-Zimmerman et al., 1973; Nakane et al., 1980; Lindhout et al., 1982, 1992a; Kaneko et al., 1988; Battino et al., 1992). In contrast, no association with maternal carbamazepine use during pregnancy was observed in studies of 10,698 or 7607 infants with congenital anomalies (Bertollini et al., 1985; Czeizel et al., 1992). Higher frequencies of congenital anomalies have been observed among infants born to mothers treated with carbamazepine in combination with other anticonvulsant agents, especially valproic acid (Lindhout et al., 1984; Kaneko et al., 1988, 1992; Shakir & Abdulwahab, 1991; Czeizel et al., 1992).

An increased frequency of neural tube defects among the children of women treated with carbamazepine during pregnancy has been suggested on the basis of clinical observations and data from one epidemiological study (Bod, 1989; Jones et al., 1989a; Rosa, 1991; Gladstone et al., 1992; Lindhout et al., 1992b). Cases of spina bifida have been observed in several other epidemiological studies of infants born to women treated with carbamazepine during pregnancy, but this putative association has not been confirmed statistically (Bertollini et al., 1985; Kallen et al., 1989; Czeizel et al., 1992; Omtzigt et al., 1992). Little et al. (1993) observed a fetus with spina bifida whose mother did not have a seizure disorder but took a large overdose of carbamazepine during the period of neural tube closure.

The existence of a fetal carbamazepine syndrome of growth and developmental delay associated with minor facial and other anomalies similar to those seen in association with maternal use of some other anticonvulsants has been suggested (Van Allen et al., 1988; Jones et al., 1989b). Features of this syndrome were seen in most of 35 children born to women treated with carbamazepine monotherapy in one study (Jones et al., 1989b). It is unclear whether these features are a result of the population evaluated or method of study or due to the medication, the maternal epilepsy, or some related factor (Dow & Riopelle, 1989; Scialli & Lione, 1989).

In one study of 20 children born to mothers who had been treated with carbamazepine alone during pregnancy, the average head circumference (but not the weight or length) was significantly decreased both at birth and at 18 months of age (Hiilesmaa et al., 1981). The head circumference among these children was not significantly decreased at 5.5 years of age, however (Gaily et al., 1990a). The average IQ of 34 5.5-year-old children whose mothers had taken carbamazepine during pregnancy was no different from controls; one other child in this study who was exposed was severely retarded, apparently for a different reason (Gaily et al., 1988). The frequency of specific cognitive dysfunction was no greater than expected among 30 of these children who were tested (Gaily et al., 1990b). Similarly, the frequencies of neurological dysfunction and school problems were no greater than expected in another study among 23 six- to 13-year-old children of epileptic women who had been treated with carbamazepine during pregnancy (van der Pol et al., 1991).

Central nervous system and other malformations have been observed among the offspring of mice treated with carbamazepine in doses 5-100 times those used clinically (Finnell & Dansky, 1991). Although maternal toxicity occurred at the higher dose levels, drug concentration in the animals' blood was within or below the range that would be considered therapeutic in humans. Results of mouse teratology studies involving doses 2-10 times those used in humans have been inconsistent (Finnell & Dansky, 1991). In rats, increased frequencies of congenital anomalies were observed among the offspring of pregnant animals treated with carbamazepine in doses 17-25 times those used in humans (Vorhees et al., 1990). Such doses produced maternal toxicity and blood levels 2-3 times greater than those considered to be therapeutic in humans. The relevance of these findings to the risks associated with therapeutic use of carbamazepine in human pregnancy is unknown.

Risk Related to Breast-feeding

Carbamazepine is excreted in breast milk. Based on data from 54 lactating women, the amount of carbamazepine that the nursing infant would be expected to ingest is between 2-7.2% of the lowest weight-adjusted therapeutic dose (Pynnonen & Sillanpaa, 1975; Pynnonen et al., 1977; Kaneko et al., 1979; Kok et al., 1982; Kuhnz et al., 1983; Froescher et al., 1984; Merlob et al., 1992).*

Infant serum levels of carbamazepine have been observed to range between 25-45% of the lowest therapeutic serum level in adults (Kok et al., 1982; Kuhnz et al., 1983; Merlob et al., 1992).[†]

No adverse effects that could be attributed to carbamazepine were noted among the nursing infants in any of these studies, with the exception of one case of transient direct hyperbilirubinemia and a high concentration of γ-glutamyltransferase in a 41-week-old infant whose mother had ingested carbamazepine throughout pregnancy and lactation (Merlob et al., 1992). The hepatic dysfunction spontaneously resolved even though the mother continued with carbamazepine therapy and "occasional" breast-feeding. Cholestatic hepatitis was observed in a three-week-old infant whose mother had taken carbamazepine per day throughout pregnancy and lactation (Frey et al., 1990). Breast milk and plasma levels were not reported. The cholestasis resolved after breast-feeding was terminated.

Both the American Academy of Pediatrics (Committee on Drugs, American Academy of Pediatrics, 1994), and the WHO Working Group on Drugs and Human Lactation (1988) regard carbamazepine to be safe to use while breast-feeding.

Key References

Battino D, Binelli S, Caccamo ML, et al.: Malformations in offspring of 305 epileptic women: A prospective study. Acta Neurol Scand 85(3):204-207, 1992.

Bertollini R, Mastroiacovo P, Segni G: Maternal epilepsy and birth defects: A case-control study in the Italian Multicentric Registry of Birth Defects (IPIMC). Eur J Epidemiol 1(1):67-72, 1985.

Bod M: Teratogenic evaluation of anticonvulsants in a population based Hungarian material. Teratology 40(3):277, 1989.

Committee on Drugs, American Academy of Pediatrics: The transfer of drugs and other chemicals into human milk. Pediatrics 93(1):137-150, 1994.

---

*This calculation is based on the following assumptions: milk concentration of carbamazepine: 1.3-4.8 mcg/mL; milk intake by the nursing infant: 150 mL/kg/d; estimated amount of carbamazepine ingested by the nursing infant: 0.2-0.7 mg/kg/d; lowest therapeutic dose of carbamazepine in children: 10 mg/kg/d.

†Infant serum levels of carbamazepine: <1-1.8 mcg/mL; lowest therapeutic serum level in adults: 4 mcg/mL.

Czeizel AE, Bod M, Halasz P: Evaluation of anticonvulsant drugs during pregnancy in a population-based Hungarian study. Eur J Epidemiol 8(1):122-127, 1992.

Dansky LV, Finnell RH: Parental epilepsy, anticonvulsant drugs and reproductive outcome: Epidemiologic and experimental findings spanning three decades; 2: Human studies. Reprod Toxicol 5(4):301-335, 1991.

Delgado-Escueta AV, Janz D: Consensus guidelines: Preconception counseling, management, and care of the pregnant woman with epilepsy. Neurology 42(Suppl 5):149-160, 1992.

Dow KE, Riopelle RJ: Teratogenic effects of carbamazepine. N Engl J Med 321:1480-1481, 1989.

Finnell RH, Dansky LV: Parental epilepsy, anticonvulsant drugs and reproductive outcome: Epidemiologic and experimental findings spanning three decades; 1: Animal studies. Reprod Toxicol 5(4):281-299, 1991.

Frey B, Schubiger G, Musy JP: Transient cholestatic hepatitis in a neonate associated with carbamazepine exposure during pregnancy and breast-feeding. Eur J Pediatr 150:136-138, 1990.

Froescher W, Echelbaum M, Niesen M, et al.: Carbamazepine levels in breast milk. Ther Drug Monit 6:266-271, 1984.

Gaily E, Kantola-Sorsa E, Granstrom M-L: Intelligence of children of epileptic mothers. J Pediatr 113:677-684, 1988.

Gaily E, Kantola-Sorsa E, Granstrom M-L: Specific cognitive dysfunction in children with epileptic mothers. Dev Med Child Neurol 32:403-414, 1990b.

Gaily EK, Granstrom M-L, Hiilesmaa VK, Bardy AH: Head circumference in children of epileptic mothers: Contributions of drug exposure and genetic background. Epilepsy Res 5:217-222, 1990a.

Gladstone DJ, Bologa M, Maguire C, et al.: Course of pregnancy and fetal outcome following maternal exposure to carbamazepine and phenytoin: A prospective study. Reprod Toxicol 6:257-261, 1992.

Hiilesmaa VK, Teramo K, Granstrom ML, Bardy AH: Fetal head growth retardation associated with maternal antiepileptic drugs. Lancet 2:165-167, 1981.

Jones KL, Johnson KA, Adams J, Lacro RV: Teratogenic effects of carbamazepine. N Engl J Med 321:1480-1481, 1989a.

Jones KL, Lacro RV, Johnson KA, Adams J: Pattern of malformations in the children of women treated with carbamazepine during pregnancy. N Engl J Med 320:1661-1666, 1989b.

Kallen B, Robert E, Mastroiacovo P, et al.: Anticonvulsant drugs and malformations. Is there a drug specificity? Eur J Epidemiol 5(1):31-36, 1989.

Kaneko S, Otani K, Fukushima Y, et al.: Teratogenicity of antiepileptic drugs: Analysis of possible risk factors. Epilepsia 29(4):459-467, 1988.

Kaneko S, Otani K, Kondo T, et al.: Malformation in infants of mothers with epilepsy receiving antiepileptic drugs. Neurology 42(Suppl 5):68-74, 1992.

Kaneko S, Sato T, Suzuki K: The levels of anticonvulsants in breast milk. Br J Clin Pharmacol 7:624-627, 1979.

Kok THHG, Taitz LS, Bennett MJ, Holt DW: Drowsiness due to clemastine transmitted in breast milk. Lancet 1:914-915, 1982.

Kuhnz W, Jager-Roman E, Deichl A, et al.: Carbamazepine and carbamazepine-10,11-epoxide during pregnancy and postnatal period in epileptic mothers and their nursed infants: Pharmacokinetics and clinical effects. Pediatr Pharmacol 3:199-208, 1983.

Lindhout D, Hoppener RJEA, Meinardi H: Teratogenicity of antiepileptic drug combinations with special emphasis on epoxidation (of carbamazepine). Epilepsia 25:77-83, 1984.

Lindhout D, Meinardi H, Barth PG: Hazards of fetal exposure to drug combinations. In: Jantz D, Bossi L, Dam M, Richens A, Schmidt D (eds). *Epilepsy, Pregnancy and the Child.* New York: Raven Press, 1982, pp 275-281.

Lindhout D, Meinardi H, Meijer JWA, Nau H: Antiepileptic drugs and teratogenesis in two consecutive cohorts: Changes in prescription policy paralleled by changes in pattern of malformations. Neurology 42(Suppl 5):94-110, 1992a.

Lindhout D, Omtzigt JGC: Teratogenic effects of antiepileptic drugs: Implications for the management of epilepsy in women of childbearing age. Epilepsia 35(Suppl 4):S19-S28, 1994.

Lindhout D, Omtzigt JGC, Cornel MC: Spectrum of neural-tube defects in 34 infants prenatally exposed to antiepileptic drugs. Neurology 42(Suppl 5):111-118, 1992b.

Little B, Santos-Ramos R, Newell JF, Maberry MC: Megadose carbamazepine during the period of neural tube closure. Obstet Gynecol 82:705-708, 1993.

Merlob P, Mor N, Litwin A: Transient hepatic dysfunction in an infant of an epileptic mother treated with carbamazepine during pregnancy and breastfeeding. Ann Pharmacother 26:1563-1565, 1992.

Nakane Y, Okkuma T, Takahashi R, et al.: Multi-institutional study on the teratogenicity and fetal toxicity of antiepileptic drugs: A report of a collaborative study group in Japan. Epilepsia 21:663-680, 1980.

Oakeshott P: Prevention of neural tube defects. Lancet 343:123-124, 1994.

Omtzigt JGC, Los FJ, Grobbee DE, et al.: The risk of spina bifida aperta after first-trimester exposure to valproate in a prenatal cohort. Neurology 42(Suppl 5):119-125, 1992.

Pynnonen S, Kanto J, Sillanpaa M, Erkkola R: Carbamazepine: Placental transport, tissue concentrations in foetus and newborn, and level in milk. Acta Pharmacol Toxicol 41:244-253, 1977.

Pynnonen S, Sillanpaa M: Carbamazepine and mother's milk. Lancet 2:563, 1975.

Rosa FW: Spina bifida in infants of women treated with carbamazepine during pregnancy. N Engl J Med 324(10):674-677, 1991.

Scialli AR, Lione A: Teratogenic effects of carbamazepine. N Engl J Med 321:1480-1481, 1989.

Shakir RA, Abdulwahab B: Congenital malformations before and after the onset of maternal epilepsy. Acta Neurol Scand 84:153-156, 1991.

Starreveld-Zimmerman AAE, van der Kolk WJ, Meinardi H, Elshove J: Are anticonvulsants teratogenic? Lancet 2:48-49, 1973.

Van Allen MI, Yerby M, Leavitt A, et al.: Increased major and minor malformations in infants of epileptic mothers: Preliminary results of the pregnancy and epilepsy study. Am J Hum Genet 43(Suppl):A73, 1988.

Van der Pol MC, Hadders-Algra M, Huisjes HJ, Touwen BCL: Antiepileptic medication in pregnancy: Late effects on the children's central nervous system development. Am J Obstet Gynecol 164:121-128, 1991.

Vorhees CV, Acuff KD, Weisenburger WP, Minck DR: Teratogenicity of carbamazepine in rats. Teratology 41:311-317, 1990.

WHO Working Group on Drugs and Human Lactation. In: Bennet PN (ed): *Drugs and Human Lactation*. Amsterdam: Elsevier, 1988, pp 335-336.

Yerby MS, Devinsky O: Epilepsy and pregnancy. Adv Neurol 64:45-63, 1994.

CARBINOXAMINE
(Allergefon®, Histex®, Ziritron®)

Carbinoxamine is an antihistaminic agent of the ethanolamine class. It is used orally to treat allergic conditions and in cough and cold preparations. The usual dose is 12-32 mg/d.

Teratogenic Risk

Magnitude of teratogenic risk to child born after exposure during gestation:	*Undetermined*
Quality and quantity of data on which risk estimate is based:	*Very poor*

No epidemiologic studies of malformations in the infants of women who took carbinoxamine during pregnancy have been published.

Studies in rats and mice suggest that treatment of pregnant women with carbinoxamine in usual therapeutic doses is unlikely to increase the children's risk of malformations greatly (Maruyama & Yoshida, 1968).

Please see agent summary on diphenhydramine for information on a related drug that has been more thoroughly studied.

Risk Related to Breast-feeding

No information regarding the distribution of carbinoxamine in breast milk has been published.

Key References

Maruyama H, Yoshida S: [Pharmacology of a new antihistamine, carbinoxamine diphenyldisulfonate. (2) Toxicity and influence on fetuses.] J Med Soc Toho Univ (Jpn) 15:367-374, 1968.

CARBOLITH® *See* Lithium

CARDIOQUIN® *See* Quinidine

CARDIZEM CD® *See Diltiazem*

CATAPRES® *See Clonidine*

CECLOR® *See Cefaclor*

CECON® *See Ascorbic Acid*

CEFACLOR
(Ceclor®)

Cefaclor is a cephalosporin antibiotic that is given orally in doses of 750-4000 mg/d.

Teratogenic Risk

Magnitude of teratogenic risk to child born after exposure during gestation:	*Undetermined*
Quality and quantity of data on which risk estimate is based:	*Very poor*

No epidemiological studies of infants of women treated with cefaclor during pregnancy have been reported.

Studies in mice, rats, rabbits and ferrets suggest that treatment of pregnant women with cefaclor in usual therapeutic doses is unlikely to increase the children's risk of malformations greatly (Markham et al., 1978; Furuhashi et al., 1979; Nomura et al., 1979).

Risk Related to Breast-feeding

Cefaclor is excreted in breast milk in very low concentrations. The amount of cefaclor that the nursing infant would be expected to ingest is <1% of the lowest therapeutic dose of cefaclor in children (Takase, 1979).*

The WHO Working Group on Drugs and Human Lactation (1988) regards cefaclor to be safe to use during breast-feeding.

Key References

Furuhashi T, Nomura A, Uehara, et al.: Reproduction studies on cefaclor (CCL). 2. Fertility study and perinatal-postnatal study in rats. Chemotherapy 27:865-880, 1979.

Markham JK, Hanasono GK, Adams ER, Owen NV: Reproduction studies on cefaclor. Toxicol Appl Pharmacol 45:292, 1978.

Nomura A, Furuhashi T, Ikeya E, et al: Reproduction study of cefaclor (CCL). 1. Teratological study in mice, rats and rabbits. Chemotherapy 27:846-864, 1979.

Takase A: Clinical and laboratory studies of cefaclor in the field of obstetrics and gynecology. Chemotherapy (Tokyo) 27(Suppl):666-671, 1979.

WHO Working Group on Drugs and Human Lactation. In: Bennet PN (ed): *Drugs and Human Lactation*. Amsterdam: Elsevier, 1988, pp 229-230.

*This calculation is based on the following assumptions: maternal dose of cefaclor: 250-500 mg; milk concentration of cefaclor: 0.12-0.35 mcg/mL; milk intake by the nursing infant: 150 mL/kg/d; estimated dose of cefaclor ingested by the nursing infant: 0.02-0.05 mg/kg/d; lowest therapeutic dose of cefaclor in children: 20 mg/kg/d.

CEFADROXIL
(Duricef®, Ultracef®)

Cefadroxil is a cephalosporin antibiotic that is given orally in doses of 1000-4000 mg/d.

Teratogenic Risk

*Magnitude of teratogenic
risk to child born after
exposure during gestation:*   *Undetermined*

*Quality and quantity of data
on which risk estimate is based:*   *Very poor*

No epidemiological studies of congenital anomalies in infants born to women treated with cefadroxil during pregnancy have been reported.

Studies in rats, mice, and rabbits suggest that treatment of pregnant women with cefadroxil in usual therapeutic doses is unlikely to increase the children's risk of malformations greatly (Hickey et al., 1978; Tauchi et al., 1980a, b).

Risk Related to Breast-feeding

Cefadroxil is excreted in breast milk. Based on data obtained from six lactating mothers, the amount of cefadroxil that the nursing infant would be expected to ingest is equivalent to 0.6-1.2% of the lowest therapeutic dose of cefadroxil on a weight-adjusted basis (Kafetzis et al., 1981).*

Both the American Academy of Pediatrics (Committee on Drugs, American Academy of Pediatrics, 1994) and the WHO Working Group on Drugs and Human Lactation (1988) regard cefadroxil to be safe to use during breast-feeding.

Key References

Committee on Drugs, American Academy of Pediatrics: The transfer of drugs and other chemicals into human milk. Pediatrics 93(1):137-150, 1994.

Hickey TE, Botta JA Jr, Clemento AJ Jr: Cefadroxil - A new antibiotic with low toxicity potential. Curr Ther Res 23(5):608-616, 1978.

Kafetzis, DA, Siafas CA, Georgakopoulos PA, Papadatos CJ: Passage of cephalosporins and amoxicillin into the breast milk. Acta Paediatr Scand 70:285-288, 1981.

Tauchi K, Kawanishi H, Igarashi N, et al.: Studies on the toxicity of cefadroxil (S-578). VI. Teratogenic study in rats. Jpn J Antibiot 33:487-496, 1980a.

Tauchi K, Kawanishi H, Igarashi N, et al.: Studies on the toxicity of cefadroxil (S-578). VII. Teratogenic study in rabbits. Jpn J Antibiot 33:497-502, 1980b.

*This calculation is based on the following assumptions: maternal dose of cefadroxil: 1 g; milk concentration of cefadroxil: 1.2-2.4 mcg/mL; milk intake by the nursing infant: 150 mL/kg/d; estimated dose of cefadroxil ingested by the nursing infant: 0.18-0.36 mg/kg/d; lowest pediatric dose of cefadroxil: 30 mg/kg/d.

WHO Working Group on Drugs and Human Lactation. In: Bennet PN (ed). *Drugs and Human Lactation.* Amsterdam: Elsevier, 1988, pp 231-232.

CEFANEX® *See* Cephalexin

CEFTIN® *See* Cefuroxime

CEFUROXIME
(Ceftin®, Kefurox®, Zinacef®)

Cefuroxime is a cephalosporin antibiotic. It is administered orally in a dose of 250-1000 mg/d or parenterally in a dose of 2250-4500 mg/d.

Teratogenic Risk

*Magnitude of teratogenic
risk to child born after
exposure during gestation:*   *Undetermined*

*Quality and quantity of data
on which risk estimate is based:*   *Very poor*

A small risk cannot be excluded, but there is no indication that the risk of congenital anomalies in children of women treated with cefuroxime during pregnancy is likely to be great.

No epidemiological studies of congenital anomalies in children of women treated with cefuroxime during pregnancy have been reported.

Studies in mice and rabbits suggest that treatment of pregnant women with cefuroxime in usual therapeutic doses is unlikely to increase the children's risk of malformations greatly (Brogden et al., 1979; Capel-Edwards et al., 1979).

Risk Related to Breast-feeding

No information regarding the distribution of cefuroxime in breast milk has been published.

Key References

Brogden RN, Heel RC, Speight TM, Avery GS: Cefuroxime: A review of its antibacterial activity, pharmacological properties and therapeutic use. Drugs 17:233-266, 1979.

Capel-Edwards K, Atkinson RM, Pratt DAH: Toxicological studies on cefuroxime sodium. Toxicology 13:1-5, 1979.

C-LEXIN® *See* Cephalexin

CENTRAX® *See* Prazepam

CEPHALEXIN
(Cefanex®, C-Lexin®, Keflex®)

Cephalexin is a cephalosporin antibiotic that is administered orally in the treatment of bacterial infections. The usual dose is 1000-4000 mg/d.

Teratogenic Risk

Magnitude of teratogenic risk to child born after exposure during gestation:	*Undetermined*
Quality and quantity of data on which risk estimate is based:	*Poor*

There are no published epidemiological studies of congenital anomalies among the children of women treated with cephalexin during pregnancy.

Studies in rats and rabbits provide no consistent evidence that treatment of pregnant women with cephalexin in usual therapeutic doses is likely to increase the children's risk of malformations greatly (Aoyama et al., 1969; Welles et al., 1969).

Risk Related to Breast-feeding

Cephalexin is excreted in small quantities in breast milk. The amount of cephalexin that the nursing infant would be expected to ingest is <1% of the lowest pediatric dose, based on data obtained from six lactating women (Kafetzis et al., 1981).*

The WHO Working Group on Drugs and Human Lactation (1988) considers cephalexin to be safe to use during breast-feeding.

Key References

Aoyama T, Furuoka R, Hasegawa N, Nemoto K: Teratologic studies of cephalexin in mice and rats. Oyo Yakuri 3:249-263, 1969.

Kafetzis DA, Siafas CA, Georgakopoulos PA, Papadatos CJ: Passage of cephalosporins and amoxicillin into the breast milk. Acta Paediatr Scand 70:285-288, 1981.

Welles JS, Froman RO, Gibson WR, et al.: Toxicology and pharmacology of cephalexin in laboratory animals. Antimicrob Agents Chemother 1968:489-496, 1969.

WHO Working Group on Drugs and Human Lactation: In: Bennet PN (ed). *Drugs and Human Lactation.* Amsterdam: Elsevier, 1988, pp 219-220.

* This calculation is based on the following assumptions: maternal dose of cephalexin: 1 gm; milk concentration of cephalexin: 0.24-0.85 mcg/mL; milk intake by the nursing infant: 150 mL/kg/d; estimated dose of cephalexin ingested by the nursing infant: 0.04-0.13 mg/kg/d; lowest pediatric dose of cephalexin: 25 mg/kg/d.

CETAMIDE® *See* Sulfacetamide

CETIRIZINE
(Reactine®, Zirtek®)

Cetirizine is an H_1 antihistamine that is used to treat allergies. Cetirizine is given orally in doses of 5-20 mg/d.

Teratogenic Risk

*Magnitude of teratogenic
risk to child born after
exposure during gestation:*   *Undetermined*

*Quality and quantity of data
on which risk estimate is based:*   *Very poor*

A small risk cannot be excluded, but a high risk of congenital anomalies in the children of women treated with cetirizine during pregnancy is unlikely.

No epidemiological studies of congenital anomalies among the children of women who were treated with cetirizine during pregnancy have been reported.

Studies in rats and rabbits suggest that treatment of pregnant women with cetirizine in usual therapeutic doses is unlikely to increase the children's risk of malformations greatly (Kamijima et al., 1994).

Please see agent summary on hydroxyzine for information on a similarly used agent that has been more thoroughly studied.

Risk Related to Breast-feeding

No information regarding the distribution of cetirizine in breast milk has been published.

Key References

Kamijima M, Sakai Y, Kinoshita K, et al.: Reproductive and developmental toxicity studies of cetirizine in rats and rabbits. Clin Rep 28:1877-1903, 1994.

CHINA WHITE *See* Heroin

CHLORAMPHENICOL
(Chloromycetin®)

Chloramphenicol is an antibiotic used orally, parenterally and topically to treat bacterial infections. The usual systemic dose is 2500-4000 mg/d, up to 6000 mg/d.

Teratogenic Risk

*Magnitude of teratogenic
risk to child born after
exposure during gestation:*   *Unlikely*

*Quality and quantity of data
on which risk estimate is based:*   *Poor to fair*

Therapeutic doses of chloramphenicol are unlikely to pose a sub-stantial teratogenic risk, but the data are insufficient to state that there is no risk.

Maternal treatment with chloramphenicol late in pregnancy may be associated with vascular collapse in the newborn infant (see below).

The frequency of congenital anomalies was no greater than expected among the children of 98 women treated with chloramphenicol during the first four lunar months or among the children of 348 women treated with the drug anytime in pregnancy in one epidemiological study (Heinonen et al., 1977).

The frequency of congenital anomalies was not increased among the offspring of mice or rabbits treated with chloramphenicol during pregnancy in doses 10-40 times those used in humans (Fritz & Hess, 1971). Similarly, no teratogenic effect was observed in rats after maternal treatment with 2-4 times the usual human dose (Prochazka et al., 1964), although various fetal anomalies were induced by maternal treatment with 10-40 times the human dose of chloramphenicol (Takaya, 1965; Fritz & Hess, 1971). An increased frequency of fetal death and decreased fetal weight were seen after such treatment in all three species. Behavioral alterations have been reported among adult rats born to dams treated during pregnancy with chloramphenicol in doses similar to those used in human therapy (Bertolini et al., 1980). The relevance of these observations to the risks associated with therapeutic use of chloramphenicol in human pregnancy is unknown.

Indirect evidence and one human case report (Oberheuser, 1971) suggest that maternal chloramphenicol treatment late in pregnancy may produce vascular collapse ("the Grey Baby Syndrome") in the newborn infant. Grey baby syndrome is a well-known complication of chloramphenicol therapy in neonates (Sutherland, 1959; Weiss et al., 1960), and the drug freely crosses the placenta at term (Scott & Warner, 1950). Thus, it is reasonable to suspect that this condition could occur after maternal chloramphenicol treatment shortly before delivery.

Risk Related to Breast-feeding

Chloramphenicol is excreted in breast milk in low concentrations. The amount of chloramphenicol that the nursing infant would be expected to ingest is between 0.2-3.6% of the lowest neonatal dose of chloramphenicol and between 0.05-0.9% of the lowest dose known to be associated with the "Grey baby syndrome" (Havelka et al., 1968; Plomp et al., 1983).*

Although chloramphenicol has the potential to cause dose-related bone marrow depression in nursing infants (USP DI, 1995), this effect has not been reported. Because of this potential, the American Academy of Pediatrics regards chloramphenicol to be a drug whose effect on the nursing infant may be a concern (Committee on Drugs, American Academy of Pediatrics, 1994).

Key References

Bertolini A, Poggioli R, Bernardi M, et al.: Pharmacological interferences in the protein synthesis during the fetal or neonatal period, in the rat: Behavioral outcomes in the adulthood. Pharmacol Res Commun 12:227-232, 1980.

Committee on Drugs, American Academy of Pediatrics: The transfer of drugs and other chemicals into human milk. Pediatrics 93(1):137-150, 1994.

Fritz H, Hess R: The effect of chloramphenicol on the prenatal development of rats, mice, and rabbits. Toxicol Appl Pharmacol 19:667-674, 1971.

Havelka J, Heizlar M, Popov V et al.: Excretion of chloramphenicol in human milk. Chemotherapy 13:204-211, 1968.

Heinonen OP, Slone D, Shapiro S: *Birth Defects and Drugs in Pregnancy.* Littleton, Mass.: John Wright-PSG, 1977, pp 297, 301, 435.

Oberheuser F: Praktische erfahrungen mit medikamenten in der schwangerschaft. Therapiewoche 31:2198-2202, 1971.

Plomp TA, Thiery M, Maes RAA: The passage of thiamphenicol and chloramphenicol into human milk after single and repeated oral administration. Vet Hum Toxicol 25(3):167-172, 1983.

Prochazka J, Simkova V, Havelka J, et al.: [Concerning the penetration of the placenta by chloramphenicol.] Pediatriia 19:311-314, 1964.

Scott WC, Warner RF: Placental transfer of chloramphenicol (chloromycetin). JAMA 142:1331-1332, 1950.

*This calculation is based on the following assumptions: maternal dose of chloramphenicol: 0.5-2 gm/d; milk concentration of chloramphenicol: 0.31-6.1 mcg/mL; milk intake by the nursing infant: 150 mL/kg/d; estimated dose of chloramphenicol ingested by the nursing infant: 0.05-0.91 mg/kg/d; lowest neonatal dose of chloramphenicol: 25 mg/kg/d; lowest dose of chloramphenicol associated with the Grey baby syndrome: 100 mg/kg/d.

Sutherland JM: Fatal cardiovascular collapse of infants receiving large amounts of chloramphenicol. Am J Dis Child 97:761-767, 1959.

Takaya M: [Teratogenic effects of antibiotics.] J Osaka City Med Cent 14:107-115, 1965.

USP DI: Chloramphenicol. In: *USP DI (USP Dispensing Information), Volume 1. Drug Information for the Health Care Professional*, 15th ed. Rockville, Md.: The US Pharmacopeial Convention, 1995, p 720.

Weiss CF, Glazko AJ, Weston JK: Chloramphenicol in the newborn infant. A physiologic explanation of its toxicity when given in excessive doses. N Engl J Med 262:787-794, 1960.

CHLORDIAZEPOXIDE
(Libritabs®, Librium®)

Chlordiazepoxide is a widely used benzodiazepine tranquilizer. It also has sedative, anticonvulsant, and muscle relaxant properties. The usual oral or parental dose of chlordiazepoxide is 15-100 mg/d, although doses as large as 400 mg/d are sometimes used to treat alcohol withdrawal symptoms.

Teratogenic Risk

Magnitude of teratogenic risk to child born after exposure during gestation:	*Unlikely*
Quality and quantity of data on which risk estimate is based:	*Fair to good*

Therapeutic doses of chlordiazepoxide are unlikely to pose a substantial teratogenic risk, but the data are insufficient to state that there is no risk.

The risk associated with maternally toxic doses is unknown but likely to be greater.

The frequency of malformations was no greater than expected among the children of women who took chlordiazepoxide during the first trimester of pregnancy in four epidemiological studies involving respectively 38, 98, 89, and 257 infants (Crombie et al., 1975; Kullander & Kallen, 1976; Heinonen et al., 1977). An association between congenital anomalies (loosely defined) in children and maternal use of chlordiazepoxide early in pregnancy was suggested in a study that included 35 women who were prescribed this medication in the first 42 days following their last menstrual period (Milkovich & van den Berg, 1974). No specificity of the anomalies present in the affected children was apparent. Studies such as this one that include multiple comparisons between maternal drug exposures and various birth defect outcomes are expected to show occasional associations with nominal statistical significance purely by chance.

No association was found with maternal use of chlordiazepoxide during the first trimester of pregnancy in a study of 1427 infants with congenital anomalies (Bracken & Holford, 1981). Similarly, no association was observed with maternal chlordiazepoxide treatment early in pregnancy in studies of 390 children with congenital heart disease (Rothman et al., 1979) or 1201 children with cleft lip and/or palate (Czeizel, 1988).

The frequency of congenital anomalies was no greater than expected among the children of 175 and 740 women who took chlordiazepoxide anytime in pregnancy in two studies (Milkovich & van den Berg, 1974; Heinonen et al., 1977). In one of these investigations, mental and motor status scores at eight months of age and IQ scores at four years of age did not differ between children born to mothers who had taken chlordiazepoxide during pregnancy and those who did not (Hartz et al., 1975).

An increase in the frequency of central nervous system malformations was observed among the offspring of hamsters treated with chlordiazepoxide in doses 45-500 times those used clinically (Guram et al., 1982). Maternal toxicity was also seen with this treatment. The frequency of malformations was not increased among the offspring of rats treated during pregnancy with chlordiazepoxide in doses 1.5-16 times those used in humans, although skeletal variants, growth retardation, and fetal death were more common at the higher doses (Buttar, 1980; Saito et al., 1984). Decreased postnatal weight gain has been observed among the offspring of pregnant mice and rats treated respectively with 2-5 or <1-3 times the human dose of chlordiazepoxide (Buttar, 1980; Adams, 1982; Pankaj & Brain, 1991; Kurishingal et al., 1992). Both neonatal and long-lasting behavioral alterations are seen among the offspring of rats and mice treated respectively with <1-7 and 2-5 times the human dose of chlordiazepoxide during pregnancy (Avnimelech-Gigus et al., 1986; Pankaj et al., 1991; Kurishingal et al., 1992). The relevance of these observations to the risks associated with therapeutic use of chlordiazepoxide in human pregnancy is unknown.

Risk Related to Breast-feeding

Chlordiazepoxide is excreted in the breast milk (USP DI, 1995); although this has not been quantitated in published reports.

Key References

Adams PM: Effects of perinatal chlordiazepoxide exposure on rat preweaning and postweaning behavior. Neurobehav Toxicol Teratol 4:279-282, 1982.

Avnimelech-Gigus N, Feldon J, Tanne Z, Gavish M: The effects of prenatal chlordiazepoxide administration on avoidance behavior and benzodiazepine receptor density in adult albino rats. Eur J Pharmacol 129:185-188, 1986.

Bracken MB, Holford TR: Exposure to prescribed drugs in pregnancy and association with congenital malformations. Obstet Gynecol 58:336-344, 1981.

Buttar HS: Effects of chlordiazepoxide on the pre- and postnatal development of rats. Toxicology 17:311-321, 1980.

Crombie DL, Pinsent RJ, Fleming DM, et al.: Fetal effects of tranquilizers in pregnancy. N Engl J Med 293:198-199, 1975.

Czeizel A: Lack of evidence of teratogenicity of benzodiazepine drugs in Hungary. Reprod Toxicol 1(3):183-188, 1988.

Guram MS, Gill TS, Geber WF: Comparative teratogenicity of chlordiazepoxide, amitriptyline, and a combination of the two compounds in the fetal hamster. Neurotoxicology 3:83-90, 1982.

Hartz SC, Heinonen OP, Shapiro S, et al.: Antenatal exposure to meprobamate and chlordiazepoxide in relation to malformations, mental development, and childhood mortality. N Engl J Med 292:726-728, 1975.

Heinonen OP, Slone D, Shapiro S: *Birth Defects and Drugs in Pregnancy*. Littleton, Mass.: John Wright-PSG, 1977, p 491.

Kullander S, Kallen B: A prospective study of drugs and pregnancy. I. Psychopharmaca. Acta Obstet Gynecol Scand 55:25-33, 1976.

Kurishingal H, Palanza P, Brain PF: Effects of exposure of pregnant mice to chlordiazepoxide (CDP) on the development and ultrasound production of their offspring. Gen Pharmacol 23(1):49-53, 1992.

Milkovich L, van den Berg BJ: Effects of prenatal meprobamate and chlordiazepoxide hydrochloride on human embryonic and fetal development. N Engl J Med 291:1268-1271, 1974.

Pankaj V, Brain PF: Effects of prenatal exposure to benzodiazepine-related drugs on early development and adult social behaviour in Swiss mice--I. Agonists. Gen Pharmacol 22(1):33-41, 1991.

Rothman KJ, Fyler DC, Goldblatt A, Kreidberg MB: Exogenous hormones and other drug exposures of children with congenital heart disease. Am J Epidemiol 109:433-439, 1979.

Saito H, Kobayashi H, Takeno S, Sakai T: Fetal toxicity of benzodiazepines in rats. Res Commun Chem Pathol Pharmacol 46:437-447, 1984.

USP DI: Benzodiazepines. In: *USP DI (USP Dispensing Information), Volume 1. Drug Information for the Health Care Professional*, 15th ed. Rockville, Md.: The US Pharmacopeial Convention, 1995, p 460.

CHLOROMYCETIN® *See* Chloramphenicol

CHLOROQUINE
(Aralen®)

Chloroquine is a quinine derivative used to treat malarial and amoebic infections and inflammatory diseases. Chloroquine is administered orally in a dose of 500 mg every seven days to suppress malaria or in a dose of 1000-1500 mg/d to treat parasitic diseases. Smaller doses are used to treat inflammatory and autoimmune diseases and when the drug is given parenterally.

Teratogenic Risk

*Magnitude of teratogenic
risk to child born after
exposure during gestation*
    Daily dose: *Minimal*
    Weekly dose: *Unlikely*

*Quality and quantity of data
on which risk estimate is based*
    Daily dose: *Poor to fair*
    Weekly dose: *Poor to fair*

> *Therapeutic doses of chloroquine are unlikely to pose a substantial teratogenic risk, but the data are insufficient to state that there is no risk.*
>
> *Malaria during pregnancy may be life-threatening to both the mother and fetus, although symptoms more often are mild (Nathwani et al., 1992; Mutabingwa, 1994).*

The frequency of major malformations was no greater than expected among 169 infants born to women who took chloroquine weekly for malaria supression (Wolfe & Cordero, 1985). No malformations were observed among four children born to women treated daily with chloroquine for systemic lupus erythematosus in one series (Parke, 1988); these women miscarried or had stillbirths in four other pregnancies while on this treatment, but such outcomes are a recognized complication of lupus. In another series of pregnancies in women who were treated with chloroquine during the first trimester, there were 14 liveborn infants, none of whom had congenital anomalies (Levy et al., 1991).

Anecdotal observations have suggested an association between maternal use of chloroquine during pregnancy and auditory, vestibular, retinal, or other neurologic dysfunction in children (Roubenoff et al., 1988; Cook, 1992). Although such problems appear to be uncommon among children born to women treated with chloroquine during pregnancy (Roubenoff et al., 1988; Levy et al., 1991), a causal relationship seems possible. Chloroquine treatment occasionally produces similar toxic manifestations in adults (Tanenbaum & Tuffanelli, 1980), and a radio-labelled chloroquine analog administered to the mother has been shown to concentrate in the uveal tract of the eye and in the cochlea and ampulla of the inner ear in a macaque fetus (Dencker et al., 1975).

In areas where malaria is endemic, weekly chloroquine prophylaxis of pregnant women does not negatively affect their infants' birth weights (Cot et al., 1992; Nyirjesy et al., 1993).

Increased frequencies of fetal death and ocular malformations were observed among the offspring of pregnant rats treated with chloroquine in doses 100 times greater than those used in humans (Udalova, 1967). Fetal growth retardation and skeletal anomalies were noted with increased frequency among the offspring of pregnant rats treated with 70 times the human therapeutic dose of chloroquine (Sharma & Rawat, 1989). The relevance of these observations to the therapeutic use of chloroquine in human pregnancy is unknown.

Risk Related to Breast-feeding

Chloroquine is excreted in the breast milk in low concentrations. The amount of chloroquine that the nursing infant would be expected to ingest is <1% of the minimum preventive pediatric dose, based on data obtained from three lactating women who were given a single oral dose of 300 mg of chloroquine and six lactating women injected intramuscularly with 5 mg/kg of chloroquine (Edstein et al., 1986; Akintonwa et al., 1988;).*

Both the American Academy of Pediatrics (Committee on Drugs, American Academy of Pediatrics, 1994) and the WHO Working Group on Drugs and Human Lactation (1988) regard chloroquine to be safe to use while breast-feeding.

Key References

Akintonwa A, Gbajumo SA, Mabadeje AFB: Placental and milk transfer of chloroquine in humans. Ther Drug Monitor 10:147-149, 1988.

Committee on Drugs, American Academy of Pediatrics: The transfer of drugs and other chemicals into human milk. Pediatrics 93(1):137-150, 1994.

Cook GC: Use of antiprotozoan and anthelmintic drugs during pregnancy: Side-effects and contra-indications. J Infect 25:1-9, 1992.

Cot M, Roisin A, Barro D, et al.: Effect of chloroquine chemoprophylaxis during pregnancy on birth weight: Results of a randomized trial. Am J Trop Med Hyg 46(1):21-27, 1992.

Dencker L, Lindquist NG, Ullberg S: Distribution of an ^{125}I-labelled chloroquine analogue in a pregnant macaca monkey. Toxicology 5:255-264, 1975.

Edstein MD, Veenendaal JR, Newman K, Hyslop R: Excretion of chloroquine, dapsone and pyrimethamine in human milk. Br J Clin Pharmacol 22:733-735, 1986.

Levy M, Buskila D, Gladman DD, et al.: Pregnancy outcome following first trimester exposure to chloroquine. Am J Perinatol 8(3):174-178, 1991.

Mutabingwa TK: Malaria and pregnancy: Epidemiology, pathophysiology and control options. Acta Trop 57:239-254, 1994.

---

*This calculation is based on the following assumptions: milk concentration of chloroquine: 0.04-0.32 mcg/mL; milk intake by the nursing infant: 150 mL/kg/d; estimated dose of chloroquine ingested by the nursing infant: 0.01-0.05 mg/kg/d; minimum preventive pediatric dose of chloroquine: 8.3 mg/kg/d.

Nathwani D, Currie PF, Douglas JG, et al.: *Plasmodium falciparum* malaria in pregnancy: A review. Br J Obstet Gynaecol 99:118-121, 1992.

Nyirjesy P, Kavasya T, Axelrod P, Fischer PR: Malaria during pregnancy: Neonatal morbidity and mortality and the efficacy of chloroquine chemoprophylaxis. Clin Infect Dis 16(1):127-132, 1993.

Parke A: Antimalarial drugs and pregnancy. Am J Med 85(Suppl 4A):30-33, 1988.

Roubenoff R, Hoyt J, Petri M, et al.: Effects of anti-inflammatory and immunosuppressive drugs on pregnancy and fertility. Semin Arthritis Rheum 18(2):88-110, 1988.

Sharma A, Rawat AK: Toxicological consequences of chloroquine and ethanol on the developing fetus. Pharmacol Biochem Behav 34:77-82, 1989.

Tanenbaum L, Tuffanelli DL: Antimalarial agents: Chloroquine, hydroxychloroquine, and quinacrine. Arch Dermatol 116:587-591, 1980.

Udalova LD: [The effect of chloroquine on the embryonal development of rats.] Pharmacol Toxical (Russian) 2:226-228, 1967.

WHO Working Group on Drugs and Human Lactation. In: Bennet PN (ed). *Drugs and Human Lactation*. Amsterdam: Elsevier, 1988, pp 293-294.

Wolfe MS, Cordero JF: Safety of chloroquine in chemosuppression of malaria during pregnancy. Br Med J 290:1466-1467, 1985.

CHLOROTHIAZIDE
(Diuril®)

Chlorothiazide is a thiazide diuretic used in the treatment of edema and hypertension. It is given orally or intravenously in doses of 125-2000 mg/d.

Teratogenic Risk

*Magnitude of teratogenic
risk to child born after
exposure during gestation:*   *Unlikely*

*Quality and quantity of data
on which risk estimate is based:*   *Poor to fair*

Therapeutic doses of chlorothiazide are unlikely to pose a sub-stantial teratogenic risk, but the data are insufficient to state that there is no risk.

The frequency of congenital anomalies was no greater than ex-pected among the children of 63 women who took chlorothiazide dur-ing the first four lunar months of pregnancy or among the children of 5283 women who took the drug anytime in pregnancy in one epidemi-ological study (Heinonen et al., 1977). The frequency of congenital anomalies was no greater than expected among the children of 506 women treated with chlorothiazide during the second and third trimes-ters of pregnancy in another study (Kraus et al., 1966).

Studies in rats suggest that treatment of pregnant women with chlorothiazide in usual therapeutic doses is unlikely to increase the children's risk of malformations greatly (Maren & Ellison, 1972). Treatment of rats with about 30 times the human therapeutic dose of chlorothiazide during pregnancy produced chronic hypertension in the offspring in one study (Grollman & Grollman, 1962). This effect has not been investigated in humans.

Neonatal thrombocytopenic purpura has been reported in several children whose mothers received treatment with chlorothiazide late in pregnancy (Rodriguez et al., 1964); thrombocytopenia is a rare compli-cation of thiazide therapy in adults. The frequency of symptomatic neonatal thrombocytopenia in the children of women who take chlorothiazide late in pregnancy is probably very small (Finnerty & Assali, 1964; Kraus et al., 1966).

Risk Related to Breast-feeding

Chlorothiazide is excreted in breast milk in low concentrations. The amount of chlorothiazide that the nursing infant would be expected to ingest is <1% of the lowest neonatal dose, based on data obtained from 11 lactating women (Werthmann & Krees, 1972).*

Inhibition of lactation has been reported for other thiazide diuretics (Healy, 1961), but not for chlorothiazide. The American Academy of Pediatrics regards chlorothiazide to be safe to use during breast-feeding (Committee on Drugs, American Academy of Pediatrics, 1994).

*This calculation is based on the following assumptions: maternal dose of chlorothiaz-ide: 500 mg; milk concentration of chlorothiazide: <1 mcg/mL; milk intake by the nursing infant: 150 mL/kg/d; estimated dose of chlorothiazide ingested by the nursing infant: 0.15 mg/kg/d; lowest neonatal dose of chlorothiazide: 20 mg/kg/d.

Key References

Committee on Drugs, American Academy of Pediatrics: The transfer of drugs and other chemicals into human milk. Pediatrics 93(1):137-150, 1994.

Finnerty FA Jr, Assali NS: Thiazide and neonatal thrombocytopenia. N Engl J Med 271:160-161, 1964.

Grollman A, Grollman EF: The teratogenic induction of hypertension. J Clin Invest 41:710-714, 1962.

Healy M: Suppressing lactation with oral diuretics. Lancet 1:1353, 1961.

Heinonen OP, Slone D, Shapiro S: *Birth Defects and Drugs in Pregnancy.* Littleton, Mass.: John Wright-PSG, 1977, pp 372, 441, 495.

Kraus GW, Marchese JR, Yen SSC: Prophylactic use of hydrochlorothiazide in pregnancy. JAMA 198:1150-1154, 1966.

Maren TH, Ellison AC: The teratological effect of certain thiadiazoles related to acetazolamide, with a note on sulfanilamide and thiazide diuretics. Johns Hopkins Med J 130:95-104, 1972.

Rodriguez SU, Leikin SL, Hiller MC: Neonatal thrombocytopenia associated with ante-partum administration of thiazide drugs. N Engl J Med 270:881-884, 1964.

Werthmann MW Jr, Krees SV: Excretion of chlorothiazide in human breast milk. J Pediatr 81:781, 1972.

CHLORPHENIRAMINE
(Aller-Chlor, Chlor-Trimeton®)

Chlorpheniramine is an antihistamine commonly used to treat rhinitis and allergic disorders. It is administered orally in doses of 12-36 mg/d, often in combination with other ingredients in cough and cold medicines. Chlorpheniramine may also be given parenterally in single doses of 5-40 mg.

Teratogenic Risk

*Magnitude of teratogenic
risk to child born after
exposure during gestation:*   *Unlikely*

*Quality and quantity of data
on which risk estimate is based:*   Fair to good

Therapeutic doses of chlorpheniramine are unlikely to pose a sub-stantial teratogenic risk, but the data are insufficient to state that there is no risk.

The frequencies of major malformations, minor anomalies, and congenital anomalies in general were no greater than expected among the infants of 1070 women who took chlorpheniramine during the first four lunar months of pregnancy in one epidemiological study (Heinonen et al., 1977). Small but statistically significant associations were seen between maternal use of chlorpheniramine during the first four lunar months of pregnancy and both inguinal hernia and eye or ear anomalies among the children. Studies such as this one that include multiple comparisons between maternal drug exposures and various birth defect outcomes are expected to show occasional associations with nominal statistical significance purely by chance. The frequency of congenital anomalies was no greater than expected among the children of 3931 women who took chlorpheniramine anytime during pregnancy in this investigation (Heinonen et al., 1977).

No increase in the frequency of congenital anomalies was observed among more than 275 infants born to women who took chlorpheniramine during the first trimester of pregnancy in two sequential cohorts of another study (Jick et al., 1981; Aselton et al., 1985).

Increased frequencies of embryonic, fetal, and neonatal death were seen in one study among the offspring of pregnant mice treated with 65-650 times the usual human dose of chlorpheniramine (Naranjo & de Naranjo, 1968). The relevance of this observation to the therapeutic use of chlorpheniramine in human pregnancy is unknown.

Risk Related to Breast-feeding

No information regarding the distribution of chlorpheniramine in breast milk has been published.

Key References

Aselton P, Jick H, Milunsky A, et al: First-trimester drug use and congenital disorders. Obstet Gynecol 65:451-455, 1985.

Heinonen OP, Slone D, Shapiro S: *Birth Defects and Drugs in Pregnancy*. Littleton, Mass.: John Wright-PSG, 1977, pp 323-324, 437.

Jick H, Holmes LB, Hunter JR, et al.: First-trimester drug use and congenital disorders. JAMA 246:343-346, 1981.

Naranjo P, de Naranjo E: Embryotoxic effects of antihistamines. Arzneimittelforsch 18:188-195, 1968.

CHLORPROMAZINE
(Thorazine®, Thor-Prom®)

Chlorpromazine is a widely used phenothiazine. It is employed as a tranquilizer and sedative in the treatment of psychoses and as a pre-medication for operations and diagnostic procedures. Chlorpromazine is also used as an antiemetic. The drug is given orally, parenterally, or rectally in doses of 20-2000 mg/d.

Teratogenic Risk

Magnitude of teratogenic risk to child born after exposure during gestation:	*Unlikely*
Quality and quantity of data on which risk estimate is based:	*Fair to good*

Therapeutic doses of chlorpromazine are unlikely to pose a substantial teratogenic risk, but the data are insufficient to state that there is no risk.

Transient neurological dysfunction may occur among newborn infants of women who were treated with chlorpromazine late in pregnancy.

The frequency of congenital anomalies was no greater than expected among the children of 142 women treated with chlorpromazine during the first four lunar months of pregnancy or the children of 284 women treated with this drug anytime during pregnancy in one epidemiological study (Heinonen et al., 1977). Similarly, the frequency of congenital anomalies was not increased among the infants of 264 women treated with a low dose of chlorpromazine in the first trimester of pregnancy in another study (Farkas & Farkas, 1971).

In most investigations, the frequency of malformations was no greater than expected among the offspring of rats treated with chlorpromazine during pregnancy in doses 1-6 times those used in humans (Robertson et al., 1980; Jones-Price et al., 1983a). Increased fetal loss, decreased fetal weight gain, and maternal toxicity were often observed, especially at the higher doses. Increased frequencies of skeletal, central nervous system, and other anomalies have also been reported among the offspring of pregnant rats treated with chlorpromazine in doses 2-10 times those used in humans (Brock & von Kreybig, 1964; Singh & Padmanabhan, 1978). In mice, increased frequencies of eye, palate, skeletal, and other anomalies as well as of fetal death have been observed among the offspring of animals treated with chlorpromazine in doses <1-2 times those used in humans (Jones-Price et al., 1983b; Yu et al., 1988). These doses also produce maternal toxicity in mice. The relevance of these studies with respect to maternal use of chlorpromazine in human pregnancy is uncertain.

Many behavioral studies in the offspring of mice and rats treated with chlorpromazine during pregnancy have been published. A variety of long-lasting alterations of behavior and neurological function have been observed in the offspring with maternal treatment using <1-3 times the usual human dose of chlorpromazine (Robertson et al., 1980; Saillenfait & Vannier, 1988). The design and results of these studies vary, and their relevance to the therapeutic use of chlorpromazine in human pregnancy is unknown.

Neurological dysfunction with extrapyramidal signs has been reported in several infants born to women treated with chlorpromazine during pregnancy (Hill et al., 1966; Tamer et al., 1969; Hammond & Toseland, 1970; Levy & Wisniewski, 1974). The muscle rigidity, hypertonia, and tremor seen in these children is quite unusual among newborns. Although the abnormalities appear to be transient, they may last for months. It seems likely that the neurological dysfunction in these infants is related to their mothers' drug therapy because similar signs of extrapyramidal dysfunction may occur as a side effect of chlorpromazine administration in adults. The frequency of this complication among infants born to women treated with chlorpromazine during pregnancy appears to be low. More commonly, the infants of women treated with chlorpromazine late in pregnancy exhibit hypertonia, tremulousness, and poor motor maturity suggestive of a neonatal withdrawal syndrome (Auerbach et al., 1992).

Risk Related to Breast-feeding

Chlorpromazine is excreted in breast milk in low concentrations. The amount of chlorpromazine that the nursing infant would be expected to ingest is between 0.03-1.3% of the lowest pediatric dose, based on data obtained from five lactating women (Blacker et al., 1962; Wiles et al., 1978).* No adverse effects were observed in two of the infants that were breast-fed, although one infant was said to be drowsy and lethargic after nursing.

The American Academy of Pediatrics lists chlorpromazine as a drug whose effect on the nursing infant may be of concern because of its potential to alter central nervous system functioning (Committee on Drugs, American Academy of Pediatrics, 1994).

Key References

Auerbach JG, Hans SL, Marcus J, Maeir R: Maternal psychotropic medication and neonatal behavior. Neurotoxicol Teratol 14(6):399-406, 1992.

Blacker KH, Weinstein BJ, Ellman GL: Mother's milk and chlorpromazine. Am J Psychiatry 119:178-179, 1962.

Brock N, von Kreybig T: [Experimental contribution to the testing of the teratogenic effect of drugs on the laboratory rat.] Naunyn Schmiedebergs Arch Exp Pathol Pharmakol 249:117-145, 1964.

Committee on Drugs, American Academy of Pediatrics: The transfer of drugs and other chemicals into human milk. Pediatrics 93(1):137-150, 1994.

Farkas VG, Farkas G Jr: [Teratogenic action of hyperemesis in pregnancy and of medication used to treat it.] Zentralbl Gynakol 10:325-330, 1971.

Hammond JE, Toseland PA: Placental transfer of chlorpromazine. A case report. Arch Dis Child 45:139-140, 1970.

Heinonen OP, Slone D, Shapiro S: *Birth Defects and Drugs in Pregnancy.* Littleton, Mass.: John Wright-PSG, 1977, pp 323, 437.

Hill RM, Desmond MM, Kay JL: Extrapyramidal dysfunction in an infant of a schizophrenic mother. J Pediatr 69:589-595, 1966.

*This calculation is based on the following assumptions: maternal dose of chlorpromazine: 19 mg/kg/d; milk concentration of chlorpromazine: 0.007-0.29 mcg/mL; milk intake by the nursing infant: 150 mL/kg/d; estimated dose of chlorpromazine ingested by the nursing infant: 0.001-0.04 mg/kg/d; lowest pediatric dose of chlorpromazine: 3.3 mg/kg/d.

Jones-Price C, Wolkowski-Tyl R, Marr MC: Teratologic evaluation of chlorpromazine hydrochloride (CAS No. 69-09-0) administered to CD-1 mice on gestational days 6 through 15. NTIS (National Technical Information Services) Report/PB83-179846, 1983b.

Jones-Price C, Wolkowski-Tyl R, Marr MC: Teratologic evaluation of chlorpromazine hydrochloride (CAS No. 69-09-0) administered to Fischer 344 rats on gestational days 6 through 15. NTIS (National Technical Information Services) Report/PB83-191080, 1983a.

Levy W, Wisniewski K: Chlorpromazine causing extrapyramidal dysfunction. In newborn infant of psychotic mother. NY State J Med 74:684-685, 1974.

Robertson RT, Majka JA, Peter CP, Bokelman DL: Effects of prenatal exposure to chlorpromazine on postnatal development and behavior of rats. Toxicol Appl Pharmacol 53:541-549, 1980.

Saillenfait AM, Vannier B: Methodological proposal in behavioural teratogenicity testing: Assessment of propoxyphene, chlorpromazine, and vitamin A as positive controls. Teratology 37:185-199, 1988.

Singh S, Padmanabhan R: Teratogenic effects of chlorpromazine hydrochloride in rat foetuses. Indian J Med Res 67:300-309, 1978.

Tamer A, McKey R, Arias D, et al.: Phenothiazine-induced extrapyramidal dysfunction in the neonate. J Pediatr 75:479-480, 1969.

Wiles DH, Orr MW, Kolakowska T: Chlorpromazine levels in plasma and milk of nursing mothers. Br J Clin Pharmacol 5:272-273, 1978.

Yu J-F, Yang Y-S, Wang W-Y, et al.: Mutagenicity and teratogenicity of chlorpromazine and scopalamine. Chin Med J 101:339-345, 1988.

CHLORPROPAMIDE
(Apo-Chlorpropamide, Diabanese®)

Chlorpropamide is an oral hypoglycemic agent. The usual dose is 250-750 mg/d.

Teratogenic Risk

Magnitude of teratogenic risk to child born after exposure during gestation:　　　*Minimal to small*

Interpretation of available data on this agent is difficult because almost all women who take this medication have diabetes which itself can alter embryonic and fetal development.

Ten of 20 infants born to women who had noninsulin dependent diabetes mellitus and were treated with oral hypoglycemic agents, usually chlorpropamide, during the first trimester of pregnancy had minor or major congenital anomalies in one study; this frequency was greater than that observed in a comparison group of infants born to women with noninsulin dependent diabetes who were untreated in early pregnancy (Piacquadio et al., 1991). Two of the infants whose mothers took chlorpropamide early in pregnancy had cardiac and vertebral malformations; both of these children and three others born to women who took chlorpropamide early in pregnancy had auricular malformations. In contrast, only one infant with congenital anomalies was observed in a clinical series of 41 born to women with noninsulin dependent diabetes mellitus treated with chlorpropamide during the first trimester of pregnancy (Coetzee & Jackson, 1984). This child had multiple malformations including sacral agenesis.

Chronic maternal chlorpropamide therapy late in pregnancy was associated with very high perinatal mortality rates in some early studies (Jackson et al., 1962), but this association appears to have been due to poor control of the maternal diabetes rather than to the drug (Anonymous, 1974; Sutherland et al., 1974; Fraser, 1982).

Neonatal hypoglycemia may occur in infants born to diabetic mothers who take chlorpropamide in pregnancy (Zucker & Simon, 1968; Piacquadio et al., 1991), but it is difficult to determine if this is an effect of the drug, the disease, or both.

No congenital anomalies were observed among the offspring of rats treated during pregnancy with chlorpropamide in doses 200-300 times those usually employed in humans (Tuchmann-Duplessis & Mercier-Parot, 1959), but malformations were noted among embryos of one strain of pregnant rats treated with a single high therapeutic dose of chlorpropamide prior to implantation (Brock & von Kreybig, 1964). The relevance of this observation to the clinical use of chlorpropamide in pregnant diabetic women is unknown.

Risk Related to Breast-feeding

Chlorpropamide is excreted in breast milk in large amounts (USP DI, 1995). Based on data that has only been published in abstract form, the amount of chlorpropamide that a nursing infant would be expected to ingest is approximately 48% of the lowest weight-adjusted therapeutic dose.* Hypoglycemia has not been reported in nursing infants whose mothers who were treated with chlorpropamide, but the occurrence of this pharmacological effect is a concern if the estimate of the amount of drug transfered in milk is correct.

Key References

Anonymous: Chlorpropamide in diabetic pregnancy. Lancet 2:32, 1974.

Brock N, von Kreybig T: [Experiments regarding the testing of teratogenic drugs in the laboratory rat.] Naunyn-Schmiedebergs Arch Pathol Pharmacol 249:117-145, 1964.

Coetzee EJ, Jackson WPU: Oral hypoglycaemics in the first trimester and fetal outcome. S Afr Med J 65:635-637, 1984.

Fraser RB: The fate of the pregnant diabetic in a developing country: Kenya. Diabetologia 22:21-24, 1982.

Jackson WPU, Campbell GD, Notelovitz M, Blumsohn D: Tolbutamide and chlorpropamide during pregnancy in human diabetics. Diabetes 2(Suppl):98-101, 1962.

Piacquadio K, Hollingsworth DR, Murphy H: Effects of in-utero exposure to oral hypoglycaemic drugs. Lancet 338:866-869, 1991.

Sutherland HW, Bewsher PD, Cormack JD, et al.: Effect of moderate dosage of chlorpropamide in pregnancy on fetal outcome. Arch Dis Child 49:283-291, 1974.

Tuchmann-Duplessis MH, Mercier-Parot L: [Action of chlorpropamide on gestation and fetal development of the rat.] C R Acad Sci (Paris) 249:1160-1162, 1959.

USP DI: Chlorpropamide. In: *USP DI (USP Dispensing Information), Volume 1. Drug Information for the Health Care Professional,* 15th ed. Rockville, Md.: The US Pharmacopeial Convention, 1995, p 269.

*This calculation is based on the following assumptions: milk concentration of chlorpropamide: 5 mcg/mL; milk intake by the nursing infant: 150 mL/kg/d; estimated dose of chlorpropamide ingested by the nursing infant: 0.75 mg/kg/d; lowest adult therapeutic dose of chlorpropamide: 1.6 mg/kg/d.

Zucker P, Simon G: Prolonged symptomatic neonatal hypoglycemia associated with maternal chlorpropamide therapy. Pediatrics 42:824-825, 1968.

CHLORTETRACYCLINE
(Aureomycin®)

Chlortetracycline is a broad-spectrum antibiotic. It is used topically to treat skin and ocular infections.

Teratogenic Risk

*Magnitude of teratogenic
risk to child born after
exposure during gestation*
    Malformations: *Undetermined*
    Dental staining: *Undetermined*

*Quality and quantity of data
on which risk estimate is based*
    Malformations: *None*
    Dental staining: *None*

A small risk cannot be excluded, but there is no indication that the risk of malformations in children of women treated with chlortetracycline during pregnancy is likely to be great.

Chlortetracycline is chemically similar to other tetracyclines that cause staining of the primary dentition in fetuses exposed during the second or third trimesters of pregnancy. It is likely that chlortetracycline can also cause such staining if it is sufficiently absorbed after topical administration.

No epidemiological studies of congenital anomalies in children of women treated with chlortetracycline during pregnancy have been reported.

No mammalian teratology studies of chlortetracycline have been published.

Please see agent summary on tetracycline for information on a closely related drug that has been studied.

Risk Related to Breast-feeding

Chlortetracycline is excreted in breast milk in low concentrations. The amount of chlortetracycline that the nursing infant would be expected to ingest is approximately 1% of the lowest weight-adjusted therapeutic dose, based on data obtained from eight lactating women (Guilbeau et al., 1950).*

Although permanent incisor staining, enamel hypoplasia, or inhibition of linear skeletal growth in nursing infants are possible with the use of tetracyclines during breast-feeding (USP DI, 1995), no such effects have been reported.

Key References

Guilbeau JA Jr, Schoenbach EB, Schaub IG, Latham DV: Aureomycin in obstetrics: Therapy and prophylaxis. JAMA 143(6):520-526, 1950.

USP DI: Tetracyclines. In: *USP DI (USP Dispensing Information), Volume 1. Drug Information for the Health Care Professional*, 15th ed. Rockville, Md.: The US Pharmacopeial Convention, 1995, pp 2634, 2642.

*This calculation is based on the following assumptions: maternal dose of chlortetracycline: 31 mg/kg/d; milk concentration of chlortetracycline: 1-2 mcg/mL; milk intake by the nursing infant: 150 mL/kg/d; estimated dose of chlortetracycline ingested by the nursing infant: 0.15-0.2 mg/kg/d; lowest adult therapeutic dose of chlortetracycline: 16 mg/kg/d.

CHLORTHALIDONE
(Apo-Chlorthalidone, Hygroton®)

Chlorthalidone is a diuretic used in the treatment of hypertension and edema. Chlorthalidone is given orally in doses of 12.5-200 mg/d.

Teratogenic Risk

Magnitude of teratogenic risk to child born after exposure during gestation:	*Unlikely*
Quality and quantity of data on which risk estimate is based:	*Fair*

132

Therapeutic doses of chlorthalidone are unlikely to pose a substantial teratogenic risk, but the data are insufficient to state that there is no risk.

The frequency of congenital anomalies was slightly increased among the children of 1310 women who were treated with chlorthalidone anytime during pregnancy in one epidemiological study (Heinonen et al., 1977). Only 20 of these women took chlorthalidone within the first four lunar months of pregnancy. Studies such as this one that include multiple comparisons between maternal drug exposures and various birth defect outcomes are expected to show occasional associations with nominal statistical significance purely by chance.

In a randomized controlled trial, the average weight and length of 108 infants born to mothers who took chlorthalidone from 16 weeks of pregnancy through term to prevent toxemia were not significantly different from controls (Tervila & Vartianen, 1971).

Studies in rats, mice, hamsters, and rabbits suggest that treatment of pregnant women with chlorthalidone in usual therapeutic doses is unlikely to increase the children's risk of malformations greatly (Fratta et al., 1965).

Risk Related to Breast-feeding

Chlorthalidone is excreted in breast milk. The amount of chlorthalidone that the nursing infant would be expected to ingest is between 1.3-13% of the lowest pediatric dose, based on data obtained from nine lactating women (Mulley et al., 1978).*

Chlorthalidone is a thiazide diuretic and suppression of lactation in the first month postpartum has been reported for some thiazide diuretics (USP DI, 1995). The American Academy of Pediatrics regards chlorthalidone to be safe to use while breast-feeding (Committee on Drugs, American Academy of Pediatrics, 1994).

*This calculation is based on the following assumptions: maternal dose of chlorthalidone: 0.8 mg/kg/d; milk concentration of chlorthalidone: 0.09-0.86 mcg/mL; milk intake by the nursing infant: 150 mL/kg/d; estimated dose of chlorthalidone ingested by the nursing infant: 0.01-0.13 mg/kg/d; lowest pediatric dose of chlorthalidone: 1 mg/kg/d.

Key References

Committee on Drugs, American Academy of Pediatrics: The transfer of drugs and other chemicals into human milk. Pediatrics 93(1):137-150, 1994.

Fratta I, Harper KH, Stenger EG, Sigg EB: Effect of chlorthalidone on embryonic development. Med Pharmacol Exp 12:245-253, 1965.

Heinonen OP, Slone D, Shapiro S: *Birth Defects and Drugs in Pregnancy.* Littleton, Mass.: John Wright-PSG, 1977, pp 372-373, 441.

Mulley BA, Parr GD, Pau WK, et al.: Placental transfer of chlorthalidone and its elimination in maternal milk. Eur J Clin Pharmacol 13:129-131, 1978.

Tervila L, Vartianen E: The effects and side effects of diuretics in the prophylaxis of toxaemia of pregnancy. Acta Obstet Gynecol Scand 50:351-356, 1971.

USP DI: Diruretics, thiazide. In: *USP DI (USP Dispensing Information), Volume 1. Drug Information for the Health Care Professional,* 15th ed. Rockville, Md.: The US Pharmacopeial Convention, 1995, p 1161.

CHLOR-TRIMETON® *See* Chlorpheniramine

CHLORZOXAZONE
(Paraflex®, Parafon Forte DSC®)

Chlorzoxazone is a centrally acting muscle relaxant. Chlorzoxazone is given orally in doses of 750-3000 mg/d.

Teratogenic Risk

Magnitude of teratogenic risk to child born after exposure during gestation:	*Undetermined*
Quality and quantity of data on which risk estimate is based:	*None*

No epidemiological studies of malformations in children born to women who used chlorzoxazone during pregnancy have been reported.

No animal teratology studies of chlorzoxazone have been published.

Risk Related to Breast-feeding

No information regarding the distribution of chlorzoxazone in breast milk has been published.

Key References

None available.

CIDOMYCIN® *See* Gentamicin

CIGARETTE SMOKING
(Tobacco)

Tobacco is the leaf of the plant *Nicotiana tabacum*. It is widely used by smoking, chewing, and dipping. Cigarette smoke contains several hundred different chemicals; nicotine and carbon monoxide are among the most abundant. Many studies of the reproductive effects of cigarette smoking have been performed. Extensive reviews are available on this subject (Stillman et al., 1986; Rosenberg, 1987; Fredricsson & Gilljam, 1992).

Teratogenic Risk

*Magnitude of teratogenic
risk to child born after
exposure during gestation*
    Malformations: *None to minimal*
    Fetal growth retardation: *Moderate to high*
    Intrauterine death: *Small to moderate*

*Quality and quantity of data
on which risk estimate is based*
    Malformations: *Good*
    Fetal growth retardation: *Good to excellent*
    Intrauterine death: *Good*

These risks are greatest for heavy smokers and may be less in women who stop smoking during pregnancy.

The relationship of maternal smoking and congenital anomalies has been examined in many epidemiological studies involving thousands of children (McIntosh, 1984a; Stillman et al., 1986). In most studies, no association between the frequency of major congenital anomalies and maternal smoking has been observed. Some studies have found associations between maternal smoking and various congenital anomalies, including gastroschisis, limb reduction defects, strabismus, and congenital heart disease, but such associations have generally been weak and not consistently reproducible in other investigations. A weak association between maternal smoking and facial clefts has been reported in several studies (Andrews & McGarry, 1972; Ericson et al., 1979; Khoury et al., 1989), but remains controversial.

Dozens of studies involving hundreds of thousands of pregnancies have examined the association between maternal cigarette smoking and infant birth weight (McIntosh, 1984a; Stillman et al., 1986; Hjortdal et al., 1989). Low birth weight is unequivocally associated with maternal smoking in a dose-related fashion. This effect seems to be due primarily to fetal growth retardation rather than to prematurity. Controversy exists regarding whether the fetal growth retardation seen among the infants of women who smoke is caused by the smoking or due to other correlated factors. The preponderance of evidence favors the former view. Persistent mild reduction of growth has been observed among the children of women who smoked during pregnancy (Rush & Callahan, 1989). The adverse effect of cigarette smoking on infant birth weight is eliminated in women who stop smoking during pregnancy (Olsen, 1992; Ahlsten et al., 1993; Li et al., 1993). Some studies suggest that birth weight is also decreased slightly among the children of nonsmoking women exposed to tobacco smoke in their environment (Haddow et al., 1989; Ogawa et al., 1991; Seidman & Mashiach, 1991; Mathai et al., 1992; Bardy et al., 1993).

An association between maternal cigarette smoking during pregnancy and slightly lower than expected measured intelligence levels has been observed in some studies (Fried, 1992, 1993; Fried et al., 1992a; Olds et al., 1994). Behavioral abnormalities have also been found more often than expected among the children of women who smoked cigarettes during pregnancy (Fried, 1992, 1993; Fried et al., 1992b; Rantakallio et al., 1992; Weitzman et al., 1992; Fergusson et al., 1993). The effects of postnatal factors as well as other prenatal factors confound such investigations so that a causal inference is not

136

possible (Baghurst et al., 1992; Fried, 1992; Naeye, 1992; Tong & McMichael, 1992).

Well-controlled studies involving thousands of women have generally shown that the frequency of spontaneous abortion is 20-80% higher than expected among women who smoke cigarettes during pregnancy (McIntosh, 1984b; Stillman et al., 1986). The risks appear to be greater for heavy smokers than for light smokers. Some studies suggest that perinatal mortality and other complications of pregnancy may also be increased among the infants of women who smoke cigarettes during pregnancy (English & Eskenazi, 1992; Little & Weinberg, 1993; Raymond & Mills, 1993; Wilcox, 1993).

Some epidemiological studies suggest that maternal smoking during pregnancy slightly increases the risk of subsequent development of childhood cancer among the offspring (Golding et al., 1990; John et al., 1991; Schwartzbaum et al., 1991; Schwartzbaum, 1992; Stjernfeldt et al., 1992), but other studies show no such effect or only an inconsistent effect (John et al., 1991; Pershagen et al., 1992; Gold et al., 1993; Olshan et al., 1993; McCredie et al., 1994). These investigations may be confounded by a variety of other factors that correlate with maternal smoking during pregnancy.

Experimental teratology studies of simulated tobacco use in experimental animals are of little value in defining the risks of cigarette smoking in pregnant women, but such studies may be very useful in identifying the underlying pathophysiologic mechanisms (Abel, 1980; Mactutus, 1989; Slotkin, 1992).

Risk Related to Breast-feeding

Nicotine and its major active metabolite, cotinine, are excreted in the breast milk of smoking mothers in a dose-response fashion (Trundle & Skellern, 1983; Luck & Nau, 1984; Woodward et al., 1986; Piazza et al., 1987). Much smaller concentrations of nicotine and cotinine are present in the breast milk of women who are passively exposed to cigarette smoke (Hardee et al., 1983; Piazza et al., 1987). The amount of nicotine and cotinine that the nursing infant would be expected to receive is between 1-100% of the lowest adult dose in nicotine chewing gum. The highest estimated amount received by the infant is

10% more than the dose obtained by smoking one cigarette (Dahlstrom et al., 1990).*

Cigarette smoking while breast-feeding has been associated with significantly lower milk volumes and shortened duration of breast-feeding (Hakansson & Cars, 1991; Vio et al., 1991; Hakansson & Carlsson, 1992; Hopkinson et al., 1992). One case of nicotine poisoning (insomnia, spastic vomiting, diarrhea, rapid pulse, and circulatory disturbance) has been described in a six-week-old infant whose mother smoked 20 cigarettes per day (Bisdom, 1937).

The American Academy of Pediatrics strongly recommends that nursing mothers refrain from smoking during the lactation period since smoking is detrimental to the health of both the mother and the infant (Committee on Drugs, American Academy of Pediatrics, 1994).

Key References

Abel EL: Smoking during pregnancy: A review of effects on growth and development of offspring. Hum Biol 52:593-626, 1980.

Ahlsten G, Cnattingius S, Lindmark G: Cessation of smoking during pregnancy improves foetal growth and reduces infant morbidity in the neonatal period. A population-based prospective study. Acta Paediatr 82:177-181, 1993.

Andrews J, McGarry JM: A community study of smoking in pregnancy. J Obstet Gynaecol Br Commonw 79(12):1057-1073, 1972.

Baghurst PA, Tong S-l, Woodward A, McMichael AJ: Effects of maternal smoking upon neuropsychological development in early childhood: Importance of taking account of social and environmental factors. Paediatr Perinat Epidemiol 6:403-415, 1992.

Bardy AH, Seppala T, Lillsunde P, et al.: Objectively measured tobacco exposure during pregnancy: Neonatal effects and relation to maternal smoking. Br J Obstet Gynaecol 100:721-726, 1993.

Bisdom W: Alcohol and ncotine poisonings in nurslings. JAMA 109:178, 1937.

*This calculation is based on the following assumptions: milk concentration of nicotine and cotinine of smoking mothers: 0.002-0.2 mcg/mL and 0.005-0.339 mcg/mL, respectively; milk concentration of nicotine and cotinine from passive exposure to smoking: 0.0005-0.02 mcg/mL and 0.0005-0.01 mcg/mL, respectively; milk intake by the nursing infant: 150 mL/kg/d; estimated dose of nicotine and cotinine ingested by the nursing infant: 0.0003-0.03 mg/kg/d and 0.0007-0.05 mg/kg/d, respectively; lowest dose of nicotine in chewing gum: 0.03 mg/kg/d; amount of nicotine obtained from smoking one cigarette: 0.02 mg/kg.

Committee on Drugs, American Academy of Pediatrics: The transfer of drugs and other chemicals into human milk. Pediatrics 93(1):137-150, 1994.

Dahlstrom A, Lundell B, Curvall M, Thapper L: Nicotine and cotinine concentrations in the nursing mother and her infant. Acta Paediatr Scand 79:142-147, 1990.

English PB, Eskenazi B: Reinterpreting the effects of maternal smoking on infant birthweight and perinatal mortality: A multivariate approach to birthweight standardization. Int J Epidemiol 21:1097-1105, 1992.

Ericson A, Kallen B, Westerholm P: Cigarette smoking as an etiologic factor in cleft lip and palate. Am J Obstet Gynecol 135:348-351, 1979.

Fergusson DM, Horwood LJ, Lynskey MT: Maternal smoking before and after pregnancy: Effects on behavioral outcomes in middle childhood. Pediatrics 92:815-822, 1993.

Fredricsson B, Gilljam H: Smoking and reproduction. Short and long term effects and benefits of smoking cessation. Acta Obstet Gynecol Scand 71:580-592, 1992.

Fried PA: Clinical implications of smoking: Determining long-term teratogenicity. In: Zagon IS, Slotkin TA (eds). *Maternal Substance Abuse and the Developing Nervous System.* San Diego, Calif..: Academic Press, 1992, pp 77-96.

Fried PA: Prenatal exposure to tobacco and marijuana: Effects during pregnancy, infancy, and early childhood. Clin Obstet Gynecol 36(2):319-337, 1993.

Fried PA, O'Connell CM, Watkinson B: 60- and 72-month follow-up of children prenatally exposed to marijuana, cigarettes and alcohol: Cognitive and language assessment. J Dev Behav Pediatr 13:383-391, 1992a.

Fried PA, Watkinson B, Gray R: A follow-up study of attentional behavior in 6-year-old children exposed prenatally to marihuana, cigarettes, and alcohol. Neurotoxicol Teratol 14(5):299-311, 1992b.

Gold EB, Leviton A, Lopez R, et al.: Parental smoking and risk of childhood brain tumors. Am J Epidmiol 137:620-628, 1993.

Golding J, Paterson M, Kinlen LJ: Factors associated with childhood cancer in a national cohort study. Br J Cancer 62:304-308, 1990.

Haddow JE, Knight GJ, Palomaki GE, et al.: Serum cotinine levels in pregnant nonsmokers in relation to birthweight. Ann NY Acad Sci 562:370-371, 1989.

Hakansson A, Cars H: Maternal cigarette smoking, breast-feeding, and respiratory tract infections in infancy. A matched-pairs study. Scand J Prim Health Care 9:115-119, 1991.

Hakansson A, Carlsson B: Maternal cigarette smoking, breast-feeding, and respiratory tract infections in infancy. A population-based cohort study. Scand J Prim Health Care 10:60-65, 1992.

Hardee GE, Stewart T, Capomacchia AC: Tobacco smoke xeno-biotic compound appearance in mothers' milk after involuntary smoke exposures. I. Nicotine and cotinine. Toxicol Lett 15:109-112, 1983.

Hjortdal JO, Hjortdal VE, Foldspang A: Tobacco smoking and fetal growth. A review. Scand J Soc Med Suppl 0(45):I-II, 1-22, 1989.

Hopkinson JM, Schanler RJ, Fraley K, Garza C: Milk production by mothers of premature infants: Influence of cigarette smoking. Pediatrics 90(6):934-938, 1992.

John EM, Savitz DA, Sandler DP: Prenatal exposure to parents' smoking and childhood cancer. Am J Epidemiol 133(2):123-132, 1991.

Khoury MJ, Gomez-Farias M, Mulinare J: Does maternal cigarette smoking during pregnancy cause cleft lip and palate in offspring? Am J Dis Child 143:333-337, 1989.

Li CQ, Windsor RA, Perkins L, et al.: The impact on infant birth weight and gestational age of cotinine-validated smoking reduction during pregnancy. JAMA 269:1519-1524, 1993.

Little RE, Weinberg CR: Risk factors for antepartum and intrapartum stillbirth. Am J Epidmiol 137:1177-1189, 1993.

Luck W, Nau H: Exposure of the fetus, neonate, and nursed infant to nicotine and cotinine from maternal smoking. N Engl J Med 311:672, 1984.

Mactutus CF: Developmental neurotoxicity of nicotine, carbon monoxide, and other tobacco smoke constituents. Ann NY Acad Sci 562:105-122, 1989.

Mathai M, Vijayasri R, Babu S, Jeyaseelan L: Passive maternal smoking and birthweight in a South Indian population. Br J Obstet Gynaecol 99:342-343, 1992.

McCredie M, Maisonneuve P, Boyle P: Antenatal risk factors for malignant brain tumours in New South Wales children. Int J Cancer 56:6-10, 1994.

McIntosh ID: Smoking and pregnancy: I. Maternal and placental risks. Public Health Rev 12:1-28, 1984b.

McIntosh ID: Smoking and pregnancy: II. Offspring risks. Public Health Rev 12:29-63, 1984a.

Naeye RL: Cognitive and behavioral abnormalities in children whose mothers smoked cigarettes during pregnancy. J Dev Behav Pediatr 13(6):425-428, 1992.

Ogawa H, Tominaga S, Hori K, et al.: Passive smoking by pregnant women and fetal growth. J Epidemiol Community Health 45:164-168, 1991.

Olds DL, Henderson CR, Tatelbaum R: Intellectual impairment in children of women who smoke cigarettes during pregnancy. Pediatrics 93:221-227, 1994.

Olsen J: Cigarette smoking in pregnancy and fetal growth. Does the type of tobacco paly a role? Int J Epidemiol 21:279-284, 1992.

Olshan AF, Breslow NE, Falletta JM, et al.: Risk factors for Wilms tumor. Report from the National Wilms Tumor Study. Cancer 72:938-944, 1993.

Pershagen G, Ericson A, Otterblad-Olausson P: Maternal smoking in pregnancy: Does it increase the risk of childhood cancer? Int J Epidemiol 21(1):1-5, 1992.

Piazza SF, Haley NJ, Clark DA, et al.: Human milk contamination with nicotine and cotinine. Pediatr Res 21(4 Part 2):401A, 1987.

Rantakallio P, Laara E, Isohanni M, Moilanen I: Maternal smoking during pregnancy and delinquency of the offspring: An association without causation? Int J Epidemiol 21:1106-1113, 1992.

Raymond EG, Mills JL: Placental abruption. Maternal risk factors and associated fetal conditions. Acta Obstet Gynecol Scand 72:633-639, 1993.

Rosenberg MJ (ed): *Smoking and Reproductive Health.* Littleton, Mass.: John Wright-PSG, 1987.

Rush D, Callahan KR: Exposure to passive cigarette smoking and child development. A critical review. Ann NY Acad Sci 562:74100, 1989.

Schwartzbaum JA: Influence of the mother's prenatal drug consumption on risk of neuroblastoma in the child. Am J Epidemiol 135:1358-1367, 1992.

Schwartzbaum JA, George SL, Pratt CB, Davis B: An exploratory study of environmental and medical factors potentially related to childhood cancer. Med Pediatr Oncol 19:115-121, 1991.

Seidman DS, Mashiach S: Involuntary smoking and pregnancy. Eur J Obstet Gynecol Reprod Biol 41:105-116, 1991.

Slotkin TA: Prenatal exposure to nicotine: What can we learn from animal models? In: Zagon IS, Slotkin TA (eds). *Maternal Substance Abuse and the Developing Nervous System.* San Diego, Calif.: Academic Press, 1992, pp 97-124.

Stillman RJ, Rosenberg MJ, Sachs BP: Smoking and reproduction. Fertil Steril 46(4):545-566, 1986.

Stjernfeldt M, Berglund K, Lindsten J, Ludvigsson J: Maternal smoking and irradiation during pregnancy as risk factors for child leukemia. Cancer Detect Prev 16:129-135, 1992.

Tong S, McMichael AJ: Maternal smoking and neuropsychological development in childhood: A review of the evidence. Dev Med Child Neurol 34:191-197, 1992.

Trundle JI, Skellern GG: Gas chromatographic determination of nicotine in human breast milk. J Clin Hosp Pharm 8:289-293, 1983.

Vio F, Salazar G, Infante C: Smoking during pregnancy and lactation and its effects on breast-milk volume. Am J Clin Nutr 54:1011-1016, 1991.

Weitzman M, Gortmaker S, Sobol A: Maternal smoking and behavior problems of children. Pediatrics 90:342-349, 1992.

Wilcox AJ: Birth weight and perinatal mortality: The effect of maternal smoking. Am J Epidemiol 137:1098-1104, 1993.

Woodward A, Grgurinovich N, Ryan P: Breast feeding and smoking hygiene: Major influences on cotinine in urine of smokers' infants. J Epidemiol Community Health 40:309-315, 1986.

CILOXAN® *See* Ciprofloxacin

CIMETIDINE
(Novocimetine®, Peptol®, Tagamet®)

Cimetidine is a histamine receptor antagonist that raises gastric pH. It is widely used in the treatment of peptic ulcer disease. Cimetidine is given orally or parenterally; the usual dose is 400-2400 mg/d.

Teratogenic Risk

Magnitude of teratogenic risk to child born after exposure during gestation:	*Undetermined*
Quality and quantity of data on which risk estimate is based:	*Very poor*

No epidemiological studies of congenital anomalies among infants born to women treated with cimetidine during pregnancy have been reported. No malformations were observed in one series of eight infants born to women who had been treated with cimetidine during the first trimester of pregnancy (Koren & Zemlickis, 1991).

Studies in rats, mice, and rabbits suggest that treatment of pregnant women with cimetidine in usual therapeutic doses is unlikely to increase the children's risk of malformations greatly (Leslie & Walker, 1977; Hirakawa et al., 1980; Kitao et al., 1983; Brimblecombe et al., 1985). Increased frequencies of fetal growth retardation and death were often seen at doses many times greater than those used in humans. Male offspring of rats treated with <1-3 times the usual human dose of cimetidine during pregnancy have been noted to have decreased virilization in some studies (Anand & Van Thiel, 1982; Parker et al., 1984) but not others (Leslie & Walker, 1977; Walker et al., 1987; Shapiro et al., 1988; Hoie et al., 1994). Sexual development has not been studied in boys born to women treated with cimetidine during pregnancy, and the clinical relevance of the animal studies is unknown.

No neonatal complications attributable to maternal cimetidine therapy just prior to delivery were observed in infants born by elective or emergency caesarean section (Johnston et al., 1982a, b).

Risk Related to Breast-feeding

Cimetidine is excreted in breast milk in low concentrations. The amount of cimetidine that the nursing infant would be expected to ingest is between <1-4.5% of the lowest pediatric dose, based on data from a single patient (Somogyi & Gugler, 1979).*

The American Academy of Pediatrics regards cimetidine to be safe to use while breast-feeding (Committee on Drugs, American Academy of Pediatrics, 1994).

Key References

Anand S, Van Thiel DH: Prenatal and neonatal exposure to cimetidine results in gonadal and sexual dysfunction in adult males. Science 218:493-494, 1982.

*This calculation is based on the following assumptions: maternal dose of cimetidine: 0.4-1g; milk concentration of cimetidine: 1-6 mcg/mL; milk intake by the nursing infant: 150 mL/kg/d; estimated dose of cimetidine ingested by the nursing infant: 0.15-0.9 mg/kg/d; lowest pediatric dose of cimetidine: 20 mg/kg/d.

Brimblecombe RW, Leslie GB, Walker TF: Toxicology of cimetidine. Hum Toxicol 4:13-25, 1985.

Committee on Drugs, American Academy of Pediatrics: The transfer of drugs and other chemicals into human milk. Pediatrics 93(1):137-150, 1994.

Hirakawa T, Suzuki T, Hayashizaki A, et al.: [Reproduction studies of cimetidine.] Kiso To Rinsho (Clin Rep) 14:2819-2831, 1980.

Hoie EB, Swigart SA, Nelson RM, Leuschen MP: Development of secondary sex characteristics in male rats after fetal and perinatal cimetidine exposure. J Pharm Sci 83(1):107-109, 1994.

Johnston JR, McCaughey W, Moore J, Dundee JW: A field trial of cimetidine as the sole oral antacid in obstetric anaesthesia. Anaesthesia 37:33-38, 1982a.

Johnston JR, McCaughey W, Moore J, Dundee JW: Cimetidine as an oral antacid before elective Caesarean section. Anaesthesia 37:26-32, 1982b.

Kitao T, Yamamoto M, Morimoto T, Ueshita S: [Reproduction studies of FPF 1002 (cimetidine) 2. Teratogenicity study in rats.] Yakuri To Chiryo (Basic Pharm Ther) 11:1727-1741, 1983.

Koren G, Zemlickis DM: Outcome of pregnancy after first trimester exposure to H_2 receptor antagonists. Am J Perinatol 8(1):37-38, 1991.

Leslie GB, Walker TF: A toxicological profile of cimetidine. Int Congr Ser Excerpta Med 416:24-37, 1977.

Parker S, Schade RR, Pohl CR, et al.: Prenatal and neonatal exposure of male rat pups to cimetidine but not ranitidine adversely affects subsequent adult sexual functioning. Gastroenterology 86:675-680, 1984.

Shapiro BH, Hirst SA, Babalola GO, Bitar MS: Prospective study on the sexual development of male and female rats perinatally exposed to maternally administered cimetidine. Toxicol Lett 44:315-329, 1988.

Somogyi A, Gugler R: Cimetidine excretion into breast milk. Br J Clin Pharmacol 7:627-629, 1979.

Walker TF, Bott JH, Bond BC: Cimetidine does not demasculinize male rat offspring exposed in utero. Fundam Appl Toxicol 8:188-197, 1987.

CIPRO® *See* Ciprofloxacin

CIPROFLOXACIN
(Ciloxan®, Cipro®)

Ciprofloxacin is a fluoroquinolone antibiotic. It is administered orally or parenterally in the treatment of bacterial infections. Ciprofloxacin is given orally in doses of 100-2250 mg/d. An ophthalmic preparation is also available, from which systemic absorption is limited.

Teratogenic Risk

Magnitude of teratogenic risk to child born after exposure during gestation:	*Undetermined*
Quality and quantity of data on which risk estimate is based:	*Very poor*

No congenital anomalies were observed among ten infants born to women who had been treated with ciprofloxacin during pregnancy in one series; most of the women were treated during the first trimester (Berkovitich et al., 1994).

No adverse effect is said to have occurred in unpublished studies among the offspring of mice or rats treated during pregnancy with ciprofloxacin in doses up to 6 times greater than those usually employed in humans (USP DI, 1995). No teratogenic effect is reported to have been seen among the offspring of pregnant rabbits treated with 1-3 times the maximum human therapeutic dose of ciprofloxacin, although maternal toxicity and increased rates of fetal death did occur (USP DI, 1995).

Risk Related to Breast-feeding

Ciprofloxacin is excreted in the breast milk. The amount of ciprofloxacin that the nursing infant would be expected to ingest is between 2-8% of the lowest pediatric dose, based on data obtained from 12 lactating women, one of which was being treated for acute renal failure

(Giamarellou et al., 1989; Cover & Mueller, 1990; Gardner et al., 1992).*

Ciprofloxacin could not be detected in serum collected from one infant (Gardner et al., 1992). No adverse effects of ciprofloxacin were noted in the infant.

The USP DI (1995) recommends that ciprofloxacin not be taken during breast-feeding since fluoroquinolones have been found to produce arthropathy in immature animals. Four cases of ciprofloxacin-induced arthropathy, which resolved following discontinuation of the drug, have been reported in adolescent cystic fibrosis patients (Fulton & Moore, 1990). Although the risk of this effect is probably low, nursing infants should nevertheless be monitored for signs of arthropathy, such as tenderness or instability in the joints (Taddio & Ito, 1994).

Key References

Berkovitch M, Pastuszak A, Gazarian M, et al.: Safety of the new quinolones in pregnancy. Obstet Gynecol 84(4):535-538, 1994.

Cover DL, Mueller BA: Ciprofloxacin penetration into human breast milk: A case report. DICP Ann Pharmacother 24:703-704, 1990.

Fulton B, Moore, LL: Comment: Ciprofloxacin excretion into breast milk. DICP Ann Pharmacother 24:1122, 1990.

Gardner DK, Gabbe SG, Harter C: Simultaneous concentrations of ciprofloxacin in breast milk and in serum in mother and breast-fed infant. Clin Pharm 11:352-354, 1992.

Giamarellou H, Kolokythas E, Petrikkos G, et al.: Pharmacokinetics of three newer quinolones in pregnant and lactating women. Am J Med 87(Suppl 5A):49S-51S, 1989.

Taddio A, Ito S: Drug use during lactation. In: Koren G (ed). *Maternal-Fetal Toxicology. A Clinician's Guide*, 2nd ed. New York: Marcel Dekker, 1994, pp 147-148.

USP DI: Fluoroquinolones. In: *USP DI (USP Dispensing Information), Volume 1. Drug Information for the Health Care Professional*, 15th ed. Rockville, Md.: The US Pharmacopeial Convention, 1995, pp 1348, 1350.

*This calculation is based on the following assumptions: maternal dose of ciprofloxacin: 7.8-11.7 mg/kg/d; milk concentration of ciprofloxacin: 0.98-3.79 mcg/mL; milk intake by the nursing infant: 150 mL/kg/d; estimated dose of ciprofloxacin ingested by the nursing infant: 0.15-0.57 mg/kg/d; lowest pediatric dose of ciprofloxacin: 7.5 mg/kg/d.

CITRACAL® *See* Calcium Salts

CITRATE
(Citric Acid, Polycitra®)

Citrate is an organic anion involved in normal intermediary metabolism. It is contained in a variety of beverages, mouth washes, effervescing mixtures, and eye lotions. Citrate is administered orally as a systemic and urinary alkalinizing agent and to prevent the development of renal stones. Therapeutic oral doses are variable but may be as high as 10.8 g of potassium citrate or 15 g of sodium citrate per day.

Teratogenic Risk

*Magnitude of teratogenic
risk to child born after
exposure during gestation:*   *Undetermined*

*Quality and quantity of data
on which risk estimate is based:*   *Very poor*

A small risk cannot be excluded, but a substantial risk of congenital anomalies in the children of women treated with citrate during pregnancy is unlikely.

No epidemiological studies of malformations in infants born to women who took large doses of citrate during pregnancy have been reported.

Studies in mice, rats, hamsters, and rabbits provide no evidence that treatment of pregnant women with citrate in usual therapeutic doses is likely to increase the children's risk of malformations greatly (Food and Drug Research Labs, 1973).

Risk Related to Breast-feeding

No information regarding the distribution of citrate in breast milk has been published.

Key References

Food and Drug Research Labs: Teratologic evaluation of FDA 71-54 (citric acid). NTIS (National Technical Information Services) Report/PB-223 814, 1973.

CITRIC ACID *See* Citrate

CLEMASTINE
(Tavist®)

Clemastine is an antihistaminic agent used to treat allergic rhinitis, urticaria, and angioedema. Clemastine is given orally in doses of 1-8 mg/d.

Teratogenic Risk

Magnitude of teratogenic risk to child born after exposure during gestation:	*Undetermined*
Quality and quantity of data on which risk estimate is based:	*None*

No epidemiological studies of congenital anomalies among infants born to women treated with clemastine during pregnancy have been reported.

No animal teratology studies of clemastine have been published.

Please see agent summary on diphenhydramine for information on a related agent that has been studied.

Risk Related to Breast-feeding

Clemastine is excreted in breast milk in low concentrations. The amount of clemastine that the nursing infant would be expected to ingest is between 2.4-4.8% of the lowest adult therapeutic dose, based on data from a single patient (Kok et al., 1982).* Infant serum levels of clemastine were undetectable.

The nursing infant was admitted to the hospital for drowsiness, irritability, neck stiffness, and refusal to nurse. Although the mother took other anticonvulsants for epilepsy, the infant's symptoms resolved one day after termination of clemastine therapy. No causal inference can be made on the basis of this anecdotal report. However, because of this one case, the American Academy of Pediatrics recommend that caution be used when giving clemastine to breast-feeding mothers (Committee on Drugs, American Academy of Pediatrics, 1994).

Key References

Committee on Drugs, American Academy of Pediatrics: The transfer of drugs and other chemicals into human milk. Pediatrics 93(1):137-150, 1994.

Kok THHG, Taitz LS, Bennett MJ, Holt DW: Drowsiness due to clemastine transmitted in breast milk. Lancet 1:914-915, 1982.

*This calculation is based on the following assumptions: maternal dose of clemastine: 0.03 mg/kg/d; milk concentration of clemastine: 0.005-0.01 mcg/mL; milk intake by the nursing infant: 150 mL/kg/d; estimated dose of clemastine ingested by the nursing infant: 0.0007-0.001 mg/kg/d; lowest adult therapeutic dose of clemastine: 0.03 mg/kg/d.

CLEOCIN® *See* Clindamycin

C-LEXIN® *See* Cephalexin

CLIDINIUM BROMIDE
(Quarzan®)

Clidinium bromide is an anticholinergic agent used in the treatment of peptic ulcer disease and other gastrointestinal disorders. Clidinium bromide is given orally; the usual dosage is 7.5-20 mg/d.

Teratogenic Risk

*Magnitude of teratogenic
risk to child born after
exposure during gestation:*   *Undetermined*

Quality and quantity of data
on which risk estimate is based: *None*

No epidemiological studies of malformations in infants born to women treated with clidinium bromide during pregnancy have been reported.

No animal teratology studies of clidinium bromide have been published.

Please see agent summary on atropine for information on a related agent that has been studied.

Risk Related to Breast-feeding

No information regarding the distribution of clidinium bromide in breast milk has been published.

Key References

None available.

CLINDAMYCIN
(Cleocin®, Dalacin ®)

Clindamycin is an antibiotic used to treat infections of anaerobic bacteria, malaria, *Pneumocystis*, and *Toxoplasma*. The drug may be given orally or parenterally in a dose that usually ranges from 600-2700 mg/d, with doses up to 4800 mg/d. Vaginal and topical preparations are poorly absorbed.

Teratogenic Risk

Magnitude of teratogenic
risk to child born after
exposure during gestation: *Undetermined*

Quality and quantity of data
on which risk estimate is based: *Poor*

A small risk cannot be excluded, but there is no indication that the risk of congenital anomalies in the children of women treated with clindamycin during pregnancy is likely to be great.

No epidemiological studies of congenital anomalies in infants born to women who were treated with clindamycin early in pregnancy have been reported. The frequency of congenital anomalies was no greater than expected among the infants of 104 women treated with clindamycin in the second or third trimester of pregnancy as part of a controlled trial of therapy to prevent low birth weight (McCormack et al., 1987).

Studies in mice and rats suggest that treatment of pregnant women with clindamycin in usual therapeutic doses is unlikely to increase the children's risk of malformations greatly (Gray et al., 1972; Bollert et al., 1974).

Risk Related to Breast-feeding

Clindamycin is excreted in the breast milk. The amount of clindamycin that the nursing infant would be expected to ingest is between <1-7% of the lowest neonatal therapeutic dose (Smith et al., 1975; Steen & Rane, 1982).*

Bloody stools were observed in one nursing infant whose mother was given 2400 mg of clindamycin and 240 mg of gentamicin intravenously per day for several days following parturition (Mann, 1980). The stools cleared rapidly once breast-feeding was discontinued and the symptoms did not reappear when breast-feeding was resumed following termination of maternal treatment. Enterocolitis is a possible side effect of clindamycin treatment in adults (USP DI, 1995), and may have been responsible for the bloody stools in this baby.

The American Academy of Pediatrics regards clindamycin to be safe to use while breast-feeding (Committee on Drugs, American Academy of Pediatrics, 1994).

Key References

Bollert JA, Gray JE, Highstrete JD, et al.: Teratogenicity and neonatal toxicity of clindamycin 2-phosphate in laboratory animals. Toxicol Appl Pharmacol 27:322-329, 1974.

*This calculation is based on the following assumptions: maternal dose of clindamycin: 2400 mg, IV and 450-1200 mg, orally; milk concentration of clindamycin: 0.5-3.18 mcg/mL; milk intake by the nursing infant: 150 mL/kg/d; estimated dose of clindamycin ingested by the nursing infant: 0.07-0.6 mg/kg/d; lowest neonatal dose of clindamycin: 8 mg/kg/d.

Committee on Drugs, American Academy of Pediatrics: The transfer of drugs and other chemicals into human milk. Pediatrics 93(1):137-150, 1994.

Gray JE, Weaver RN, Bollert JA, Feenstra ES: The oral toxicity of clindamycin in laboratory animals. Toxicol Appl Pharmacol 21:516-531, 1972.

Mann CF: Clindamycin and breast-feeding. Pediatrics 66(6):1030-1031, 1980.

McCormack WM, Rosner B, Lee YH, et al.: Effect on birth weight of erythromycin treatment of pregnant women. Obstet Gynecol 69:202-207, 1987.

Smith JA, Morgan JR, Rachlis AR, Papsin FR: Clindamycin in human breast milk. Can Med Assoc 112:806, 1975.

Steen B, Rane A: Clindamycin passage into human milk. Br J Clin Pharmacol 13:661-664, 1982.

USP DI: Clindamycin. In: *USP DI (USP Dispensing Information), Volume 1. Drug Information for the Health Care Professional*, 15th ed. Rockville, Md.: The US Pharmacopeial Convention, 1995, pp 777-778.

CLINORIL® *See Sulindac*

CLOMIPRAMINE
(Anafranil®)

Clomipramine is a tricyclic antidepressant. It is used orally in doses of 25-300 mg/d.

Teratogenic Risk

*Magnitude of teratogenic
risk to child born after
exposure during gestation:*   *Undetermined*

*Quality and quantity of data
on which risk estimate is based:*   *Poor*

Transient abnormalities of perinatal adaptation and seizures have been reported among infants of women treated with clomipramine late

No controlled epidemiological studies of congenital anomalies among the infants of women treated with clomipramine during pregnancy have been reported. None of the four children born to women who had taken clomipramine early in pregnancy in one series had malformations (Schimmell et al., 1991).

Increased frequencies of central nervous system and other malformations have been observed among the offspring of mice treated with 36 times the human therapeutic dose of clomipramine during pregnancy (Jurand, 1980). Persistent alterations of behavior occur in the offspring of pregnant rats treated with clomipramine in doses equivalent to or greater than those used therapeutically in humans (File & Tucker, 1983; de Ceballos et al., 1985; Drago et al., 1985). The relevance of these observations to the therapeutic use of clomipramine in human pregnancy is unknown.

Please see agent summary on amitriptyline for information on a related agent that has been more thoroughly studied.

Risk Related to Breast-feeding

Clomipramine is excreted in the breast milk. The amount of clomipramine that the nursing infant would be expected to ingest is between 2.5-7.5% of the lowest weight-adjusted therapeutic dose for an infant, based on data from a single patient (Schimmell et al., 1991).[*]

Serum clomipramine levels in this infant were 7-60% of the lowest therapeutic serum levels.[†] Neither clomipramine nor its metabolites could be detected in the serum of four nursing infants whose mothers were treated with 75-125 mg/d of clomipramine in another study (Wisner et al., 1995).

The American Academy of Pediatrics regards clomipramine to be safe to use while breast-feeding (Committee on Drugs, American Academy of Pediatrics, 1994).

[*]This calculation is based on the following assumptions: maternal dose of clomipramine: 125-150 mg/d; milk concentration of clomipramine: 0.22-0.62; milk intake by the nursing infant: 150 mL/kg/d; estimated dose of clomipramine ingested by the nursing infant: 0.03-0.09 mg/kg/d; lowest adult therapeutic dose of clomipramine: 1.2 mg/kg/d.

[†]This calculation is based on the following assumptions: infant serum levels of clomipramine: 0.01-0.09 mcg/mL; lowest adult therapeutic serum level of clomipramine: 0.15 mcg/mL.

Key References

Bromiker R, Kaplan M: Apparent intrauterine fetal withdrawal from clomipramine hydrochloride. JAMA 272(22):1722-1723, 1994.

Committee on Drugs, American Academy of Pediatrics: The transfer of drugs and other chemicals into human milk. Pediatrics 93(1):137-150, 1994.

Cowe L, Lloyd DJ, Dawling S: Neonatal convulsions caused by withdrawal from maternal clomipramine. Br Med J 284:1837-1838, 1982.

de Ceballos ML, Benedi A, de Felipe C, del Rio J: Prenatal exposure of rats to antidepressants enhances agonist affinity of brain dopamine receptors and dopamine-mediated behaviour. Eur J Pharmacol 116:257-262, 1985.

Drago F, Continella G, Alloro MC, Scapagnini U: Behavioral effects of perinatal administration of antidepressant drugs in the rat. Neurobehav Toxicol Teratol 7:493-497, 1985.

File SE, Tucker JC: Neonatal clomipramine treatment in the rat does not effect social, sexual and exploratory behaviors in adulthood. Neurobehav Toxicol Teratol 5(1):3-8, 1983.

Jurand A: Malformations of the central nervous system induced by neurotropic drugs in mouse embryos. Dev Growth Differ 22:61-78, 1980.

Musa AB, Smith CS: Neonatal effects of maternal clomipramine therapy. Arch Dis Child 54(5):405, 1979.

Ostergaard GZ, Pedersen SE: Neonatal effects of maternal clomipramine treatment. Pediatrics 69(2):233-234, 1982.

Schimmell MS, Katz EZ, Shaag Y, et al.: Toxic neonatal effects following maternal clomipramine therapy. Clin Toxicol 29(4):479-484, 1991.

Singh S, Gulati S, Narang A, Bhakoo ON: Non-narcotic withdrawal syndrome in a neonate due to maternal clomipramine therapy. J Paediatr Child Health 26(2):110, 1990.

Wisner KL, Perel JM, Foglia JP: Serum clomipramine and metabolite levels in four nursing mother-infant pairs. J Clin Psychiatry 56:17-20, 1995.

CLONAZEPAM
(Klonopin®, Rivotril®)

Clonazepam is a benzodiazepine that is used as an anticonvulsant. Clonazepam is given orally in doses of 1.5-20 mg/d.

Teratogenic Risk

*Magnitude of teratogenic
risk to child born after
exposure during gestation:*   None to minimal

*Quality and quantity of data
on which risk estimate is based:*   Poor to fair

*The frequency of congenital anomalies may be increased among
the children of women with epilepsy, regardless of anticonvulsant
medication (Kelly, 1984; Koch et al., 1992).*

Maternal use of clonazepam during pregnancy was not significantly increased in a study of 10,698 infants with congenital anomalies
(Czeizel et al., 1992). Congenital anomalies have been reported among
the children of epileptic women who took clonazepam during pregnancy, but the features have not been described sufficiently to determine if these represent a pattern of anomalies similar to that seen with
other anticonvulsants (Lander & Eadie, 1990; Czeizel et al., 1992;
Eskazan & Aslan, 1992).

Studies in rats, mice, and rabbits suggest that treatment of pregnant women with clonazepam in usual therapeutic doses is unlikely to
increase the children's risk of malformations greatly (Blum et al., 1973;
Sullivan & McElhatton, 1977; Takeuchi et al., 1977; Jurand, 1980;
Saito et al., 1984). Altered T-lymphocyte responsiveness has been observed among the offspring of rats treated with 8 times the human dose
of clonazepam during pregnancy (Schlumpf et al., 1990). The relevance of this observation to the use of clonazepam in therapeutic doses
in human pregnancy is unknown.

*Please see agent summary on diazepam for information on a
related drug that has been more thoroughly studied.*

Risk Related to Breast-feeding

Clonazepam is excreted in the breast milk. The amount of
clonazepam that the nursing infant would be expected to ingest is ap-

proximately 16% of the lowest pediatric dose of clonazepam, based on data from a single mother (Fisher et al., 1985).*

At 14 days of age, the infant's serum level of clonazepam was 5% of the lowest therapeutic serum level in adults.[†]

Key References

Blum VJE, Haefely W, Jalfre M, et al.: [Pharmacology and toxicology of the antiepileptic drug clonazepam.] Arzneimittelforsch 23:377-389, 1973.

Czeizel AE, Bod M, Halasz P: Evaluation of anticonvulsant drugs during pregnancy in a population-based Hungarian study. Eur J Epidemiol 8(1):122-127, 1992.

Eskazan E, Aslan S: Antiepileptic therapy and teratogenicity in Turkey. Int J Clin Pharmacol Ther Toxicol 30(8):261-264, 1992.

Fisher JB, Edgren BE, Mammel MC, Coleman JM: Neonatal apnea associated with maternal clonazepam therapy: A case report. Obstet Gynecol 66(Suppl):34S-35S, 1985.

Jurand A: Malformations of the central nervous system induced by neurotropic drugs in mouse embryos. Dev Growth Differ 22:61-78, 1980.

Kelly TE: Teratogenicity of anticonvulsant drugs. I: Review of the literature. Am J Med Genet 19:413-434, 1984.

Koch S, Losche G, Jager-Roman E, et al.: Major and minor birth malformations and antiepileptic drugs. Neurology 42(Suppl 5):83-88, 1992.

Lander CM, Eadie MJ: Antiepileptic drug intake during pregnancy and malformed offspring. Epilepsy Res 7:77-82, 1990.

Saito H, Kobayashi H, Takeno S, Sakai T: Fetal toxicity of benzodiazepines in rats. Res Commun Chem Pathol Pharmacol 46:437-447, 1984.

Schlumpf M, Parmar R, Ramseier HR, Lichtensteiger W: Prenatal benzodiazepine immunosuppression: Possible involvement of peripheral benzodiazepine site. Dev Pharmacol Ther 15:178-185, 1990.

*This calculation is based on the following assumptions:; milk concentration of clonazepam: 0.011-0.013 mcg/mL; milk intake by the nursing infant: 150 mL/kg/d; estimated dose of clonazepam ingested by the nursing infant: 0.002 mg/kg/d; lowest pediatric dose of clonazepam: 0.01 mg/kg/d.

†This calculation is based on the following assumptions: infant serum level of clonazepam: 0.001 mcg/mL; lowest therapeutic serum level of clonazepam in adults: 0.02 mcg/mL.

Sullivan FM, McElhatton PR: A comparison of the teratogenic activity of the antiepileptic drugs carbamazepine, clonazepam, ethosuximide, phenobarbital, phenytoin, and primidone in mice. Toxicol Appl Pharmacol 40:365-378, 1977.

Takeuchi Y, Shiozaki U, Noda A, et al.: [Studies on the toxicity of clonazepam. Part 3. Teratogenicity tests in rabbits.] Yakuri To Chiryo 5:2457-2466, 1977.

CLONIDINE
(Catapres®, Dixarit®)

Clonidine is an α_2-adrenergic agonist. It is given orally or transdermally in a dose of 0.1-2.4 mg/d to treat hypertension. Small oral doses are also used to treat dysmenorrhea and to prevent vascular headaches.

Teratogenic Risk

*Magnitude of teratogenic
risk to child born after
exposure during gestation:*   *Undetermined*

*Quality and quantity of data
on which risk estimate is based:*   *Poor*

A small risk cannot be excluded, but there is no indication that the risk of congenital anomalies in the children of women treated with clonidine during pregnancy is likely to be great.

No adverse effect of maternal clonidine therapy was apparent among the infants of 47 hypertensive women treated during the last half of pregnancy in a therapeutic trial (Horvath et al., 1985). No difference in head size, neurological examination, or school performance compared to matched controls was found among 22 three- to nine-year-old children of women who had been treated with clonidine in pregnancy, usually after the end of the first trimester (Huisjes et al., 1986). Sleep disturbances were reported more often among the exposed children, but no other behavioral abnormalities were noted. The clinical importance of this observation is uncertain.

157

Transient neonatal hypertension has been reported among the infants of women treated with clonidine late in pregnancy (Boutroy et al., 1988), but this complication appears to be uncommon (Horvath et al., 1985).

Studies in rats, mice, and rabbits suggest that treatment of pregnant women with clonidine in usual therapeutic doses is unlikely to increase the children's risk of malformations greatly (von Delbruck, 1966; Angelova et al., 1975; Shirota et al., 1993; Wada et al., 1993). Inconsistent reductions of fetal and maternal body weight occurred when pregnant rats were treated during pregnancy with clonidine in doses 2-13 times the maximum dose used in humans (Pizzi et al., 1988; Ryan & Pappas, 1990; Shirota et al., 1993). Behavioral alterations were observed among the offspring of rats treated during pregnancy with 1-4 times the maximum human dose of clonidine (Feenstra, 1992; Shirota et al., 1993). The relevance of these observations to the therapeutic use of clonidine in human pregnancy is unknown.

Risk Related to Breast-feeding

Clonidine is excreted in breast milk at levels twice those found in maternal serum (Hartikainen-Sorri et al., 1987; Boutroy et al., 1988; Bunjes et al., 1993). The amount of clonidine that the nursing infant would be expected to ingest is between 3-14% of the lowest therapeutic neonatal dose (Boutroy et al., 1988; Bunjes et al., 1993).*

The serum level of clonidine in an infant whose mother was treated with a small dose of clonidine (70 mcg/d) was undetectable in one study (Bunjes et al., 1993), but infant serum levels were similar to therapeutic serum levels in two other studies in which the mothers were treated with large doses of clonidine (242-450 mcg/d) (Hartikainen-Sorri et al., 1987; Boutroy et al., 1988).[†] Hypotension was not observed in the infants in these studies; however, raised arterial blood pressure was seen in four infants (Boutroy et al., 1988). Transitory neonatal hypertension has been associated with prenatal exposure to clonidine (see above).

*This calculation is based on the following assumptions: maternal doses of clonidine: 1.2-7 mcg/kg/d; milk concentration of clonidine: 0.6-2.8 ng/mL; milk intake by the nursing infant: 150 mL/kg/d; estimated dose of clonidine ingested by the nursing infant: 0.09-0.42 mcg/kg/d; lowest therapeutic neonatal dose of clonidine: 3 mcg/kg/d.

†Therapeutic serum levels of clonidine in adults: 0.7 ng/mL.

Key References

Angelova O, Gendzhev Z, Ilieva J, Ivanov K: Investigations on the reproductive function of rats treated with high doses of clonidine. Zentralbl Pharmkother Laboratoriumsdiagn 114:251-255, 1975.

Boutroy MJ, Gisonna CR, Legagneur M: Clonidine: Placental transfer and neonatal adaption. Early Hum Dev 17:275-286, 1988.

Bunjes R, Schaefer C, Holzinger D: Clonidine and breast-feeding. Clin Pharm 12:178-179, 1993.

Feenstra MGP: Functional neuroteratology of drugs acting on adrenergic receptors. Neurotoxicology 13:55-64, 1992.

Hartikainen-Sorri A-L, Heikkinen JE, Koivisto M: Pharmacokinetics of clonidine during pregnancy and nursing. Obstet Gynecol 69:598-600, 1987.

Horvath JS, Phippard A, Korda A, et al.: Clonidine hydrochloride - A safe and effective antihypertensive agent in pregnancy. Obstet Gynecol 66(5):634-638, 1985.

Huisjes HJ, Hadders-Algra M, Touwen BCL: Is clonidine a behavioural teratogen in the human? Early Hum Dev 14:43-48, 1986.

Pizzi WJ, Ali SF, Holson RR: Behavioral evaluation of rats prenatally exposed to the adrenergic agonists clonidine and lofexidine. Neurotoxicology 9(3):559-566, 1988.

Ryan CL, Pappas BA: Prenatal exposure to antiadrenergic antihypertensive drugs: Effects on neurobehavioral development and the behavioral consequences of enriched rearing. Neurotoxicol Teratol 12:359-366, 1990.

Shirota M, Watanabe C, Nagao T, et al.: Reproductive and developmental toxicity studies of clonidine. (II) Teratogenicity study by subcutaneous administration in rats. Iyakuhin Kenkyu 24(9):935-952, 1993.

von Delbruck VO: The results of toxicologic and teratologic animal trials with 2-(2,6-dichlorophenylamino)-2-imidazoline-hydrochloride. Arzneimittelforsch 16:1053-1055, 1966.

Wada K, Hashimoto Y, Shirota M, et al.: Reproductive and developmental toxicity studies of clonidine. (IV) Teratogenicity study by subcutaneous administration in rabbits. Iyakuhin Kenkyu 24(9):969-976, 1993.

CLOPRA® *See* Metoclopramide

CLORAZEPATE
(Tranxene®)

Clorazepate is a benzodiazepine that is given orally in doses up to 90 mg/d to treat anxiety and alcohol withdrawal. Clorazepate is also in patients with seizure disorders as an adjunct to anticonvulsant medications.

Teratogenic Risk

Magnitude of teratogenic risk to child born after exposure during gestation:	*Undetermined*
Quality and quantity of data on which risk estimate is based:	*Very Poor*

No epidemiological studies of congenital anomalies in infants born to women who took clorazepate during pregnancy have been published. There is one report of an infant with multiple congenital anomalies whose mother took clorazepate early in pregnancy, but a cause and effect relationship seems unlikely (Patel & Patel, 1980).

Studies in mice, rats, and rabbits suggest that treatment of pregnant women with clorazepate in usual therapeutic doses is unlikely to increase the children's risk of malformations greatly (Brunaud et al., 1970; Corwin & DeMeyer, 1980; Jackson et al., 1980).

Transient neonatal neurological depression has been observed among children born to women who took clorazepate late in pregnancy (Bavoux et al., 1981).

Risk Related to Breast-feeding

Nordiazepam, the active metabolite of clorazepate, is excreted in breast milk in low concentrations (Rey et al., 1979). The amount of nordiazepam that the nursing infant would be expected to ingest is equivalent to <1% of the lowest weight-adjusted therapeutic dose of clorazepate.*

*This calculation is based on the following assumptions: Maternal dose of clorazepate: 20 mg; milk concentration of nordiazepam: 0.007-0.015 mcg/mL; milk intake by the nursing infant: 150 mL/kg/d; estimated dose of nordiazepam ingested by the nursing infant: 0.001-0.002 mg/kg/d; lowest oral adult dose of clorazepate: 0.23 mg/kg/d.

Infant serum levels of nordiazepam were 15-30% of maternal serum levels in this study.

The WHO Working Group on Drugs and Human Lactation (1988) regards small doses of clorazepate to be safe to use while breast-feeding.

Key References

Bavoux F, Lanfranchi C, Olive G, et al.: Adverse effects on newborns from intra uterine exposure to benzodiazepines and other psychotropic agents. Therapie 36:305-312, 1981.

Brunaud M, Navarro J, Salle J, Siou G: Pharmacological, toxicological, and teratological studies on dipotassium-7-chloro-3-carboxy-1,3-dihydro-2,2-dihydroxy-5-phenyl-2H-1,4-benzodiazepine-chloroazepate (dipotassium chlorazepate, 4306 CB), a new tranquillizer. Arzneimittelforsch 20:123-125, 1970.

Corwin H, DeMyer W: Failure of clorazepate to cause malformations or fetal wastage in the rat. Arch Neurol 37:347-349, 1980.

Jackson VP, DeMyer W, Hingtgen J: Delayed maze-learning in rats after prenatal exposure to clorazepate. Arch Neurol 37:350-351, 1980.

Patel DA, Patel AR: Clorazepate and congenital malformations. JAMA 244:135-136, 1980.

Rey E, Giraux P, d'Athis Ph, et al.: Pharmacokinetics of the placental transfer and distribution of clorazepate and its metabolite nordiazepam in the feto-placental unit and in the neonate. Eur J Clin Pharmacol 15:181-185, 1979.

Who Working Group on Human Lactation: In: Bennet PN (ed): *Drugs and Human Lactation.* Amsterdam: Elsevier, 1988, pp 363-364.

CLOTRIMAZOLE
(Lotrimin®, Mycelex Cream®)

Clotrimazole is an antifungal agent that is used in topical preparations that are absorbed poorly through skin or mucous membranes. Clotrimazole is also used orally for treatment of candidiasis; systemic absorption occurs erratically with this route of administration. The dose employed varies from 30-50 mg/d (orally) to as much as 500 mg/d (vaginally).

Teratogenic Risk

Magnitude of teratogenic risk to child born after exposure during gestation:	Unlikely
Quality and quantity of data on which risk estimate is based:	Poor to fair

Topical use of clotrimazole during pregnancy is unlikely to pose a substantial teratogenic risk, but the data are insufficient to state that there is no risk.

The frequency of maternal use of vaginal clotrimazole early in pregnancy was no greater than expected among 6564 infants diagnosed as having a "birth defect" in one study (Rosa et al., 1987). Similar negative results were obtained in subgroups of infants with oral clefts, cardiovascular defects, and spina bifida. A weak but statistically significant association was observed between maternal vaginal treatment with clotrimazole and spontaneous abortion in this study, but the association was only seen in comparison with one of two control groups and may have resulted from confounding factors (Rosa et al., 1987). Studies such as this one that include multiple comparisons between maternal drug exposures and various birth defect outcomes are expected to show occasional associations with nominal statistical significance purely by chance.

The frequency of malformations was not significantly increased, but fetal death, skeletal and visceral variations, and growth retardation were seen more often than expected among the offspring of pregnant rats treated subcutaneously with 25 times the maximum human vaginal dose of clotrimazole (Hasegawa et al., 1984). This treatment also produced maternal toxicity. Decreased numbers of embryos developed in pregnant rats treated subcutaneously with 5 times the maximum human vaginal dose of clotrimazole prior to implantation (Kobayashi & Hara, 1984). In another study, no teratogenic effects were reportedly observed among the offspring of mice, rats, or rabbits given clotrimazole in oral doses up to 200 times that used in humans (Tettenborn, 1974), but this investigation has not been published in sufficient detail to permit independent assessment of the data. The relevance of these observations to the therapeutic use of clotrimazole in human pregnancy is unknown.

Risk Related to Breast-feeding

No information regarding the distribution of clotrimazole in breast milk has been published.

Key References

Hasegawa Y, Takegawa Y, Yoshida T: [Subcutaneous administration of antifungal drug, 710674-S during organogenesis period in rats.] Kiso To Rinsho (Clin Rep) 18:4937-4968, 1984.

Kobayashi F, Hara K: [Preconceptional and prenatal administration of antifungal drug, 710674-S in rats.] Kiso To Rinsho (Clin Rep) 18:4917-4935, 1984.

Rosa FW, Baum C, Shaw M: Pregnancy outcomes after first-trimester vaginitis drug therapy. Obstet Gynecol 69:751-755, 1987.

Tettenborn D: Toxicity of clotrimazole. Postgrad Med J (July Suppl):17-20, 1974.

CLOXACILLIN
(Cloxapen®, Tegopen®)

Cloxacillin is a penicillin derivative used to treat infections by penicillinase-resistant bacteria. The drug is administered orally or parenterally in doses of 1000-6000 mg/d.

Teratogenic Risk

Magnitude of teratogenic risk to child born after exposure during gestation:	*Undetermined*
Quality and quantity of data on which risk estimate is based:	*Very poor*

A small risk cannot be excluded, but a substantial risk of congenital anomalies in the children of women treated with cloxacillin during pregnancy is unlikely.

No epidemiological studies of congenital anomalies among infants born to women treated with cloxacillin during pregnancy have been reported.

No teratogenic effect is said to have occurred in rabbits treated with cloxacillin in doses similar to those used in humans in a study reported only as an abstract (Brown et al., 1968).

Please see agent summary on penicillin for information on a related drug that has been more thoroughly studied.

Risk Related to Breast-feeding

Cloxacillin is excreted into breast milk (Matsuda, 1984). The amount of cloxacillin that the nursing infant is expected to ingest is <1% of the maternal dose (Taddio & Ito, 1994).

Key References

Brown DM, Harper KH, Palmer AK, Tesh SA: Effect of antibiotics upon pregnancy in the rabbit. Toxicol Appl Pharmacol 12:295, 1968.

Matsuda S: Transfer of antibiotics into maternal milk. Biol Res Pregnancy Perinatol 5:57-60, 1984.

Taddio A, Ito S: Drug use during lactation. In: Koren G (ed). *Maternal-Fetal Toxicology. A Clinician's Guide*, 2nd ed. New York: Marcel Dekker, 1994, pp 133-219.

CLOXAPEN® *See* Cloxacillin

COCAINE
(Blow, Coke, Crack)

Cocaine is a topical anesthetic, local vasoconstrictor, and central nervous system (CNS) stimulant that is widely abused recreationally. The maximum dose of topically administered cocaine for local anesthesia range from 1-3 mg/kg.

Teratogenic Risk

Magnitude of teratogenic risk to child born after exposure during gestation:

Placental abruption and other serious pregnancy complications:	*Moderate*
Congenital anomalies:	*Small to moderate*

Quality and quantity of data
on which risk estimate is based:

Placental abruption and other serious pregnancy complications:	*Fair to good*
Congenital anomalies:	*Fair to good*

Vascular disruption in the fetus appears to be associated with maternal cocaine use and may be a particular hazard in the second or third trimester of pregnancy.

The extensive medical literature on the effects of maternal cocaine use in pregnancy must be interpreted with great caution. Confounding factors are present in human studies that often make it difficult to attribute abnormalities observed directly to a teratogenic effect of cocaine (Coles & Platzman, 1993; Ellis et al., 1993; Frank et al., 1993; Hutchings, 1993; Snodgrass, 1994). Documentation of the frequency, timing, and dosage of the mothers' use of cocaine, other illicit drugs, and alcohol is usually poor. Moreover, there appears to be a systematic publication bias in favor of studies that show an association between maternal cocaine use and untoward pregnancy outcomes and against studies that do not (Koren et al., 1989; Coles, 1993).

Increased frequencies of CNS infarction, disruption, or malformations have been observed in neuroimaging studies of infants born to women who had abused cocaine during pregnancy (Dixon & Bejar, 1989; Heier et al., 1991; Cohen et al., 1994; Dogra et al., 1994a, b; Singer et al., 1994). These studies each included between 19 and 43 exposed infants. No such association was seen in another study of 86 very-low-birth-weight infants whose mothers had used the drug during pregnancy (Dusick et al., 1993). Similar brain lesions have been noted among infants of women who used cocaine during pregnancy in other series (Volpe, 1992; Gieron-Korthals et al., 1994; Suchet, 1994). Such defects may represent residua of cocaine-induced CNS hemorrhage or ischemia at various gestational ages (Volpe, 1992).

Other congenital anomalies thought to be due to vascular disruption have been reported anecdotally among children of mothers who abused cocaine during pregnancy. These abnormalities include segmental intestinal atresia, gastroschisis, sirenomelia, limb-body wall complex, and limb reduction defects (MacGregor et al., 1987; Chasnoff et al., 1988; Hoyme et al., 1990; Drongowski et al., 1991; Hannig & Phillips, 1991; van den Anker et al., 1991; Sarpong & Headings, 1992; Sheinbaum & Badell, 1992; Spinazzola et al., 1992; Viscarello et al., 1992; Hume et al., 1994; Martinez et al., 1994). No association with maternal cocaine use during pregnancy was seen in a study of 110 infants with gastroschisis (Torfs et al., 1994). Moreover, the prevalence of cases with multiple vascular disruption defects seen in the Metropolitan Atlanta Congenital Defects Program did not change significantly between 1968 and 1989, a period marked by a substantial increase in cocaine abuse (Martin et al., 1992). This suggests that cocaine abuse did not produce a major increase in the overall frequency of such birth defects in this population.

The occurrence of neonatal necrotizing enterocolitis seems to be associated with maternal cocaine use during pregnancy (Czyrko et al., 1991; Porat & Brodsky, 1991; Sehgal et al., 1993), and neonatal myocardial infarction has been reported in the infant of a woman who abused cocaine throughout pregnancy (Bulbul et al., 1994). Such anomalies may be caused by the vasoconstrictive and hypertensive actions of cocaine.

Data suggesting an association between maternal cocaine use during pregnancy and the occurrence of congenital anomalies of the genitourinary system in infants have been reported. Several infants with the rare prune belly anomaly have been born to women who used cocaine during pregnancy (Chasnoff et al., 1985, 1989; Bingol et al., 1986). A small but statistically significant increase in the frequency of congenital anomalies of the urinary, but not of the genital, tract was found in one epidemiological study (Chavez et al., 1989). Nine of 52 infants born to women who chronically abused cocaine had genitourinary tract anomalies in another study (Chasnoff et al., 1988, 1989). In contrast, congenital urogenital anomalies were no more frequent than expected in a cohort of 1324 children of women who abused cocaine during pregnancy (Rajegowda et al., 1991). Several other investigations also have found no increase in the frequency of urinary tract anomalies among the children of women who used cocaine during pregnancy (Bingol et al., 1987; Little et al., 1989; Neerhof et al., 1989; Rosenstein et al., 1990), but the sample sizes involved (50-100 exposed infants) are too small to rule out even a substantial increase in the rate.

An increased frequency of cardiovascular malformations was observed among 214 infants with neonatal toxicology screens showing the presence of cocaine in one study (Lipshultz et al., 1991), but meta-analysis of six other epidemiological studies revealed no significant association between maternal cocaine use in pregnancy and fetal cardiovascular malformations (Lutiger et al., 1991).

Significantly increased frequencies of congenital anomalies in general have been reported in studies of 138, 53, and 50 infants of women who abused cocaine during pregnancy (Bingol et al., 1987; Little et al., 1989; Neerhof et al., 1989), but not in other studies of similar or larger size (Hadeed & Siegel, 1989; Gillogley et al., 1990; Handler et al., 1991; Slutsker, 1992; Eyler et al., 1994).

A distinctive pattern of minor anomalies (i.e., a "fetal cocaine syndrome") has been recognized among infants born to women who used cocaine during pregnancy (Fries et al., 1993). Frequent features include low birth weight, prematurity, irritability, microcephaly, large fontanelles, prominent glabella, marked periorbital and eyelid edema, low nasal bridge, short nose, and small toenails. The clinical importance of this syndrome is currently unclear; further delineation of the characteristics and natural history is necessary.

Growth retardation involving weight, length, and head circumference has consistently been noted among infants born to women who abused cocaine during pregnancy; although much of this effect may be due to concomitant exposure to alcohol or cigarette smoking (Bateman et al., 1993; Behnke & Eyler, 1993; Singer et al., 1993; Weathers et al., 1993; Burkett et al., 1994; Eyler et al., 1994; Jacobson et al., 1994a, b; Kliegman et al., 1994; Knight et al., 1994; Richardson & Day, 1994). Data on subsequent growth and development of these children are limited, but few differences were observed by three years of age between 93 infants whose mothers used cocaine and a group of infants whose mothers did not use cocaine but had similar use of alcohol, cigarettes, and marijuana during pregnancy (Azuma & Chasnoff, 1993; Griffith et al., 1994). In another study of 59 infants born to women who abused cocaine and other drugs during pregnancy, catch-up growth was observed for weight but not for length or head circumference at 6.5 and 13 months of age, after correcting for the effects of maternal smoking, alcohol use and opiate use during pregnancy (Jacobson et al., 1994).

Lower than expected Bayley developmental scores were achieved at a corrected gestational age of about 17 months in a series of 30 children born to women who used cocaine during pregnancy, but prenatal exposure to alcohol and other drugs was not controlled in the analysis (Singer et al., 1994). Development at about 20 months of age was similar to controls in a group of 30 children born to women who used cocaine "socially" during the first trimester of pregnancy in another study (Graham et al., 1992). No difference in global IQ but significantly decreased language development and head circumference were found in comparison to controls within a group of 23 children born to women who abused cocaine during pregnancy (Nulman et al., 1994). The children, who had all been adopted into other families, were studied at a mean age of 34 months.

Prematurity and abnormalities of neonatal cardiorespiratory and neurological function are often observed among infants born to women who used cocaine during pregnancy (Black et al., 1993; Dusick et al., 1993; Forman et al., 1993; Mayes et al., 1993; Singer et al., 1993; Eyler et al., 1994; Frassica et al., 1994; Kliegman et al., 1994). Structural and functional abnormalities of the eyes have been described in these infants in some studies but not others (Dominguez et al., 1991; Good et al., 1992; Stafford et al., 1994). Persistent arterial hypertension may be relatively frequent among children born to women who abuse cocaine during pregnancy (Horn, 1992).

An increased frequency of SIDS was observed in one study of almost 1000 infants and another of 8868 infants whose mothers had used cocaine during pregnancy (Durand et al., 1990; Kandall et al., 1993). The rate of SIDS among the infants of women who had used cocaine during pregnancy was 4.6 per 1000 in the latter study, but very much higher rates were reported in two smaller series of infants born to women who chronically abused cocaine during pregnancy (Chasnoff et al., 1988; Cordero & Custard, 1990). Other investigations have found no association between maternal cocaine use during pregnancy and SIDS (Bauchner et al., 1988; Silvestri et al., 1991).

Abruptio placentae, often with fetal death, has been associated with cocaine use during pregnancy (Slutsker, 1992; Dusick et al., 1993; Burkett et al., 1994). The occurrence of abruption in these cases is probably due to the vasoconstrictive and hypertensive effects of the drug.

An increase in the frequency of limb and tail reduction defects was observed among the offspring of pregnant rats treated with 2.5-4 times the usual human dose of cocaine (Webster & Brown-Woodman, 1990). Some of the fetuses with limb defects were also found to have CNS anomalies of a type associated with vascular disruption (Webster et al., 1991). In another study, urinary tract anomalies were observed with increased frequency among the offspring of rats injected with cocaine in doses similar to those used recreationally in humans (El-Bizri et al., 1991). Increased frequencies of congenital anomalies, including brain, eye, urinary tract, and cardiovascular defects, have been observed in some studies among the offspring of mice given <1-3 times the usual human recreational dose of cocaine during pregnancy (Finnell et al., 1990; Gressens et al., 1992; Mahalik & Hitner, 1992; Fisher et al.,

1994). This was not seen in other studies using similar doses in mice, rats, or rabbits (Fantel & MacPhail, 1982; Church et al., 1988; Henderson & McMillen, 1990; Weese-Mayer et al., 1991). Various behavioral abnormalities have been noted among the offspring of rats and mice treated with cocaine during pregnancy (Kunko et al., 1993; Johns et al., 1994; Kosofsky et al., 1994; Molina et al., 1994; Wood et al., 1994).

Risk Related to Breast-feeding

Cocaine is excreted into breast milk in low concentrations (Chasnoff et al., 1987). Cocaine intoxication (vomiting, diarrhea, seizures, irritability, tachycardia, tachypnea, and tremulousness) has been described in two infants breast-fed by mothers who either used cocaine intranasally or topically prior to breast-feeding (Chasnoff et al., 1987; Chaney et al., 1988). In the latter case, the mother denied using cocaine other than for treatment of nipple soreness.

The American Academy of Pediatrics regards cocaine to be contraindicated during breast-feeding because it can be detrimental to the health of both the nursing infant and the mother (Committee on Drugs, American Academy of Pediatrics, 1994).

Key References

Azuma SD, Chasnoff IJ: Outcome of children prenatally exposed to cocaine and other drugs: A path analysis of three-year data. Pediatrics 92:396-402, 1993.

Bateman DA, Ng SKC, Hansen CA, Heagarty MC: The effects of intrauterine cocaine exposure in newborns. Am J Public Health 83(2):190-193, 1993.

Bauchner H, Zuckerman B, McClain M, et al.: Risk of sudden infant death syndrome among infants with in utero exposure to cocaine. J Pediatr 113:831-834, 1988.

Behnke M, Eyler FD: The consequences of prenatal substance use for the developing fetus, newborn, and young child. Int J Addict 28(13):1341-1391, 1993.

Bingol N, Fuchs M, Diaz V, et al.: Teratogenicity of cocaine in humans. J Pediatr 110:93-96, 1987.

Bingol N, Fuchs M, Holipas N, et al.: Prune belly syndrome associated with maternal cocaine abuse. Am J Hum Genet 39:A51, 1986.

Black M, Schuler M, Nair P: Prenatal drug exposure: Neurodevelopmental outcome and parenting environment. J Pediatr Psychol 18(5):605-620, 1993.

Bulbul ZR, Rosenthal DN, Kleinman CS: Myocardial infarction in the perinatal period secondary to maternal cocaine abuse. A case report and literature review. Arch Pediatr Adolesc Med 148:1092-1096, 1994.

Burkett G, Yasin SY, Palow D, et al.: Patterns of cocaine binging: Effect on pregnancy. Am J Obstet Gynecol 171:372-379, 1994.

Chaney NE, Franke J, Wadlington WB: Cocaine convulsions in a breast-feeding baby. J Pediatr 112:134-135, 1988.

Chasnoff IJ, Lewis DE, Squires L: Cocaine intoxication in a breast-fed infant. Pediatrics 80(6):836-838, 1987.

Chasnoff IJ, Burns WJ, Schnoll SH, Burns KA: Cocaine use in pregnancy. N Engl J Med 313:666-669, 1985.

Chasnoff IJ, Chisum GM, Kaplan WE: Maternal cocaine use and genitourinary tract malformations. Teratology 37:201-204, 1988.

Chasnoff IJ, Griffith DR, MacGregor S, et al.: Temporal patterns of cocaine use in pregnancy. Perinatol outcome. JAMA 261:1741-1744, 1989.

Chavez GF, Mulinare J, Cordero JF: Maternal cocaine use during early pregnancy as a risk factor for congenital urogenital anomalies. JAMA 262:795-798, 1989.

Church MW, Dintcheff BA, Gessner PK: Dose-dependent consequences of cocaine on pregnancy outcome in the Long-Evans rat. Neurotoxicol Teratol 10:51-58, 1988.

Cohen HL, Sloves JH, Laungani S, et al.: Neurosonographic findings in full-term infants born to maternal cocaine abusers: Visualization of subependymal and periventricular cysts. J Clin Ultrasound 22:327-333, 1994.

Coles CD: Saying "goodbye" to the "crack baby." Neurotoxicol Teratol 15:290-292, 1993.

Coles CD, Platzman KA: Behavioral development in children prenatally exposed to drugs and alcohol. Int J Addict 28(13):1393-1433, 1993.

Committee on Drugs, American Academy of Pediatrics: The transfer of drugs and other chemicals into human milk. Pediatrics 93(1):135-150, 1994.

Cordero L, Custard M: Effects of maternal cocaine abuse on perinatal and infant outcome. Ohio Med 86(5):410-412, 1990.

Czyrko C, Del Pin CA, O'Neill JA, et al.: Maternal cocaine abuse and necrotizing enterocolitis: Outcome and survival. J Pediatr Surg 26(4):414-421, 1991.

Dixon SD, Bejar R: Echoencephalographic findings in neonates associated with maternal cocaine and methamphetamine use: Incidence and clinical correlates. J Pediatr 115:770-778, 1989.

Dogra VS, Menon PA, Poblete J, Smeltzer JS: Neurosonographic imaging of small-for-gestational-age neonates exposed and not exposed to cocaine and cytomegalovirus. J Clin Ultrasound 22:93-102, 1994a.

Dogra VS, Shyken JM, Menon PA, et al.: Neurosonographic abnormalities associated with maternal history of cocaine use in neonates of appropriate size for their gestational age. AJNR Am J Neuroradiol 15:697-702, 1994b.

Dominguez R, Vila-Coro AA, Slopis JM, et al.: Brain and ocular abnormalities in infants with in utero exposure to cocaine and other street drugs. Am J Dis Child 145:688-695, 1991.

Drongowski RA, Smith RK Jr, Coran AG, Klein MD: Contribution of demographic and environmental factors to the etiology of gastroschisis: A hypothesis. Fetal Diagn Ther 6:14-27, 1991.

Durand DJ, Espinoza AM, Nickerson BG: Association between prenatal cocaine exposure and sudden infant death syndrome. J Pediatr 117(6):909-911, 1990.

Dusick AM, Covert RF, Schreiber MD, et al.: Risk of intracranial hemorrhage and other adverse outcomes after cocaine exposure in a cohort of 323 very low birth weight infants. J Pediatr 122:438-445, 1993.

El-Bizri H, Guest I, Varma DR: Effects of cocaine on rat embryo development in vivo and in cultures. Pediatr Res 29(2):187-190, 1991.

Ellis JE, Byrd LD, Sexson WR, Patterson-Barnett CA: In utero exposure to cocaine: A review. South Med J 86:725-731, 1993.

Eyler FD, Behnke M, Conlon M, et al.: Prenatal cocaine use: A comparison of neonates matched on maternal risk factors. Neurotoxicol Teratol 16(1):81-87, 1994.

Fantel AG, MacPhail BJ: The teratogenicity of cocaine. Teratology 26:17-19, 1982.

Finnell RH, Toloyan S, van Waes M, Kalivas PW: Preliminary evidence for a cocaine-induced embryopathy in mice. Toxicol Appl Pharmacol 103:228-237, 1990.

Fisher JE, Potturi RB, Collins M, et al.: Cocaine-induced embryonic cardiovascular disruption in mice. Teratology 49:182-191, 1994.

Forman R, Klein J, Meta D, et al.: Maternal and neonatal characteristics following exposure to cocaine in Toronto. Reprod Toxicol 7:619-622, 1993.

Frank DA, Bresnahan K, Zuckerman BS: Maternal cocaine use: Impact on child health and development. Adv Pediatr 40:65-99, 1993.

171

Frassica JJ, Orav EJ, Walsh EP, Lipshultz SE: Arrhythmias in children prenatally exposed to cocaine. Arch Pediatr Adolesc Med 148:1163-1169, 1994.

Fries MH, Kuller JA, Norton ME, et al.: Facial features of infants exposed prenatally to cocaine. Teratology 48:413-420, 1993.

Gieron-Korthals MA, Helal A, Martinez CR: Expanding spectrum of cocaine induced central nervous system malformations. Brain Dev 16:253-256, 1994.

Gillogley KM, Evans AT, Hansen RL, et al.: The perinatal impact of cocaine, amphetamine, and opiate use detected by universal intrapartum screening. Am J Obstet Gynecol 163(5):1535-1542, 1990.

Good WV, Ferriero DM, Golabi M, Kobori JA: Abnormalities of the visual system in infants exposed to cocaine. Ophthalmology 99:341-346, 1992.

Graham K, Feigenbaum A, Pastuszak A, et al.: Pregnancy outcome and infant development following gestational cocaine use by social cocaine users in Toronto, Canada. Clin Invest Med 15(4):384-394, 1992.

Gressens P, Kosofsky BE, Evrard P: Cocaine-induced disturbances of corticogenesis in the developing murine brain. Neurosci Lett 140:113-116, 1992.

Griffith DR, Azuma SD, Chasnoff IJ: Three-year outcome of children exposed prenatally to drugs. J Am Acad Child Adolesc Psychiatry 33(1):20-27, 1994.

Hadeed AJ, Siegel SR: Maternal cocaine use during pregnancy: Effect on the newborn infant. Pediatrics 84:205-210, 1989.

Handler A, Kistin N, Davis F, Ferre C: Cocaine use during pregnancy: Perinatal outcomes. Am J Epidemiol 133(8):818-825, 1991.

Hannig VL, Phillips JA III: Maternal cocaine abuse and fetal anomalies: Evidence for teratogenic effects of cocaine. South Med J 84(4):498-499, 1991.

Heier LA, Carpanzano CR, Mast J, et al.: Maternal cocaine abuse: The spectrum of radiologic abnormalities in the neonatal CNS. AJNR Am J Neuroradiol 12(5):951-956, 1991.

Henderson MG, McMillen BA: Effects of prenatal exposure to cocaine or related drugs on rat developmental and neurological indices. Brain Res Bull 24:207-212, 1990.

Horn PT: Persistent hypertension after prenatal cocaine exposure. J Pediatr 121:288-291, 1992.

Hoyme HE, Jones KL, Dixon SD, et al.: Prenatal cocaine exposure and fetal vascular disruption. Pediatrics 85:743-747, 1990.

Hume RF Jr, Gingras JL, Martin LS, et al.: Ultrasound diagnosis of fetal anomalies associated with in utero cocaine exposure: Further support for cocaine-induced vascular disruption teratogenesis. Fetal Diagn Ther 9:239-245, 1994.

Hutchings DE: The puzzle of cocaine's effects following maternal use during pregnancy: Are there reconcilable differences? Neurotoxicol Teratol 15(5):281-286, 1993.

Jacobson JL, Jacobson SW, Sokol RJ: Effects of prenatal exposure to alcohol, smoking, and illicit drugs on postpartum somatic growth. Alcohol Clin Exp Res 18(2):317-323, 1994a.

Jacobson JL, Jacobson SW, Sokol RJ, et al.: Effects of alcohol use, smoking, and illicit drug use on fetal growth in black infants. J Pediatr 124:757-764, 1994b.

Johns JM, Means MJ, Bass EW, et al.: Prenatal exposure to cocaine: Effects on aggression in Sprague-Dawley rats. Dev Psychobiol 27:227-239, 1994.

Kandall SR, Gaines J, Habel L, et al.: Relationship of maternal substance abuse to subsequent sudden infant death syndrome in offspring. J Pediatr 123:120-126, 1993.

Kliegman RM, Madura D, Kiwi R, et al.: Relation of maternal cocaine use to the risks of prematurity and low birth weight. J Pediatr 124:751-756, 1994.

Knight EM, James H, Edwards CH, et al.: Relationships of serum illicit drug concentrations during pregnancy to maternal nutritional status. J Nutr 124:973S-980S, 1994.

Koren G, Graham K, Shear H, Einarson T: Bias against the null hypothesis: The reproductive hazards of cocaine. Lancet 2:1440-1442, 1989.

Kosofsky BE, Wilkins AS, Gressens P, Evrard P: Transplacental cocaine exposure: A mouse model demonstrating neuroanatomic and behavioral abnormalities. J Child Neurol 9:234-241, 1994.

Kunko PM, Moyer D, Robinson SE: Intravenous gestational cocaine in rats: Effects on offspring development and weanling behavior. Neurotoxicol Teratol 15:335-344, 1993.

Lipshultz SE, Frassica JJ, Orav EJ: Cardiovascular abnormalities in infants prenatally exposed to cocaine. J Pediatr 118(1):44-51, 1991.

Little BB, Snell LM, Klein VR, Gilstrap LC III: Cocaine abuse during pregnancy: Maternal and fetal implications. Obstet Gynecol 73:157-160, 1989.

Lutiger B, Graham K, Einarson TR, Koren G: Relationship between gestational cocaine use and pregnancy outcome: A metaanalysis. Teratology 44:405-414, 1991.

MacGregor SN, Keith LG, Chasnoff IJ, et al.: Cocaine use during pregnancy: Adverse perinatal outcome. Am J Obstet Gynecol 157:686-690, 1987.

Mahalik MP, Hitner HW: Antagonism of cocaine-induced fetal anomalies by prazosin and diltiazem in mice. Reprod Toxicol 6:161-169, 1992.

Martin ML, Khoury MJ, Cordero JF, Waters GD: Trends in rates of multiple vascular disruption defects, Atlanta, 1968-1989: Is there evidence of a cocaine teratogenic epidemic? Teratology 45:647-653, 1992.

Martinez JM, Fortuny A, Comas C, et al.: Body stalk anomaly associated with maternal cocaine abuse. Prenat Diagn 14:669-672, 1994.

Mayes LC, Granger RH, Frank MA, et al.: Neurobehavioral profiles of neonates exposed to cocaine prenatally. Pediatrics 91(4):778-783, 1993.

Molina VA, Wagner JM, Spear LP: The behavioral response to stress is altered in adult rats exposed prenatally to cocaine. Physiol Behav 55(5):941-945, 1994.

Neerhof MG, MacGregor SN, Retzky SS, Sullivan TP: Cocaine abuse during pregnancy: Peripartum prevalence and perinatal outcome. Am J Obstet Gynecol 161(3):633-638, 1989.

Nulman I, Rovet J, Altmann D, et al.: Neurodevelopment of adopted children exposed in utero to cocaine. Can Med Assoc J 151(111)1591-1597, 1994.

Porat R, Brodsky N: Cocaine: A risk factor for necrotizing enterocolitis. J Perinatol 11(1):30-32, 1991.

Rajegowda B, Lala R, Nagaraj A, et al.: Does cocaine (CO) increase congenital urogenital abnormalities (CUGA) in newborns? Pediatr Res 29(4):71A, 1991.

Richardson GA, Day NL: Detrimental effects of prenatal cocaine exposure: Illusion or reality? J Am Acad Child Adolesc Psychiatry 33(1):28-34, 1994.

Rosenstein BJ, Wheeler JS, Heid PL: Congenital renal abnormalities in infants with in utero cocaine exposure. J Urol 144:110-112, 1990.

Sarpong S, Headings V: Sirenomelia accompanying exposure of the embryo to cocaine. South Med J 85:545-547, 1992.

Sehgal S, Ewing C, Waring P, et al.: Morbidity of low-birthweight infants with intrauterine cocaine exposure. J Natl Med Assoc 85(1):20-24, 1993.

Sheinbaum KA, Badell A: Physiatric management of two neonates with limb deficiencies and prenatal cocaine exposure. Arch Phys Med Rehabil 73:385-388, 1992.

Silvestri JM, Long JM, Weese-Mayer DE, Barkov GA: Effect of prenatal cocaine on respiration, heart rate, and sudden infant death syndrome. Pediatr Pulmonol 11:328-334, 1991.

Singer L, Arendt R, Minnes S: Neurodevelopmental effects of cocaine. Clin Perinatol 20(1):245-262, 1993.

Singer LT, Yamashita TS, Hawkins S, et al.: Increased incidence of intraventricular hemorrhage and developmental delay in cocaine-exposed, very low birth weight infants. J Pediatr 124:765-771, 1994.

Slutsker L: Risks associated with cocaine use during pregnancy. Obstet Gynecol 79:778-789, 1992.

Snodgrass SR: Cocaine babies: A result of multiple teratogenic influences. J Child Neurol 9:227-233, 1994.

Spinazzola R, Kenigsberg K, Usmani SS, Harper RG: Neonatal gastrointestinal complications of maternal cocaine abuse. NY State J Med 92(1):22-23, 1992.

Stafford JR Jr, Rosen TS, Zaider M, Merriam JC: Prenatal cocaine exposure and the development of the human eye. Ophthalmology 101:301-308, 1994.

Suchet IB: Schizencephaly: Antenatal and postnatal assessment with colour-flow Doppler imaging. Can Assoc Radiol J 45(3):193-200, 1994.

Torfs CP, Velie EM, Oechsli FW, et al.: A population-based study of gastroschisis: Demographic, pregnancy, and lifestyle risk factors. Teratology 50:44-53, 1994.

van den Anker JN, Cohen-Overbeek TE, Wladimiroff JW, Sauer PJJ: Prenatal diagnosis of limb-reduction defects due to maternal cocaine use. Lancet 338:1332, 1991.

Viscarello RR, Ferguson DD, Nores J, Hobbins JC: Limb-body wall complex associated with cocaine abuse: Further evidence of cocaine's teratogenicity. Obstet Gynecol 80:523-526, 1992.

Volpe JJ: Effect of cocaine use on the fetus. N Engl J Med 327(6):399-407, 1992.

Weathers WT, Crane MM, Sauvain KJ, Blackhurst DW: Cocaine use in women from a defined population: Prevalence at delivery and effects on growth in infants. Pediatrics 91(2):350-354, 1993.

Webster WS, Brown-Woodman PDC: Cocaine as a cause of congenital malformations of vascular origin: Experimental evidence in the rat. Teratology 41:689-697, 1990.

Webster WS, Brown-Woodman PDC, Lipson AH, Ritchie HE: Fetal brain damage in the rat following prenatal exposure to cocaine. Neurotoxicol Teratol 13:621-626, 1991.

Weese-Mayer DE, Klemka-Walden LM, Chan MK, Gingras JL: Effects of prenatal cocaine exposure on perinatal morbidity and postnatal growth in the rabbit. Dev Pharmacol Ther 4:221-230, 1991.

Wood RD, Bannoura MD, Johanson IB: Prenatal cocaine exposure: Effects on play behavior in the juvenile rat. Neurotoxicol Teratol 16(2):139-144, 1994.

(Codipertussin®, Methylmorphine Phosphate, Tricodein®)

Codeine is a commonly used narcotic analgesic often encountered as a constituent of multiple agent preparations. It may be given orally, subcutaneously, or intramuscularly in doses of 9-360 mg/d to treat mild to moderate pain. Oral doses of 40-120 mg/d are also used to treat cough, and doses up to 200 mg/d are used to treat diarrhea.

Teratogenic Risk

Magnitude of teratogenic
risk to child born after
exposure during gestation: *Unlikely*

Quality and quantity of data
on which risk estimate is based: *Fair to good*

Therapeutic doses of codeine are unlikely to pose a substantial teratogenic risk, but the data are insufficient to state that there is no risk.

The frequencies of congenital anomalies in general, of major malformations, and of minor anomalies were no greater than expected among the children of 563 women who took codeine during the first four lunar months of pregnancy in a large epidemiological study (Heinonen et al., 1977). The frequency of congenital anomalies was no greater than expected among the children of 2522 women who took codeine anytime during pregnancy in this study. No increase in congenital anomalies was observed among the children of more than 630 women who took medications containing codeine during the first trimester of pregnancy in another large investigation (Jick et al., 1981; Aselton et al., 1985). Three epidemiological studies involving respectively 390, 298, and 330 children with congenital heart disease have reported an association with maternal codeine use during the first trimester of pregnancy (Rothman et al., 1979; Zierler & Rothman, 1985; Bracken, 1986), but methodological limitations of these studies raise serious questions regarding the validity of this association. No association was observed between cardiac malformations and maternal codeine use during early pregnancy in two other epidemiological studies (Heinonen et al., 1977; Shaw et al., 1990, 1992).

Associations between maternal use of codeine and various other congenital anomalies in the offspring have been observed in individual studies but not independently confirmed. These associations include a slight but statistically significant excess of respiratory tract malformations among the children of 563 women who took codeine during the first four lunar months of pregnancy (Heinonen et al., 1977) and an association of first-trimester maternal codeine use in 1427 children with a variety of malformations (Bracken & Holford, 1981). Saxen found an association with maternal use of narcotic analgesics (mostly codeine) during pregnancy in one study among 599 children with cleft lip and/or palate (Saxen, 1975a) but not in a later study of 194 affected children (Saxen, 1975b).

The frequency of malformations was not significantly increased among the offspring of mice, rats, hamsters, or rabbits treated during pregnancy with codeine in doses many times larger than those employed in humans (Geber & Schramm, 1975; Lehman, 1976; Ching & Tang, 1986; Price, 1987; Sleet et al., 1987; Williams et al., 1991). Fetal growth retardation was seen among the offspring of treated animals in most species.

Narcotic withdrawal symptoms have been reported in neonates born to mothers who used codeine chronically late in pregnancy (Ruggins et al., 1992).

Please see agent summary on heroin for information regarding the chronic use and abuse of narcotics.

Risk Related to Breast-feeding

Codeine and its active metabolite, morphine, are excreted into breast milk in low concentrations following usual therapeutic doses (Anderson, 1977; Pagliaro & Levin, 1979; Findlay et al., 1981). The amount of codeine that the nursing infant would be expected to ingest is between <1-7% of the lowest pediatric dose of codeine, based on data obtained from eight lactating women (Findlay et al., 1981; Meny et al.,

1993).* Corresponding serum levels of codeine in the infants ranged between 6-35% of the lowest therapeutic serum level for codeine (Meny et al., 1993).[†]

Morphine was also detected in the breast milk following maternal ingestion of codeine (Meny et al., 1993). On the basis of this data, the estimated amount of morphine that the nursing infant would receive is <1% of the lowest therapeutic dose of morphine in adults.[‡] The amount of morphine measured in the serum of the infants was between 7-31% of the lowest therapeutic serum level of morphine.[§]

The American Academy of Pediatrics considers codeine to be safe to use during breastfeeding (Committee on Drugs, American Academy of Pediatrics, 1994).

Key References

Anderson PO: Drugs and Breast-feeding--a review. Drug Intell Clin Pharm 11:208, 1977.

Aselton P, Jick H, Milunsky A, et al.: First-trimester drug use and congenital disorders. Obstet Gynecol 65:451-455, 1985.

Bracken MB: Drug use in pregnancy and congenital heart disease in offspring. N Engl J Med 314:1120, 1986.

Bracken MG, Holford TR: Exposure to prescribed drugs in pregnancy and association with congenital malformations. Obstet Gynecol 58:336-344, 1981.

Ching M, Tang L: Neuroleptic drug-induced alterations on neonatal growth and development. I. Prenatal exposure influences birth size, mortality rate, and the neuroendocrine system. Biol Neonate 49:261-269, 1986.

Committee on Drugs, American Academy of Pediatrics: The transfer of drugs and other chemicals into human milk. Pediatrics 93(1):137-150, 1994.

Findlay JWA, DeAngelis RL, Kearney MF, et al.: Analgesic drugs in breast milk and plasma. Clin Pharmacol Ther 29:625-633, 1981.

*This calculation is based on the following assumptions: maternal dose of codeine: 60 mg; milk concentration of codeine: <33.8-314 ng/mL; milk intake by the nursing infant: 150 mL/kg/d; estimated dose of codeine ingested by the nursing infant: <0.005-0.07 mg/kg/d; lowest pediatric dose of codeine: 1 mg/kg/d.

[†]Infant serum levels of codeine: 0.8-4.5 ng/mL; lowest therapeutic serum level in adults: 13 ng/mL.

[‡]This calculation is based on the following assumptions: milk concentration of morphine: 0.002-0.02 mcg/mL; estimated dose of morphine ingested by the nursing infant: 0.003 mg/kg/d; lowest therapeutic dose of morphine in adults: 0.75 mg/kg/d.

[§]Infant serum levels of morphine: 0.5-2.2 ng/mL; lowest therapeutic serum level of morphine in adults: 7 ng/mL.

Geber WF, Schramm LC: Congenital malformations of the central nervous system produced by narcotic analgesics in the hamster. Am J Obstet Gynecol 123:705-713, 1975.

Heinonen OP, Slone D, Shapiro S: *Birth Defects and Drugs in Pregnancy*. Littleton, Mass.: John Wright-PSG, 1977, pp 287-288, 434.

Jick H, Holmes LB, Hunter JR, et al.: First-trimester drug use and congenital disorders. JAMA 246:343-346, 1981.

Lehmann VH: [Teratologic studies in rabbits and rats with the morphine derivative codeine.] Arzneimittelforsch 26:551-554, 1976.

Meny RG, Naumburg EG, Alger LS, et al.: Codeine and the breastfed neonate. J Hum Lact 9(4):237-240, 1993.

Pagliaro LA, Levin RH: *Problems in Pediatric Drug Therapy*. Hamilton, Il.: Drug Intell Publ, 1979.

Price CJ: Teratologic evaluation of codeine (CAS No. 76-57-3) administered to CD-1 mice on gestational days 6 through 15. NTIS (National Technical information Service) Report/PB87-209524, 1987.

Rothman KJ, Fyler DC, Goldblatt A, Kreidberg MB: Exogenous hormones and other drug exposures of children with congenital heart disease. Am J Epidemiol 109:433-439, 1979.

Ruggins NR, Watkins S, Rutter N: An unusual cause of convulsions in a newborn infant. Eur J Pediatr 151:918, 1992.

Saxen I: Associations between oral clefts and drugs taken during pegnancy. Int J Epidemiol 4:37-44, 1975a.

Saxen I: Epidemiology of cleft lip and palate. Br J Prev Soc Med 29:103-110, 1975b.

Shaw GM, Malcoe LH, Swan SH, et al.: Congenital cardiac anomalies relative to selected maternal exposures and conditions during early pregnancy. Eur J Epidemiol 8:(5):757-760, 1992.

Shaw GM, Malcoe LH, Swan SH, et al.: Risks for congenital cardiac anomalies relative to selected maternal exposures during early pregnancy. Teratology 41(5):590, 1990.

Sleet RB, Price CJ, George JD, et al.: Teratologic evaluation of codeine (CAS No. 76-57-3) administered to LVG hamsters on gestational days 5 through 13. NTIS (National Technical Information Service) Report/PB88-131040, 1987.

Williams J, Price CJ, Sleet RB et al: Codeine: Developmental toxicity in hamsters and mice. Fundam Appl Toxicol 16:401-413, 1991.

Zierler S, Rothman KJ: Congenital heart disease in relation to maternal use of bendectin and other drugs in early pregnancy. N Engl J Med 313:347-352, 1985.

CODIPERTUSSIN® *See* Codeine

COKE *See* Cocaine

COMPAZINE® *See* Prochlorperazine

CORGARD® *See* Nadolol

CORTEF® *See* Hydrocortisone

CORTELAN® *See* Cortisone

CORTISOL® *See* Hydrocortisone

CORTISONE
(Acetisone®, Cortelan®, Cortone®)

Cortisone is a glucocorticoid normally excreted by the adrenal cortex. It is administered orally or parenterally for replacement therapy and to treat allergic and inflammatory diseases. The dose used varies from 20-300 mg/d.

Teratogenic Risk

Magnitude of teratogenic
risk to child born after
exposure during gestation: *Unlikely*

Quality and quantity of data
on which risk estimate is based: *Fair to good*

Therapeutic doses of cortisone are unlikely to pose a substantial teratogenic risk, but the data are insufficient to state that there is no risk.

The frequency of congenital anomalies was no greater than expected among the children of 34 women treated with cortisone during the first four lunar months of pregnancy in one epidemiological study

(Heinonen et al., 1977). Four of 27 infants born to women treated with cortisone for hyperemesis gravidarum during the first half of pregnancy in another study had congenital anomalies, all of which were different from each other (Wells, 1953). The fact that the anomalies were all different suggests that they were not related to the maternal cortisone therapy.

Cortisone in doses substantially greater than those usually employed in humans is definitely teratogenic in several animal species. An increased frequency of cleft palate is seen among the offspring of pregnant mice or hamsters treated during pregnancy with cortisone in doses many times greater than those used in humans (Walker, 1971; Biddle & Fraser, 1976; Shah & Kilistoff, 1976; Kalter, 1981; Mosier et al., 1982). Cleft palate has been observed in rabbits after maternal treatment with cortisone in doses comparable to those used therapeutically in humans (Walker, 1967). A variety of malformations occurs in the offspring of beagle dogs treated with about 25 times the usual human dose of cortisone during pregnancy (Nakayama et al., 1978). The relevance, if any, of these observations to the therapeutic use of cortisone in human pregnancy is unknown.

Please see agent summary on prednisone/prednisolone for information on a related agent that has been more thoroughly studied.

Risk Related to Breast-feeding

No information regarding the distribution of cortisone in breast milk has been published. The USP DI (1995) states that administration of cortisone at doses of 25 mg/d or less to breast-feeding mothers should be safe for the nursing infant.

Key References

Biddle FG, Fraser FC: Genetics of cortisone-induced cleft palate in the mouse--embryonic and maternal effects. Genetics 84:743-754, 1976.

Heinonen OP, Slone D, Shapiro S: *Birth Defects and Drugs in Pregnancy.* Littleton, Mass.: John Wright-PSG, 1977, pp 389, 391.

Kalter H: Dose-response studies with genetically homogeneous lines of mice as a teratology testing and risk-assessment procedure. Teratology 24:79-86, 1981.

Mosier HD Jr, Dearden LC, Jansons RA, et al.: Disproportionate growth of organs and body weight following glucocorticoid treatment of the rat fetus. Dev Pharmacol Ther 4:89-105, 1982.

Nakayama T, Hirayama M, Esaki K: Effects of cortisone acetate in the beagle fetus. Teratology 18:149, 1978.

Shah RM, Kilistoff A: Cleft palate induction in hamster fetuses by glucocorticoid hormones and their synthetic analogues. J Embryol Exp Morphol 36:101-108, 1976.

USP DI: Corticosteroids/corticotropin--glucocorticoid effects. In: *USP DI (USP Dispensing Information), Volume 1. Drug Information for the Health Care Professional*, 15th ed. Rockville, Md.: The US Pharmacopeial Convention, 1995, p 881.

Walker BE: Induction of cleft palate in rabbits by several glucocorticoids. Proc Soc Exp Biol Med 125:1281-1284, 1967.

Walker BE: Induction of cleft palate in rats with anti-inflammatory drugs. Teratology 4:39-42, 1971.

Wells CN: Treatment of hyperemesis gravidarum with cortisone. I. Fetal results. Am J Obstet Gynecol 66:598-601, 1953.

CORTONE® *See Cortisone*

COUMADIN® *See Warfarin*

CRACK *See Cocaine*

CROMOLYN
(Gastrocrom®, Nalcrom®, Sodium Cromoglycate)

Cromolyn is used in the prevention of allergic diseases and related conditions. It is administered by inhalation, and in oral, nasal, and ophthalmic preparations. Systemic absorption from all of these routes is poor, ranging from <1% for ophthalmic administration to 8-10% after inhalation. Doses are also quite variable, ranging from 6.4-800 mg/d, depending on route and preparation.

Teratogenic Risk

Magnitude of teratogenic risk to child born after exposure during gestation:	*Unlikely*
Quality and quantity of data on which risk estimate is based:	*Poor to fair*

> *Therapeutic doses of cromolyn are unlikely to pose a substantial teratogenic risk, but the data are insufficient to state that there is no risk.*

The frequency of congenital anomalies did not appear to be increased in a series of 296 children of asthmatic women treated with cromolyn throughout pregnancy (Wilson, 1982).

Studies in mice, rats, and rabbits suggest that treatment of pregnant women with cromolyn in usual therapeutic doses is unlikely to increase the children's risk of malformations greatly (Cox et al., 1970). Treatment of pregnant mice with cromolyn in doses more than 38 times that used in humans did increase the teratogenic effect produced by concurrent administration of isoproterenol (Cox et al., 1970). The relevance of this observation to therapeutic use of cromolyn and isoproterenol in pregnant women is unknown.

Risk Related to Breast-feeding

No information regarding the distribution of cromolyn in breast milk has been published. Cromolyn is found in very low concentrations in maternal serum and therefore very little would be expected to reach the nursing infant (USP DI, 1995).

Doses up to 20 mg/kg/d have been administered to infants to treat resistant allergies (Daglish, 1983).

Key References

Cox JSG, Beach JE, Blair AMJN, et al.: Disodium Cromoglycate (Intal®). Adv Drug Res 5:115-196, 1970.

Daglish MS: Breastfeeding and allergy. Can Pharm J 116:304-336, 1983.

USP DI: Cromolyn. In: USP DI (USP Dispensing Information), Volume 1. Drug Informtion for the Health Care Professional, 15th ed. Rockville, Md.: The US Pharmacopeial Convention, 1995, p 991.

Wilson J: Utilisation du cromoglycate de sodium au cours de la grossesse: Resultats sur 296 femmes asthmatiques. Acta Therap 8(Suppl):45-51, 1982.

C-SPAN® *See Ascorbic Acid*

CYANOCOBALAMIN
(Anacobin®, Bedoz®, Rubion®)

Cyanocobalamin is one form of vitamin B_{12}, a water-soluble vitamin. The US RDA of vitamin B_{12} is 2.2 mcg/d in pregnancy (NRC, 1989). Cyanocobalamin is administered orally in doses of 1-25 mcg/d and parenterally in doses up to 100 mcg/d to treat deficiency states.

Teratogenic Risk

Magnitude of teratogenic risk to child born after exposure during gestation:	*Undetermined*
Quality and quantity of data on which risk estimate is based:	*Very poor*

A small risk cannot be excluded, but a high risk of congenital anomalies in the children of women who cyanocobalamin in usual therapeutic doses during pregnancy is unlikely.

No adequate epidemiological studies of congenital anomalies among infants born to women treated with large doses of cyanocobalamin during pregnancy have been reported.

Studies in mice suggest that treatment of pregnant women with cyanocobalamin in usual therapeutic doses is unlikely to increase the children's risk of malformations greatly (Mitala et al., 1978).

Risk Related to Breast-feeding

Cyanocobalamin is a normal constituent of breast milk (Samson & McClelland, 1980; Sandberg et al., 1981; Sneed et al., 1981; Ford et al., 1983). Concentrations of cyanocobalamin have been found to be much higher in colostrum than in mature milk (Sneed et al., 1981; Ford et al., 1983).

Several cases of megaloblastic anemia in breast-fed infants of strict vegetarians or mothers with cyanocobalamin deficiency (Jadhav et al., 1962; Lampkin & Saunders, 1969; Frader et al., 1978; Hoey et al., 1982; Gambon et al., 1986; Sklar, 1986; Kuhne et al., 1991) have been reported.

The breast milk levels of cyanocobalamin in ten nursing mothers taking supplements of cyanocobalamin were increased in some studies but unchanged in others (Thomas et al., 1979; Sandberg et al., 1981; Sneed et al., 1981).

The American Academy of Pediatrics regards cyanocobalamin to be safe to take while breast-feeding (Committee on Drugs, American Academy of Pediatrics, 1994).

Key References

Committee on Drugs, American Academy of Pediatrics: The transfer of drugs and other chemicals into human milk. Pediatrics 93(1):137-150, 1994.

Ford JE, Zechalko A, Murphy J, Brooke OG: Comparison of the B vitamin composition of milk from mothers of preterm and term babies. Arch Dis Child 58:367-372, 1983.

Frader J, Reibman B, Turkewitz D: Vitamin B_{12} deficiency in strict vegetarians. N Engl J Med 299:1319, 1978.

Gambon RC, Lentze MJ, Rossi E: Megaloblastic anaemia in one of monozygous twins breast fed by their vegetarian mother. Eur J Pediatr 145:570-571, 1986.

Hoey H, Linnell JC, Oberholzer VG, Laurance BM: Vitamin B_{12} deficiency in a breastfed infant of a mother with pernicious anaemia. J R Soc Med 75:656-658, 1982.

Jadhav M, Webb JKG, Vaishnava S, Baker SJ: Vitamin-B_{12} deficiency in Indian infants. A clinical syndrome. Lancet 2:903-907, 1962.

Kuhne T, Bubl R, Baumgartner R: Maternal vegan diet causing a serious infantile neurological disorder due to vitamin B_{12} deficiency. Eur J Pediatr 150:205-208, 1991.

Lampkin BC, Saunders EF: Nutritional vitamin B_{12} deficiency in an infant. J Pediatr 75:1053-1055, 1969.

Mitala JJ, Mann DE Jr, Gautieri RF: Influence of cobalt (dietary), cobalamins, and inorganic cobalt salts on phenytoin- and cortisone-induced teratogenesis in mice. J Pharm Sci 67:377-380, 1978.

NRC (National Research Council): *Recommended Dietary Allowances, 10th ed. Report of the Subcommittee on the Tenth Edition of the RDAs, Food and Nutrition Board, Commission on Life Sciences.* Washington, DC: National Academy Press, 1989, p 262.

Samson RR, McClelland DBL: Vitamin B_{12} in human colostrum and milk. Acta Paediatr Scand 69:93-99, 1980.

Sandberg D P, Begley JA, Hall CA: The content, binding, and forms of vitamin B_{12} in milk. Am J Clin Nutr 34:1717-1724, 1981.

Sklar R: Nutritional vitamin B_{12} deficiency in a breast-fed infant of a vegan-diet mother. Clin Pediatr 25:219-221, 1986.

Sneed SM, Zane C, Thomas MR: The effects of ascorbic acid, vitamin B_6, vitamin B_{12}, and folic acid supplementation on the breast milk and maternal nutritional status of low socioeconomic lactating women. Am J Clin Nutr 34:1338-1346, 1981.

Thomas MR, Kawamoto J, Sneed SM, Eakin R: The effects of vitamin C, vitamin B_6, and vitamin B_{12} supplementation on the breast milk and maternal status of well-nourished women. Am J Clin Nutr 32:1679-1685, 1979.

CYCLOBENZAPRINE
(Cycloflex®, Flexeril®)

Cyclobenzaprine is a centrally acting muscle relaxant used for relief of muscle spasms. The drug is given orally in doses of 20-60 mg/d.

Teratogenic Risk

Magnitude of teratogenic risk to child born after exposure during gestation:	*Undetermined*
Quality and quantity of data on which risk estimate is based:	*None*

No epidemiological studies of congenital anomalies among infants born to women treated with cyclobenzaprine during pregnancy have been reported.

A child with a very unusual pattern of anomalies consisting of imperforate oropharynx, abnormal facies and vertebral defects, whose mother took cyclobenzaprine early in the first trimester of pregnancy has been reported (Flannery, 1989). No causal relationship can be established on the basis of this single anecdotal observation.

Unpublished studies in mice, rats, and rabbits are said to suggest that treatment of pregnant women with cyclobenzaprine in usual therapeutic doses is unlikely to increase the children's risk of malformations greatly (USP DI, 1995).

Risk Related to Breast-feeding

No information regarding the distribution of cyclobenzaprine in breast milk has been published.

Key References

Flannery DB: Syndrome of imperforate oropharynx with costovertebral and auricular anomalies. Am J Med Genet 32:189-191, 1989.

USP DI: Cyclobenzaprine. In: *USP DI (USP Dispensing Information), Volume 1. Drug Information for the Health Care Professional,* 15th ed. Rockville, Md.: The US Pharmacopeial Convention, 1995, p 1088.

CYCLOFLEX® *See* Cyclobenzaprine

CYCLOSPAR® *See* Tetracycline

CYCLOSPORINE
(Sandimmune®)

Cyclosporine is a cyclic polypeptide of fungal origin. It is used as an immunosuppressant in the prevention and treatment of allograft rejection and also in the treatment of some autoimmune disorders. The usual oral dose is 5-10 mg/kg of body weight per day, although up to 25 mg/kg/d may be used immediately preceding or following transplantation and somewhat smaller doses may be given intravenously.

Teratogenic Risk

Magnitude of teratogenic
risk to child born after
exposure during gestation:
    Malformations: *Minimal*
    Fetal growth retardation: *Small to moderate*

Quality and quantity of data
on which risk estimate is based:
    Malformations: *Fair*
    Fetal growth retardation: *Fair*

Women who are treated with cyclosporine during pregnancy have serious medical problems and often are treated with other medications concomitantly. It is impossible to separate the effects of cyclosporine from the effects of other medication and maternal illness in available human studies of cyclosporine teratogenicity.

It is unclear whether the growth retardation and malformations that have been reported in infants born to women treated with cyclosporine during pregnancy are manifestations of the same or different pathogenic processes.

More than 200 pregnancies have been reported among women who were treated with cyclosporine, often in combination with other drugs, throughout pregnancy (Armenti et al., 1993, 1994, 1995; Claris et al., 1993; Crawford et al., 1993; Salmela et al., 1993; Wagoner et al., 1993; Burrows et al., 1994; Ha et al., 1994; Haugen et al., 1994; Pilarski et al., 1994; Takahashi et al., 1994; Radomski et al., 1995). It is impossible to determine what the total number of reported cases is because the series overlap. Most of the reports are of single cases or small groups of cases, and many are not described in sufficient detail to interpret fully.

Congenital anomalies have been described in at least 13 children of women who were treated with cyclosporine during pregnancy, but no recurrent pattern of anomalies has been noted (Kossoy et al., 1988; Niesert et al., 1988; Cockburn et al., 1989; Pujals et al., 1989; Zeidan et al., 1991; Crawford et al., 1993; Framarino di Malatesta et al., 1993; Armenti et al., 1994; Ha et al., 1994). It is impossible to determine which, if any, of the reported malformations are related to the maternal cyclosporine therapy.

Most children born to women treated with cyclosporine during pregnancy do not have malformations, but few cases have been followed beyond infancy. Malformations were observed in only two of 107 newborns of renal transplant recipients treated with cyclosporine during pregnancy and reported to the National Transplantation Pregnancy Register (Armenti et al., 1994). In another group of 21 children born to women who had been treated with cyclosporine and other immunosuppressants during pregnancy because of a previous organ transplant, there were two infants with major congenital anomalies and unexpectedly high rates of fetal growth retardation and prematurity (Crawford et al., 1993). No malformations were observed among the infants of 23 female heart transplant recipients who were treated with cyclosporine during pregnancy in another series (Wagoner et al., 1993).

Fetal growth retardation and prematurity are unusually frequent among the children of women treated with cyclosporine during pregnancy (Muirhead et al., 1992; Crawford et al., 1993; Wagoner et al., 1993; Armenti et al., 1994, 1995; Haugen et al., 1994; Olshan et al., 1994; Radomski et al., 1995), but these appear to be related, at least in part, to the mothers' underlying illnesses or other aspects of their treatment. Of 137 liveborn infants of renal transplant recipients reported to the National Transplantation Pregnancy Register who were treated with cyclosporine during pregnancy, 54% were premature (<37 weeks gestation) and 50% had low birth weights (<2500 g) (Armenti et al., 1995; Radomski, et al., 1995). Women with reduced renal function or with hypertension requiring drug treatment before conception were more likely to have low birth weight infants (Armenti et al., 1994, 1995). The number of cases of twins described seems high (Burrows et al., 1988; Prieto et al., 1989; Grow et al., 1991; Wagoner et al., 1993), but this may be a reporting bias.

There was no evidence of nephrotoxicity in 26 children followed in one study to an average age of 39 months after their birth to women who were treated with cyclosporine during pregnancy (Shaheen et al., 1993).

Transient neonatal thrombocytopenia, neutropenia, and lymphopenia have occasionally been reported in the infants of women treated with cyclosporine during pregnancy (Grischke et al., 1986; Grow et al., 1991; Baarsma & Kamps, 1993). Lower than expected numbers of B-lymphocytes were found in the cord blood of six infants whose mothers had been treated with cyclosporine and other immunosuppressive agents during pregnancy (Takahashi et al., 1994). This deficiency of B-cells persisted for at least the first six months of life in most cases. No abnormality of immunological function was found among five one- to six-year-old children whose mothers had been treated with cyclosporine during pregnancy in another series, but these children did exhibit a slight delay in T-cell development (Pilarski et al., 1994).

Alterations of immunological function have been observed among the offspring of pregnant mice treated with cyclosporine in doses similar to those used therapeutically in humans (Classen & Shevach, 1991). Studies in rats, mice, and rabbits suggest that treatment of pregnant women with cyclosporine in usual therapeutic doses is unlikely to increase the children's risk of malformations greatly (Ryffel et al., 1983; Brown et al., 1985; Fein et al., 1989). Fetal growth retardation and death were increased in all of these species at doses at or just above the maximum used therapeutically in humans; such doses were often toxic to the mothers as well (Ryffel et al., 1983; Brown et al., 1985; Mason et al., 1985; Fein et al., 1989; Classen & Shevach, 1991; Olshan et al., 1994).

Risk Related to Breast-feeding

Cyclosporine is excreted into breast milk in low concentrations. The amount of cyclosporine that the nursing infant would be expected to ingest is <1% of the lowest pediatric dose, based on data obtained from two lactating women (Lewis et al., 1983; Flechner et al., 1985).*

The American Academy of Pediatrics recommends that women on cyclosporine refrain from breast-feeding because of a theoretical risk of growth retardation, nephrotoxicity, and malignancy in the infant (Committee on Drugs, American Academy of Pediatrics, 1994).

Key References

Armenti VT, Ahlswede KM, Ahlswede BA, et al.: National Transplantation Pregnancy Registry--outcomes of 154 pregnancies in cyclosporine-treated female kidney transplant recipients. Transplantation 57:502-506, 1994.

Armenti VT, Ahlswede KM, Ahlswede BA, et al.: The National Transplantation Pregnancy Registry: Outcomes of 414 pregnancies in female transplant recipients. Teratology 47(5):393, 1993.

Armenti VT, Ahlswede KM, Ahlswede BA, et al.: Variables affecting birthweight and graft survival in 197 pregnancies in cyclosporine-treated female kidney transplant recipients. Transplantation 59:476-479, 1995.

Baarsma R, Kamps WA: Immunological responses in an infant after cyclosporine A exposure during pregnancy. Eur J Pediatr 152:476-477, 1993.

Brown PAJ, Gray ES, Whiting PH, et al.: Effects of cyclosporin A on fetal development in the rat. Biol Neonate 48:172-180, 1985.

Burrows DA, O'Neil TJ, Sorrells TL: Successful twin pregnancy after renal transplant maintained on cyclosporine A immunosuppression. Obstet Gynecol 72(3):459-461, 1988.

Burrows L, Knight R, Thomas A, Panico M: Cyclosporine levels during pregnancy. Transplant Proc 26(5):2820-2821, 1994.

*This calculation is based on the following assumptions: maternal dose of cyclosporine: 325-450 mg/d; milk concentration of cyclosporine: 0.02-0.26 mcg/mL; milk intake by the nursing infant: 150 mL/kg/d; estimated dose of cyclosporine ingested by the nursing infant: 0.003-0.04 mg/kg/d; lowest pediatric dose of cyclosporine: 5 mg/kg/d.

Claris O, Picaud J-C, Brazier J-L, Salle BL: Pharmacokinetics of cyclosporin A in 16 newborn infants of renal or cardiac transplant mothers. Dev Pharmacol Ther 20:180-185, 1993.

Classen JB, Shevach EM: Evidence that cyclosporine treatment during pregnancy predisposes offspring to develop autoantibodies. Transplantation 51(5):1052-1057, 1991.

Cockburn I, Krupp P, Monka C: Present experience of Sandimmun® in pregnancy. Transplant Proc 21(4):3730-3732, 1989.

Committee on Drugs, American Academy of Pediatrics: The transfer of drugs and other chemicals into human milk. Pediatrics 93(1):137-150, 1994.

Crawford JS, Johnson K, Jones KL: Pregnancy outcome after transplantation in women maintained on cyclosporine immunosuppression. Reprod Toxicol 7(2):156, 1993.

Fein A, Vechoropoulos M, Nebel L: Cyclosporin-induced embryotoxicity in mice. Biol Neonate 56:165-173, 1989.

Flechner SM, Katz AR, Rogers AJ, et al.: The presence of cyclosporine in body tissues and fluids during pregnancy. Am J Kidney Dis 5:60-63, 1985.

Framarino di Malatesta ML, Poli L, Pierucci F, et al.: Pregnancy and kidney transplantation: Clinical problems and experience. Transplant Proc 25(3):2188-2189, 1993.

Grischke E, Kaufmann M, Dreikorn K, et al.: [Successful pregnancy with kidney transplant and cyclosporin A.] Geburtshilfe Frauenheilkd 46:176-179, 1986.

Grow DR, Simon NV, Liss J, Delp WT: Twin pregnancy after orthotopic liver transplantation, with exacerbation of chronic graft rejection. Am J Perinatol 8(2):135-138, 1991.

Ha J, Kim SJ, Kim ST: Pregnancy following renal transplantation. Transplant Proc 26:2117-2118, 1994.

Haugen G, Fauchald P, Sodal G, et al.: Pregnancy outcome in renal allograft recipients in Norway. Acta Obstet Gynecol Scand 73:541-546, 1994.

Kossoy LR, Herbert CM III, Wentz AC: Management of heart transplant recipients: Guidelines for the obstetrician-gynecologist. Am J Obstet Gynecol 159(2):490-499, 1988.

Lewis GJ, Lamont CAR, Lee HA, Slapak M: Successful pregnancy in a renal transplant recipient taking cyclosporin A. Br Med J 286:603, 1983.

Mason RJ, Thomson AW, Whiting PH, et al.: Cyclosporine-induced fetotoxicity in the rat. Transplantation 39(1):9-12, 1985.

Muirhead N, Sabharwal AR, Rieder MJ, et al.: The outcome of pregnancy following renal transplantation--the experience of a single center. Transplantation 54(3):429-432, 1992.

Niesert S, Gunter H, Frei U: Pregnancy after renal transplantation. Br Med J 296:1736, 1988.

Olshan AF, Mattison DR, Zwanenburg TSB: Cyclosporine A: Review of genotoxicity and potential for adverse human reproductive and developmental effects. Mutat Res 317:163-173, 1994.

Pilarski LM, Yacyshyn BR, Lazarovits AI: Analysis of peripheral blood lymphocyte populations and immune function from children exposed to cyclosporine or to azathioprine in utero. Transplantation 57(1):133-144, 1994.

Prieto C, Errasti P, Olaizola JI, et al.: Successful twin pregnancies in renal transplant recipients taking cyclosporine. Transplantation 48(6):1065-1067, 1989.

Pujals JM, Figueras G, Puig JM, et al.: Osseous malformation in baby born to woman on cyclosporin. Lancet 1:667, 1989.

Radomski BA, Ahlswede BE, Jarrell J, et al.: Outcomes of 500 pregnancies in 335 female kidney, liver, and heart transplant recipients. Transplant Proc 27(1):1089-1090, 1995.

Ryffel B, Donatsch P, Madorin M, et al.: Toxicologic evaluation of cyclosporin A. Arch Toxicol 53:107-141, 1983.

Salmela KT, Kyllonen LEJ, Holmberg C, Gronhagen-Riska C: Impaired renal function after pregnancy in renal transplant recipients. Transplantation 56(6):1372-1375, 1993.

Shaheen FAM, Al-Sulaiman MH, Al-Khader AA: Long-term nephrotoxicity after exposure to cyclosporine in utero. Transplantation 56(1):224-225, 1993.

Takahashi N, Nishida H, Hoshi J: Severe B cell depletion in newborns from renal transplant mothers taking immunosuppressive agents. Transplantation 57(11):1617-1621, 1994.

Wagoner LE, Taylor DO, Olsen SL et al.: Immunosuppressive therapy, management, and outcome of heart transplant recipients during pregnancy. J Heart Lung Transplant 12:993-1000, 1993. [Erratum: J Heart Lung Transplant 13(2):342, 1994.]

Zeidan BS, Waltzer WC, Monheit AG, Rapaport FT: Anemia associated with pregnancy in a cyclosporine-treated renal allograft recipient. Transplant Proc 23(4):2301-2303, 1991.

CYSTOSPAZ® *See Hyoscyamine*

DALACIN C® *See* Clindamycin

DALMANE® *See* Flurazepam

DARVON® *See* Propoxyphene

DATRIL® *See* Acetaminophen

DECADERM® *See* Dexamethasone

DECADRON® *See* Dexamethasone

DELFEN® *See* Nonoxynols

DELTALIN® *See* Vitamin D

DELTASONE® *See* Prednisone/Prednisolone

DEMEROL® *See* Meperidine

DEMULEN® *See* Ethynodiol Diacetate

DEPAKENE® *See* Valproic Acid

DEPAKOTE® *See* Valproic Acid

DEPO-PROVERA® *See* Medroxyprogesterone

DES *See* Diethylstilbestrol

DESOXIMETASONE
(Actiderm®, Desoxymethasone, Topicort®)

Desoximetasone is a synthetic corticosteroid used topically to treat dermatologic disorders. Systemic absorption of desoximetasone occurs after topical application.

Teratogenic Risk

Magnitude of teratogenic risk to child born after exposure during gestation:	*Undetermined*
Quality and quantity of data on which risk estimate is based:	*Very poor*

No epidemiological studies of congenital anomalies in infants born to women who were treated with desoximetasone during pregnancy have been published.

The frequency of malformations was not increased among the offspring of rats and mice born of mothers subcutaneously injected with about 1-2 times the usual human topical dose of desoximetasone during pregnancy. At doses about 8 times that used topically in humans, cleft palate was induced in mice, but such doses were toxic to the mothers (Miyamoto et al., 1975). The relevance of these findings to topical use of desoximetasone in human pregnancy is unknown.

Please see agent summary on cortisone for information on a related drug that has been more thoroughly studied.

Risk Related to Breast-feeding

No information regarding the distribution of desoximetasone in breast milk has been published. Application of desoximetasone to the breasts prior to nursing is not recommended (USP DI, 1995).

Key References

Miyamoto M, Ohtsu M, Sugisaki T, Sakaguchi T: [Teratogenic effect of 9-fluoro-11-β, 21-dihydroxy-16-α-methylpregna-1, 4-diene-3, 20-dione (A 41 304), a new anti-inflammatory agent, and of dexamethasone in rats and mice.] Nippon Yakurigaku Zasshi (Folia Pharmacol Jpn) 71:367-378, 1975.

USP DI: Corticosteroids. In: *USP DI (USP Dispensing Information), Volume 1. Drug Information for the Health Care Professional*, 15th ed. Rockville, Md.: The US Pharmacopeial Convention, 1995, p 860.

DESOXYMETHASONE *See* Desoximetasone

DESOXYN® *See* Methamphetamine

DESYREL® *See* Trazodone

DETENSOL® *See* Propranolol

DEXAMETHASONE
(Aeroseb®, Decadron®, Hexadrol®)

Dexamethasone is a synthetic adrenocortical steroid that is used to treat a variety of inflammatory and allergic disorders. The usual oral dose is 0.5-9 mg/d, but intravenous doses as large as 80 mg/d are sometimes used to treat shock. Dexamethasone is also given by injection into joints, soft tissues, and lesions as well as in nasal, opthalmic, otic, and topical preparations. Substantial systemic absorption of dexamethasone may occur after administration by any route.

Teratogenic Risk

Magnitude of teratogenic risk to child born after exposure during gestation: *Unlikely*

Quality and quantity of data on which risk estimate is based: *Poor to fair*

Therapeutic doses of dexamethasone are unlikely to pose a substantial teratogenic risk, but the data are insufficient to state that there is no risk.

No epidemiological studies of congenital anomalies among infants born to women treated with dexamethasone early in pregnancy have been reported.

Dexamethasone treatment of pregnant women has been used to provide fetal therapy for congenital virilizing adrenal hyperplasia due to a genetic deficiency of 21-hydroxylase. Such therapy appears to prevent virilization of most female fetuses affected with this disease (Pang et al., 1990; Forest & David, 1992; Karaviti et al., 1992; Couper et al., 1993; Nivelon et al., 1993). No adverse effect of this therapy has been noted among these children, some of whom were treated in the first trimester of gestation.

Maternal dexamethasone therapy in the late second or third trimester of pregnancy has been used to accelerate fetal lung maturation and prevent respiratory distress syndrome in prematurely born infants (Cosmi & DiRenzo, 1989; Roberts & Morrison, 1991). No growth, physical, motor, or developmental deficiencies attributable to such prenatal therapy were observed in a three-year follow-up study of 200 children delivered to treated women (Collaborative Group on Antenatal Steroid Therapy, 1984). Normal spontaneous closure of the ductus arteriosus occurred more frequently in infants born before 31 weeks gestation whose mothers had been treated with dexamethasone just prior to delivery than in those whose mothers had not been so treated in a randomized controlled trial (Eronen et al., 1993).

Scalp aplasia was observed among the offspring of rhesus monkeys treated in early pregnancy with dexamethasone in doses similar to or several times greater than those used in humans (Jerome & Hendrickx, 1988). Cranium bifidum occurred in one of the monkeys with scalp defects. Fetal weight and head circumference were reduced and alterations of brain histology were observed among the offspring of rhesus monkeys treated late in pregnancy with dexamethasone in doses within the human therapeutic range (Novy & Walsh, 1983; Uno et al., 1990).

Increased frequency of cleft palate occurs among the offspring of mice treated during pregnancy with 4-10 times the maximal human dose of dexamethasone (Pinsky & DiGeorge, 1965; Natsume et al., 1986). Fetal growth retardation and neonatal immune deficiency have been reported among the offspring of mice treated during pregnancy with dexamethasone in doses similar to those used in the treatment of asthma and inflammatory diseases in humans (Eishi et al., 1983).

Increased frequencies of palatal, cardiac, and abdominal wall defects were observed among the offspring of rats treated during pregnancy with dexamethasone in doses within the human therapeutic range or several times greater (Vannier & Bremaud, 1985; LaBorde et al., 1992).

Fetal and neonatal growth retardation have also been observed among the offspring of pregnant rats treated with dexamethasone in doses within the human therapeutic range (LaBorde et al., 1992; Benediktsson et al., 1993; Bian et al., 1993). An increased frequency of fetal growth retardation was observed among the offspring of pregnant rabbits treated dermally with dexamethasone ointment in a dose that was within the human therapeutic range but caused maternal toxicity in the rabbits (Esaki et al., 1981). Fetal growth retardation and congenital myopathy were found among the offspring of minipigs treated during pregnancy with dexamethasone in doses similar to those used in the treatment of asthma and inflammatory diseases in humans (Jirmanova & Lojda, 1985).

Please see agent summary on prednisone/prednisolone for information on a related agent that has been more thoroughly studied.

Risk Related to Breast-feeding

No information regarding the distribution of dexamethasone in breast milk has been published. Although it is not known whether topical preparations containing dexamethasone contain enough of the drug to produce detectable amounts of dexamethasone in the breast milk, application of creams containing dexamethasone to the breasts prior to nursing should be avoided.

Key References

Benediktsson R, Lindsay RS, Nobel J, et al.: Glucocorticoid exposure in utero: New model for adult hypertension. Lancet 341:339-341, 1993. [Erratum: Lancet 341:572, 1993.]

Bian X, Seidler FJ, Slotkin TA: Fetal dexamethasone exposure interferes with establishment of cardiac noradrenergic innervation and sympathetic activity. Teratology 47:109-117, 1993.

Collaborative Group on Antenatal Steroid Therapy: Effects of antenatal dexamethasone administration in the infant: Long-term follow-up. J Pediatr 104(2):259-267, 1984.

Cosmi EV, Di Renzo GC: Prevention and treatment of fetal lung immaturity. Fetal Ther 4(Suppl 1):52-62, 1989.

Couper JJ, Hutson JM, Warne GL: Hydrometrocolpos following prenatal dexamethasone treatment for congenital adrenal hyperplasia (21-hydroxylase deficiency). Eur J Pediatr 152:9-11, 1993.

Eishi Y, Hirokawa K, Hatakeyama S: Long-lasting impairment of immune and endocrine systems of offspring induced by injection of dexamethasone into pregnant mice. Clin Immunol Immunopathol 26:335-349, 1983.

Eronen M, Kari A, Pesonen E, Hallman M: The effect of antenatal dexamethasone administration on the fetal and neonatal ductus arteriosus. Am J Dis Child 147:187-192, 1993.

Esaki K, Shikata Y, Yanagita T: Effects of dermal administration of dexamethasone 17-valerate in rabbit fetuses. Jitchuken Zenrinsho Kenkyuho 7:245-256, 1981.

Forest MG, David M: Prenatal treatment of congenital adrenal hyperplasia due to 21-hydroxylase deficiency: A 10 year experience. Indian J Pediatr 59:515-522, 1992.

Jerome CP, Hendrickx AG: Comparative teratogenicity of triamcinolone acetonide and dexamethasone in the rhesus monkey (*Macaca mulatta*). J Med Primatol 17:195-203, 1988.

Jirmanova I, Lojda L: Dexamethasone applied to pregnant minisows induces splayleg in minipiglets. Zentralbl Veterinarmed [A] 32:445-458, 1985.

Karaviti LP, Mercado AB, Mercado MB, et al.: Prenatal diagnosis/treatment in families at risk for infants with steroid 21-hydroxylase deficiency (congenital adrenal hyperplasia). J Steroid Biochem Mol Biol 41:445-451, 1992.

LaBorde JB, Hansen DK, Young JF, et al.: Prenatal dexamethasone exposure in rats: Effects of dose, age at exposure, and drug-induced hypophagia on malformations and fetal organ weights. Fundam Appl Toxicol 19:545-554, 1992.

Natsume N, Narukawa T, Kawai T: Teratogenesis of dexamethasone and preventive effect of vitamin B_{12}. Int J Oral Maxillofac Surg 15:752-755, 1986.

Nivelon JL, Chouchane M, Forest MG, et al.: [Prenatal treatment of congenital adrenal hyperplasia due to 21-hydroxylase deficiency. A review of nine cases.] Ann Pediatr (Paris) 40(7):421-425, 1993.

Novy MJ, Walsh SW: Dexamethasone and estradiol treatment in pregnant rhesus macaques: Effects on gestational length, maternal plasma hormones, and fetal growth. Am J Obstet Gynecol 145(8):920-931, 1983.

Pang S, Pollack MS, Marshall RN, Immken L: Prenatal treatment of congenital adrenal hyperplasia due to 21-hydroxylase deficiency. N Engl J Med 322(2):111-115, 1990.

Pinsky L, DiGeorge AM: Cleft palate in the mouse: A teratogenic index of glucocorticoid potency. Science 147:402-403, 1965.

Roberts WE, Morrison JC: Pharmacologic induction of fetal lung maturity. Clin Obstet Gynecol 34(2):319-327, 1991.

Uno H, Lohmiller L, Thieme C, et al.: Brain damage induced by prenatal exposure to dexamethasone in fetal rhesus macaques. I. Hippocampus. Dev Brain Res 53:157-167, 1990.

Vannier B, Bremaud R: Induction of heart defects in the rat foetus with dexamethasone. Teratology 32(2):35A, 1985.

DEXATRIM® *See* Phenylpropanolamine

DEXEDRINE® *See* Dextroamphetamine

DEXTROAMPHETAMINE
(Dexedrine®, DextroStat®)

Dextroamphetamine is a sympathomimetic agent and central nervous system stimulant. It is used as a stimulant, an anorectic, and in the treatment of narcolepsy. Dextroamphetamine is given orally in a dose of 5-60 mg/d.

Teratogenic Risk

Magnitude of teratogenic risk to child born after exposure during gestation:	*Minimal*
Quality and quantity of data on which risk estimate is based:	*Fair to good*

The frequencies of congenital anomalies, of major malformations, and of minor anomalies were no greater than expected among the children of 367 women who took dextroamphetamine during the first four lunar months of pregnancy in one epidemiological study (Heinonen et al., 1977). No association was observed with congenital anomalies in other studies involving 52 children born to mothers who took dextroamphetamine or 347 children born to mothers who took some drug in the amphetamine group early in pregnancy (Nora et al., 1967; Milkovich & van den Berg, 1977). The frequency of congenital anomalies was not increased among the children of 1069 women who took dextroamphetamine anytime during pregnancy or 1694 children of women who took a drug of the amphetamine class anytime during pregnancy (Heinonen et al., 1977; Milkovich & van den Berg, 1977). No association with maternal use of amphetamines as a recreational drug during the first trimester of pregnancy was found in a study of 110 infants with gastroschisis (Torfs et al., 1994).

In contrast, use of dextroamphetamine during early pregnancy was found more frequently than expected among the mothers of 458 infants with a variety of congenital anomalies in one study (Nelson & Forfar, 1971) and among the mothers of 184 children with cardiovascular malformations in another investigation (Nora et al., 1970). A history of maternal dextroamphetamine use during the period of fetal bile duct formation was observed with unusually high frequency among 11 infants with primary biliary atresia (Levin, 1971). The clinical importance of these observations is brought into question by their inconsistency with other epidemiological studies.

Eriksson & Zetterstrom (1981, 1994) observed for up to ten years of age 71 infants of women who abused dextroamphetamine during pregnancy. Two of these infants had intestinal atresia and one had a cardiovascular malformation. Premature delivery was frequent, and four of the infants died in the perinatal period. All of the children had normal intellectual capacity, but significant associations were observed between the amount and duration of maternal dextroamphetamine abuse during pregnancy and lower scores on tests of intelligence and behavior in the children at eight years of age (Billing et al., 1994). Interpretation of these associations is complicated by the mothers' concomitant abuse of alcohol and other drugs as well as by various other adverse social factors in these women (Eriksson & Zetterstrom, 1994).

Increased frequencies of fetal death and cardiac, skeletal, eye, and other malformations have been reported among the offspring of mice treated with 80-160 times the dose of dextroamphetamine used in humans (Nora et al., 1965; Fein et al., 1987), but such doses are also toxic to the mothers. Persistent behavioral alterations occured among the offspring of mice and rats treated with dextroamphetamine during pregnancy in doses equivalent to and greater than those used in humans (Holson et al., 1985; Lyon & McClure, 1994). The relevance of these findings to the clinical use of dextroamphetamine in human pregnancy is uncertain.

Risk Related to Breast-feeding

Dextroamphetamine is excreted in the breast milk. The amount of dextroamphetamine that the nursing infant would be expected to ingest is between 10-25% of the lowest therapeutic dose in adults, based on data obtained from a single patient (Steiner et al., 1984).* No adverse effects were observed in the nursed infant, and neurobehavioral development of the infant was normal at two years of age.

Since amphetamines are potential drugs of abuse, the American Academy of Pediatrics regards amphetamines to be contraindicated during breast-feeding even though no adverse effects on the nursing infant have been published (Committee on Drugs, American Academy of Pediatrics, 1994).

Key References

Billing L, Eriksson M, Jonsson B, et al.: The influence of environmental factors on behavioural problems in 8-year-old children exposed to amphetamine during fetal life. Child Abuse Negl 28:3-9, 1994.

Committee on Drugs, American Academy of Pediatrics: The transfer of drugs and other chemicals into human milk. Pediatrics 93(1):137-150, 1994.

Eriksson M, Zetterstrom R: Amphetamine addiction during pregnancy: 10-year follow-up. Acta Paediatr Suppl 404:27-31, 1994.

Eriksson M, Zetterstrom R: The effect of amphetamine-addiction on the fetus and child. Teratology 24:39A, 1981.

Fein A, Shviro Y, Manoach M, Nebel L: Teratogenic effects of d-amphetamine sulphate: Histodifferentiation and electrocardiogram pattern of mouse embryonic heart. Teratology 35:27-34, 1987.

Heinonen OP, Slone D, Shapiro S: *Birth Defects and Drugs in Pregnancy.* Littleton, Mass.: John Wright-PSG, 1977, pp 346, 347, 350, 353, 355, 459, 491.

---

*This calculation is based on the following assumptions: maternal dose of dextroamphetamine: 20 mg/d; milk concentration of dextroamphetamine: 0.055-0.138 mcg/mL; milk intake by the nursing infant: 150 mL/kg/d; estimated dose of dextroamphetamine by the nursing infant: 0.008-0.02 mg/kg/d; lowest therapeutic dose of dextroamphetamine in adults: 0.08 mg/kg/d.

Holson R, Adams J, Buelkje-Sam J, et al.: d-amphetamine as a behavioral teratogen: Effects depend on dose, sex, age and task. Neurobehav Toxicol Teratol 7:753-758, 1985.

Levin JN: Amphetamine ingestion with biliary atresia. J Pediatr 79(1):130-131, 1971.

Lyon M, McClure WO: Investigations of fetal development models for prenatal drug exposure and schizophrenia. Prenatal d-amphetamine effects upon early and late juvenile behavior in the rat. Psychopharmacology 116:226-236, 1994.

Milkovich L, van den Berg BJ: Effects of antenatal exposure to anorectic drugs. Am J Obstet Gynecol 129:637-642, 1977.

Nelson MM, Forfar JO: Associations between drugs administered during pregnancy and congenital abnormalities of the fetus. Br Med J 1:523-527, 1971.

Nora JJ, McNamara DG, Fraser FC. Dexamphetamine sulfate and human malformations. Lancet 1:570-571, 1967.

Nora JJ, Trasler DG, Fraser FC: Malformations in mice induced by dexamphetamine sulphate. Lancet 2:1021-1022, 1965.

Nora JJ, Vargo TA, Nora AH, et al.: Dexamphetamine: A possible environmental trigger in cardiovascular malformations. Lancet 1:1290-1291, 1970.

Steiner E, Villen T, Hallberg M, Rane A: Amphetamine secretion in breast milk. Eur J Clin Pharmacol 27:123-124, 1984.

Torfs CP, Velie EM, Oechsli FW, et al.: A population-based study of gastroschisis: Demographic, pregnancy and lifestyle risk factors. Teratology 50:44-53, 1994.

DEXTROMETHORPHAN
(Drixoral®, Pertussin CS®, Vicks Formula 44®)

Dextromethorphan is an antitussive that is a component of many widely used cough medicines. Dextromethorphan is taken orally in doses of 60-120 mg/d.

Teratogenic Risk

*Magnitude of teratogenic
risk to child born after
exposure during gestation:*   *None*

The frequencies of congenital anomalies in general, of major malformations, and of minor anomalies were no greater than expected among the children of 300 women who used dextromethorphan during the first four lunar months of pregnancy in one epidemiological study (Heinonen et al., 1977). There was also no increase in the frequency of congenital anomalies among the children of 580 women who took dextromethorphan anytime during pregnancy in this study. The frequency of malformations was no greater than expected among the children of 59 women who used dextromethorphan during the first trimester of pregnancy in another study (Aselton et al., 1985). The anecdotal observation that four of five women who gave birth to infants with agenesis of the cloacal membrane in one series may have taken a cough medicine containing dextromethorphan during first trimester of pregnancy probably represents an unusual coincidence (Robinson & Tross, 1984).

No teratology studies of dextromethorphan in experimental animals have been published.

Risk Related to Breast-feeding

No information regarding the distribution of dextromethorphan in breast milk has been published.

Key References

Aselton P, Jick H, Milunsky A, et al.: First-trimester drug use and congenital disorders. Obstet Gynecol 65:451-455, 1985.

Heinonen OP, Slone D, Shapiro S: *Birth Defects and Drugs in Pregnancy*. Littleton, Mass.: John Wright-PSG, 1977, pp 379, 496.

Robinson HB Jr, Tross K: Agenesis of the cloacal membrane. A probable teratogenic anomaly. Perspect Pediatr Pathol 8:79-96, 1984.

DEXTROSTAT® *See* Dextroamphetamine

DIABENESE® *See* Chlorpropamide

DIACETYLMORPHINE *See* Heroin

DIAMOX® *See* Acetazolamide

DIAZEPAM
(Valium®)

Diazepam is a widely used benzodiazepine. It is employed as a tranquilizer, skeletal muscle relaxant, preoperative medication, and adjunct to anticonvulsants in the treatment of seizures. Diazepam is administered orally, parenterally, or rectally, usually in doses of 4-40 mg/d.

Teratogenic Risk

*Magnitude of teratogenic
risk to child born after
exposure during gestation:*   Minimal

*Quality and quantity of data
on which risk estimate is based:*   Good

Neonatal behavioral alterations have been observed in infants born to women treated with diazepam during pregnancy, but it is not known what, if any, implications this has for long-term development of these children (see below).

Available epidemiological data regarding the risk of malformations among children born to women who took diazepam during pregnancy are inconsistent. The frequency of congenital anomalies was not increased among the infants of more than 150 women who took diazepam during the first trimester of pregnancy in two cohorts of one study or among the infants of 60 women so treated in another study (Crombie et al., 1975; Jick et al., 1981; Aselton et al., 1985). No association with maternal use of diazepam during pregnancy was seen in a study involving 417 children with multiple congenital anomalies (Czeizel, 1988). In contrast, maternal use of diazepam during the first trimester of pregnancy was reported almost 3 times more frequently than expected in a study involving 1427 children with various congenital anomalies (Bracken & Holford, 1981) and almost 8 times more frequently than expected in another study involving 222 similarly-affected children (Restrepo et al., 1990).

No association with maternal use of diazepam during the first trimester of pregnancy was found among 611 children with oral clefts in a study that was designed specifically to test the hypothesis that first-trimester exposure to diazepam increases the risk of cleft lip with or without cleft palate or of cleft palate alone (Rosenberg et al., 1983). This finding is supported by three other studies involving 194, 522, and 1201 children with oral clefts, respectively (Saxen, 1975b; Czeizel, 1988), and by a study of the children of 854 women who took diazepam during the first trimester of pregnancy (Shiono & Mills, 1984). The negative results in these studies make it unlikely that maternal use of diazepam during the first trimester of pregnancy substantially increases the risk of cleft lip or palate in infants despite the previously reported associations found in 111, 49, and 599 children with oral clefts (Aarskog, 1975; Safra & Oakley, 1975; Saxen, 1975a).

Two studies involving 383 and 390 children with cardiovascular malformations have suggested an association with maternal use of diazepam or related drugs during the first trimester of pregnancy (Rothman et al., 1979; Bracken & Holford, 1981). However, Bracken (1986) reanalyzed the data from his study and failed to find a significant association, and Rothman reported that no association was found in a follow-up study of another 298 children with congenital heart disease (Zierler & Rothman, 1985). No association with maternal use of diazepam during the first trimester of pregnancy was seen in other studies involving 150 children with ventricular septal defect or 90 children with conotruncal malformations (Tikkanen & Heinonen, 1991, 1992).

Decreased birth weight and head circumference were observed in a series of 17 infants born to women who took diazepam or other benzodiazepines during pregnancy (Laegreid et al., 1992a). The weights of these children had become normal by ten months of age, but the head circumferences were still smaller than expected at 18 months (Laegreid et al., 1992b).

The suggestion that there exists a "benzodiazepine embryofetopathy" comprised of typical facial features, neurological dysfunction, and other anomalies (Laegreid et al., 1987, 1989, 1990, 1992b) is not generally accepted.

Treatment of pregnant women with diazepam during the third trimester of pregnancy or during delivery has resulted in apnea, hypotonia, and hypothermia in the newborn (Gillberg, 1977; Speight, 1977; Laegreid et al., 1992a). Tremors, irritability, and hypertonia reminiscent of neonatal narcotic withdrawal occur in some babies whose mothers were treated with diazepam chronically in the third trimester (Rementeria & Bhatt, 1977). In one study of 17 children born to mothers who took diazepam or other benzodiazepines during pregnancy, delayed gross motor development was observed at six and ten months, but at 18 months few differences from controls were apparent (Laegreid et al., 1992b; Viggedal et al., 1993).

A few apparently normal infants have been reported whose mothers took toxic doses of diazepam during pregnancy (Cerqueira et al., 1988; Czeizel, 1988). In most of these cases, the toxic ingestion occurred after the first trimester.

An increased frequency of malformations has been demonstrated among the offspring of mice and hamsters treated with diazepam during pregnancy, but only at doses hundreds of times larger than those used in humans (Weber, 1985). Cleft palate is the abnormality most commonly seen in affected mice; neural tube defects are most common in hamsters. Studies in rats and rabbits have generally not shown an increased frequency of malformations after maternal treatment with diazepam during pregnancy in doses as much as 150 times those usually employed in humans (Esaki et al., 1981; Weber, 1985). Diazepam treatment of rats, mice, and cats late in gestation causes persistent abnormalities of central nervous system biochemistry and function in the offspring (Weber, 1985; Kellogg et al., 1993; Rodriguez-Zafra et al., 1993; Perez-Laso et al., 1994). The relevance of these observations to the therapeutic use of diazepam in human pregnancy is unknown.

Risk Related to Breast-feeding

Diazepam and its active metabolite, desmethyldiazepam are excreted in breast milk. The amount of diazepam and desmethyldiazepam that the nursing infant would be expected to ingest is equivalent to <1-6% of the lowest therapeutic dose of diazepam in infants (Erkkola & Kanto, 1972; Cole & Hailey, 1975; Brandt, 1976; Wesson et al., 1985; Dusci et al., 1990).*

*This calculation is based on the following assumptions: maternal dose of diazepam: 6-80 mg/d; milk concentrations of diazepam and desmethyldiazepam: 0.01-0.31 mcg/mL and 0.01-0.14 mcg/mL, respectively; milk intake by the nursing infant: 150 mL/kg/d; estimated dose of both diazepam and desmethyldiazepam ingested by the nursing infant, assuming similar bioavailability, activity, and molecular weights: 0.003-0.07 mg/kg/d; lowest therapeutic dose of diazepam in infants: 1.2 mg/kg/d.

Observed levels of diazepam in infant serum varied from <0.01-0.2 mcg/mL (Erkkola & Kanto, 1972; Cole & Hailey, 1975; Brandt, 1976; Wesson et al., 1985; Dusci et al., 1990). The maximum concentration observed in infant serum is within the range of therapeutic serum concentrations found in adults.[†] Infant serum concentrations of desmethyldiazepam were similar to those of diazepam.

Sedation was observed in one of the infants when nursed shortly after taking diazepam (Wesson et al., 1985), and mild jaundice was reported in three other infants (Cole & Hailey, 1975). Lethargy and weight loss that resolved after discontinuation of breast-feeding were described in a nursing infant whose mother had taken diazepam (Patrick et al., 1972).

The American Academy of Pediatrics lists diazepam as a drug whose effect on the nursing infant may be of concern because of its potential to alter central nervous system functioning (Committee on Drugs, American Academy of Pediatrics, 1994). However, the WHO Working Group on Drugs and Human Lactation (1988) recommends that small acute doses of diazepam can be safely used by nursing mothers.

Key References

Aarskog D: Association between maternal intake of diazepam and oral clefts. Lancet 2:921, 1975.

Aselton P, Jick H, Milunsky A, et al.: First-trimester drug use and congenital disorders. Obstet Gynecol 65:451-455, 1985.

Bracken MB: Drug use in pregnancy and congenital heart disease in offspring. N Engl J Med 314:1120, 1986.

Bracken MB, Holford TR: Exposure to prescribed drugs in pregnancy and association with congenital malformations. Obstet Gynecol 58:336-344, 1981.

Brandt R: Passage of diazepam and desmethyldiazepam into breast milk. Arzneimittelforsch 26:454-457, 1976.

Cerqueira MJ, Olle C, Bellart J, et al.: Intoxication by benzodiazepines during pregnancy. Lancet 1:1341, 1988.

Cole AP, Hailey DM: Diazepam and active metabolite in breast milk and their transfer to the neonate. Arch Dis Child 50:741-742, 1975.

[†]Therapeutic serum levels of diazepam in adults: (0.07-2.8 mcg/mL).

Committee on Drugs, American Academy of Pediatrics: The transfer of drugs and other chemicals into human milk. Pediatrics 93(1):137-150, 1994.

Crombie DL, Pinsent RJ, Fleming DM, et al.: Fetal effects of tranquilizers in pregnancy. N Engl J Med 293:198-199, 1975.

Czeizel A: Lack of evidence of teratogenicity of benzodiazepine drugs in Hungary. Reprod Toxicol 1:183-188, 1988.

Dusci LJ, Good SM, Hall RW, Ilett KF: Excretion of diazepam and its metabolites in human milk during withdrawal from combination high dose diazepam and oxazepam. Br J Clin Pharmacol 29:123-126, 1990.

Erkkola R, Kanto J: Diazepam and breast-feeding. Lancet 1:1235-1236, 1972.

Esaki K, Sakai Y, Yanagita T: Effects of oral administration of alprazolam (TUS-1) on rabbit fetus. Jitchuken Zenrinsho Kenkyuho 7:79-90, 1981.

Gillberg C: "Floppy infant syndrome" and maternal diazepam. Lancet 2:244, 1977.

Jick H, Holmes LB, Hunter JR, et al.: First-trimester drug use and congenital disorders. JAMA 246:343-346, 1981.

Kellogg CK, Taylor MK, Rodriguez-Zafra, Pleger GL: Altered stressor-induced changes in GABA(A) receptor function in the cerebral cortex of adult rats exposed in utero to diazepam. Pharmacol Biochem Behav 44(2):267-273, 1993.

Laegreid L, Hagberg G, Lundberg A: The effect of benzodiazepines on the fetus and the newborn. Neuropediatrics 23:18-23, 1992a.

Laegreid L, Hagberg G, Lundberg A: Neurodevelopment in late infancy after prenatal exposure to benzodiazepines--A prospective study. Neuropediatrics 23:60-67, 1992b.

Laegreid L, Olegard R, Conradi N, et al.: Congenital malformations and maternal consumption of benzodiazepines: A case-control study. Dev Med Child Neurol 32:432-441, 1990.

Laegreid L, Olegard R, Wahlstrom J, Conradi N: Abnormalities in children exposed to benzodiazepines in utero. Lancet 1:108-109, 1987.

Laegreid L, Olegard R, Walstrom J, Conradi N: Teratogenic effects of benzodiazepine use during pregnancy. J Pediatr 114:126-131, 1989.

Patrick MJ, Tilstone WJ, Reavey P: Diazepam and breast-feeding. Lancet 1:542-543, 1972.

Perez-Laso C, Valencia A, Rodriguez-Zafra M, et al.: Perinatal administration of diazepam alters sexual dimorphism in the rat accessory olfactory bulb. Brain Res 634:1-6, 1994.

Rementeria JL, Bhatt K: Withdrawal symptoms in neonates from intrauterine exposure to diazepam. J Pediatr 90:123-126, 1977.

Restrepo M, Munoz N, Day N, et al.: Birth defects among children born to a population occupationally exposed to pesticides in Colombia. Scand J Work Environ Health 16:239-246, 1990.

Rodriguez-Zafra M, de Blas MR, Perez-Laso C, et al.: Effects of perinatal diazepam exposure on the sexually dimorphic rat locus coeruleus. Neurotoxicol Teratol 15:139-144, 1993.

Rosenberg L, Mitchell AA, Parsells JL, et al.: Lack of relation of oral clefts to diazepam use during pregnancy. N Engl J Med 309:1282-1285, 1983.

Rothman KJ, Fyler DC, Goldblatt A, Kreidberg MB: Exogenous hormones and other drug exposures of children with congenital heart disease. Am J Epidemiol 109:433-439, 1979.

Safra MJ, Oakley GP Jr: Association between cleft lip with or without cleft palate and prenatal exposure to diazepam. Lancet 2:478-479, 1975.

Saxen I: Associations between oral clefts and drugs taken during pregnancy. Int J Epidemiol 4:37-44, 1975a.

Saxen I: Epidemiology of cleft lip and palate. Int J Prev Soc Med 29:103-110, 1975b.

Shiono PH, Mills JL: Oral clefts and diazepam use during pregnancy. N Engl J Med 311:919-920, 1984.

Speight ANP: Floppy-infant syndrome and maternal diazepam and/or nitrazepam. Lancet 2:878, 1977.

Tikkanen J, Heinonen OP: Risk factors for conal malformations of the heart. Eur J Epidemiol 8(1):48-57, 1992.

Tikkanen J, Heinonen OP: Risk factors for ventricular septal defect in Finland. Public Health 105:99-112, 1991.

Viggedal G, Hagberg BS, Laegreid L, Aronsson M: Mental development in late infancy after prenatal exposure to benzodiazepines--a prospective study. J Child Psychol Psychiatry 34(3):295-305, 1993.

Weber LWD: Benzodiazepines in pregnancy--academical debate or teratogenic risk? Biol Res Pregnancy 6:151-167, 1985.

Wesson DR, Camber S, Harkey M, Smith DE: Diazepam and desmethyldiazepam in breast milk. J Psychoactive Drugs 17:55-56, 1985.

WHO Working Group on Drugs and Human Lactation. In: Bennet PN (ed). *Drugs and Human Lactation*. Amsterdam: Elsevier, 1988, p 358-359.

Zierler S, Rothman KJ: Congenital heart disease in relation to maternal use of Bendectin and other drugs in early pregnancy. N Engl J Med 313:347-352, 1985.

DICOUMARIN *See* Dicumarol

DICUMAROL
(Dicoumarin)

Dicumarol is a coumarin anticoagulant that is administered orally in doses of 25-300 mg/d.

Teratogenic Risk

*Magnitude of teratogenic
risk to child born after
exposure during gestation:*   *Moderate*

*Quality and quantity of data
on which risk estimate is based:*   *Fair to good*

It seems likely that maternal use of dicumarol during pregnancy is associated with teratogenic and perinatal risks similar to those of warfarin. Please see agent summary on warfarin for information on this closely related drug that has been more thoroughly studied.

In a series of 78 pregnancies in women who were treated with dicumarol for cardiac valve prostheses, there were 35 (45%) abortions and 43 liveborn infants (Quaini et al., 1986). Among the latter, four infants had petechiae or cutaneous hematomas; one child had cleft lip and palate; and another had abnormal occipital calcification, hypoplasia of the nasal cartilage, choanal stenosis, and fatal respiratory insufficiency. The features in this last infant are typical of those that may be caused by maternal use during pregnancy of warfarin, a closely related drug (Hall et al., 1980). Among 29 infants born to women treated with dicumarol during pregnancy and reported prior to 1965, there were six fetal deaths, three of which were demonstrably associated with hemorrhage, and two liveborn infants who had intracranial hemorrhage (Villasanta, 1965). In addition, one child had optic atrophy, microcephaly, and cerebral agenesis, but it is uncertain which anticoagulant this mother took during pregnancy (Quenneville et al., 1959). In another series of 20 pregnancies among women treated with dicumarol, four of the infants were stillborn (Fillmore & McDevitt, 1970).

Fatal neonatal hemorrhage was often observed among the offspring of dogs and rabbits treated during pregnancy with dicumarol in doses similar to those used in humans (Quick, 1946; Kraus et al., 1949). Fetal death occurred frequently among the offspring of rabbits and mink treated during pregnancy with dicumarol in doses within or below the human therapeutic range (Kraus et al., 1949; Kangas & Makela, 1974).

Risk Related to Breast-feeding

No information regarding the distribution of dicumarol in breast milk has been published. No anticoagulant effect or evidence of toxicity was observed in the infants of 125 breast-feeding mothers who were given dicumarol for three weeks following delivery (Brambel & Hunter, 1950). Nursing infants whose mothers are taking dicumarol should be monitored for signs of hypothrombinemia.

Key References

Brambel CE, Hunter RE: Effect of dicumarol on the nursing infant. Am J Obstet Gynecol 59:1153-1159, 1950.

Fillmore SJ, McDevitt E: Effects of coumarin compounds on the fetus. Ann Intern Med 73:731-735, 1970.

Hall JG, Pauli RM, Wilson KM: Maternal and fetal sequelae of anticoagulation during pregnancy. Am J Med 68:122-140, 1980.

Kangas J, Makela J: Dikumarols abortframkallande effekt hos mink. Nord Veteriaermed 26:444-447, 1974.

Kraus AP, Perlow S, Singer K: Danger of dicumarol treatment in pregnancy. JAMA 139:758-762, 1949.

Quaini E, Vitali E, Colombo T, Donatelli F: Complicanze materne e fetali in 105 gravidanze di portatrici di protesi valvolari cardiache. Minerva Ginecol 38:217-224, 1986.

Quenneville G, Barton B, McDevitt E, et al.: The use of anticoagulants for thrombophlebitis during pregnancy. Am J Obstet Gynecol 77:1135-1149, 1959.

Quick AJ: Experimentally induced changes in the prothrombin level of the blood. III. Prothrombin concentration of new-born pups of a mother given dicumarol before parturition. J Biol Chem 164:371-376, 1946.

Villasanta U: Thromboembolic disease in pregnancy. Am J Obstet Gynecol 93:142-160, 1965.

DICYCLOMINE
(Antispas®, Bentyl®, Spasmoban®)

Dicyclomine is an anticholinergic agent with peripheral effects similar to, but considerably weaker than, those of atropine. Dicyclomine is given orally or parenterally in doses of 30-160 mg/d to treat irritable bowel syndrome.

Teratogenic Risk

Magnitude of teratogenic risk to child born after exposure during gestation:	*None*
Quality and quantity of data on which risk estimate is based:	*Good*

Most human studies of dicyclomine were undertaken when the drug was a component of Bendectin, a medication that is no longer on the market. These data are not summarized here, but several comprehensive reviews of the extensive teratology studies on Bendectin are available (MacMahon, 1982; Cordero & Oakley, 1983; Holmes, 1983; Sheffield & Batagol, 1985) The studies indicate that maternal use of Bendectin early in pregnancy did not measurably increase the risk of congenital anomalies in children. (Dicyclomine was removed from Bendectin in 1976 in the US when Bendectin was reformulated.)

The frequency of congenital anomalies was no greater than expected among the infants of 97 women who took dicyclomine during the first trimester of pregnancy in one study (Aselton et al., 1985). An increased frequency of phocomelia was observed among 1327 children of women who took dicyclomine during the first trimester of pregnancy in a Tasmanian cohort study (Correy et al., 1991). This association is of marginal statistical significance and is based on only two cases in the exposed group. Studies such as this one that include multiple comparisons between maternal drug exposures and various birth defect outcomes are expected to show occasional associations with nominal statistical significance purely by chance. Moreover, the finding is inconsistent with studies of Bendectin use during pregnancy that do not show such an association.

Studies in rats and rabbits suggest that treatment of pregnant women with dicyclomine in usual therapeutic doses is unlikely to increase the children's risk of malformations greatly (Gibson et al., 1968).

Risk Related to Breast-feeding

No information regarding the distribution of dicyclomine in breast milk has been published.

Key References

Aselton P, Jick H, Milunsky A, et al.: First-trimester drug use and congenital disorders. Obstet Gynecol 65:451-455, 1985.

Cordero JF, Oakley GP: Drug exposure during pregnancy: Some epidemiologic considerations. Clin Obstet Gynecol 26:418-428, 1983.

Correy JF, Newman NM, Collins JA, et al.: Use of prescription drugs in the first trimester and congenital malformations. Aust NZ J Obstet Gynaecol 31(4):340-344, 1991.

Gibson JP, Staples RE, Larson EJ, et al.: Teratology and reproduction studies with an antinauseant. Toxicol Appl Pharmacol 13:439-447, 1968.

Holmes LB: Teratogen update: Bendectin. Teratology 27:277-281, 1983.

MacMahon B: More on Bendectin. JAMA 246:371-372, 1982.

Sheffield LJ, Batagol R: The creation of therapeutic orphans--or, what have we learnt from the debendox fiasco? Med J Aust 143:143-147, 1985.

DIETHYLSTILBESTROL
(DES, Stilboestrol)

Diethylstilbestrol (DES) is a nonsteroidal synthetic estrogen that is used in the palliative treatment of breast carcinoma. It is usually given orally in a dose of 15 mg/d. Doses up to 50 mg/d have been prescribed for postcoital contraception.

Teratogenic Risk

Magnitude of teratogenic
risk to child born after
exposure during gestation:
    For clear cell carcinoma
      of the cervix: *Minimal to small*
    For genital tract anomalies
      in females: *Small to moderate*
    For genital tract anomalies
      in males: *Minimal*
    For nongenital congenital
      anomalies: *None to minimal*

Quality and quantity of data
on which risk estimate is based:
    For clear cell carcinoma
      of the cervix: *Good*
    For genital tract anomalies
      in females: *Fair to good*
    For genital tract anomalies
      in males: *Poor to fair*
    For nongenital congenital
      anomalies: *Fair to good*

Adenosis and other abnormalities of the vagina are very common among the daughters of women who were treated with diethylstilbestrol in pregnancy. Gross structural abnormalities of the cervix or vagina occur in about one-fourth and histological abnormalities of the vaginal epithelium in at least one-third to one-half of women whose mothers took DES during gestation (Kaufman et al., 1984; Robboy et al., 1984; Vessey, 1989). Malformations, such as T-shaped uterus, constricting bands of the uterine cavity, uterine hypoplasia, or para-ovarian cysts, also occur with increased frequency.

Several studies suggest that development of clear cell adenocarcinoma, a rare tumor of the vagina or cervix, is associated with in utero exposure to DES (Herbst et al., 1971; Marselos & Tomatis, 1992; Emens, 1994; Giusti et al., 1995). In a registry that includes more than 500 cases of clear cell adenocarcinoma of the vagina diagnosed in the

US since 1971, prenatal exposure to DES was reported in 60% of patients in whom maternal history was available (Melnick et al., 1987; Herbst & Anderson, 1990). The median age at which malignancy was diagnosed was 19 years. The risk that a woman whose mother took DES during pregnancy will develop clear cell adenocarcinoma of the vagina or cervix by age 34 is estimated to be about 1/1000. The risk of vaginal or cervical squamous cell intraepithelial neoplasia has been estimated to be about twice as great as expected among women who were exposed in utero to DES (Robboy et al., 1984; Bornstein et al., 1988). Available data on genital tract neoplasms among women exposed to DES in utero are subject to several potential biases, and some authors question whether the observed associations between prenatal DES exposure and malignancy are causal (McFarlane et al., 1986; Bornstein et al., 1988; Edelman, 1989).

Ectopic implantation, miscarriage, and premature delivery are more common than expected among the pregnancies of women whose mothers took DES during gestation (Linn et al., 1988; de Hass et al., 1991; Heffner et al., 1993; Giusti et al., 1995). Some studies have also shown an increased frequency of infertility among these women (Herbst et al., 1980; Senekjian et al., 1988). This may be a result of the uterine abnormalities associated with prenatal DES exposure (Berger & Alper, 1986; Kaufman et al., 1986).

Most studies suggest that epididymal cysts, hypoplastic testes, cryptorchidism, and abnormalities on semen analysis are more frequent than expected among the sons of mothers treated with DES during pregnancy (Bibbo et al., 1977; Gill et al., 1979; Shy et al., 1984; Giusti et al., 1995; Wilcox et al., 1995). However, men who were exposed to DES in utero do not appear to have any impairment of fertility or sexual function even if they do have such genital anomalies (Wilcox et al., 1995). An association between maternal treatment with DES during pregnancy and subsequent development of testicular cancer in their sons has been suggested, but the data are inconsistent (Gershman & Stolley, 1988; Vessey, 1989; Giusti et al., 1995).

In a large epidemiological study in which genital abnormalities of the type discussed above would not be detected, the frequencies of congenital anomalies in general, of major malformations, and of minor anomalies were no greater than expected among the children of 164 women treated with DES during the first four lunar months of pregnancy (Heinonen et al., 1977). Similarly, the frequency of congenital anomalies was not increased among the children of 233 women treated with this drug anytime during pregnancy.

Depression, anxiety, eating disorders, altered psychosexual behavior, and variations in cognitive function have been reported with increased frequency among adult children of women treated with DES during pregnancy (Gustavson et al., 1991; Lish et al., 1991; Reinisch & Sanders, 1992; Newbold, 1993; Pillard et al., 1993; Giusti et al., 1995). The effects observed have varied in different studies and may be related, at least in part, to the perceived burden of being a "DES daughter or son" rather than to prenatal exposure to DES per se.

Gross and microscopic genital tract abnormalities similar to those found in humans have been observed among the offspring of monkeys treated during pregnancy with DES in doses within the human therapeutic range (Walker, 1989). Similar findings have been reported in mice, rats, hamsters, guinea pigs, and ferrets (Walker, 1989; Marselos & Tomatis, 1993). Neoplasms of the uterus, vagina, breast, pituitary gland, rete testis, and testis have been found among the offspring of DES-treated rodents in some studies (Walker, 1989; Walker & Kurth, 1993).

Risk Related to Breast-feeding

No information on the distribution of DES in breast milk has been published.

Key References

Berger MJ, Alper MM: Intractable primary infertility in women exposed to diethylstilbestrol in utero. J Reprod Med 31(4):231-235, 1986.

Bibbo M, Gill WB, Azizi F, et al.: Follow-up study of male and female offspring of DES-exposed mothers. Obstet Gynecol 49(1):1-8, 1977.

Bornstein J, Adam E, Adler-Storthz K, Kaufman RH: Development of cervical and vaginal squamous cell neoplasia as a late consequence of in utero exposure to diethylstilbestrol. Obstet Gynecol Surv 43(1):15-21, 1988.

de Haas I, Harlow BL, Cramer DW, Frigoletto FD Jr: Spontaneous preterm birth: A case-control study. Am J Obstet Gynecol 165:1290-1296, 1991.

Edelman DA: Diethylstilbestrol exposure and the risk of clear cell cervical and vaginal adenocarcinoma. Int J Fertil 34(4):251-255, 1989.

Emens JM: Continuing problems with diethylstilboestrol. Br J Obstet Gynaecol 101:748-750, 1994.

Gershman ST, Stolley PD: A case-control study of testicular cancer using Connecticut tumour registry data. Int J Epidemiol 17(4):738-742, 1988.

Gill WB, Schumacher GFB, Bibbo M, et al.: Association of diethylstilbestrol exposure in utero with cryptorchidism, testicular hypoplasia and semen abnormalities. J Urol 122:36-39, 1979.

Giusti RM, Iwamoto K, Hatch EE: Diethylstilbestrol revisited: A review of the long-term health effects. Ann Intern Med 122:778-788, 1995.

Gustavson CR, Gustavson JC, Noller KL, et al.: Increased risk of profound weight loss among women exposed to diethylstilbestrol in utero. Behav Neural Biol 55:307-312, 1991.

Heffner LJ, Sherman CB, Speizer FE, Weiss ST: Clinical and environmental predictors of preterm labor. Obstet Gynecol 81:750-757, 1993.

Heinonen OP, Slone D, Shapiro S: *Birth Defects and Drugs in Pregnancy.* Littleton, Mass.: John Wright-PSG, 1977, pp 389-391, 433.

Herbst AL, Anderson D: Clear cell adenocarcinoma of the vagina and cervix secondary to intrauterine exposure to diethylstilbestrol. Semin Surg Oncol 6(6):343-346, 1990.

Herbst AL, Hubby MM, Blough RR, Azizi F: A comparison of pregnancy experience in DES-exposed and DES-unexposed daughters. J Reprod Med 24:62-69, 1980.

Herbst AL, Ulfelder H, Poskanzer DC: Adenocarcinoma of the vagina. Association of maternal stilbestrol therapy with tumor appearance in young women. N Engl J Med 284(16):878-881, 1971.

Kaufman RH, Adam E, Noller K, et al.: Upper genital tract changes and infertility in diethylstilbestrol-exposed women. Am J Obstet Gynecol 154(6):1312-1318, 1986.

Kaufman RH, Noller K, Adam E, et al.: Upper genital tract abnormalities and pregnancy outcome in diethylstilbestrol-exposed progeny. Am J Obstet Gynecol 148:973-984, 1984.

Linn S, Lieberman E, Schoenbaum SC, et al.: Adverse outcomes of pregnancy in women exposed to diethylstilbestrol in utero. J Reprod Med 33(1):3-7, 1988.

Lish JD, Ehrhardt AA, Meyer-Bahlburg HFL, et al.: Gender-related behavior development in females exposed to diethylstilbestrol (DES) in utero: An attempted replication. J Am Acad Child Adolesc Psychiatry 30(1):29-37, 1991.

Marselos M, Tomatis L: Diethylstilboestrol: I, Pharmacology, toxicology and carcinogenicity in humans. Eur J Cancer 28A(6/7):1182-1189, 1992.

Marselos M, Tomatis L: Diethylstilboestrol: II, Pharmacology, toxicology and carcinogenicity in experimental animals. Eur J Cancer 29A(1):149-155, 1993.

McFarlane MJ, Feinstein AR, Horwitz RI: Diethylstilbestrol and clear cell vaginal carcinoma. Reappraisal of the epidemiologic evidence. Am J Med 81:855-863, 1986.

Melnick S, Cole P, Anderson D, Herbst A: Rates and risks of diethylstilbestrol-related clear-cell adenocarcinoma of the vagina and cervix. N Engl J Med 316(9):514-516, 1987.

Newbold RR: Gender-related behavior in women exposed prenatally to diethylstilbestrol. Environ Health Perspect 101:208-213, 1993.

Pillard RC, Rosen LR, Meyer-Bahlburg H, et al.: Psychopathology and social functioning in men prenatally exposed to diethylstilbestrol (DES). Psychosom Med 55:485-491, 1993.

Reinisch JM, Sanders SA: Effects of prenatal exposure to diethylstilbestrol (DES) on hemispheric laterality and spatial ability in human males. Horm Behav 25:62-75, 1992.

Robboy SJ, Noller KL, O'Brien P, et al.: Increased incidence of cervical and vaginal dysplasia in 3,980 diethylstilbestrol-exposed young women. Experience of the National Collaborative Diethylstilbestrol Adenosis Project. JAMA 252:2979-2983, 1984.

Senekjian EK, Potkul RK, Frey K, Herbst AL: Infertility among daughters either exposed or not exposed to diethylstilbestrol. Am J Obstet Gynecol 158:493-498, 1988.

Shy KK, Stenchever MA, Karp LE, et al.: Genital tract examinations and zona-free hamster egg penetration tests from men exposed in utero to diethylstilbestrol. Fertil Steril 42(5):772-778, 1984.

Vessey MP: Epidemiological studies of the effects of diethylstilboestrol. IARC Sci Publ (96):335-348, 1989.

Walker BE: Animal models of prenatal exposure to diethylstilboestrol. IARC Sci Publ (96):349-364, 1989.

Walker BE, Kurth LA: Pituitary tumors in mice exposed prenatally to diethylstilbestrol. Cancer Res 53:1546-1549, 1993.

Wilcox AJ, Baird DD, Weinberg CR, et al.: Fertility in men exposed prenatally to diethylstilbestrol. N Engl J Med 332:1411-1416, 1995.

DIFLUCAN® *See* Fluconazole

DIFLUNISAL
(Dolobid®)

Diflunisal is a salicylate analgesic in the treatment of arthritis. Diflunisal is given orally in doses of 500-1500 mg/d.

Teratogenic Risk

*Magnitude of teratogenic
risk to child born after
exposure during gestation:*   *Undetermined*

*Quality and quantity of data
on which risk estimate is based:*   *Poor*

A small risk cannot be excluded, but there is no indication that the risk of congenital anomalies in the children of women treated with diflunisal during pregnancy is likely to be great.

No epidemiological studies of congenital anomalies in children of women who took diflunisal during pregnancy have been reported.

No teratogenic effect was observed among the offspring of cynomolgus monkeys treated with 1-3 times the human therapeutic dose of diflunisal during pregnancy (Rowland et al., 1987). The frequency of malformations was not increased among the offspring of rats or rabbits treated during pregnancy with diflunisal in doses, respectively, 1-4 and 1-2 times those used in humans (Nakatsuka & Fujii, 1979; Clark et al., 1984). In rabbits, increases in fetal death and vertebral anomalies were observed with higher doses, but these were toxic to the mothers.

Please see agent summary on aspirin for information on a related agent that has been more thoroughly studied.

Risk Related to Breast-feeding

Diflunisal is excreted in breast milk at concentrations ranging from 2-7% of the maternal plasma concentration (USP DI, 1995). On the basis of this data, the amount of diflunisal that the nursing infant would be expected to ingest is between 3.8-13% of the lowest weight-adjusted therapeutic dose of diflunisal.*

Key References

Clark RL, Robertson RT, Minsker DH, et al.: Diflunisal-induced maternal anemia as a cause of teratogenicity in rabbits. Teratology 30:319-332, 1984.

Nakatsuka T, Fujii T: Comparative teratogenicity study of diflunisal (MK-647) and aspirin in the rat. Oyo Yakuri 17:551-557, 1979.

Rowland JM, Robertson RT, Cukierski M, et al.: Evaluation of the teratogenicity and pharmacokinetics of diflunisal in cynomolgus monkeys. Fundam Appl Toxicol 8:51-58, 1987.

USP DI: Nonsteroidal anti-inflammatory drugs. In: *USP DI (USP Dispensing Information), Volume 1. Drug Information for the Health Care Professional*, 15th ed. Rockville, Md.: The US Pharmacopeial Convention, 1995, p 2002.

*This calculation is based on the following assumptions: therapeutic serum concentration of diflunisal in adults: 100 mcg/mL; milk concentration of diflunisal: 2-7 mcg/mL; milk intake by the nursing infant: 150 mL/kg/d; estimated dose of diflunisal ingested by the nursing infant: 0.3-1 mg/kg/d; lowest therapeutic dose of diflunisal in adults: 7.8 mg/kg/d.

DIGOXIN
(Lanoxicaps®, Lanoxin®)

Digoxin is a cardiac glycoside used in the treatment of heart failure and cardiac arrhythmias. The usual maintenance dose is 0.125-0.5 mg/d; somewhat larger loading doses are often administered when beginning treatment. Digoxin may be given orally or intravenously. Therapeutic serum concentrations are 0.8-2 ng/mL; serum levels above 2 ng/mL are considered to be toxic.

Teratogenic Risk

*Magnitude of teratogenic
risk to child born after
exposure during gestation:*   *Unlikely*

*Quality and quantity of data
on which risk estimate is based:*   *Fair*

Therapeutic doses of digoxin are unlikely to pose a substantial teratogenic risk, but the data are insufficient to state that there is no risk.

The frequency of congenital anomalies was no greater than expected among the infants of 142 women who were treated with digoxin in the first trimester of pregnancy in one epidemiological study (Aselton et al., 1985). Similarly, the frequency of congenital anomalies was not increased among the children of 52 women treated with cardiac glycosides in the first four lunar months of pregnancy or of 129 women treated with these agents anytime in pregnancy in another large study (Heinonen et al., 1977).

Studies in rats and rabbits suggest that treatment of pregnant women with cardiac glycosides in usual therapeutic doses is unlikely to increase the children's risk of malformations greatly (Hatano, 1976; Nagaoka et al., 1976).

Fetal cardiac arrhythmia and hydrops have been treated successfully during the second half of pregnancy by administration of digoxin to the mother or directly to the fetus (Weiner et al., 1988; Maeda et al., 1992; Cox & Gardner, 1993).

Maternal digitalis toxicity may cause serious or even fatal arrhythmias in the fetus or neonate (Sherman & Locke, 1960; Potondi, 1966).

Risk Related to Breast-feeding

Digoxin is excreted into breast milk in small amounts. The amount of digoxin that the nursing infant would be expected to receive is <1% of the lowest infant dose, based on data from eight lactating women (Levy, 1977; Loughnan, 1978; Finley et al., 1979).*

Infant plasma levels of digoxin were measured in three of the infants and found to range between <12-25% of the lowest therapeutic plasma level of digoxin (Loughnan, 1978; Finley et al., 1979).[†]

The American Academy of Pediatrics regards digoxin to be safe to use while breast-feeding (Committee on Drugs, American Academy of Pediatrics, 1994).

---

*This calculation is based on the following assumptions: maternal dose of digoxin: 0.25-0.75 mg/d; milk concentration of digoxin: 0.0003-0.002 mcg/mL; milk intake by the nursing infant: 150 mL/kg/d; estimated dose of digoxin ingested by the nursing infant: 0.045-0.28 mcg/kg/d; lowest dose of digoxin in infants: 0.2 mg/kg/d.

†Infant serum levels of digoxin: <0.1-0.2 ng/mL; lowest therapeutic plasma level of digoxin in children: 0.8 ng/mL.

Key References

Aselton P, Jick H, Milunsky A, et al.: First-trimester drug use and congenital disorders. Obstet Gynecol 65:451-455, 1985.

Committee on Drugs, American Academy of Pediatrics: The transfer of drugs and other chemicals into human milk. Pediatrics 93(1):137-150, 1994.

Cox JL, Gardner MJ: Treatment of cardiac arrhythmias during pregnancy. Prog Cardiovasc Dis 36(2):137-178, 1993.

Finley JP, Waxman MB, Wong PY, Lickrish GM: Digoxin excretion in human milk. J Pediatr 94:339, 1979.

Hatano M, Nagaoka T, Osuka F, Shigemura T: Reproduction studies of beta-methyldigoxin. 1. Teratogenicity study in rats. Kiso To Rinsho (Clin Rep) 10:579-593, 1976.

Heinonen OP, Slone D, Shapiro S: *Birth Defects and Drugs in Pregnancy.* Littleton, Mass.: John Wright-PSG, 1977, pp 441, 496.

Levy M, Granit L, Laufer N: Excretion of drugs in human milk. N Engl J Med 297(14):789, 1977.

Loughnan PM: Digoxin excretion in human breast milk. J Pediatr 92:1019-1020, 1978.

Maeda H, Koyanagi T, Nakano H: Intrauterine treatment on non-immune hydrops fetalis. Early Hum Dev 29:241-249, 1992.

Nagaoka T, Osuka F, Shigemura T, Hatano M: Teratogenicity test of β-methyldigoxin (β-MD). Kiso To Rinsho (Clin Rep) 10:405-411, 1976.

Potondi A: Congenital rhabdomyoma of the heart and intrauterine digitalis poisoning. J Forensic Sci 11:81-88, 1966.

Sherman JL Jr, Locke RV: Transplacental neonatal digitalis intoxication. Am J Cardiol 6:834-837, 1960.

Weiner CP, Thompson MIB: Direct treatment of fetal supraventricular tachycardia after faile transplacental therapy. Am J Obstet Gynecol 158:570-573, 1988.

DIHYDROCODEINE
(Hydrocodeine)

Dihydrocodeine is a narcotic analgesic. It is usually given orally in doses of 40-60 mg/d as a cough suppressant and in doses of 120-180 mg/d for relief of pain.

Teratogenic Risk

*Magnitude of teratogenic
risk to child born after
exposure during gestation:*   *Undetermined*

*Quality and quantity of data
on which risk estimate is based:*   *None*

No epidemiological studies of congenital anomalies in infants born to women who used dihydrocodeine during pregnancy have been reported.

No animal teratology studies of dihydrocodeine have been published.

Please see agent summary on codeine for information on a closely related dru gthat has been more thoroughly studied.

Risk Related to Breast-feeding

No information regarding the distribution of dihydrocodeine in breast milk has been published.

Key References

None available.

DILACOR® *See* Diltiazem

DILANTIN® *See* Phenytoin

DILTIAZEM
(Cardizem CD®, Dilacor®)

Diltiazem is a calcium channel-blocking agent used in the management of hypertension, angina pectoris, and cardiac arrhythmias. Diltiazem is given orally or intravenously in doses of 90-540 mg/d.

Teratogenic Risk

*Magnitude of teratogenic
risk to child born after
exposure during gestation:*   *Undetermined*

*Quality and quantity of data
on which risk estimate is based:*   *Very poor*

No epidemiological studies of congenital anomalies among infants born to women treated with diltiazem during pregnancy have been reported.

An increased frequency of embryonic loss was observed among pregnant rabbits, mice, and rats treated with diltiazem in doses respectively 2, 2, and 6 or more times those used in humans (Ariyuki, 1975). Malformations of the limbs and tail were observed in the offspring of rabbits and rats, but not mice, treated with similar doses. No significant teratogenic effect was observed among the offspring of animals of these three species treated with smaller doses of diltiazem during pregnancy. In another study, the frequency of fetal anomalies, primarily palatal defects, and hydrocephalus, was increased among the offspring of pregnant mice treated with diltiazem in doses similar to those used in humans (Mahalik & Hitner, 1992). The relevance, if any, of these findings to the therapeutic use of diltiazem in human pregnancy is unknown.

Diltiazem, in doses 7 times those used clinically, inhibits labor in rats at term (Hahn et al., 1984). This effect has not been studied in humans.

Risk Related to Breast-feeding

Diltiazem is excreted into breast milk in amounts similar to those found in maternal serum (Okada et al., 1985). The amount of diltiazem that the nursing infant would be expected to ingest is approximately 1% of the lowest weight-adjusted therapeutic dose, based on data from a single patient (Okada et al., 1985).*

*This calculation is based on the following assumptions: maternal dose of diltiazem: 240 mg/d; milk concentration of diltiazem: <0.05-0.2 mcg/mL; milk intake by the nursing infant: 150 mL/kg/d; estimated dose of diltiazem ingested by the nursing infant: 0.007-0.03 mg/kg/d; lowest therapeutic dose of diltiazem in adults: 1.5 mg/kg/d.

No adverse effects were found in breast-fed twins of a woman who was treated diltiazem throughout pregnancy and during breast-feeding (Lubbe, 1987). Breast milk and infant serum levels were not measured.

The American Academy of Pediatrics regards diltiazem to be safe to use during breast-feeding (Committee on Drugs, American Academy of Pediatrics, 1994).

Key References

Ariyuki F: Effects of diltiazem hydrochloride on embryonic development: Species differences in the susceptibility and stage specificity in mice, rats, and rabbits. Okajimas Folia Anat Jpn 52:103-117, 1975.

Committee on Drugs, American Academy of Pediatrics: The transfer of drugs and other chemicals into human milk. Pediatrics 93(1):137-150, 1994.

Hahn DW, McGuire JL, Vanderhoof M, et al.: Evaluation of drugs for arrest of premature labor in a new animal model. Am J Obstet Gynecol 148:775-778, 1984.

Lubbe WF: Use of diltiazem during pregnancy. NZ Med J 100:121, 1987.

Mahalik MP, Hitner HW: Antagonism of cocaine-induced fetal anomalies by prazosin and diltiazem in mice. Reprod Toxicol 6:161-169, 1992.

Okada M, Inoue H, Nakamura Y, et al.: Excretion of diltiazem in human milk. N Engl J Med 312(15):992-993, 1985.

DIPHENHYDRAMINE
(Allergan®, Benadryl®, Sleep-EZE D®)

Diphenhydramine is an ethanolamine antihistamine. It is used orally and parenterally to treat allergic reactions and nausea and vomitting. Diphenhydramine is also given orally as a hypnotic and to treat coughs, colds, and Parkinson's disease. Daily doses vary from 50-400 mg, depending on indication and frequency of administration.

Teratogenic Risk

*Magnitude of teratogenic
risk to child born after
exposure during gestation:*   *Unlikely*

225

Quality and quantity of data
on which risk estimate is based: *Fair to good*

Therapeutic doses of diphenhydramine are unlikely to pose a substantial teratogenic risk, but the data are insufficient to state that there is no risk.

The frequencies of congenital anomalies in general, of major malformations, minor anomalies, and major categories of congenital anomalies were no greater than expected among the children of 595 women who took diphenhydramine during the first four lunar months of pregnancy in one large epidemiological study (Heinonen et al., 1977). The frequency of congenital anomalies among the children of 2948 women who took this drug anytime during pregnancy was also no greater than expected. Similarly, the frequency of malformations was no greater than expected among the infants of a total of 631 women who used diphenhydramine during the first trimester of pregnancy in two cohorts of another large epidemiological study (Jick et al., 1981; Aselton et al., 1985).

An association with maternal first-trimester use of diphenhydramine was observed in a study of 590 children with oral clefts (Saxen, 1974), but no relationship between oral clefts and maternal use of diphenhydramine early in pregnancy was apparent in another investigation (Heinonen et al., 1977). A causal basis for the association does not seem likely on the basis of available data.

Studies in mice, rats, and rabbits suggest that treatment of pregnant women with diphenhydramine in usual therapeutic doses is unlikely to increase the children's risk of malformations greatly (Iuliucci & Gautieri, 1971; Schardein et al., 1971; Jones-Price et al., 1982a, b, 1983).

Uterine hyperstimulation and associated fetal compromise have been reported in women given diphenhydramine during labor (Hay & Wood, 1967; Hara et al., 1980).

Risk Related to Breast-feeding

No information on the distribution of diphenhydramine in breast milk has been published.

The American Academy of Pediatrics regards antihistamines to be safe to use during breast-feeding (Committee on Drugs, American Academy of Pediatrics, 1994).

Key References

Aselton P, Jick H, Milunsky A, et al.: First-trimester drug use and congenital disorders. Obstet Gynecol 65:451-455, 1985.

Committee on Drugs, American Academy of Pediatrics: The transfer of drugs and other chemicals into human milk. Pediatrics 93(1):137-150, 1994.

Hara GS, Carter RP, Krantz KE: Dramamine in labor: Potential boon or a possible bomb? J Kans Med Soc 81:134-136, 155, 1980.

Hay TB, Wood C: The effect of dimenhydrinate on uterine contractions. Aust NZ J Obstet Gynaecol 7:81-89, 1967.

Heinonen OP, Slone D, Shapiro S: *Birth Defects and Drugs in Pregnancy.* Littleton, Mass.: John Wright-PSG, 1977, pp 437, 475.

Iuliucci JD, Gautieri RF: Morphine-induced fetal malformation. II: Influence of histamine and diphenhydramine. J Pharm Sci 60:420-424, 1971.

Jick H, Holmes LB, Hunter JR, et al.: First-trimester drug use and congenital disorders. JAMA 246:343-346, 1981.

Jones-Price C, Ledoux TA, Reel JR, et al.: Teratologic evaluation of diphenhydramine hydrochloride (CAS No. 147-24-0) administered to CD-1 mice on gestational days 11 through 14. NTIS (National Technical Information Service) Report/PB83-148684, 1982a.

Jones-Price C, Ledoux TA, Reel JR, Langhoff-Paschke L: Teratologic evaluation of diphenhydramine hydrochloride (CAS No. 147-24-0) in CD rats. NTIS (National Technical Information Service) Report/PB83-180612, 1983.

Jones-Price C, Ledoux TA, Reel JR, Langhoff-Paschke L: Teratologic evaluation of diphenhydramine hydrochloride (CAS No. 147-24-0) in CD-1 mice. NTIS (National Technical Information Service) Report/PB83-163055, 1982b.

Saxen I: Cleft palate and maternal diphenhydramine intake. Lancet 1:407-408, 1974.

Schardein JL, Hentz DL, Petrere JA, Kurtz SM: Teratogenesis studies with diphenhydramine HCl. Toxicol Appl Pharmacol 18:971-976, 1971.

DIPHENOXYLATE
(Lomocot®, Lomotil®)

Diphenoxylate is chemically related to narcotics but has no analgesic action. It decreases intestinal motility and is used to treat acute and chronic diarrhea. Diphenoxylate is given orally in doses of 5-20 mg/d. The drug is formulated with atropine to prevent abuse.

Teratogenic Risk

Magnitude of teratogenic risk to child born after exposure during gestation:	*Undetermined*
Quality and quantity of data on which risk estimate is based:	*Very poor*

No adequate epidemiological study of malformations in infants born to women who used diphenoxylate during pregnancy has been reported.

Fetal death was increased among pregnant rats that were treated with 75-125 times the maximum human dose of diphenoxylate (Wang et al., 1987). The relevance of this observation to the therapeutic use of diphenoxylate in human pregnancy is uncertain.

Risk Related to Breast-feeding

No information regarding the distribution of diphenoxylate in breast milk has been published; however, its metabolite, diphenoxylic acid, is known to be excreted in breast milk (USP DI, 1995).

Key References

USP DI: Diphenoxylate and Atropine. In: *USP DI (USP Dispensing Information), Volume 1. Drug Information for the Health Care Professional*, 15th ed. Rockville, Md.: The US Pharmacopeial Convention, 1995, p 1125.

Wang NG, Guan MZ, Lei HP: [Studies on the effect of the combined use of dl-15methyl-prostaglandin $F_2\alpha$ methyl ester with diphenoxylate hydrochloride in early pregnancy in rats.] Chung Kuo I Hsueh Ko Hsueh Yuan Hsueh Pao 9:414-417, 1987.

DIPYRIDAMOLE
(Persantine®, Pyridamole®)

Dipyridamole is an antithrombotic agent. It has been used in pregnancy to prevent fetal growth retardation and fetal death. It is also employed in the long-term management of angina pectoris. Dipyridamole is given orally or intravenously in doses of 60-400 mg/d.

Teratogenic Risk

Magnitude of teratogenic risk to child born after exposure during gestation:	*Unlikely*
Quality and quantity of data on which risk estimate is based:	*Poor to fair*

Therapeutic doses of dipyridamole are unlikely to pose a substantial teratogenic risk, but the data are insufficient to state that there is no risk.

Maternal therapy with dipyridamole and aspirin may prevent recurrence of fetal growth retardation and fetal death in women who have had previously affected pregnancies (Beaufils et al., 1985; Wallenburg & Rotmans, 1987; Uzan et al., 1991). No increase in congenital anomalies or other adverse effects among the infants was observed in controlled trials of 119, 48, and 30 high-risk pregnancies in women who were treated with dipyridamole and aspirin in the second and third trimesters (Beaufils et al., 1985, 1986; Wallenburg & Rotmans, 1987; Uzan et al., 1991). Although a variety of congenital anomalies have been observed in children whose mothers were treated with dipyridamole during pregnancy, no consistent pattern of malformations is apparent, and the frequency of anomalies in these series does not seem unusually high (Tejani, 1973; Ibarra-Perez et al., 1976; Chen et al., 1982).

Fetal loss is frequent among women with artificial heart valves who are treated during pregnancy with warfarin and may be even higher in those treated with both warfarin and dipyridamole (Ibarra-Perez et al., 1976; Sareli et al., 1989). The clinical significance of this observation is unclear.

Unpublished studies in mice, rats, and rabbits are said to suggest that treatment of pregnant women with dipyridamole in usual therapeutic doses is unlikely to increase the children's risk of malformations greatly (USP DI, 1995).

Risk Related to Breast-feeding

Dipyridamole is excreted into breast milk (USP DI, 1995), although this has not been quantitated in published reports.

Key References

Beaufils M, Donsimoni R, Uzan S, Colau JC: Prevention of preeclampsia early antiplatelet therapy. Lancet 1:840-842, 1985.

Beaufils M, Uzan S, Donsimoni R, Colau JC: Prospective controlled study of early antiplatelet therapy in prevention of preeclampsia. Adv Nephrol 15:87-94, 1986.

Chen WWC, Chan CS, Lee PK, et al.: Pregnancy in patients with prosthetic heart valves: An experience with 45 pregnancies. Q J Med 51:358-365, 1982.

Ibarra-Perez C, Arevalo-Toledo N, Alvarez-De La Cadena O, Noriega-Guerra L: The course of pregnancy in patients with artificial heart valves. Am J Med 61:504-512, 1976.

Sareli P, England MJ, Berk MR, et al.: Maternal and fetal sequelae of anticoagulation during pregnancy in patients with mechanical heart valve prostheses. Am J Cardiol 63:1462-1465, 1989.

Tejani N: Anticoagulant therapy with cardiac valve prosthesis during pregnancy. Obstet Gynecol 42:785-793, 1973.

USP DI: Dipyridamole. In: *USP DI (USP Dispensing Information), Volume 1. Drug Information for the Health Care Professional*, 15th ed. Rockville, Md.: The US Pharmacopeial Convention, 1995, p 1135.

Uzan S, Beaufils M, Breart G, et al.: Prevention of fetal growth retardation with low-dose aspirin: Findings of the EPREDA trial. Lancet 337(8755):1427-1431, 1991.

Wallenburg HCS, Rotmans N: Prevention of recurrent idiopathic fetal growth retardation by low-dose aspirin and dipyridamole. Am J Obstet Gynecol 157(5):1230-1235, 1987.

DISOPYRAMIDE
(Norpace®, Rythmodon®)

Disopyramide is an oral cardiac antiarrhythmic agent with anticholinergic and local anesthetic properties. Disopyramide is given orally or intravenously, usually in doses of 300-800 mg/d.

Teratogenic Risk

Magnitude of teratogenic risk to child born after exposure during gestation:	*Undetermined*
Quality and quantity of data on which risk estimate is based:	*Very poor*

No epidemiological studies of congenital anomalies in children born to women treated with disopyramide during pregnancy have been reported.

Studies in mice, rats, and rabbits suggest that treatment of pregnant women with disopyramide in usual therapeutic doses is unlikely to increase the children's risk of malformations greatly (Jequier et al., 1970; Esaki and Yanagita, 1981; Umemura et al., 1981; 1984, Esaki et al., 1983).

Disopyramide induces uterine contractions and delivery when administered to pregnant women at term (Tadmor et al., 1990). Administration of disopyramide at 32 weeks gestation to a woman with cardiac arrhythmia was associated with premature onset of labor (Leonard et al., 1978).

Risk Related to Breast-feeding

Excretion of disopyramide and its active metabolite, N-monodesalkyl disopyramide, are excreted in the breast milk. The amount of disopyramide and N-monodesalkyl disopyramide that the nursing infant would be expected to ingest is equivalent to 3.6-26.5% of the lowest therapeutic dose of disopyramide for infants, based on data from four lactating women (Barnett et al., 1982; MacKintosh & Buchanan, 1985; Hoppu et al., 1986; Ellsworth et al., 1989).*

Measurable serum levels of disopyramide were found for only one infant (Hoppu et al., 1986). These levels were 5-7% of the lowest therapeutic serum levels of disopyramide reported in infants.[†] N-monodesalkyl disopyramide was not detected in the serum of three of the infants from which samples were obtained. No adverse effects were reported in any of the nursing infants studied above, with the exception of restlessness and excessive crying in one (Hoppu et al., 1986). The relationship, if any, of this observation to the maternal treatment is unknown.

The American Academy of Pediatrics regards disopyramide to be safe to use while breast-feeding (Committee on Drugs, American Academy of Pediatrics, 1994).

Key References

Barnett DB, Hudson SA, McBurney A: Disopyramide and its N-monodesalkyl metabolite in breast milk. Br J Clin Pharmacol 14:310-312, 1982.

Committee on Drugs, American Academy of Pediatrics: The transfer of drugs and other chemicals into human milk. Pediatrics 93(1):137-150, 1994.

Ellsworth AJ, Horn JR, Raisys VA, et al.: Disopyramide and N-monodesalkyl disopyramide in serum and breast milk. Drug Intell Clin Pharm 23:56-57, 1989.

Esaki K, Umemura T, Yanagita T: Teratogenicity of intragastric administration of disopyramide phosphate in rabbits. Jitchuken Zenrinsho Kenkyuho (Preclin Rep Cent Inst Ext Animal) 9(1):83-92, 1983.

Esaki K, Yanagita T: Effects of intravenous administration of disopyramide phosphate on the rabbit fetus. Jitchuken Zenrinsho Kenkyuho (Preclin Rep Cent Inst Exp Animal) 7:189-198, 1981.

Hoppu K, Neuvonen P, Korte T: Disopyramide and breast feeding. Br J Clin Pharmacol 21:553, 1986.

*This calculation is based on the following assumptions: maternal dose of disopyramide: 400-1350 mg/d; milk concentrations of disopyramide and N-monodesalkyl disopyramide: 0.58-5.7 mcg/mL and 1.8-12.3 mcg/mL, respectively; milk intake by the nursing infant: 150 mL/kg/d; estimated dose of both disopyramide and N-mondesalkyl disopyramide ingested by the nursing infant, assuming similar bioavailability, activity, and molecular weights: 0.36-2.65 mg/kg/d; lowest therapeutic dose of disopyramide in infants: 10 mg/kg/d.

†This calculation is based on the following assumptions: infant serum levels of disopyramide: 0.1-0.14 mcg/mL; lowest therapeutic serum level in infants: 2 mcg/mL.

Jequier R, Deraedt R, Plongeron R, Vannier B: [Pharmacology and toxicology of disopiramide.] Minerva Med 61 (Suppl):3689-3693, 1970.

Leonard RF, Braun TE, Levy AM: Initiation of uterine contractions by disopyramide during pregnancy. N Engl J Med 299:84-85, 1978.

MacKintosh D, Buchanan N: Excretion of disopyramide in human breast milk. Br J Clin Pharmacol 19:856-857, 1985.

Tadmor OP, Keren A, Rosenak D, et al.: The effect of disopyramide on uterine contractions during pregnancy. Am J Obstet Gynecol 162:482-486, 1990.

Umemura T, Esaki K, Ando K, et al.: Effects of intragastric administration of disopyramide phosphate on reproduction in rats. III. Experiment on drug administration during the organogenesis period. CIEA (Preclin Rep Cent Inst Ext Animal) 10:87-110, 1984.

Umemura T, Sasa H, Esaki K, Takada K, et al.: Effects of disopyramide phosphate on reproduction in the rats. II. Experiments on drug administration during the organogenesis periods. Jitchuken Zenrinsho Kenkyuho (Preclin Rep Cent Inst Exp Animal) 7:157-173, 1981.

DIULO® *See* Metolazone

DIURIL® *See* Chlorothiazide

DIXARIT® *See* Clonidine

DOLOBID® *See* Diflunisal

DOPAMET® *See* Methyldopa

DOXAPHENE® *See* Propoxyphene

DOXEPIN
(Adapin®, Sinequan®, Triadapin®)

Doxepin is a tricyclic antidepressant with strong sedative action. It is given orally to treat depression, panic disorder, neurogenic pain, vascular headaches, and peptic ulcer disease. The usual starting dose is 75 mg/d, but doses up to 150 mg/d may be used in outpatients and up to 500 mg/d in hospitalized patients. Because most adverse effects are dose-related, occasional low-dose use is likely to be safer than chronic high-dose use.

Teratogenic Risk

Magnitude of teratogenic risk to child born after exposure during gestation:	*Undetermined*
Quality and quantity of data on which risk estimate is based:	*Poor*

There are no published epidemiological studies of congenital anomalies among the children of women treated with doxepin during pregnancy.

Studies in rats and rabbits suggest that treatment of pregnant women with doxepin in usual therapeutic doses is unlikely to increase the children's risk of malformations greatly (Owaki et al., 1971a, b).

Risk Related to Breast-feeding

Doxepin and its active metabolite, N-desmethyldoxepin, are excreted in breast milk. The amount of doxepin and N-desmethyldoxepin that the nursing infant would be expected to ingest is equivalent to <1-21% of the lowest weight-adjusted therapeutic dose of doxepin, based on data obtained from two lactating women (Kemp et al., 1985; Matheson et al., 1985).*

Serum levels of N-desmethyldoxepin in one infant, who experienced respiratory depression, were found to be 3 times as high as the lowest therapeutic serum level of N-desmethyldoxepin in adults.[†] No measurable levels of doxepin were found in the infant's serum. (Matheson et al., 1985).

*This calculation is based on the following assumptions: maternal dose of doxepin: 75-150 mg/d; milk concentrations of doxepin and N-desmethyldoxepin: 0.01-0.08 mcg/mL and <0.01-0.14 mcg/mL; milk intake by the nursing infant: 150 mL/kg/d; estimated infant dose of both doxepin and N-desmethyldoxepin, assuming similar bioavailability, activity, and molecular weights: <0.002-0.033 mg/kg/d; lowest therapeutic dose of doxepin in adults: 0.16 mg/kg/d.

[†]Lowest therapeutic serum level of N-desmethyldoxepin in adults: 0.02 mcg/mL.

The American Academy of Pediatrics considers chronic use of doxepin to be a concern when given to nursing mothers (Committee on Drugs, American Academy of Pediatrics, 1994). The WHO Working Group on Drugs and Human Lactation (1988) regards doxepin to be contraindicated during breast-feeding.

Key References

Committee on Drugs, American Academy of Pediatrics: The transfer of drugs and other chemicals into human milk. Pediatrics 93(1):137-150, 1994.

Kemp J, Ilett KF, Booth J, Hackett LP: Excretion of doxepin and N-desmethyldoxepin in human milk. Br J Clin Pharmacol 20:497-499, 1985.

Matheson I, Pande H, Alertsen AR: Respiratory depression caused by N-desmethyldoxepin in breast milk. Lancet 2:1124, 1985.

Owaki Y, Momiyama H, Onodera N: Effects of doxepin hydrochloride administered to pregnant rabbits upon the fetuses. Oyo Yakuri 5:905-912, 1971a.

Owaki Y, Momiyama H, Onodera N: Effects of doxepin hydrochloride administered to pregnant rats upon the fetuses and their postnatal development. Oyo Yakuri 5:913-924, 1971b.

WHO Working Group on Drugs and Human Lactation. In: Bennet PN (ed). *Drugs and Human Lactation.* Amsterdam: Elsevier, 1988, pp 393-394.

DOXINE® *See* Pyridoxine

DOXYCIN® *See* Doxycycline

DOXYCYCLINE
(Doxycin®, Monodox®, Vibramycin®)

Doxycycline is a tetracycline antibiotic used in the treatment of a wide variety of infections. Doxycycline is given orally or parenterally, usually in doses of 100-300 mg/d, although doses as high as 600 mg/d are employed in the treatment of gonorrhea.

Teratogenic Risk

Magnitude of teratogenic
risk to child born after
exposure during gestation
    Malformations: *Undetermined*
    Dental staining: *High*

Quality and quantity of data
on which risk estimate is based
    Malformations: *Very poor*
    Dental staining: *Excellent*

A small risk cannot be excluded, but there is no indication that the risk of malformations in the children of women treated with doxycycline during pregnancy is likely to be great.

Tetracyclines cause staining of the primary dentition in fetuses exposed during the second or third trimester of pregnancy (Toaff & Ravid, 1966; Cohlan, 1977).

No epidemiological studies of malformations in infants born to women who took doxycycline during pregnancy have been reported.

Studies in mice, rats, and rabbits suggest that treatment of pregnant women with doxycycline in usual therapeutic doses is unlikely to increase the children's risk of malformations greatly (Cahen & Fave, 1972).

Please see agent summary on tetracycline for information on a related drug that has been more thoroughly studied.

Risk Related to Breast-feeding

Doxycycline is excreted in the breast milk. The amount of doxycycline that the nursing infant would be expected to ingest is between 3-5% of the lowest pediatric dose of doxycycline, based on data obtained from 15 lactating women (Morganti et al., 1968).*

    *This calculation is based on the following assumptions: maternal dose of doxycycline: 100 and 200 mg; milk concentrations of doxycycline: 0.38-0.77 mcg/mL; milk intake by the nursing infant: 150 mL/kg/d; estimated dose of doxycycline ingested by the nursing infant: 0.06-0.12 mg/kg/d; lowest pediatric dose of doxycycline: 2.2 mg/kg/d.

Dental staining or inhibition of bone growth associated with ingestion of doxycycline through the breast milk is a theoretical possibility with chronic maternal treatment, but these effects have not been documented. The WHO Working Group on Drugs and Human Lactation (1988) regards doxycycline to be safe to use during breast-feeding for brief periods of time.

Key References

Cahen RL, Fave A: Absence of teratogenic effect of 6-α-deoxy-5 oxytetracycline. Fed Proc Fed Am Soc Exp Biol 31:238, 1972.

Cohlan SQ: Tetracycline staining of teeth. Teratology 15:127-130, 1977.

Morganti G, Ceccarelli G, Ciaffi G: Comparative concentrations of a tetracycline antibiotic in serum and maternal milk. Antibiotica 6:216-223, 1968.

Toaff R, Ravid R: Tetracyclines and the teeth. Lancet 2:281-282, 1966.

WHO Working Group on Drugs and Human Lactation. In: Bennet PN (ed). *Drugs and Human Lactation*. Amsterdam: Elsevier, 1988.

DOXYLAMINE
(Unisom®)

Doxylamine is given orally in doses of 30-75 mg/d as an antihistaminic agent and in a single dose of 25 mg as a hypnotic.

Teratogenic Risk

*Magnitude of teratogenic
risk to child born after
exposure during gestation:*   *None*

*Quality and quantity of data
on which risk estimate is based:*   *Good to excellent*

Most human studies of doxylamine were undertaken when the drug was a component of Bendectin, a medication that is no longer on the market. These data are not summarized here, but several comprehensive reviews of the extensive teratology studies on Bendectin are available (MacMahon, 1982; Cordero & Oakley, 1983; Holmes, 1983; Sheffield & Batagol, 1985). The studies indicate that maternal use of Bendectin early in pregnancy did not measurably increase the risk of congenital anomalies in children.

The frequencies of congenital anomalies in general, of major malformations, of minor anomalies, and of major classes of anomalies were no greater than expected among the children of 1169 women who took doxylamine as an antinauseant during the first four lunar months of pregnancy in one study (Heinonen et al., 1977). Similarly, the frequency of congenital anomalies was not increased among the children of 1700 women who took doxylamine anytime during pregnancy in this study. No association with maternal use of doxylamine during the first trimester of pregnancy was observed in a study of 298 children with congenital heart disease (Zierler & Rothman, 1985).

The frequency of malformations was not increased among the offspring of rats or rabbits treated with 3-33 times the maximum human dose of doxylamine during pregnancy in one study (Gibson et al., 1968). In contrast, McBride reported increased frequencies of eye, limb, and other malformations among the offspring of rabbits treated with doxylamine in doses 7-111 times the maximum used in humans (McBride, 1984; McBride & Hicks, 1987); maternal death was frequent with such doses. Limb and tail malformations were reported among the offspring of a marmoset monkey treated during pregnancy with 38 times the maximum human dose of doxylamine; abortion was consistently induced by higher doses (McBride, 1985). The validity of these studies by McBride has been cast into doubt by evidence that he engaged in scientific fraud.

Risk Related to Breast-feeding

No information regarding the distribution of doxylamine in breast milk has been published.

Key References

Cordero JF, Oakley GP: Drug exposure during pregnancy: Some epidemiologic considerations. Clin Obstet Gynecol 26:418-428, 1983.
Gibson JP, Staples RE, Larson EJ, et al.: Teratology and reproduction studies with an antinauseant. Toxicol Appl Pharmacol 13:439-447, 1968.

Heinonen OP, Slone D, Shapiro S: *Birth Defects and Drugs in Pregnancy*. Littleton, Mass.: John Wright-PSG, 1977, pp 323, 437.

Holmes LB: Teratogen update: Bendectin. Teratology 27:277-281, 1983.

MacMahon B: More on Bendectin. JAMA 246:371-372, 1982.

McBride WG: Doxylamine succinate induced dysmorphogenesis in the marmoset (*Callithrix jacchus*). IRCS Med Sci 13:225-226, 1985.

McBride WG: Teratogenic effect of doxylamine succinate in New Zealand white rabbits. IRCS Med Sci 12:536-537, 1984.

McBride WG, Hicks LJ: Acetylcholine and choline levels in rabbit fetuses exposed to anticholinergics. Int J Dev Neurosci 5:117- 125, 1987.

Sheffield LJ, Batagol R: The creation of therapeutic orphans--or, what have we learnt from the debendox fiasco? Med J Aust 143:143-147, 1985.

Zierler S, Rothman KJ: Congenital heart disease in relation to maternal use of Bendectin and other drugs in early pregnancy. N Engl J Med 313:347-352, 1985.

DRIXORAL® *See* Dextromethorphan

DULCAINE® *See* Lidocaine

DURAQUIN® *See* Quinidine

DURAZEPAM® *See* Oxazepam

DURICEF® *See* Cefadroxil

D-VERT® *See* Meclizine

DYRENIUM® *See* Triamterene

ECOTRIN® *See* Aspirin

ELAVIL® *See* Amitriptyline

ELTROXIN® *See* Levothyroxine

EMEX® *See* Metoclopramide

E-MYCIN® *See* Erythromycin

ENALAPRIL
(Vasotec®)

Enalapril is an angiotensin-converting enzyme (ACE) inhibitor that is administered orally in the treatment of hypertension. Enalapril is usually given orally in doses of 2.5-40 mg/d; the drug may also be given intravenously in a dose of 5 mg/d.

Teratogenic Risk

Magnitude of teratogenic
risk to child born after
exposure during gestation:
    First-trimester use: *Undetermined*
    Use later in pregnancy: *Moderate*

Quality and quantity of data
on which risk estimate is based:
    First-trimester use: *Poor*
    Use later in pregnancy   *Fair to good*

A small risk cannot be excluded, but a high risk of congenital anomalies in the children of women treated with enalapril during pregnancy is unlikely.

There is a substantial risk of oligohydramnios and fetal distress or death in hypertensive women treated with enalapril in the latter part of pregnancy. The effect may be related to the pharmacological action of this drug on the fetus (see below).

The risk associated with maternal use of enalapril during the second or third trimester of pregnancy increases with the duration of treatment.

One malformed infant was observed among 12 in one series of infants born to women treated with enalapril or another ACE inhibitor during the first trimester of pregnancy (Piper et al., 1992). This child, whose mother had been treated with enalapril, had an occipital encephalocele.

Two cases have been reported in which hypocalvaria, an unusual underdevelopment of the skull bones, and other skeletal anomalies occurred in the infants of women treated with enalapril throughout pregnancy (Mehta & Modi, 1989; Cunniff et al., 1990). Five infants with similar unusual skull defects have been observed after maternal treatment throughout pregnancy with other ACE inhibitors (Duminy & Berger, 1981; Rothberg & Lorenz, 1984; Barr & Cohen, 1991; Bhatt-Mehta & Deluga, 1993; Pryde et al., 1993).

Oligohydramnios, fetal growth retardation and neonatal renal failure, hypotension, pulmonary hypoplasia, joint contractures, and death have been repeatedly observed after maternal treatment with enalapril or related drugs during pregnancy (Hanssens et al., 1991; Bhatt-Mehta & Deluga, 1993; Pryde et al., 1993; Shotan et al., 1994). One infant among 15 born to women treated with enalapril or other ACE inhibitors during the second or third trimester of pregnancy in one series had oligohydramnios and neonatal hypotension and anuria (Piper et al., 1992). It is important to note that these effects do not appear to reflect abnormal embryogenesis but rather a pharmacologic response of the fetus to enalapril during the second half of gestation (Beckman & Brent, 1990; Brent & Beckman, 1991).

Multicystic, dysplastic kidneys were found in an infant born at 37 weeks after a pregnancy complicated by long-standing oligohydramnios and maternal enalapril treatment throughout pregnancy (Thorpe-Beeston et al., 1993). No causal inference is possible on the basis of this single case report, but renal tubular dysplasia has been observed among other infants who died in the neonatal period with anuria after maternal treatment during pregnancy with enalapril or other ACE inhibitors (Cunniff et al., 1990; Pryde et al., 1993).

The frequency of malformations was no greater than expected but fetal growth retardation was increased among the offspring of rats treated with 4-1500 times the usual human dose of enalapril during pregnancy (Fujii et al., 1985; Robertson et al., 1986; Al-Harbi et al., 1992; Valdes et al., 1992). Incomplete skull ossification was also reported in two of these studies (Al-Harbi et al., 1992; Valdes et al., 1992). Increased frequencies of fetal death but not of malformations were observed among the offspring of rabbits treated during pregnancy with 4-40 times the human dose of enalapril (Minsker et al., 1990).

Fetal death occurred only when the drug was administered during the last portion of pregnancy. Fetal hypotension has been demonstrated when pregnant sheep were given 2.5 times the human dose of enalapril (Broughton Pipkin & Wallace, 1986).

Risk Related to Breast-feeding

Enalapril and its active metabolite, enalaprilat, are excreted in the breast milk in low concentrations. The amount of enalapril and enalaprilat that the nursing infant would be expected to receive is approximately 0-3% of the lowest pediatric dose of enalapril, based on data from six lactating women (Redman et al., 1990; Rush et al., 1991).* Enalaprilat was not detected in the breast milk of three lactating women in another study (Huttunen et al. 1989).

The American Academy of Pediatrics regards enalapril to be safe to use while breast-feeding (Committee on Drugs, American Academy of Pediatrics, 1994).

Key References

Al-Harbi MM, Al-shabanah OA, Al-Gharably NMA, Islam MW: The effect of maternal administration of enalapril on fetal development in the rat. Res Commun Chem Pathol Pharmacol 77(3):347-358, 1992.

Barr M Jr, Cohen MM Jr: ACE inhibitor fetopathy and hypocalvaria: The kidney-skull connection. Teratology 44:485-495, 1991.

Beckman DA, Brent RL: Teratogenesis: Alcohol, angiotensin-converting-enzyme inhibitors, and cocaine. Curr Opin Obstet Gynecol 2(2):236-245, 1990.

Bhatt-Mehta V, Deluga KS: Fetal exposure to lisinopril: Neonatal manifestations and management. Pharmacotherapy 13(5):515-518, 1993.

Brent RL, Beckman DA: Angiotensin-converting enzyme inhibitors, an embryopathic class of drugs with unique properties: Information for clinical teratology counselors. Teratology 43:543-546, 1991.

*This calculation is based on the following assumptions: maternal dose of enalapril: 5-20 mg/d; milk concentration of enalapril and enalaprilat: 0.0-0.006 mcg/mL and 0.0-0.002 mcg/mL, respectively; milk intake by the nursing infant: 150 mL/kg/d; estimated dose of both enalapril and enalaprilat ingested by the nursing infant: 0.001 mg/kg/d; lowest pediatric dose of enalapril: 0.04 mg/kg/d.

Broughton Pipkin F, Wallace CP: The effect of enalapril (MK421), an angiotensin converting enzyme inhibitor, on the conscious pregnant ewe and her foetus. Br J Pharmacol 87:533-542, 1986.

Committee on Drugs, American Academy of Pediatrics: The transfer of drugs and other chemicals into human milk. Pediatrics 93(1):137-150, 1994.

Cunniff C, Jones KL, Phillipson J, et al.: Oligohydramnios sequence and renal tubular malformation associated with maternal enalapril use. Am J Obstet Gynecol 162:187-189, 1990.

Duminy PC, Burger P du T: Fetal abnormality associated with the use of captopril during pregnancy. S Afr Med J 60:805, 1981.

Fujii T, Nakatsuka T, Hanada S, et al.: MK-421: Oral teratogenicity study in the rat. Yakuri To Chiryo 13:519-528, 1985.

Hanssens M, Keirse MJNC, Vankelecom F, Van Assche FA: Fetal and neonatal effects of treatment with angiotensin-converting enzyme inhibitors in pregnancy. Obstet Gynecol 78:128-135, 1991.

Huttunen K, Gronhagen-Riska C, Fybrquist F: Enalapril treatment of a nursing mother with slightly impaired renal function. Clin Nephrol 31:278, 1989.

Mehta N, Modi N: Ace inhibitors in pregnancy. Lancet 2:96, 1989.

Minsker DH, Bagdon WJ, MacDonald JS, et al.: Maternotoxicity and fetotoxicity of an angiotensin-converting enzyme inhibitor, enalapril, in rabbits. Fundam Appl Toxicol 14:461-470, 1990.

Piper JM, Ray WA, Rosa FW: Pregnancy outcome following exposure to angiotensin-converting enzyme inhibitors. Obstet Gynecol 80:429-432, 1992.

Pryde PG, Sedman AB, Nugent CE, Barr M Jr: Angiotensin-converting enzyme inhibitor fetopathy. J Am Soc Nephrol 3:1575-1582, 1993.

Redman CWG, Kelly JG, Cooper WD: The excretion of enalapril and enalaprilat in human breast milk. Eur J Clin Pharmacol 38:99, 1990.

Robertson RT, Minsker DA, Bokelman DL, Fujii T: MK-421 (enalapril maleate): Fertility study in male and female rats. Yakuri To Chiryo 14(1):25-41, 1986.

Rothberg AD, Lorenz R: Can captopril cause fetal and neonatal renal failure? Pediatr Pharmacol 4:189-192, 1984.

Rush JE, Snyder DL, Barrish A, Hichens M: Comment. Clin Nephrol 35:234, 1991.

Shotan A, Widerhorn J, Hurst A, Elkayam U: Risks of angiotensin-converting enzyme inhibition during pregnancy: Experimental and clinical evidence, potential mechanisms, and recommendations for use. Am J Med 96:451-456, 1994.

Thorpe-Beeston JG, Armar NA, Dancy M, et al.: Pregnancy and ACE inhibitors. Br J Obstet Gynaecol 100:692-693, 1993.

Valdes G, Marinovic D, Falcon C, et al.: Placental alterations, intrauterine growth retardation and teratogenicity associated with enalapril use in pregnant rats. Biol Neonate 61:124-130, 1992.

ENDURON® *See* Methyclothiazide

ENGERIX-B® *See* Hepatitis B Vaccine

EPHEDRINE
(Fedrine®, Neorespin®, Stopasthme®)

Ephedrine is a sympathomimetic drug used to treat nasal congestion and bronchospasm. Ephedrine is a component of many cough and cold medicines. The usual oral dose is 75-250 mg/d; similar doses may be given parenterally. Ophthalmic preparations containing ephedrine are used to relieve blood-shot eyes, and ephedrine nasal sprays are used to treat nasal congestion.

Teratogenic Risk

*Magnitude of teratogenic
risk to child born after
exposure during gestation:*   *Unlikely*

*Quality and quantity of data
on which risk estimate is based:*   *Poor to fair*

Therapeutic doses of ephedrine are unlikely to pose a substantial teratogenic risk, but the data are insufficient to state that there is no risk.

The frequencies of congenital anomalies in general, of major malformations, and of minor anomalies were no greater than expected among the children of 373 women who used ephedrine during the first four lunar months of pregnancy in one epidemiological study (Heinonen et al., 1977). The frequency of congenital anomalies was not increased among the children of 873 women who used ephedrine anytime during pregnancy in this study. No association with maternal ephedrine use during the first trimester of pregnancy was seen in studies of 76 children with gastroschisis and 416 children with various congenital anomalies thought to have a vascular pathogenesis (Werler et al., 1992).

Increased fetal heart rate and beat-to-beat variability have been observed in association with maternal ephedrine treatment during labor (Wright et al., 1981).

An increased frequency of cardiac anomalies, primarily ventricular septal defects, was observed among the offspring of rats treated during pregnancy with ephedrine in doses 3-1700 times the single dose used in humans (or 1-420 times the human daily dose) in a study that has only been published in abstract form (Kanai et al., 1986). The relevance of this observation to the therapeutic use of ephedrine in human pregnancy is unknown.

Risk Related to Breast-feeding

No information regarding the distribution of ephedrine in breast milk has been published.

Key References

Heinonen OP, Slone D, Shapiro S: *Birth Defects and Drugs in Pregnancy.* Littleton, Mass.: John Wright-PSG, 1977, pp 346, 347, 439, 491.

Kanai T, Nishikawa T, Satoh A, Kajita A: Cardiovascular teratogenicity of ephedrine in rats. Teratology 34:469, 1986.

Werler MM, Mitchell AA, Shapiro S: First trimester maternal medication use in relation to gastroschisis. Teratology 45:361-367, 1992.

Wright RG, Shnider SM, Levinson G, et al.: The effect of maternal administration of ephedrine on fetal heart rate and variability. Obstet Gynecol 57:734-738, 1981.

EPINEPHRINE
(Bronkaid Mist®, Primatene Mist®)

Epinephrine is a direct-acting sympathomimetic hormone released from the adrenal medulla in response to stress. Epinephrine is administered therapeutically to alleviate bronchospasm and other allergic conditions. Epinephrine is given parenterally in doses of 0.2-1.5 mg which may be repeated frequently. Epinephrine is also given by inhalation in doses of 0.16-0.55 mg which may be repeated every three hours.

Teratogenic Risk

Magnitude of teratogenic risk to child born after exposure during gestation:	*Unlikely*
Quality and quantity of data on which risk estimate is based:	*Fair*

Therapeutic doses of epinephrine are unlikely to pose a substantial teratogenic risk, but the data are insufficient to state that there is no risk.

The frequency of congenital anomalies was increased among the children of 189 women treated with epinephrine during the first four lunar months of pregnancy in one epidemiological study, but this increase was due entirely to mild defects that had highly variable rates of occurrence at participating institutions (Heinonen et al., 1977). Studies such as this one that include multiple comparisons between maternal drug exposures and various birth defect outcomes are expected to show occasional associations with nominal statistical significance purely by chance. The frequency of congenital anomalies was not increased among the children of 508 women who were treated with epinephrine anytime during pregnancy in this investigation.

Disruptions of limb development can be produced by injection of epinephrine directly into rat or rabbit fetuses in doses thousands of times greater than those used clinically (Jost et al., 1964, 1969). Cataracts can be induced in rat fetuses under similar conditions (Pitel & Lerman, 1962). No teratogenic effect was observed among the offspring of pregnant rats given continuous infusions of epinephrine at a dose about 8 times that used in humans (Trend & Bruce, 1989). An increased frequency of cleft palate was observed in the offspring of one strain of mice, but not another, treated during pregnancy with epinephrine in doses 40-80 times those used in humans (Loevy & Roth, 1968; Blaustein et al., 1971). An increased frequency of fetal loss was reported in pregnant mice and rabbits given, respectively, 200 and 85 times the human therapeutic dose of epinephrine (Loevy & Roth, 1968; Auletta, 1971). The frequency of malformations was not increased among the offspring of hamsters treated during pregnancy with 25 times the human subcutaneous dose of epinephrine (Hirsch & Fritz, 1981). Behavioral alterations have been noted in the offspring of rats treated with epinephrine during pregnancy in doses 140-430 times those used in humans (Thompson et al., 1963). Fetal asphyxia can be produced in term rhesus monkey fetuses by administration of epinephrine to their mothers in doses similar to those used in human therapy (Adamsons et al., 1971). The relevance of these observations to therapeutic use of epinephrine in human pregnancy is unknown.

Risk Related to Breast-feeding

Epinephrine is excreted into breast milk (USP DI, 1995), although this has not been quantitated in published reports.

Key References

Adamsons K, Mueller-Heubach E, Myers RE: Production of fetal asphyxia in the rhesus monkey by administration of catecholamines to the mother. Am J Obstet Gynecol 109:248-262, 1971.

Auletta FJ: Effect of epinephrine on implantation and foetal survival in the rabbit. J Reprod Fertil 27:281-282, 1971.

Blaustein FM, Feller R, Rosenzweig S: Effect of ACTH and adrenal hormones on cleft palate frequency in CD-1 mice. J Dent Res 50:609-612, 1971.

Heinonen OP, Slone D, Shapiro S: *Birth Defects and Drugs in Pregnancy*. Littleton, Mass.: John Wright-PSG, 1977, pp 346-347, 439.

Hirsch KS, Fritz HI: Teratogenic effects of mescaline, epinephrine, and norepinephrine in the hamster. Teratology 23:287-291, 1981.

Jost A, Petter C, Duval G, et al.: [Effect of adrenalin on the division of blood between the fetus and placenta: Hemodynamic factors of certain congenital lesions of the limbs.] CR Acad Sci Paris 259:3086-3088, 1964.

Jost A, Roffi J, Courtat M: Congenital amputations determined by the BR gene and those induced by adrenalin injection in the rabbit fetus. In: Swinyard CA (ed). *Limb Development and Deformity: Problems of Evaluation and Rehabilitation*. Springfield, Ill.: Charles C Thomas, 1969, pp 187-199.

Loevy H, Roth BF: Induced cleft palate development in mice: Comparison between the effect of epinephrine and cortisone. Anat Rec 160:386, 1968.

Pitel M, Lerman S: Studies on the fetal rat lens. Effects of intrauterine adrenalin and noradrenalin. Invest Ophthalmol 1:406-412, 1962.

Thompson WR, Goldenberg L, Watson J, Watson M: Behavioral effects of maternal adrenalin injection during pregnancy in rat offspring. Psychol Rep 12:279-284, 1963.

Trend SG, Bruce NW: Resistance of the rat embryo to elevated maternal epinephrine concentrations. Am J Obstet Gynecol 160:498-501, 1989.

USP DI: Bronchodilators, Adrenergic. In: *USP DI (USP Dispensing Information), Volume 1. Drug Information for the Health Care Professional*, 15th ed. Rockville, Md.: The US Pharmacopeial Convention, 1995, p 536.

EPITOL® *See* Carbamazepine

EPIVAL® *See* Valproic Acid

EQUAL® *See* Aspartame

ERGOSTAT® *See* Ergotamine

ERGOTAMINE
(Ergostat®, Medihaler-Ergotamine®)

Ergotamine is an ergot alkaloid that acts as a vasoconstrictor. The drug is used in the treatment of migraine headaches and premenstrual tension. Ergotamine is given orally in a dose of 1-6 mg/d, by aerosol in a dose of 0.36-2.16 mg/d, or by rectal suppository in a dose of 0.5-4 mg/d.

Teratogenic Risk

*Magnitude of teratogenic
risk to child born after
exposure during gestation:*   *Minimal*

*Quality and quantity of data
on which risk estimate is based:*   *Fair to good*

*This risk assessment is for therapeutic use of ergotamine; the risk
is probably greater with maternally toxic doses.*

In one study of 9460 children with various congenital anomalies, maternal use of ergotamine was no more frequent than expected during the first trimester or anytime in pregnancy (Czeizel, 1989). An association of neural tube defects with maternal use of ergotamine was seen in this study, but this observation is based on only three cases with first trimester exposure and requires confirmation. The frequency of congenital anomalies was not increased among the children of 25 women who were treated with ergotamine during the first four lunar months of pregnancy in another investigation (Heinonen et al., 1977).

Various congenital anomalies attributed to vascular disruption have been reported in individual infants whose mothers took ergotamine during pregnancy; no causal inference can be made on the basis of these anecdotal observations (Peeden et al., 1979; Graham et al., 1983; Hughes & Goldstein, 1988; Verloes et al., 1990).

Intrauterine death has been observed in a pregnant woman who took a toxic overdose of ergotamine in a suicide attempt (Au et al., 1985).

Frequent severe uterine contractions and fetal tachycardia occurred in a term pregnancy after the mother took ergotamine in a therapeutic dose (de Groot et al., 1993). This may have resulted from ergotamine's potent oxytocic activity.

Increased frequencies of embryonic and fetal death were found among pregnant mice, rats, and rabbits treated during pregnancy with 830-2500, 83-830, and 8-250 times the usual human dose of ergotamine, respectively (Grauwiler & Schon, 1973). An increased frequency of malformations was found only among the offspring of pregnant rabbits treated with the highest dose of ergotamine. No teratogenic effect was noted among the offspring of pregnant pigs treated with about 5 times the human therapeutic dose of ergotamine (Bailey et al., 1973).

Risk Related to Breast-feeding

In one study, chronic ergot poisoning (vomiting, diarrhea, weak pulse) occurred in 90% of the nursing infants of women who had ingested a number of ergot alkaloids, including ergotamine (Fomina, 1934). On the basis of this study, the American Academy of Pediatrics regards ergotamine to be contraindicated during breast-feeding (Committee on Drugs, American Academy of Pediatrics, 1994).

Key References

Au KL, Woo JSK, Wong VCW: Intrauterine death from ergotamine overdosage. Eur J Obstet Gynecol Reprod Biol 19:313-315, 1985.

Bailey J, Wrathall AE, Mantle PG: The effect of feeding ergot to gilts during early pregnancy. Br Vet J 129:127-133, 1973.

Committee on Drugs, American Academy of Pediatrics: The transfer of drugs and other chemicals into human milk. Pediatrics 93(1):137-150, 1994.

Czeizel A: Teratogenicity of ergotamine. J Med Genet 26:69-71, 1989.

de Groot ANJA, van Dongen PWH, van Roosmalen J, Eskes TAKB: Ergotamine-induced fetal stress: Review of side effects of ergot alkaloids during pregnancy. Eur J Obstet Gynecol Reprod Biol 51:73-77, 1993.

Fomina PI: Untersuchungen uber den Ubergang des aktiven agens des Mutterkorns in die milch stillender Mutter. Arch Gynecol 157:275, 1934.

Graham JM Jr, Marin-Padilla M, Hoefnagel D: Jejunal atresia associated with Cafergot® ingestion during pregnancy. Clin Pediatr (Phila) 22(3):226-228, 1983.

Grauwiler J, Schon H: Teratological experiments with ergotamine in mice, rats, and rabbits. Teratology 7:227-235, 1973.

Heinonen OP, Slone D, Shapiro S: *Birth Defects and Drugs in Pregnancy.* Littleton, Mass.: John Wright-PSG, 1977, pp 358-360.

Hughes HE, Goldstein DA: Birth defects following maternal exposure to ergotamine, beta blockers, and caffeine. J Med Genet 25:396-399, 1988.

Peeden JN Jr, Wilroy RS Jr, Soper RG: Prune perineum. Teratology 20:233-236, 1979.

Verloes A, Emonts P, Dubois M, et al.: Paraplegia and arthrogryposis multiplex of the lower extremities after intrauterine exposure to ergotamine. J Med Genet 27:213-214, 1990.

ERYBID® See Erythromycin

ERYTHROMYCIN
(E-mycin®, Erybid®)

Erythromycin is a macrolide antibiotic that is used to treat a variety of infections, especially in patients allergic to penicillin. The usual oral dose of erythromycin is 1000-2000 mg/d and the usual intravenous dose is 15-20 mg/kg/d, but doses up to 4000 mg/d are sometimes employed in very serious infections.

Teratogenic Risk

Magnitude of teratogenic risk to child born after exposure during gestation:	*None*
Quality and quantity of data on which risk estimate is based:	*Fair to Good*

The frequency of congenital anomalies was no greater than expected among the children of 79 women treated with erythromycin during the first four lunar months of pregnancy or the children of 230 women treated anytime in pregnancy in one large epidemiological study (Heinonen et al., 1977). Similarly, no increase in the frequency of congenital anomalies was observed among the children of two groups of women who had been treated with erythromycin during the first trimester of pregnancy in another epidemiological study (Jick et al., 1981; Aselton et al., 1985). One of these groups included the children of 100-200 treated women and the other group included the children of 260 treated women.

The frequency of congenital anomalies was no greater than expected among the infants of 398 women treated with erythromycin during the second or third trimester of pregnancy in a controlled trial of antibiotic therapy for vaginal infections (McCormack et al., 1987). No medication-related adverse effects have been noted among the infants of women treated with erythromycin during the second or third trimester of pregnancy in various other therapeutic trials (Mercer et al., 1992; Romero et al., 1993).

Studies in mice and rats suggest that treatment of pregnant women with erythromycin in usual therapeutic doses is unlikely to increase the children's risk of malformations greatly (Takaya, 1965; Moriguchi et al., 1972a, b).

Risk Related to Breast-feeding

Erythromycin is excreted into breast milk in low quantities (Knowles, 1972; Matsuda, 1984; Murray & Seger, 1994; USP DI, 1995). The amount of erythromycin that the nursing infant would ingest is between <1-2.4% of the lowest therapeutic dose of erythromycin in neonates (Knowles, 1972).*

Both the American Academy of Pediatrics (Committee on Drugs, American Academy of Pediatrics, 1994) and the WHO Working Group on Drugs and Human Lactation (1988) consider it safe to use erythromycin for a short period of time during breast-feeding.

Key References

Aselton P, Jick H, Milunsky A, et al.: First-trimester drug use and congenital disorders. Obstet Gynecol 65:451-455, 1985.

Committee on Drugs, American Academy of Pediatrics: The transfer of drugs and other chemicals into human milk. Pediatrics 93(1):137-150, 1994.

Heinonen OP, Slone D, Shapiro S: *Birth Defects and Drugs in Pregnancy.* Littleton, Mass.: John Wright-PSG, 1977, pp 297, 301.

Jick H, Holmes LB, Hunter JR, et al.: First-trimester drug use and congenital disorders. JAMA 246:343-346, 1981.

Knowles JA: Drugs in milk. Pediatr Currents 21:28-32, 1972.

Matsuda T: Transfer of antibiotics into maternal milk. Biol Res Pregnancy Perinatol 5:57-60, 1984.

McCormack WM, Rosner B, Lee Y-H, et al.: Effect on birth weight of erythromycin treatment of pregnant women. Obstet Gynecol 69:202-207, 1987.

Mercer BM, Moretti ML, Prevost RR, Sibai BM: Erythromycin therapy in preterm premature rupture of the membranes: A prospective, randomized trial of 220 patients. Am J Obstet Gynecol 166:794-802, 1992.

*This calculation is based upon the following assumptions: maternal dose of erythromycin: 1.2-2 g/d; milk concentration of erythromycin: 0.4-3.2 mcg/mL; milk intake by the nursing infant: 150 mL/kg/d; estimated dose of erythromycin ingested by the nursing infant: 0.06-0.48 mg/kg/d; lowest therapeutic dose of erythromycin in neonates: 20 mg/kg/d.

Moriguchi M, Fujita M, Koeda T: Teratological studies on SF-837 in mice. Jpn J Antibiot 25:193-198, 1972b.

Moriguchi M, Fujita M, Koeda T: Teratological studies on SF-837 in rats. Jpn J Antibiot 25:187-192. 1972a.

Murray L, Seger D: Drug therapy during pregnancy and lactation. Emerg Med Clin North Am 12(1):129-149, 1994.

Romero R, Sibai B, Caritis S, et al.: Antibiotic treatment of preterm labor with intact membranes: A multicenter, randomized, double-blinded, placebo-controlled trial. Am J Obstet Gynecol 169:764-774, 1993.

Takaya M: Teratogenic effects of antibodies. J Osaka City Med Cen 14:107-115, 1965.

USP DI: Erythromycin In: *USP DI (USP Dispensing Information), Volume 1. Drug Information for the Health Care Professional*, 15th ed. Rockville, Md.: The US Pharmacopeial Convention, 1995, p 1245.

WHO Working Group on Drugs and Human Lactation. In: Bennet PN (ed). *Drugs and Human Lactation*. Amsterdam: Elsevier, 1988, pp 253-254.

ESIDRIX® *See* Hydrochlorothiazide

ESKALITH® *See* Lithium

ESTINYL® *See* Ethinyl Estradiol

ETHAMBUTOL
(Etibi®, Myambutol®)

Ethambutol is used in the treatment of tuberculosis. Ethambutol is given orally in doses of 300-2500 mg/d.

Teratogenic Risk

Magnitude of teratogenic risk to child born after exposure during gestation:	*Unlikely*
Quality and quantity of data on which risk estimate is based:	*Poor to fair*

> *Therapeutic doses of ethambutol are unlikely to pose a substantial teratogenic risk, but the data are insufficient to state that there is no risk.*

The frequency of congenital anomalies was not increased among 303 children born to women treated with ethambutol during pregnancy in one series (Jentgens, 1973). Congenital anomalies were noted in 2.2% of 638 infants born to women treated with ethambutol during pregnancy in a series compiled from published cases, including those of Jentgens (Snider et al., 1980). No consistent pattern was observed among the infants who did have anomalies. Of these women, 320 were treated during the first four months of pregnancy.

Unpublished studies are said to have shown an increased frequency of congenital anomalies among the offspring of mice, rats, and rabbits treated with ethambutol during pregnancy (USP DI, 1995). The doses used are said to be "high." Neural tube defects, cleft palate, and vertebral anomalies were the most commonly observed abnormalities among mice, minor anomalies of vertebrae were most common among rats, and ocular abnormalities, cleft lip and palate, and limb reduction defects were most common among rabbits. The relevance of these studies to the therapeutic use of ethambutol in human pregnancy is unknown.

Risk Related to Breast-feeding

Ethambutol is excreted in breast milk in concentrations similar to those found in maternal serum (USP DI, 1995). The amount of ethambutol that the nursing infant would be expected to ingest is between 3-15% of the lowest pediatric therapeutic dose, based on data from two lactating women (Snider & Powell, 1984).*

Ethambutol treatment is contraindicated in children younger than six years of age because optic neuritis, a recognized side effect, is difficult to monitor in small children (USP DI, 1995). However, optic neuritis has not been reported in nursing infants of women treated with ethambutol.

The American Academy of Pediatrics regards ethambutol to be safe to use while breast-feeding (Committee on Drugs, American Academy of Pediatrics, 1994).

*This calculation is based on the following assumptions: maternal dose of ethambutol: 15 mg/kg/d; milk concentration of ethambutol: 1-5 mcg/mL.; milk intake by the nursing infant: 150 mL/kg/d; estimated dose of ethambutol ingested by the nursing infant: 0.15-0.75 mg/kg/d; lowest pediatric therapeutic dose: 5 mg/kg/d.

Key References

Committee on Drugs, American Academy of Pediatrics: The transfer of drugs and other chemicals into human milk. Pediatrics 93(1):137-150, 1994.

Jentgens H: Antituberkulose chemotherapie und schwangerschaftsabbruch. Prax Pneumol 27:479-488, 1973.

Snider DE, Layde PM, Johnson MW, et al.: Treatment of tuberculosis during pregnancy. Am Rev Respir Dis 122:65-79, 1980.

Snider DE, Powell KE: Should women taking antituberculosis drugs breast-feed? Arch Intern Med 144:589-590, 1984.

USP DI: Ethambutol. In: *USP DI (USP Dispensing Information), Volume 1. Drug Information for the Health Care Professional*, 15th ed. Rockville, Md.: The US Pharmacopeial Convention, 1995, pp 1278-1279.

ETHANOL *See* Alcohol

ETHINYL ESTRADIOL
(Estinyl®, Feminone®)

Ethinyl estradiol is a synthetic estrogen. It is a commonly used in oral contraceptives in doses of 20-50 mcg/d in combination with various progestins. Ethinyl estradiol is also given to treat menopausal symptoms and menstrual disorders in oral doses of 20-50 mcg/d. Oral doses up to 150 mcg/d are used in estrogen replacement therapy and a dose of 3000 mcg/d (3 mg/d) is used in palliative treatment of breast cancer. It is used at a daily dose of 200 mcg for postcoital contraception.

Teratogenic Risk

Magnitude of teratogenic risk to child born after exposure during gestation: *None*

Quality and quantity of data on which risk estimate is based: *Good*

255

This rating is for maternal treatment with ethinyl estradiol in doses used for contraception or estrogen replacement. The risk related to very high dose treatment, as is used in some women with breast cancer, is unknown, but such treatment is generally limited to post-menopausal women.

The frequency of congenital anomalies was not significantly increased among the infants of 89 women who took ethinyl estradiol during the first four lunar months of pregnancy or of 98 women who took this drug anytime during pregnancy in one epidemiological study (Heinonen et al., 1977). In another study, use during pregnancy of ethinyl estradiol was no more frequent than expected among the mothers of 171 infants with congenital anomalies (Spira et al., 1972). Similarly, the frequency of hormonal pregnancy tests using ethinyl estradiol during the second month of pregnancy was not increased among the mothers of 194 infants with major malformations or 551 infants with minor anomalies (Kullander & Kallen, 1976).

Studies in monkeys, mice, rats, and rabbits suggest that treatment of pregnant women with ethinyl estradiol in doses used for contraception or therapy of estrogen deficiency is unlikely to increase the children's risk of nongenital malformations greatly (Yasuda et al., 1981; Joshi et al., 1983; Hendrickx et al., 1987; Harada et al., 1991a, b; Kwarta et al., 1991a, b). Embryonic loss and genital alterations were observed at higher doses in cynomolgus monkeys, but such doses were also toxic to the mothers. Pregnancy loss occurred in rhesus monkeys treated with this drug at 100 times the human contraceptive dose (Prahalada & Hendrickx, 1983). Pregnancy loss was frequent at even higher doses in rodents. Alterations of gonadal and internal genital tract morphology were observed among the offspring of mice treated during pregnancy with 20-2000 times the human contraceptive dose of ethinyl estradiol (Yasuda et al., 1987, 1988). Cryptorchidism was found with increased frequency among the offspring of a genetically-predisposed strain of mice treated during pregnancy with 200 times the human contraceptive dose of ethinyl estradiol (Walker et al., 1990). The relevance of these observations to the use of ethinyl estradiol in human pregnancy is uncertain.

Risk Related to Breast-feeding

Ethinyl estradiol is excreted in the breast milk. The amount of ethinyl estradiol that the nursing infant would receive is between 2-14% of the lowest weight-adjusted dose used for oral contraception, based on data from eight lactating mothers who took oral contraceptives containing ethinyl estradiol (Nilsson et al., 1978a).* This amount is similar to breast milk concentrations of natural estradiol measured in mothers not taking oral contraceptives (Nilsson et al., 1978b).

No effect of maternal use of oral contraceptives containing ethinyl estradiol was observed on the physical or mental development of 48 breast-fed children followed until eight years of (Nilsson et al., 1986).

Inhibition of lactation by estrogens is dose-related so that oral contraceptives containing low doses of estrogen have little, if any, effect on milk production in well-nourished mothers (Kamal et al., 1970; Borglin & Sandholm, 1971; WHO, 1984; Brumsted & Riddick, 1994).

The American Academy of Pediatrics regards combination oral contraceptives to be safe to use while breast-feeding (Committee on Drugs, American Academy of Pediatrics, 1994).

Key References

Borglin N-E, Sandholm L-E: Effect of oral contraceptives on lactation. Fertil Steril 22:39-41, 1971.

Brumsted JR, Riddick DH: The breast during pregnancy and lactation. In: Speroff L, et al. (eds). *Gynecology and Obstetrics,* Volume 5. Philadelphia, Pa.: JB Lippincott, 1994, p 10.

Committee on Drugs, American Academy of Pediatrics: The transfer of drugs and other chemicals into human milk. Pediatrics 93(1):137-150, 1994.

Harada S, Takayama S, Miyazaki Y, et al.: Teratogenicity study of oral contraceptives DT-5061 and DT-5062 (1/35) in rabbits. Yakuri To Chiryo 19(Suppl 4):233-249, 1991b.

Harada S, Takayama S, Shibano T, et al.: Teratogenicity study of oral contraceptives DT-5061 and DT-5062 (1/35) in rats. Yakuri To Chiryo 19(Suppl 4):197-231, 1991a.

Heinonen OP, Slone D, Shapiro S: *Birth Defects and Drugs in Pregnancy.* Littleton, Mass.: John Wright-PSG, 1977, pp 389-391, 443.

*This calculation is based on the following assumptions: maternal dose of ethinyl estradiol: 50-500 mcg/d; milk concentrations of ethinyl estradiol: 0.00005-0.0003 mcg/mL; milk intake by the nursing infant: 150 mL/kg/d; estimated dose of ethinyl estradiol ingested by the nursing infant: 0.007-0.045 mcg/kg/d; lowest oral contraceptive dose of ethinyl estradiol: 0.31 mcg/kg/d.

Hendrickx AG, Korte R, Leuschner F, et al.: Embryotoxicity of sex steroidal hormone combinations in nonhuman primates: I. Norethisterone acetate + ethinylestradiol and progesterone estradiol benzoate (*Macaca mulatta, Macaca fascicularis,* and *Papio cynocephalus*). Teratology 35:119-127, 1987.

Joshi NJ, Ambani LM, Munshi SR: Evaluation of teratogenic potential of a combination of norethisterone and ethinyl estradiol in rats. Indian J Exp Biol 21:591-596, 1983.

Kamal I, Hefnawi F, Ghoneim M, et al.: Clinical, biochemical, and experimental studies on lactation. V. Clinical effects of steroids on the initiation of lactation. Am J Obstet Gynecol 108(4):655-658, 1970.

Kullander S, Kallen B: A prospective study of drugs and pregnancy. 3. Hormones. Acta Obstet Gynecol Scand 55:221-224, 1976.

Kwarta RF Jr, Hemm RD, Pollock JJ, et al.: Levonorgestrel/ethinyl estradiol: Developmental toxicity study with behavioral and reproductive assessment of the offspring (seg II-rat). Oyo Yakuri 42(4):327-340, 1991a.

Kwarta RF Jr, Hemm RD, Pollock JJ, et al.: Levonorgestrel/ethinyl estradiol: Study of developmental toxicity in rabbits. Oyo Yakuri 42(4):341-349, 1991b.

Nilsson S, Mellbin T, Hofvander Y, et al.: Long-term follow-up of children breast-fed by mothers using oral contraceptives. Contraception 34(5):443-457, 1986.

Nilsson S, Nygren K-G, Johansson EDB: Ethinyl estradiol in human milk and plasma after oral administration. Contraception 17:131-139, 1978a.

Nilsson S, Nygren K-G, Johansson EDB: Transfer of estradiol to human milk. Am J Obstet Gynecol 132:653-657, 1978b.

Prahalada S, Hendrickx AG: Embryotoxicity of norlestrin, a combined synthetic oral contraceptive, in rhesus macaques (*Macaca mulatta*). Teratology 27:215-222, 1983.

Spira N, Goujard J, Huel G, Rumeau-Rouquette C: [Investigation into the teratogenic action of sex hormones first results of an epidemiologic survey involving 20,000 women.] Rev Med 41:2683-2694, 1972.

Walker AH, Bernstein L, Warren DW, et al.: The effect of in utero ethinyl oestradiol exposure on the risk of cryptorchid testis and testicular teratoma in mice. Br J Cancer 62(4):599-602, 1990.

WHO: World Health Organization Special Programme of Research, Development and Research Training in Human Reproduction.

Task force on oral contraceptives. Effects of hormonal contraceptives on milk volume and infant growth. Contraception 30(6):505-522, 1984.

Yasuda Y, Kihara T, Nishimura H: Effect of ethinyl estradiol on development of mouse fetuses. Teratology 23:233-239, 1981.

Yasuda Y, Konishi H, Tanimura T: Ovarian follicular cell hyperplasia in fetal mice treated transplacentally with ethinyl estradiol. Teratology 36:35-43, 1987.

Yasuda Y, Ohara I, Konishi H, Tanimura T: Long-term effects on male reproductive organs of prenatal exposure to ethinyl estradiol. Am J Obstet Gynecol 159(5):1246-1250, 1988.

ETHOSUXIMIDE
(Zarontin®)

Ethosuximide is a succinimide anticonvulsant used to treat petit mal epilepsy. Ethosuximide is given orally in doses of 500-1500 mg/d.

Teratogenic Risk

*Magnitude of teratogenic
risk to child born after
exposure during gestation:*   *None to minimal*

*Quality and quantity of data
on which risk estimate is based:*   *Poor to fair*

This assessment is based on limited data. Because ethosuximide is an anticonvulsant and maternal treatment with other anticonvulsant drugs during pregnancy is associated with an increased risk of congenital anomalies, it is possible that ethosuximide may have similar teratogenic risks.

The frequency of congenital anomalies was no greater than expected among 57 children of women with seizure disorders treated with ethosuximide during pregnancy in one study (Lindhout et al., 1992). In a prospective series of children born to women who had been treated with anticonvulsants during pregnancy, maternal use of ethosuximide was no more frequent among 23 children with major or minor congenital anomalies than among unaffected children (Lander & Eadie, 1990).

Increased frequencies of skeletal, central nervous system, and other anomalies were observed among the offspring of rats, mice, hamsters, and rabbits treated during pregnancy with ethosuximide in doses, respectively, <1-25, 6-36, <1-18, and <1-7 times those used in humans (Sullivan & McElhatton, 1977; Dluzniewski et al., 1979; El-Sayed et al., 1983). Behavioral alterations were seen among the offspring of rats treated during pregnancy with ethosuximide in doses similar to those used clinically (Nakanishi & Fujii, 1990). The clinical relevance of these observations is unclear.

Risk Related to Breast-feeding

Ethosuximide is excreted in breast milk in concentrations approximating those of maternal serum (Koup et al., 1978; Kaneko et al., 1979; Rane & Tunell, 1981; Kuhnz et al., 1984). The amount of ethosuximide that the nursing infant would be expected to ingest is between 13-58% of the lowest pediatric dose, based on data from 21 lactating mothers (Koup et al., 1978; Kaneko et al., 1979; Rane & Tunell, 1981; Kuhnz et al., 1984).*

Serum levels of ethosuximide in nursing infants of treated women range between 26-100% of the lowest therapeutic serum concentration of ethosuximide in adults (Rane & Tunell, 1981; Kuhnz et al., 1984).[†]

The American Academy of Pediatrics regards ethosuximide to be safe to use while breast-feeding (Committee on Drugs, American Academy of Pediatrics, 1994); however, the WHO Working Group on Drugs and Human Lactation (1988) does not recommend breast-feeding while taking ethosuximide because of the high plasma levels found in nursing infants

Key References

Committee on Drugs, American Academy of Pediatrics: The transfer of drugs and other chemicals into human milk. Pediatrics 93(1):137-150, 1994.

*This calculation is based on the following assumptions: maternal dose of ethosuximide: 3.5-23.6 mg/kg/d; milk concentrations of ethosuximide: 18-77 mcg/mL; milk intake by the nursing infant: 150 mL/kg/d; estimated dose of ethosuximide ingested by the nursing infant: 2.7-11.5 mg/kg/d; lowest pediatric dose of ethosuximide: 20 mg/kg/d.

†Infant serum levels of ethosuximide: 10.6-40 mcg/mL; lowest therapeutic concentration of ethosuximide in adults: 40 mcg/mL.

Dluzniewski A, Gastol-Lewinska L, Kulej-Grodecka A, et al.: Teratogenic activity of ethosuximide in rats, hamsters, and rabbits. In: Benasova O, Rychter A, Jelinek R (eds). *Evaluation of Embryotoxicity, Mutagenicity and Carcinogenicity Risks in New Drugs. Proc 3rd Symp on Toxicol Test for Safety of New Drugs.* Prague: Univerzita Karlova, 1979, pp 59-68.

El-Sayed MGA, Aly AE, Kadri M, Moustafa AM: Comparative study on the teratogenicity of some antiepileptics in the rat. East Afr Med J 60:407-415, 1983.

Kaneko S, Sato T, Suzuki K: The levels of anticonvulsants in breast milk. Br J Clin Pharmacol 7:624-626, 1979.

Koup JR, Rose JQ, Cohen ME: Ethosuximide pharmacokinetics in a pregnant patient and her newborn. Epilepsia 19:535-539, 1978.

Kuhnz W, Koch S, Jakob S, et al.: Ethosuximide in epileptic women during pregnancy and lactation period. Placental transfer, serum concentrations in nursed infants and clinical status. Br J Clin Pharmacol 18:671-677, 1984.

Lander CM, Eadie MJ: Antiepileptic drug intake during pregnancy and malformed offspring. Epilepsy Res 7:77-82, 1990.

Lindhout D, Meinardi H, Meijer WJA, Nau H: Antiepileptic drugs and teratogenesis in two consecutive cohorts: Changes in prescription policy paralleled by changes in pattern of malformations. Neurology 42(Suppl 5):94-110, 1992.

Nakanishi H, Fujii T: Behavioral changes in juvenile rats after prenatal exposure to ethosuximide. Pharmacol Biochem Behav 36(1):163-168, 1990.

Rane A, Tunell R: Ethosuximide in human milk and in plasma of a mother and her nursed infant. Br J Clin Pharmacol 12:855-858, 1981.

Sullivan FM, McElhatton PR: A comparison of the teratogenic activity of the antiepileptic drugs carbamazepine, clonazepam, ethosuximide, phenobarbital, phenytoin and primidone in mice. Toxicol Appl Pharmacol 40:365-378, 1977.

WHO Working Group on Drugs and Human Lactation. In: Bennet PN (ed). *Drugs and Human Lactation.* Amsterdam: Elsevier, 1988, pp 333-334.

ETHYNODIOL DIACETATE
(Demulen®, Nelulen®)

Ethynodiol diacetate is a synthetic progestin that is used alone or in combination with an estrogenic compound as an oral contraceptive and in treatment of menstrual disorders. The oral dose of ethynodiol diacetate ranges from 0.5-2.0 mg/d.

Teratogenic Risk

*Magnitude of teratogenic
risk to child born after
exposure during gestation:*   *Unlikely*

*Quality and quantity of data
on which risk estimate is based:*   *Poor to fair*

Therapeutic doses of ethynodiol diacetate are unlikely to pose a substantial teratogenic risk, but the data are insufficient to state that there is no risk.
This risk estimate is for virilization of the genitalia in a female fetus. The estimate is based on studies involving use of other progestational hormones at doses that are often much greater than those currently employed.

Maternal use of ethynodiol diacetate was no more frequent than expected among 171 infants with congenital anomalies in one epidemiological study (Spira et al., 1972).

The frequency of malformations was no greater than expected among the offspring of rats treated during pregnancy with ethynodiol diacetate in combination with an estrogenic agent in doses 10-100 times those used in human contraception, although increased fetal loss was observed among pregnant animals treated with 24 or more times the usual human dose of ethynodiol diacetate alone (Saunders & Elton, 1967). Malformations were no more frequent than expected among the offspring of rabbits treated during pregnancy with ethynodiol diacetate alone or in combination with an estrogenic agent in doses 1-25 or more times greater than those used in human contraception (Saunders & Elton, 1967).

Risk Related to Breast-feeding

Ethynodiol diacetate, is excreted into breast milk (USP DI, 1995), although this not been quantitated in published reports.

The American Academy of Pediatrics regards oral contraceptives to be safe to use while breast-feeding (Committee on Drugs, American Academy of Pediatrics, 1994).

Key References

Committee on Drugs, American Academy of Pediatrics: The transfer of drugs and other chemicals into human milk. Pediatrics 93(1):137-150, 1994.

Saunders FJ, Elton RL: Effects of ethynodiol diacetate and mestranol in rats and rabbits, on conception, on the outcome of pregnancy and on the offspring. Toxicol Appl Pharmacol 11:229-244, 1967.

Spira N, Goujard J, Huel G, et al.: Investigation into the teratogenic action of sex hormones: First results of an epidemiologic survey involving 20,000 women. Rev Med 41:2683-2694, 1972.

USP DI: Estrogens and progestins (oral contraceptives). In: *USP DI (USP Dispensing Information), Volume 1. Drug Information for the Health Care Professional*, 15th ed. Rockville, Md.: The US Pharmacopeial Convention, 1995, p 1272.

ETIBI® *See* Ethambutol

FAMOTIDINE
(Pepcid®)

Famotidine is a histamine H$_2$-receptor antagonist used in the treatment of peptic ulcer and gastric hypersecretory states. Famotidine is given orally or parenterally; the usual dose is 20-40 mg/d, although doses as great as 640 mg/d are sometimes used in severe Zollinger-Ellison syndrome.

Teratogenic Risk

*Magnitude of teratogenic
risk to child born after
exposure during gestation:*   *Undetermined*

263

No epidemiological studies of congenital anomalies among the children of women treated with famotidine during pregnancy have been reported.

Studies in rats and rabbits suggest that treatment of pregnant women with famotidine in usual therapeutic doses is unlikely to increase the children's risk of malformations greatly (Shibata et al., 1983; Burek et al., 1985).

Please see agent summary on cimetidine for information on a related drug.

Risk Related to Breast-feeding

Famotidine is excreted in breast milk in low concentrations. The amount of famotidine that the nursing infant would be expected to ingest is approximately 1% of the lowest pediatric dose, based on data from eight lactating women (Courtney et al., 1988).*

Key References

Burek JD, Majka JA, Bokelman DL: Famotidine: Summary of preclinical safety assessment. Digestion 32(Suppl 1):7-14, 1985.

Courtney TP, Shaw RW, Cedar E, et al.: Excretion of famotidine in breast milk. Clin Pharmacol 26:639P, 1988.

Shibata M, Kawano K, Shiobara Y: Teratological study of famotidine (YM-11170) administered orally to rats. Oyo Yakuri 26:489-497, 1983.

*This calculation is based on the following assumptions: maternal dose of famotidine: 40 mg; milk concentration of famotidine: 0.02-0.07 mcg/mL; milk intake by the nursing infant: 150 mL/kg/d; estimated dose of famotidine ingested by the nursing infant: 0.002-0.01 mg/kg/d; lowest pediatric dose of famotidine: 1 mg/kg/d.

FEDRINE® *See* Ephedrine

FELDENE® *See* Piroxicam

FEMINONE® *See* Ethinyl Estradiol

FEMOTRONE® *See* Progesterone

FENOPREN
(Nalfon®)

Fenoprofen is a nonsteroidal anti-inflammatory agent with analgesic and antipyretic actions. It is given orally in doses of 900-3200 mg/d to treat dysmenorrhea, other kinds of pain, and rheumatic disorders.

Teratogenic Risk

Magnitude of teratogenic risk to child born after exposure during gestation:	*Undetermined*
Quality and quantity of data on which risk estimate is based:	*Very poor*

No epidemiological studies of congenital anomalies in the children of women who took fenoprofen during pregnancy have been reported.

In one study published only as an abstract, no teratogenic effects were noted in the offspring of rats or rabbits treated during pregnancy with fenoprofen in doses 1.5-2.5 times those used clinically (Emmerson et al., 1973).

Premature closure of the ductus arteriosus was observed among the offspring of rats treated near term with fenoprofen in doses equivalent to or slightly larger than those used in humans (Powell & Cochrane, 1978; Momma et al., 1984). Similar abnormalities of perinatal cardiovascular adaptation have been reported in human neonates whose mothers took drugs that are pharmacologically similar to fenoprofen late in pregnancy [*please see agent summary on indomethacin for further discussion*].

Several prostaglandin inhibitors have been shown to block or delay labor in women late in pregnancy (Zuckerman et al., 1974; Grella & Zanor, 1978), but such studies have not been reported for fenoprofen.

Risk Related to Breast-feeding

Fenoprofen is excreted in breast milk in very small amounts (Rubin et al., 1974).

Key References

Emmerson JL, Gibson WR, Pierce EC, Todd GC: Preclinical toxicology of fenoprofen. Toxicol Appl Pharmacol 25:444, 1973.

Grella P, Zanor P: Premature labor and indomethacin. Prostaglandins 16:1007-1017, 1978.

Momma K, Hagiwara H, Konishi T: Constriction of fetal ductus arteriosus by non-steroidal anti-inflammatory drugs: Study of additional 34 drugs. Prostaglandins 28:527-536, 1984.

Powell JG, Cochrane RL: The effects of the administration of fenoprofen or indomethacin to rat dams during late pregnancy, with special reference to the ductus arteriosus of the fetuses and neonates. Toxicol Appl Pharmacol 45:783-796, 1978.

Rubin A, Chernish SM, Crabtree R, et al.: A profile of the physiological disposition and gastro-intestinal effects of fenoprofen in man. Curr Med Res Opin 2:529-544, 1974.

Zuckerman H, Reiss U, Rubinstein I: Inhibition of human premature labor by indomethacin. Obstet Gynecol 44:787-792, 1974.

FERROUS FUMURATE *See* Iron

FERROUS GLUCONATE *See* Iron

FERROUS SULFATE *See* Iron

FIBERALL® *See* Psyllium

FLAGYL® *See* Metronidazole

FLAVITAN® *See* Riboflavin

FLETCHER'S CASTORIA *See* Senna

FLEURDIN® *See* Flunarizine

FLEXERIL® *See* Cyclobenzaprine

FLUCONAZOLE
(Diflucan®)

Fluconazole is a triazole antifungal agent used to treat serious mycotic infections. It is given orally or intravenously in doses of 100-400 mg/d. In exceptional cases, doses of up to 800 mg/d are given.

Teratogenic Risk

Magnitude of teratogenic risk to child born after exposure during gestation:	*Undetermined*
Quality and quantity of data on which risk estimate is based:	*Very Poor*

No epidemiological studies of congenital anomalies among infants born to women treated with fluconazole during pregnancy have been reported. A child with features of Antley-Bixler syndrome, an autosomal recessive condition, was born to a woman who was treated with fluconazole throughout pregnancy, but this occurrence is almost certainly coincidental (Lee et al., 1992).

In unpublished studies, the frequency of malformations was reportedly not increased among the offspring of pregnant rabbits treated with 1-9 times the usual human dose of fluconazole, although fetal loss was increased at the highest dose (USP DI, 1995). Increased fetal death is said to have occurred among pregnant rats treated with 3 times the human dose of fluconazole, and skeletal, craniofacial, and palatal anomalies were seen with doses 10-40 times those used in humans (Lee et al., 1992; USP DI, 1995). Maternal toxicity occurred at all these doses in both species, and the fetal effects may have been related to this toxicity rather than to direct teratogenicity of the agent. The relevance of these findings to the therapeutic use of fluconazole in human pregnancy is unknown.

Risk Related to Breast-feeding

Fluconazole is excreted in human milk in amounts similar to those found in maternal plasma (USP DI, 1995). Based on this data, the amount of fluconazole that the nursing infant would be expected to ingest is equivalent to the lowest pediatric dose.*

Key References

Lee BE, Feinberg M, Abraham JJ, Murthy ARK: Congenital malformations in an infant born to a woman treated with fluconazole. Pediatr Infect Dis J 11:1062-1064, 1992.

USP DI: Antifungals, Azole. In: *USP DI (USP Dispensing Information), Volume 1. Drug Information for the Health Care Professional,* 15th ed. Rockville, Md.: The US Pharmacopeial Convention, 1995, p 282.

*This calculation is based on the following assumptions: therapeutic serum level of fluconazole in adults: 6.5 mcg/mL; milk concentration of fluconazole: 6.5 mcg/mL; milk intake by the nursing infant: 150 mL/kg/d; estimated dose of fluconazole ingested by the nursing infant: 0.97 mg/kg/d; lowest therapeutic dose of fluconazole in children: 1 mg/kg/d.

FLUGERAL® *See* Flunarizine

FLU-IMMUNE® *See* Influenza Virus Vaccine

FLUNARIZINE
(Fleurdin®, Flugeral®)

Flunarizine is a calcium channel blocking agent that is used to treat migraine headache and other cerebrovascular disorders. Flunarizine is administered orally; the usual dose is 10 mg/d.

Teratogenic Risk

Magnitude of teratogenic risk to child born after exposure during gestation:	*Undetermined*
Quality and quantity of data on which risk estimate is based:	*Poor*

No epidemiological studies of congenital anomalies among infants born to women treated with flunarizine during pregnancy have been reported.

Increased fetal death and fetal growth retardation were seen in association with maternal toxicity when rats were treated with 150-400 times the human dose of flunarizine during pregnancy (Miyazaki et al., 1982). The frequency of malformations was not significantly increased among the offspring of pregnant rats treated with 150 times the human dose of flunarizine, and no teratogenic effect was seen among the offspring of rats treated during pregnancy with 15-50 times the human dose. Fetal death was also increased in association with maternal toxicity when pregnant rabbits were treated with 110-180 times the human dose of flunarizine (Miyazaki et al., 1982), but no increase in malformations was seen at these or lower doses. The relevance of these observations to the use of flunarizine in therapeutic doses in human pregnancy is unknown.

Risk Related to Breast-feeding

No information regarding the distribution of flunarizine in breast milk has been published.

Key References

Miyazaki E, Haro T, Nishikawa T, Oguro T: [Toxicologic studies of K-W-3149.] Kiso To Rinsho 16:1840-1859, 1982.

FLUNISOLIDE
(Nasalide®, Rhinalar®)

Flunisolide is a synthetic glucocorticoid used by inhalation in doses of 1-2 mg/d to treat asthma. Flunisolide is also given by nasal instillation in doses of 0.2-0.4 mg/d to treat allergic rhinitis. Systemic absorption occurs after administration by either route.

Teratogenic Risk

*Magnitude of teratogenic
risk to child born after
exposure during gestation:*   *Undetermined*

*Quality and quantity of data
on which risk estimate is based:*   *Poor*

A small risk cannot be excluded, but a high risk of congenital anomalies in the children of women treated with flunisolide during pregnancy is unlikely.

No epidemiological studies of congenital anomalies among the infants of women treated with flunisolide during pregnancy have been reported.

Increased frequencies of cleft palate and other anomalies have been observed among the offspring of mice and rats treated during pregnancy with flunisolide in doses respectively 5 and 2.5 times those used in the therapy of asthma in humans (Itabashi et al., 1982; Tamagawa et al., 1982). Teratogenic effects were not seen with lower doses in either strain. The relevance of these findings to the clinical use of flunisolide in human pregnancy is unknown.

Please see agent summary on beclomethasone for information on a related drug that has been more thoroughly studied.

Risk Related to Breast-feeding

No information regarding the distribution of flunisolide in breast milk has been published. However, high concentrations of inhaled corticosteroids in breast milk are unlikely (USP DI, 1995).

Key References

Itabashi M, Inoue T, Yokota M, et al.: Reproduction studies on flunisolide in rats. (2) Oral administration during the period of organogenesis. Oyo Yakuri (Pharmacometrics) 24(5):643-659, 1982.

Tamagawa M, Hatori M, Ooi A, et al.: Comparative teratological study of flunisolide in mice. Oyo Yakuri (Pharmacometrics) 24(6):741-750, 1982.

USP DI: Corticosteroids. In: *USP DI (USP Dispensing Information), Volume 1. Drug Information for the Health Care Professional,* 15th ed. Rockville, Md.: The US Pharmacopeial Convention, 1995, p 841.

FLUOCINONIDE
(Lidex®, Lyderm®, Metosyn®)

Fluocinonide is a synthetic glucocorticoid used topically in the treatment of dermatologic disorders. Systemic absorption occurs after topical application of fluocinonide.

Teratogenic Risk

Magnitude of teratogenic risk to child born after exposure during gestation:	*Undetermined*
Quality and quantity of data on which risk estimate is based:	*None*

No epidemiological studies of congenital anomalies in infants born to women who used fluocinonide during pregnancy have been reported. No animal teratology studies of fluocinonide have been published.

Risk Related to Breast-feeding

No information regarding the distribution of fluocinonide in breast milk has been published. Application of fluocinonide to the breasts prior to nursing is not recommended (USP DI, 1995).

Key References

USP DI: Corticosteroids. In: *USP DI (USP Dispensing Information), Volume 1. Drug Information for the Health Care Professional*, 15th ed. Rockville, Md.: The US Pharmacopeial Convention, 1995, p 860.

FLUOGEN® *See* Influenza Virus Vaccine

FLUOXETINE
(Prozac®)

Fluoxetine is an antidepressant that selectively inhibits the reuptake of serotonin. Fluoxetine is given orally in doses of 20-80 mg/d.

Teratogenic Risk

*Magnitude of teratogenic
risk to child born after
exposure during gestation:*   None

*Quality and quantity of data
on which risk estimate is based:*   Poor to fair

The frequency of congenital anomalies was no greater than expected among the infants of 98 women who took fluoxetine during the first trimester of pregnancy in one epidemiological study (Pastuszak et al., 1993). Six infants from 107 pregnancies in which the mother took fluoxetine in another series had congenital anomalies (Chambers et al., 1992). The malformations developed prior to treatment in at least two of these cases. The frequency of congenital anomalies did not appear unusual among the infants of 59 women who were pregnant while taking part in clinical trials of fluoxetine or among the children of 485 women voluntarily reported to the manufacturer during a pregnancy in which they were taking fluoxetine (Goldstein & Marvel., 1993). Among 28 infants with major congenital anomalies born to women who had taken fluoxetine during pregnancy and retrospectively reported to the manufacturer, no consistent pattern of malformations was apparent (Goldstein & Marvel, 1993).

Studies in rats and rabbits suggest that treatment of pregnant women with fluoxetine in usual therapeutic doses is unlikely to increase the children's risk of malformations greatly (Byrd et al., 1989; Hoyt et al., 1989).

Risk Related to Breast-feeding

Fluoxetine and its active metabolite, norfluoxetine, are excreted in the breast milk. The amount of fluoxetine and norfluoxetine that the nursing infant would be expected to ingest is <1-18% of the lowest weight-adjusted therapeutic dose, based on data from 13 nursing mothers (Isenberg, 1990; Burch & Wells, 1992; Lester et al., 1993; Taddio et al., 1994).*

Serum levels of fluoxetine and norfluoxetine were measured in two infants whose mothers were taking fluoxetine while breast-feeding. Although measurable serum levels of fluoxetine were not found in one infant (Taddio et al., 1994), fluoxetine and norfluoxetine serum levels well within the therapeutic range were detected in the serum of another infant (Lester et al.,1993).[†] Vomiting, excessive crying, watery stools, and decreased sleep were observed in this infant. These symptoms disappeared when the mother began bottle-feeding the infant and recurred when the infant was again permitted to breast-feed while the mother continued to take the drug.

Although similar adverse effects were not reported in the other infants studied, the American Academy of Pediatrics regards fluoxetine to be a drug that could potentially affect central nervous system function in nursing infants (Committee on Drugs, American Academy of Pediatrics, 1994).

Key References

Burch KJ, Wells BG: Fluoxetine/norfluoxetine concentrations in human milk. Pediatrics 89:676-677, 1992.

Byrd RA, Brophy GT, Markham JK: Developmental toxicology studies of fluoxetine hydrochloride (I) administered orally to rats and rabbits. Teratology 39(5):444, 1989.

Chambers CD, Johnson KA, Jones KL: Pregnancy outcome in women exposed to fluoxetine. Teratology 45(5):527, 1992.

Committee on Drugs, American Academy of Pediatrics: The transfer of drugs and other chemicals into human milk. Pediatrics 93(1):137-150, 1994.

Goldstein D, Marvel D, et al.: Psychotropic medications during pregnancy: Risk to the fetus. JAMA 270(18):2177, 1993.

*This calculation is based on the following assumptions: maternal dose of fluoxetine: 20 mg/d; milk concentration of fluoxetine and norfluoxetine: 0.02-0.18 mcg/mL and 0.01-0.2 mcg/mL, respectively; milk intake by the nursing infant: 150 mL/kg/d; estimated dose of both fluoxetine and norfluoxetine ingested by the nursing infant, assuming similar bioavailability and molecular weights and demonstrated activity similar to fluoxetine: 0.004-0.056 mg/kg/d; lowest therapeutic dose of fluoxetine in adults: 0.31 mg/kg/d.

†Infant serum levels of fluoxetine and norfluoxetine: 0.34 mcg/mL and 0.21 mcg/mL, respectively; therapeutic range of serum concentrations of fluoxetine and norfluoxetine in adults: 0.09-0.3 mcg/mL and 0.07-0.3 mcg/mL, respectively.

Hoyt JA, Byrd RA, Brophy GT, et al.: A reproduction study of fluoxetine hydrochloride. (I) Administration in the diet to rats. Teratology 39(5):459-1989.

Isenberg KE: Excretion of fluoxetine in human breast milk. J Clin Psychiatry 51(4):169, 1990.

Lester BM, Cuccca J, Andreozzi L, et al.: Possible association between fluoxetine hydrochloride and colic in an infant. J Am Acad Child Adolesc Psychiatry 32(6):1253-1255, 1993.

Pastuszak A, Schick-Boschetto B, Zuber D, et al.: Pregnancy outcome following first-trimester exposure to fluoxetine (Prozac®). JAMA 269(17):2246-2248, 1993.

Taddio A, Ito S, Koren G: Excretion of fluoxetine and its metabolite in human breast milk. Pediatr Res 35 (4 Part 2):149A, 1994.

FLURAZEPAM
(Dalmane®)

Flurazepam is a benzodiazepine derivative that is used as a hypnotic. It is given orally in doses of 15-30 mg.

Teratogenic Risk

*Magnitude of teratogenic
risk to child born after
exposure during gestation:*   *Unlikely*

*Quality and quantity of data
on which risk estimate is based:*   *Poor*

Therapeutic doses of flurazepam are unlikely to pose a substantial teratogenic risk, but the data are insufficient to state that there is no risk.

No epidemiological studies of congenital anomalies among infants born to women treated with flurazepam during pregnancy have been reported.

Studies in rats, mice, and rabbits suggest that treatment of pregnant women with flurazepam in usual therapeutic doses is unlikely to increase the children's risk of malformations greatly (Irikura et al., 1977; Noda et al., 1977).

Please see agent summary on diazepam for information on a related drug that has been more thoroughly studied.

Risk Related to Breast-feeding

No information regarding the distribution of flurazepam in breast milk has been published.

Key References

Irikura T, Hosomi J, Suzuki H, et al.: Teratological study on flurazepam free base in mice and rats. Oyo Yakuri 14:659-667, 1977.

Noda K, Hirabayashi M, Irikura T, et al.: Teratological study on flurazepam free base in rabbits. Oyo Yakuri 14:801-804, 1977.

FLUZONE® *See* Influenza Vaccine

FOLEX® *See* Methotrexate

FOLIC ACID
(Folvite®, Novo-Folacid®)

Folic acid is a water-soluble B vitamin that is required for the synthesis of DNA and the metabolism of some amino acids. Folates occur in many foods including green vegetables, potatoes, cereals, fruits, and liver. The US recommended dietary allowance (RDA) for folic acid is 0.4 mg/d during pregnancy and 0.28 during lactation (NRC, 1989; Bailey, 1992). Doses of 1 mg/d of folic acid are frequently used to treat deficiency states, and doses up to 15 mg/d are used in patients with malabsorption syndromes. Folic acid is usually given orally, but it may also be administered parenterally.

Teratogenic Risk

*Magnitude of teratogenic
risk to child born after
exposure during gestation:*   *None*

(The risk of neural tube defects is reduced in the children of women who take folic acid during early pregnancy--see below.)

Quality and quantity of data
on which risk estimate is based: *Good to excellent*

> *The current RDA for folic acid in pregnancy appears to be subop-timal because the rate of congenital anomalies, especially neural tube defects, is lower in women who take folic acid supplements during pregnancy (Oakley et al., 1994; Crandall et al., 1995; Cunningham et al., 1995).*
>
> *This rating is for maternal use of folic acid supplements in a dose of 0.4-4.0 mg/d in early pregnancy. The risk associated with maternal use of larger doses of folic acid during pregnancy is unknown.*

Maternal ingestion of 0.4-4.0 mg/d of folic acid early in pregnancy reduces the risk of neural tube defects in infants (Rose & Mennuti, 1994; Wald, 1994; Wald & Bower, 1994; Czeizel, 1995). In a random-ized controlled trial involving 2104 pregnancies in women who re-ceived multivitamin supplements containing 0.8 mg/d of folic acid be-ginning before conception, the frequency of neural tube defects was substantially reduced (Czeizel & Dudas, 1992). In another epidemiol-ogical study involving 361 infants with neural tube defects, a negative association, i.e., a protective effect, was seen with maternal daily use of multivitamins containing folic acid (usually 0.4 mg) between 28 days before and 28 days after conception of the affected pregnancy (Werler et al., 1993). A negative association was also seen with maternal use of folic acid during the first trimester of pregnancy in a study involving 287 infants with neural tube defects (Martinez-Frias & Rodriguez-Pinilla, 1992). Similar results were obtained in a study of 77 children with isolated neural tube defects when the analysis was perfomed by estimating maternal free folate intake from all sources during the first six weeks of pregnancy (Bower & Stanley, 1989). In a study of women in whom serum α-fetoprotein testing was performed, the frequency of neural tube defects was significantly lower among the infants of 10,713 women who took multivitamins containing folic acid in the first six weeks of pregnancy (Milunsky et al., 1989). No association with ma-ternal use of folate-containing multivitamins early in pregnancy was found in one study of infants with neural tube defects (Mills et al., 1989).

The protective effect of maternal folic acid supplementation early in gestation is also supported by studies of recurrence of neural tube defects in infants of women who have previously had an affected child

(Laurence et al., 1981; Smithells et al., 1983; Vergel et al., 1990; Kirke et al., 1992; MRC Vitamin Study Research Group, 1991).

The frequency of other congenital anomalies may also be decreased in the children of women who take supplemental folic acid during pregnancy. The rate of congenital anomalies in general was decreased among the infants of 2104 women who received periconceptional folic acid supplementation in a randomized controlled trial (Czeizel & Dudas, 1992; Czeizel, 1993). Maternal multivitamin and folic acid supplementation early in pregnancy has been associated with a decreased risk of recurrence for cleft lip in some studies (Conway, 1958; Briggs, 1976; Tolarova, 1982). A protective effect of higher maternal folate intake during pregnancy was seen in a case-control study of 166 children with neuroectodermal brain tumors (Bunin et al., 1993).

No teratology studies of animals fed excessive amounts of folic acid during pregnancy have been reported.

Risk Related to Breast-feeding

Folic acid is a normal constitutent of breast milk. Concentrations of folic acid in breast milk increase as lactation progresses regardless of maternal folate status (Butte & Calloway, 1981; Cooperman et al., 1982; Ford et al., 1983). The amount of total folate that the nursing infant would be expected to ingest is between <1-10 times the RDA for infants up to one year of age (Tamura et al., 1980; Ek, 1983; Smith et al., 1983).*

Only when there is a folic-acid deficiency in the mother does daily supplementation with folic acid produce an increase in breast milk folate levels (Metz, 1970; Tamura et al., 1980; Thomas et al., 1980; Sneed et al., 1981; Smith et al., 1983; Subcommittee on Nutrition & Lactation, 1991). As a result of these increased breast milk concentrations, the nursing infant would be expected to ingest folic acid in amounts that exceeded the RDA for infants. No adverse effects have been reported in nursing infants whose mothers took large amounts of folic acid.

The American Academy of Pediatrics regards folic acid to be safe to take while breast-feeding (Committee on Drugs, American Academy of Pediatrics, 1994).

*This calculation is based on the following assumptions: milk concentrations of total and free folate: 0.006-0.28 mcg/mL and 0.006-0.21 mc/gmL, respectively; milk intake by the nursing infant: 150 mL/kg/d; estimated amount of total and free folate ingested by the nursing infant: 0.001-0.04 mg/kg/d and 0.001-0.03 mg/kg/d, respectively; RDA for infants up to one year of age: 0.004 mg/kg/d.

Key References

Bailey LB: Evaluation of a new Recommended Dietary Allowance for folate.   J Am Diet Assoc 92(4):463-468, 471, 1992.

Bower C, Stanley FJ: Dietary folate as a risk factor for neural-tube defects: Evidence from a case-control study in Western Australia. Med J Aust 150:613-619, 1989.

Briggs RM: Vitamin supplementation as a possible factor in the incidence of cleft lip/palate deformities in humans.   Clin Plast Surg 3:647-652, 1976.

Bunin GR, Kuijten RR, Buckley JD, et al.:   Relation between maternal diet and subsequent primitive neuroectodermal brain tumors in young children.   N Engl J Med 329:536-541, 1993.

Butte NF, Calloway DH: Evaluation of lactational performance of Navajo women.   Am J Clin Nutr 34:2210-2215, 1981.

Committee on Drugs, American Academy of Pediatrics: The transfer of drugs and other chemicals into human milk.   Pediatrics 93(1):137-150, 1994.

Conway H: Effects of supplemental vitamin therapy on the limitation of incidence of cleft lip and cleft palate in humans.   Plast Reconstr Surg 22:450-453, 1958.

Cooperman JM, Dweck HS, Newman LJ, et al.:   The folate in human milk.   Am J Clin Nutr 36:576-580, 1982.

Crandall BF, Corson VL, Goldberg JD, et al.:   Folic acid and pregnancy.   Am J Med Genet 55:134-135, 1995.

Cunningham GC: California's public health policy on preventing neural tube defects by folate supplementation.   West J Med 162:265-267, 1995.

Czeizel AE: Folic acid in the prevention of neural tube defects.   J Pediatr Gastroenterol Nutr 20:4-16, 1995.

Czeizel AE: Prevention of congenital abnormalities by periconceptional multivitamin supplementation.   BMJ 306:1645-1648, 1993.

Czeizel AE, Dudas I: Prevention of the first occurrence of neural-tube defects by periconceptional vitamin supplementation.   N Engl J Med 327:1832-1835, 1992.

Ek J: Plasma, red cell, and breast milk folacin concentrations in lactating women.   Am J Clin Nutr 38:929-935, 1983.

Ford JE, Zechalko A, Murphy J, Brooke OG: Comparison of the B vitamin composition of milk from mothers of preterm and term babies. Arch Dis Child 58:367-372, 1983.

Kirke PN, Daly LE, Elwood H: A randomised trial of low dose folic acid to prevent neural tube defects. Arch Dis Child 67:1442-1446, 1992.

Laurence KM, James N, Miller MH, et al.: Double-blind randomised controlled trial of folate treatment before conception to prevent recurrence of neural-tube defects. Br Med J 282:1509-1511, 1981.

Martinez-Frias M-L, Rodriguez-Pinilla E: Folic acid supplementation and neural tube defects. Lancet 340:620, 1992.

Metz J: Folate deficiency conditioned by lactation. Am J Clin Nutr 23(6):843-847, 1970.

Mills JL, Rhoads GG, Simpson JL, et al.: The absence of a relation between the periconceptional use of vitamins and neural-tube defects. N Engl J Med 321:430-435, 1989.

Milunsky A, Jick H, Jick SS, et al.: Multivitamin/folic acid supplementation in early pregnancy reduces the prevalence of neural tube defects. JAMA 262:2847-2852, 1989.

MRC Vitamin Study Research Group: Prevention of neural tube defects: Results of the Medical Research Council Vitamin Study. Lancet 338:131-137, 1991.

NRC (National Research Council): *Recommended Dietary Allowances, 10th ed. Report of the Subcommittee on the Tenth Edition of RDAs, Food and Nutrition Board, Commission on Life Sciences.* Washington, DC: National Academy Press, 1989, p 262.

Oakley GP Jr, Erickson JD, James LM, et al.: Prevention of folic acid-preventable spina bifida and anencephaly. Ciba Found Symp 181:212-231, 1994.

Rose NC, Mennuti MT: Periconceptional folate supplementation and neural tube defects. Clin Obstet Gynecol 37:605-620, 1994.

Smith AM, Picciano MF, Deering RH: Folate supplementation during lactation: Maternal folate status, human milk folate content, and their relationship to infant folate status. J Pediatr Gastroenterol Nutr 2:622-628, 1983.

Smithells RW, Seller MJ, Harris R, et al.: Further experience of vitamin supplementation for prevention of neural tube defect recurrences. Lancet 1:1027-1031, 1983.

Sneed SM, Zane C, Thomas MR: The effects of ascorbic acid, vitamin B_6, vitamin B_{12}, and folic acid supplementation on the breast milk and maternal nutritional status of low socioeconomic lactating women. Am J Clin Nutr 34:1338-1346, 1981.

Subcommittee on Nutrition and Lactation: Meeting maternal nutrient needs during lactation. In: *Nutrition During Lactation.* Washington, DC: National Academy of Sciences, 1991, pp 213-235.

Tamura T, Yashimura Y, Arakawa T: Human milk folate and folate status in lactating mothers and their infants. Am J Clin Nutr 33:193-197, 1980.

Thomas MR, Sneed SM, Wei C, et al.: The effects of vitamin C, vitamin B₆, vitamin B₁₂, folic acid, riboflavin, and thiamin on the breast milk and maternal status of well-nourished women at 6 months post-partum. Am J Clin Nutr 33:2151-2156, 1980.

Tolarova M: Periconceptional supplementation with vitamins and folic acid to prevent recurrence of cleft lip. Lancet 2:217, 1982.

Vergel RG, Sanchez LR, Heredero BL, et al.: Primary prevention of neural tube defects with folic acid supplementation: Cuban experience. Prenat Diagn 10:149-152, 1990.

Wald NJ: Folic acid and neural tube defects. The current evidence and implications for prevention. Ciba Found Symp 181:192-211, 1994.

Wald NJ, Bower C: Folic acid, pernicious anaemia, and prevention of neural tube defects. Lancet 343:307, 1994.

Werler MM, Shapiro S, Mitchell AA: Periconceptional folic acid exposure and risk of occurrent neural tube defects. JAMA 269:1257-1261, 1993.

FOLLISTREL® *See* Norgestrel

FOLVITE® *See* Folic Acid

FULVICIN® *See* Griseofulvin

FURADANTIN® See Nitrofurantoin

FUROSEMIDE
(Lasix®)

Furosemide is a diuretic used in the treatment of hypertension. Furosemide is given orally or parenterally, usually in doses of 20-600 mg/d. Doses as high as 6000 mg/d are sometimes used in acute renal failure.

Teratogenic Risk

*Magnitude of teratogenic
risk to child born after
exposure during gestation:*   *Undetermined*

*Quality and quantity of data
on which risk estimate is based:*   *Poor*

> *A small risk cannot be excluded, but there is no indication that the
> risk of congenital anomalies in the children of women treated with
> furosemide is likely to be great.*
> *Possible effects on perinatal electrolyte balance are discussed
> below.*

No adequate epidemiological studies of congenital anomalies among children of women treated with furosemide during pregnancy have been reported.

An increased frequency of fetal loss has been observed in rabbits treated early in pregnancy with furosemide in a dose about 10 times that used in humans (Godde & Grote, 1975). The frequency of malformations was no greater than expected among the offspring of mice treated with 17-100 times or of rats treated with 25-50 times the human dose of furosemide during pregnancy (Robertson et al., 1981; Hayasaka et al., 1984). Skeletal anomalies occurred at 40-100 times or at 4-50 times the human therapeutic dose in mice and rats, respectively (Robertson et al., 1981; Hayasaka et al., 1984; Sterz et al., 1985; Nakatsuka et al., 1993). Decreased renal maturation has been reported among the offspring of rats treated with 6 times the human dose of furosemide during pregnancy (Mallie et al., 1985). The relevance, if any, of these observations to the clinical use of furosemide in pregnant women is unclear.

Pharmacologic effects of furosemide have been demonstrated in the fetus after maternal administration of the drug (Wladimiroff, 1975), and this has been used to assess fetal urinary obstruction (Barrett et al., 1983). Administration of furosemide to the mother has also been used to treat fetal hydrops in the third trimester of pregnancy (Harris et al., 1993).

Furosemide is cleared from the circulation considerably more slowly in the neonate, especially if born prematurely, than in adults (Guignard, 1993). *Thus, babies born to mothers who have recently taken furosemide may be at risk of developing electrolyte disturbances as a result of pharmacological actions of the drug (Vert et al., 1982.)* Furosemide can displace bilirubin from albumin and may pose a risk to prenatally exposed newborns who become jaundiced (Turmen et al., 1982).

Risk Related to Breast-feeding

Furosemide is excreted in breast milk (USP DI, 1995), although this has not been quantitated in published reports.

Key References

Barrett RJ, Rayburn WF, Barr M Jr: Furosemide (Lasix®) challenge test in assessing bilateral fetal hydronephrosis. Am J Obstet Gynecol 147:846-847, 1983.

Godde VE, Grote W: [Animal experimental investigations on the dysionic genesis of intrauterine malformations.] Arzneimittelforsch 25:809-813, 1975.

Guignard J-P: Effect of drugs on the immature kidney. Adv Nephrol 22:193-211, 1993.

Harris JP, Alexson CG, Manning JA, Thompson HO: Medical therapy for the hydropic fetus with congenital complete atrioventricular block. Am J Perinatol 10(3):217-219, 1993.

Hayasaka I, Uchiyama K, Murakami K, et al.: Teratogenicity of azosemide, a loop diuretic, in rats, mice and rabbits. Cong Anom 24:111-121, 1984.

Mallie JP, Gerard A, Gerard H: Does the in-utero exposure to furosemide delay the renal maturation? Pediatr Pharmacol 5:131-138, 1985.

Nakatsuka T, Fujikake N, Hasebe M, Ikeda H: Effects of sodium bicarbonate and ammonium chloride on the incidence of furosemide-induced fetal skeletal anomaly, wavy ribs, in rats. Teratology 48:139-147, 1993.

Robertson RT, Minsker DH, Bokelman DL, et al.: Potassium loss as a causative factor for skeletal malformations in rats produced by indacrinone: A new investigational loop diuretic. Toxicol Appl Pharmacol 60:142-150, 1981.

Sterz H, Sponer G, Neubert P, Hebold G: A postulated mechanism of β-sympathomimetic induction of rib and limb anomalies in rat fetuses. Teratology 31:401-412, 1985.

Turmen T, Thom P, Louridas AT, et al.: Protein binding and bilirubin displacing properties of bumetanide and furosemide. J Clin Pharmacol 22:551-556, 1982.

USP DI: Diuretics, Loop. In: *USP DI (USP Dispensing Information), Volume 1. Drug Information for the Health Care Professional,* 15th ed. Rockville, Md.: The US Pharmacopeial Convention, 1995, p 1149.

Vert P, Broquaire M, Legagneur M, Morselli PL: Pharmacokinetics of furosemide in neonates. Eur J Clin Pharmacol 22:39-45, 1982.

Wladimiroff JW: Effect of furosemide on fetal urine production. Br J Obstet Gynaecol 82:221-224, 1975.

GAMASOLE® *See* Sulfamethoxazole

GANTANOL® *See* Sulfamethoxazole

GANTRISIN® *See* Sulfisoxazole

GARAMYCIN® *See* Gentamicin

GASTROCOM® *See* Cromolyn

GENTACIDIN® *See* Gentamicin

GENTAMICIN
(Cidomycin®, Garamycin®, Gentacidin®)

Gentamicin is an aminoglycoside antibiotic used parenterally and in topical, ophthalmic, and otic preparations to treat infections. The usual parenteral dose is 3-5 mg/kg of body weight per day (about 150-400 mg/d for a 110 pound woman), with doses up to 8-15 mg/kg in severe cases. Ophthalmic and otic preparations are poorly absorbed, but considerable absorption of topical gentamicin can occur through denuded or burned skin.

Teratogenic Risk

Magnitude of teratogenic risk to child born after exposure during gestation:	*Undetermined*
Quality and quantity of data on which risk estimate is based:	*Poor*

A small risk cannot be excluded, but there is no indication that the risk of malformations in children of women treated with gentamicin during pregnancy is likely to be great.

Because it is an aminoglycoside, maternal gentamicin treatment during pregnancy may be associated with an increased risk for fetal auditory nerve or renal damage. This has not been demonstrated to date in humans, however.

No epidemiological studies of congenital anomalies among infants born to women treated with gentamicin during pregnancy have been reported.

Increased frequencies of fetal death were observed among the off-spring of pregnant mice treated with 1-12 times the human dose of gentamicin during pregnancy (Nishio et al., 1987). A slightly increased rate of congenital anomalies was seen at the lower but not the higher dose. Typical aminoglycoside nephrotoxicity was observed among the offspring of rats treated with 9-25 times the human dose of gentamicin during pregnancy (Gossrau et al., 1990; Gilbert et al., 1991; Smaoui et al., 1991). Maternal nephrotoxicity regularly occurred under these conditions. Hearing loss was demonstrated among the off-spring of pregnant rats fed a magnesium-deficient diet and treated with 12.5-37.5 times the human dose of gentamicin; this effect was not seen in animals treated similarly but fed a normal diet (Gunther et al., 1989). Hearing loss also occurred in the mothers in these experiments. The relevance of these findings to the clinical use of gentamicin in human pregnancy is unknown.

Please see agent summary on streptomycin for information on a related agent that has been more thoroughly studied.

Risk Related to Breast-feeding

Gentamicin is excreted in the breast milk in low concentrations. The amount of gentamicin that would be expected to be systemically absorbed by the nursing infant is <1% of the lowest therapeutic dose for infants, based on data from ten lactating women (Celiloglu et al., 1994).*

The concentration of gentamicin in the serum of infants of women who were being treated with gentamicin ranged from 7-12% of the lowest therapeutic serum level of gentamicin.[†]

Key References

Celiloglu M, Celiker S, Guven H, et al.: Gentamicin excretion and uptake from breast milk by nursing infants. Obstet Gynecol 84:263-265, 1994.

Gilbert T, Lelievre-Pegorier M, Merlet-Benichou C: Long-term effects of mild oligonephronia induced in utero by gentamicin in the rat. Pediatr Res 30(5):450-456, 1991.

Gossrau R, Graf R, Chahoud J, et al.: Enzyme histochemical and histological changes in the adult rat kidney after prenatal gentamicin exposure. Z Mikrosk Anat Forsch 104(3):385-394, 1990.

Gunther T, Rebentisch E, Ising H, Vormann J: Enhanced ototoxicity of gentamicin in maternal and fetal rats due to magnesium deficiency. Magnesium-Bull 11:19-21, 1989.

Nishio A, Ryo S, Miyao N: Effects of gentamicin, exotoxin and their combination on pregnant mice. The Bulletin of the Faculty of Agriculture, Kagoshima University 37:129-136, 1987.

Smaoui H, Mallie J-P, Cheignon M, et al.: Glomerular alterations in rat neonates after transplacental exposure to gentamicin. Nephron 59:626-631, 1991.

---

*This calculation is based on the following assumptions: maternal dose of gentamicin: 240 mg/d; milk concentration of gentamicin: 0.27-0.74 mcg/mL; milk intake by the nursing infant: 150 mL/kg/d; estimated dose of gentamicin systemically absorbed by the nursing infant (assuming that 0.2% of the oral dose is absorbed): 0.0008-0.002 mg/kg/d; lowest therapeutic parenteral dose of gentamicin in infants: 5 mg/kg/d.

†Infant serum levels of gentamicin: 0.27-0.49 mcg/mL; lowest therapeutic serum level of gentamicin in adults: 4 mcg/ml.

GESTEROL® *See Progesterone*

GRAMICIDIN
(Argicilline®)

Gramicidin is an antimicrobial polypeptide that is employed in combination with other antibiotics in ophthalmic preparations. Gramicidin is not significantly absorbed systemically after ophthalmic administration.

Teratogenic Risk

Magnitude of teratogenic risk to child born after exposure during gestation:	*None*
Quality and quantity of data on which risk estimate is based:	*Poor*

The frequency of congenital anomalies was no greater than expected among the children of 61 women treated with gramicidin during the first trimester or the children of 96 women treated anytime during gestation in one epidemiological study (Heinonen et al., 1977).

No teratology studies of gramicidin in experimental animals have been reported.

Risk Related to Breast-feeding

No information regarding the distribution of gramicidin in breast milk has been published.

Key References

Heinonen OP, Slone D, Shapiro S: *Birth Defects and Drugs in Pregnancy*. Littleton, Mass.: John Wright-PSG, 1977, pp 297, 301, 435.

GRISACTIN® *See* Griseofulvin

GRISEOFULVIN
(Fulvicin®, Grisactin®)

Griseofulvin is an antifungal agent that is given orally to treat infections of the skin, nails, and hair. The usual dose of griseofulvin is 250-1000 mg/d.

Teratogenic Risk

Magnitude of teratogenic
risk to child born after
exposure during gestation: *Undetermined*

Quality and quantity of data
on which risk estimate is based: *Poor*

A small risk cannot be excluded, but a high risk of congenital anomalies in the children of women treated with griseofulvin during pregnancy is unlikely.

No epidemiological studies of congenital anomalies among the children of women treated with griseofulvin during pregnancy have been published. Rosa et al. (1987) reported two cases in which the mother took griseofulvin early in pregnancy and gave birth to conjoined twins. In contrast, none of 86 cases of conjoined twins identified in eight birth defects registries were associated with maternal griseofulvin treatment during pregnancy (Knudsen, 1987; Metneki & Czeizel, 1987).

Fetal death was observed with increased frequency among the offspring of rats and mice treated with griseofulvin during pregnancy in doses 75-250 times those used in humans (Klein & Beall, 1972; Jindra et al., 1979). In rats, fetal growth retardation was observed with maternal griseofulvin treatment during pregnancy in doses 6-75 times those used in humans (Klein & Beall, 1972). Increased frequencies of major skeletal anomalies were observed in the offspring of pregnant rats treated with 62-75 times the human dose and among the offspring of pregnant mice treated with 250 times the human dose of griseofulvin (Klein & Beall, 1972; Jindra et al., 1979). A variety of skeletal and central nervous system malformations were observed among the offspring of cats treated during pregnancy with several times the human dose of griseofulvin (Scott et al., 1975). The relevance of these observations to the therapeutic use of griseofulvin in human pregnancy is unknown.

Risk Related to Breast-feeding

No information regarding the distribution of griseofulvin in breast milk has been published.

Key References

Jindra J, Aujezdska A, Janousek V: Embryotoxic effect of high doses of griseofulvin on the skeleton of the albino mouse. In: Benesova O, Rychter Z, Jelinek R (eds). *Evaluation of Embryotoxicity, Mutagenicity and Carcinogenicity Risks in New Drugs. Proceedings of the 3rd Symposium on "Toxicological Testing for Safety of New Drugs."* Praha, USSR: Universzita Karlova, 1979, pp 161-165.

Klein MF, Beall JR: Griseofulvin: A teratogenic agent. Science 175:1483-1484, 1972.

Knudsen LB: No association between griseofulvin and conjoined twinning. Lancet 2:1097, 1987.

Metneki J, Czeizel A: Griseofulvin teratology. Lancet 1:1042, 1987.

Rosa FW, Hernandez C, Carlo WA: Griseofulvin teratology, including two thoracopagus conjoined twins. Lancet 1:171, 1987.

Scott FW, De LaHunta A, Schultz RD, et al.: Teratogenesis in cats associated with griseofulvin therapy. Teratology 11:79-86, 1975.

GUAIFENESIN
(Anti-Tuss®, Benylin-E®, Robitussin®)

Guaifenesin, an expectorant, is a component of many proprietary cough mixtures. Guaifenesin is taken orally in doses of 1200-2400 mg/d.

Teratogenic Risk

*Magnitude of teratogenic
risk to child born after
exposure during gestation:*   None

The frequency of malformations was no greater than expected among the children of more than 925 women who took guaifenesin in the first trimester of pregnancy in one epidemiological study (Jick et al., 1981; Aselton et al., 1985). Similarly, the frequency of congenital anomalies was not increased among the infants of 197 women who used guaifenesin in the first four lunar months or in the infants of 1336 women who used the drug anytime during pregnancy in another study (Heinonen et al., 1977).

No animal teratology studies of guaifenesin have been published.

Risk Related to Breast-feeding

No information regarding the distribution of guaifenesin in breast milk has been published.

Key References

Aselton P, Jick H, Milunsky A, et al.: First-trimester drug use and congenital disorders. Obstet Gynecol 65:451-455, 1985.

Heinonen OP, Slone D, Shapiro S: *Birth Defects and Drugs in Pregnancy.* Littleton, Mass.: John Wright-PSG, 1977, pp 378-379, 496.

Jick H, Holmes LB, Hunter JR, et al.: First-trimester drug use and congenital disorders. JAMA 246:343-346, 1981.

GYNOL II® *See* Nonoxynols

HALCION® *See* Triazolam

HALDOL® *See* Haloperidol

HALOPERIDOL
(Haldol®, Peridol®)

Haloperidol is a major tranquilizer used in the treatment of psychosis, Tourette syndrome, mania, and severe hyperactivity. It is occasionally employed as an antinauseant or anxiolytic. Haloperidol is given orally or parenterally; the usual dose is 1-15 mg/d, and exceptionally, at doses up to 100 mg/d.

Teratogenic Risk

Magnitude of teratogenic risk to child born after exposure during gestation:	*Unlikely*
Quality and quantity of data on which risk estimate is based:	*Fair*

Therapeutic doses of haloperidol are unlikely to pose a substantial teratogenic risk, but the data are insufficient to state that there is no risk.

The frequency of malformations was not increased among a cohort of infants born to 98 women treated with haloperidol during pregnancy (90 in the first trimester) (van Waes & van de Velde, 1969). These women were treated for hyperemesis gravidarum; the dose of haloperidol used was substantially less than that generally employed for psychiatric illness. Two isolated cases of infants with limb reduction defects born to women who used haloperidol during the period of limb morphogenesis have been reported (Dieulangard et al., 1966; Kopelman et al., 1975). No cause-and-effect inference can be made from such anecdotal observations.

Increased frequencies of micromelia, cleft palate, and fetal death were observed among the offspring of rats treated during pregnancy with haloperidol in doses 70-80 times those used clinically (Szabo & Brent, 1974; Druga et al., 1980). Decreased fetal and postnatal growth and increased rates of cleft palate, central nervous system, and skeletal malformations were observed among the offspring of pregnant mice treated with 2.5 or more times the human dose of haloperidol (Szabo & Brent, 1974; Jurand & Martin, 1990; Sullivan-Jones et al., 1992; Williams et al., 1992). Increased rates of embryonic death and of brain and skull malformations have been observed among the offspring of hamsters treated with haloperidol during pregnancy in doses 70-130 times those used in humans (Gill et al., 1982). Long-lasting alterations of behavior have been noted among the offspring of pregnant rats treated with haloperidol in doses similar to or greater than those used in humans (Hull et al., 1984; Cuomo et al., 1985; Scalzo et al., 1989; Archer & Fredriksson, 1992). The relevance of these observations to the risks associated with therapeutic use of haloperidol in human pregnancy is unknown.

Transient neonatal tardive dyskinesia has been observed in an infant whose mother was treated with haloperidol during pregnancy (Sexson & Barak, 1989). Such neurological symptoms are a recognized complication of haloperidol therapy in children and adults.

Risk Related to Breast-feeding

Haloperidol is excreted in the breast milk. The amount of haloperidol that the nursing infant would be expected to ingest is between <1-12% of the lowest pediatric dose of gentamicin, based on data from two patients (Stewart et al., 1980; Whalley et al., 1981).* Haloperidol-induced sedation was not observed in one nursing infant whose mother was being treated with haloperidol.

Although adverse effects of haloperidol on nursing infants have not been reported, the American Academy of Pediatrics regards haloperidol to be a drug whose potential effect on the central nervous system is a concern for nursing infants when their mothers are treated with haloperidol while breast-feeding (Committee on Drugs, American Academy of Pediatrics, 1994).

Key References

Archer T, Fredriksson A: Functional changes implicating dopaminergic systems following perinatal treatments. Dev Pharmacol Ther 18:201-222, 1992.

Committee on Drugs, American Academy of Pediatrics: The transfer of drugs and other chemicals into human milk. Pediatrics 93(1):137-150, 1994.

Cuomo V, Cagiano R, Renna G, et al.: Comparative evaluation of the behavioural consequences of prenatal and early postnatal exposure to haloperidol in rats. Neurobehav Toxicol Teratol 7:489-492, 1985.

Dieulangard P, Coignet J, Vidal JC: [On a case of phocomelia: Possibly caused by medication.] Bull Fed Soc Gynecol Obstet Lang Fr 18:85-87, 1966.

*This calculation is based on the following assumptions: maternal dose: 7-29 mg/d; milk concentration of haloperidol: 0.002-0.02 mcg/mL; milk intake by the nursing infant: 150 mL/kg/d; estimated dose of haloperidol ingested by the nursing infant: 0.0003-0.003 mg/kg/d; lowest therapeutic pediatric dose of haloperidol: 0.025 mg/kg/d.

Druga A, Nyitray M, Szaszovszky E: Experimental teratogenicity of structurally similar compounds with or without piperazine-ring: A preliminary report. Pol J Pharmacol Pharm 32:199-204, 1980.

Gill TS, Guram MS, Geber WF: Haloperidol teratogenicity in the fetal hamster. Dev Pharmacol Ther 4:1-5, 1982.

Hull EM, Nishita JK, Bitran D, Dalterio S: Perinatal dopamine-related drugs demasculinize rats. Science 224:1011-1013, 1984.

Jurand A, Martin LVH: Teratogenic potential of two neurotropic drugs, haloperidol and dextromoramide, tested on mouse embryos. Teratology 42:45-54, 1990.

Kopelman AE, McCullar FW, Heggeness L: Limb malformations following maternal use of haloperidol. JAMA 231:62-64, 1975.

Scalzo FM, Ali SF, Holson RR: Behavioral effects of prenatal haloperidol exposure. Pharmacol Biochem Behav 34:727-731, 1989.

Sexson WR, Barak Y: Withdrawal emergent syndrome in an infant associated with maternal haloperidol therapy. J Perinatol 9:170-172, 1989.

Stewart RB, Karas B, Springer PK: Haloperidol excretion in human milk. Am J Psychiatry 137:849-850, 1980.

Sullivan-Jones P, Hansen DK, Sheehan DM, Holson RR: The effect of teratogens on maternal corticosterone levels and cleft incidence in A/J mice. J Craniofac Genet Dev Biol 12:183-189, 1992.

Szabo KT, Brent RL: Species differences in experimental teratogenesis by tranquillizing agents. Lancet 1:565, 1974.

van Waes A, van de Velde E: Safety evaluation of haloperidol in the treatment of hyperemesis gravidarum. J Clin Pharmacol 9:224-227, 1969.

Whalley LJ, Blain PG, Prime JK: Haloperidol secreted in breast milk. Br Med J 282:1746-1747, 1981.

Williams R, Ali SF, Scalzo FM, et al.: Prenatal haloperidol exposure: Effects on brain weights and caudate neurotransmitter levels in rats. Brain Res Bull 29(3/4):449-458, 1992.

HEPALEAN® *See* Heparin

HEPARIN
(Calcilean®, Hepalean®, Liquaemin®)

Heparin, a sulfated glycosaminoglycan prepared from mammalian tissue, is administered parenterally to prevent blood clotting. Standard heparin is a heterogeneous material with a variable number of monosaccharide side chains, variable sulfation, and a molecular weight ranging from 5000-30,000 Da. Low molecular weight heparins (1000-10,000 Da) are fractions of the native molecule with different pharmacokinetic characteristics and a modified effect on the clotting system (Greaves, 1993; Hirsh & Fuster, 1994; Nelson-Piercy, 1994). When given during pregnancy, heparin preparations cross the placenta very poorly if at all (Matzsch et al., 1991; Bajoria & Contractor, 1992; Forestier et al., 1992; Melissari et al., 1992). The dosage of heparin administered varies substantially depending on the preparation being used, the indication, and demonstrable effect on the patient's clotting system. The usual dose of standard heparin is 10,000-40,000 units/d.

Teratogenic Risk

Magnitude of teratogenic
risk to child born after
exposure during gestation: *Unlikely*

Quality and quantity of data
on which risk estimate is based: *Fair*

   Therapeutic doses of heparin are unlikely to pose a substantial teratogenic risk, but the data are insufficient to state that there is no risk.
   Because of its anticoagulant activity, there is an increased risk of maternal hemorrhage associated with the use of heparin during pregnancy.

More than 350 cases in which the mother was treated with standard heparin during pregnancy were identified in the published literature prior to 1986 (Ginsberg et al., 1989a; Ginsberg & Hirsh, 1989). The overall rate of "adverse outcomes" was 21.7%, but most of these were associated with severe toxemia, glomerulonephritis, a history of recurrent miscarriage, or other maternal factors that are known to predispose to adverse pregnancy outcome. If these cases are excluded, the rates of prematurity (6.8%) and fetal or neonatal death (2.5%) are more similar to those expected in the general population. Only three of the 317 liveborn infants in this series had congenital anomalies, which were different in each case (Ginsberg et al., 1989a). It seems likely that the maternal illnesses for which heparin was administered account for the earlier conclusions that at least one-third of pregnancies in women treated with heparin have abnormal outcomes (Hall et al., 1980;

Nageotte et al., 1981; Howie, 1986; Ginsberg et al., 1989a; Ginsberg & Hirsh, 1989).

The frequencies of miscarriage, stillbirth, prematurity, and congenital anomalies did not appear unusual in a retrospective series of 100 consecutive pregnancies in women treated with standard heparin (Ginsberg et al., 1989b); 34 of these pregnancies were treated in the first trimester. No malformations and one case of mental retardation were reported among the children of 96 women who had received cardiac valve prostheses and were treated with standard heparin during the first trimester of pregnancy in a survey of European cardiologists (Sbarouni & Oakley, 1994). The frequency of stillbirths in this study was higher among women who were treated with heparin throughout pregnancy (4/30) than among those who were treated with heparin in the first trimester and then switched to coumadin (1/66).

No teratogenic effect was observed among the offspring of rats or rabbits treated during pregnancy with standard heparin in doses <1-4 times those used clinically (Lehrer & Becker, 1974; Bertoli & Borelli, 1986). At doses 12 times those used clinically, increased rates of embryonic death were seen in both species (Lehrer & Becker, 1974). The frequency of malformations was not increased among the offspring of pregnant rats or rabbits treated with FR-860, a low molecular weight heparin preparation, in doses of 1250-10,000 units/kg and 625-40,000 units/kg, respectively (Shimazu et al., 1989; Umemura et al., 1989). Increased fetal death was observed in both species at the highest dose.

Risk Related to Breast-feeding

Because of its high molecular weight, heparin is not excreted in breast milk (USP DI, 1995).

Key References

Bajoria R, Contractor SF: Transfer of heparin across the human perfused placental lobule. J Pharm Pharmacol 44(12):952-959, 1992.

Bertoli D, Borelli G: Peri- and postnatal, teratology and reproductive studies of a low molecular weight heparin in rats. Arzneimittelforsch 36:1260-1263, 1986.

Forestier F, Sole Y, Aiach M, et al.: Absence of transplacental passage of Fragmin (Kabi) during the second and the third trimesters of pregnancy. Thromb Haemost 67(1):180-181, 1992.

Ginsberg JS, Hirsh J: Anticoagulants during pregnancy. Annu Rev Med 40:79-86, 1989.

Ginsberg JS, Hirsh J, Turner DC, et al.: Risks to the fetus of anti-coagulant therapy during pregnancy. Thromb Haemost 61(2):197-203, 1989a.

Ginsberg JS, Kowalchuk G, Hirsh J, et al.: Heparin therapy during pregnancy. Risks to the fetus and mother. Arch Intern Med 149:2233-2236, 1989b.

Greaves M: Anticoagulants in pregnancy. Pharmacol Ther 59:311-327, 1993.

Hall JG, Pauli RM, Wilson KM: Maternal and fetal sequelae of anticoagulation during pregnancy. Am J Med 68(1):122-140, 1980.

Hirsh J, Fuster V: Guide to anticoagulant therapy. Part 1: Heparin. Circulation 89:1449-1468, 1994.

Howie PW: Anticoagulants in pregnancy. Clin Obstet Gynaecol 13(2):349-363, 1986.

Lehrer SB, Becker BA: Effects of heparin on fetuses of pregnant rats and rabbits. Teratology 9:A26-A27, 1974.

Matzsch T, Bergqvist D, Bergqvist A, et al.: No transplacental passage of standard heparin or an enzymatically depolymerized low molecular weight heparin. Blood Coagul Fibrinolysis 22:273-278, 1991.

Melissari E, Parker CH, Wilson NV, et al.: Use of low molecular weight heparin in pregnancy. Thromb Haemost 68(6):652-656, 1992.

Nageotte MP, Freeman RK, Garite TJ, Block RA: Anticoagulation in pregnancy. Am J Obstet Gynecol 141:472-473, 1981.

Nelson-Piercy C: Low molecular weight heparin for obstetric thromboprophylaxis. Br J Obstet Gynaecol 101:6-8, 1994.

Sbarouni E, Oakley CM: Outcome of pregnancy in women with valve prostheses. Br Heart J 71:196-201, 1994.

Shimazu H, Ishida S, Shioda Y, et al.: Reproduction studies of low molecular weight heparin sodium (FR-860) (2nd report)--Teratological study in rats. Kiso To Rinsho 23(16):317-340, 1989.

Umemura T, Shichida O, Isachi M, et al.: Reproduction studies of low molecular weight heparin sodium (FR-860) (4th report)--Teratological study in rabbits. Kiso To Rinsho 23(16):361-370, 1989.

USP DI: Heparin. In: *USP DI (USP Dispensing Information), Volume 1. Drug Information for the Health Care Professional*, 15th ed. Rockville, Md.: The US Pharmacopeial Convention, 1995, p 1450.

HEPATITIS B VACCINE
(Engerix-B®, Recombivax HB®)

Hepatitis B vaccines contain either hepatitis B surface antigen produced by recombinant DNA technology or inactivated and purified hepatitis B viral protein obtained from human plasma. Hepatitis B vaccine is administered parenterally to impart active immunity to hepatitis B virus. Doses used vary from 2-20 mcg per injection.

Teratogenic Risk

*Magnitude of teratogenic
risk to child born after
exposure during gestation:*   *Undetermined*

*Quality and quantity of data
on which risk estimate is based:*   *Very poor*

A small risk cannot be excluded, but a high risk of congenital anomalies in the children of women who were immunized with hepatitis B vaccine during pregnancy is unlikely.

No abnormalities were found among the infants of ten women who were immunized with hepatitis B vaccine during the first trimester of pregnancy in one series (Levy & Koren, 1991). One spontaneous abortion occurred among 16 women who conceived after in vitro fertilization and were subsequently immunized with recombinant hepatitis B vaccine during pregnancy; six of these women were vaccinated in the first trimester (Grosheide et al., 1993). No "abnormal birth defects" were observed among the infants of 72 women vaccinated with hepatitis B vaccine in the third trimester of pregnancy in another study (Ayoola & Johnson, 1987).

No animal teratology studies of hepatitis B vaccine have been published.

Risk Related to Breast-feeding

No information regarding the distribution of hepatitis B vaccine in breast milk has been published. The Advisory Committee on Immunization Practices considers hepatitis B vaccine to be safe to administer during breast-feeding (ACIP, 1994).

Key References

ACIP: General recommendations on immunization. Recommendations of the Advisory Committee on Immunization Practices (ACIP). MMWR 43(RR-1):1-38, 1994.

Ayoola EA, Johnson AOK: Hepatitis B vaccine in pregnancy: Immunogenicity, safety and transfer of antibodies to infants. Int J Gynaecol Obstet 25:297-301, 1987.

Grosheide PM, Schalm SW, van Os HC, et al.: Immune response to hepatitis B vaccine in pregnant women receiving post-exposure prophylaxis. Eur J Obstet Gynecol Reprod Biol 50:53-58, 1993.

Levy M, Koren G: Hepatitis B vaccine in pregnancy: Maternal and fetal safety. Am J Perinatol 8(3):227-232, 1991.

HEROIN
(Black Tar, China White, Diacetylmorphine)

Heroin is an opiate narcotic that is widely abused. Outside of the US, heroin is used medically to relieve severe pain. Heroin is usually administered parenterally in 5-10 mg doses.

Teratogenic Risk

*Magnitude of teratogenic
risk to child born after
exposure during gestation:*   *Unlikely*

*Quality and quantity of data
on which risk estimate is based:*   *Fair*

Heroin use is unlikely to pose a substantial teratogenic risk, but the data are insufficient to state that there is no risk.

Neonatal withdrawal symptoms often occur among infants born to women who regularly use heroin during pregnancy (see below).

Epidemiological studies of malformations in the children of women who used heroin during pregnancy deal with addicted populations who take the drug illicitly. Such women often abuse other drugs, alcohol, and cigarettes and have poor nutritional and health status. Moreover, the dose of heroin taken and the period of gestation during which it was used are generally unknown. Nevertheless, the frequency of malformations does not appear unusually high in most series of infants born to heroin-addicted mothers (Levy & Koren, 1990; Little et al., 1991; Glantz & Woods, 1993). A statistically significant increase in the frequency of malformations was observed in one study of 830 infants born to narcotic-dependent mothers (Ostrea & Chavez, 1979), but the frequency of malformations in children born to addicts in this study was about what would be expected in the general population (2.4%), while the frequency in control infants was inexplicably low (0.5%). Although several anecdotal reports of children with congenital anomalies born to heroin-addicted mothers have been published, no consistent pattern of malformations has been observed (Rothstein & Gould, 1974; Glantz & Woods, 1993), and no causal inference is possible.

Intrauterine growth retardation, perinatal death, and a variety of other perinatal complications have frequently been observed in the children of narcotic-addicted mothers (Lifschitz et al., 1983; Gregg et al., 1988; Little et al., 1990, 1991; Lam et al., 1992; Glantz & Woods, 1993), but it is unclear whether these effects are due to fetal exposure to heroin or to the generally poor health of these mothers. Subsequent growth of these children appears to be normal in most cases although the head circumference may continue to be somewhat smaller than expected (Lifschitz et al., 1985; Chasnoff et al., 1986; Lifschitz & Wilson, 1991; Little et al., 1991).

Neonatal withdrawal symptoms are observed in 40-80% of infants born to heroin-addicted women (Alroomi et al., 1988; Lam et al., 1992; Levy & Spino, 1993). Although the duration of these symptoms is sometimes prolonged, it is usually less than three weeks. Sudden infant death syndrome and behavioral and intellectual deficits have been reported with increased frequency in older children whose mothers were addicted to heroin during pregnancy (van Baar, 1990; Kandall & Gaines, 1991; Wilson, 1992; Kandall et al., 1993), but the occurrence of other social and health problems in these families makes interpretation of such reports with respect to cause difficult.

Increased frequencies of central nervous system and other malformations have been observed among the offspring of mice treated during pregnancy with single doses of heroin 100-150 times those usually used in humans (Jurand, 1980, 1985). Significantly increased frequencies of central nervous system and other malformations were also observed in the offspring of hamsters injected with heroin during pregnancy in doses 200-1000 times those used by humans (Geber & Schramm,

1975). The relevance of these findings to human use of heroin during pregnancy is unknown.

Higher-than-expected frequencies of acquired chromosomal aberrations in peripheral blood lymphocytes have been reported in narcotic addicts (Kushnick et al., 1972; Amarose & Norusis, 1976). Similar findings were observed in the infants of narcotic-addicted women in one study (Amarose & Norusis, 1976) but not in another (Kushnick et al., 1972). Evidence from an investigation in rhesus monkeys supports the possibility that maternal heroin use may cause somatic cell chromosome breakage in infants (Fischman et al., 1983), but the clinical relevance of this observation is unknown.

Risk Related to Breast-feeding

No information regarding the distribution of heroin in breast milk has been published.

The American Academy of Pediatrics considers heroin to be hazardous to both the nursing infant and mother and therefore recommends against its use by breast-feeding women (Committee on Drugs, American Academy of Pediatrics, 1994).

Key References

Alroomi LG, Davidson J, Evans TJ, et al.: Maternal narcotic abuse and the newborn. Arch Dis Child 63(1):81-83, 1988.

Amarose AP, Norusis MJ: Cytogenetics of methadone-managed and heroin-addicted pregnant women and their newborn infants. Am J Obstet Gynecol 124:635-640, 1976.

Chasnoff IJ, Burns KA, Burns WJ, Schnoll SH: Prenatal drug exposure: Effects on neonatal and infant growth development. Neurobehav Toxicol Teratol 8:357-362, 1986.

Committee on Drugs, American Academy of Pediatrics: The transfer of drugs and other chemicals into human milk. Pediatrics 93(1):137-150, 1994.

Fischman HK, Roizin L, Moralishvili E, et al.: Clastogenic effects of heroin in pregnant monkeys and their offspring. Mutat Res 118:77-89, 1983.

Geber WF, Schramm LC: Congenital malformations of the central nervous system produced by narcotic analgesics in the hamster. Am J Obstet Gynecol 123:705-713, 1975.

Glantz JC, Woods JR Jr: Cocaine, heroin, and phencyclidine: Obstetric perspectives. Clin Obstet Gynecol 36(2):279-301, 1993.

Gregg JEM, Davidson DC, Weindling AM: Inhaling heroin during pregnancy: Effects on the baby. Br Med J 296:754, 1988.

Jurand A: Malformations of the central nervous system induced by neurotropic drugs in mouse embryos. Dev Growth Differ 22(1):61-78, 1980.

Jurand A: The interference of naloxone hydrochloride in the teratogenic activity of opiates. Teratology 31:235-240, 1985.

Kandall SR, Gaines J: Maternal substance use and subsequent sudden infant death syndrome (SIDS) in offspring. Neurotoxicol Teratol 13(2):235-240, 1991.

Kandall SR, Gaines J, Habel L, et al.: Relationship of maternal substance abuse to subsequent sudden infant death syndrome in offspring. J Pediatr 123:120-126, 1993.

Kushnick T, Robinson M, Tsao C: Narcotic addicts and their newborns. J Med Soc NJ 69:727-728, 1972.

Lam SK, To WK, Duthie SJ, Ma HK: Narcotic addiction in pregnancy with adverse maternal and perinatal outcome. Aust NZ J Obstet Gynaecol 32(3):216-221, 1992.

Levy M, Koren G: Obstetric and neonatal effects of drugs of abuse. Emerg Med Clin North Am 8(3):633-652, 1990.

Levy M, Spino M: Neonatal withdrawal syndrome: Associated drugs and pharmacologic management. Pharmacotherapy 13(3):202-211, 1993.

Lifschitz MH, Wilson GS: Patterns of growth and development in narcotic-exposed children. NIDA Res Monogr 114:323-339, 1991.

Lifschitz MH, Wilson GS, Smith EO, Desmond MM: Factors affecting head growth and intellectual function in children of drug addicts. Pediatrics 75:269-274, 1985.

Lifschitz MH, Wilson GS, Smith EO, Desmond MM: Fetal and postnatal growth of children born to narcotic-dependent women. J Pediatr 102:686-691, 1983.

Little BB, Snell LM, Klein VR, et al.: Maternal and fetal effects of heroin addiction during pregnancy. J Reprod Med 35(2):159-162, 1990.

Little BB, Snell LM, Knoll KA, et al.: Heroin abuse during pregnancy: Effects on perinatal outcome and early childhood growth. Am J Hum Biol 3:463-468, 1991.

Ostrea EM Jr, Chavez CJ: Perinatal problems (excluding neonatal withdrawal) in maternal drug addiction: A study of 830 cases. J Pediatr 94:292-295, 1979.

Rothstein P, Gould JB: Born with habit. Infants of drug-addicted mothers. Pediatr Clin North Am 21:307-321, 1974.

van Baar A: Development of infants of drug dependent mothers. J Child Psychol Psychiatry 31(6):911-920, 1990.

Wilson GS: Heroin use during pregnancy: Clinical studies of long-term effects. In: Sonderegger TB (ed). *Perinatal Substance Abuse: Research Findings and Clinical Implications.* Baltimore, Md.: The Johns Hopkins University Press, 1992, pp 224-238.

HEXACHLOROPHENE
(Septisol®)

Hexachlorophene is a disinfectant that is used topically. It is absorbed through the skin.

Teratogenic Risk

*Magnitude of teratogenic
risk to child born after
exposure during gestation:*   *Unlikely*

*Quality and quantity of data
on which risk estimate is based:*   *Poor to fair*

Topical use of hexachlorophene-containing soaps is unlikely to pose a substantial teratogenic risk, but the data are insufficient to state that there is no risk.

An increased frequency of a heterogenous group of congenital anomalies was reported in one study among 460 children born to women medical personnel who very frequently washed with hexachlorophene-containing soaps during the first trimester of their pregnancies (Halling, 1979). This study has been severely criticized for its methodological deficiencies (Kallen, 1978) and could not be confirmed in a partially overlapping investigation of 3007 infants born to women who had worked in hospitals where hexachlorophene was used extensively (Baltzar et al., 1979). No association with maternal exposure to hexachlorophene during early pregnancy was observed in a study involving 1047 children with various congenital anomalies (Hernberg et al., 1983). A possible association of borderline statistical significance was observed with maternal occupational exposure to hexachlorophene or phenylphenol during the sixth through ninth month of pregnancy in a study of 306 children with mental retardation of unknown etiology

(Roeleveld et al., 1993). Studies such as this one that include multiple comparisons between parental occupational exposures and birth defect outcomes are expected to show occasional associations with nominal statistical significance purely by chance.

Increased frequencies of ocular malformations, hydrocephalus, and other anomalies were observed among the offspring of rats treated intravaginally with 80-300 mg/kg/d or orally with 30 mg/kg/d of hexachlorophene during pregnancy (Kimmel et al., 1974; Kennedy et al., 1975). Similar results were observed in rabbits fed hexachlorophene in a dose of 6 mg/kg/d (Kennedy et al., 1975). No teratogenic effects were seen after vaginal treatment with 20 mg/kg/d in rabbits. Maternal toxicity occurred with the high doses in both species. The relevance of these studies to maternal occupational use of hexachlorophene in human pregnancy is uncertain.

Risk Related to Breast-feeding

No adequate studies investigating the distribution of hexachlorophene in breast milk have been published.

Key References

Baltzar B, Ericson A, Kallen B: Pregnancy outcome among women working in Swedish hospitals. N Engl J Med 300:627-628, 1979.

Halling H: Suspected link between exposure to hexachlorophene and malformed infants. Ann NY Acad Sci 320:426-436, 1979.

Hernberg S, Kurppa K, Ojajarvi J, et al.: Congenital malformations and occupational exposure to disinfectants: A case-referent study. Scand J Work Environ Health 9:55, 1983.

Kallen B: Hexachlorophene teratogenicity in humans disputed. JAMA 240(15):1585-1586, 1978.

Kennedy GL Jr, Smith SH, Keplinger ML, Calandra JC: Evaluation of the teratological potential of hexachlorophene in rabbits and rats. Teratology 12:83-88, 1975.

Kimmel CA, Moore W Jr, Hysell DK, Stara J: Teratogenicity of hexachlorophene in rats. Comparison of uptake following various routes of administration. Arch Environ Health 28:43-48, 1974.

Roeleveld N, Zielhuis GA, Gabreels F: Mental retardation and parental occupation: A study on the applicability of job exposure. Br J Ind Med 50:945-954, 1993.

HEXADROL® *See* Dexamethasone

HISTANIL® *See* Promethazine

HISTEX® *See* Carbinoxamine

HUMULIN® *See* Insulin

HYDRALAZINE
(Alazine Tabs®, Apresoline®)

Hydralazine is a peripheral vasodilator used to treat hypertension. Hydralazine is given orally or parenterally, usually in doses of 40-300 mg/d. Larger doses are sometimes used to treat congestive heart failure.

Teratogenic Risk

*Magnitude of teratogenic
risk to child born after
exposure during gestation:*   *Undetermined*

*Quality and quantity of data
on which risk estimate is based:*   *Very Poor*

Transient neonatal thrombocytopenia and fetal distress have been reported in infants born to women treated with hydralazine late in pregnancy.

The frequency of congenital anomalies was not significantly increased among the children of 136 women treated with hydralazine anytime during pregnancy in one epidemiological study (Heinonen et al., 1977). Only eight of these women were treated during the first four lunar months of pregnancy.

Digital anomalies were observed with increased frequency among the offspring of rabbits treated during pregnancy with 12.5-25 times the maximum human dose of hydralazine (Danielsson et al., 1989). Unpublished studies in pregnant mice and rabbits given, respectively, 20-

30 times and 10-15 times the maximum human dose of hydralazine reportedly showed an increased frequency of craniofacial defects among the offspring (USP DI, 1995). The frequency of malformations was not increased among the offspring of pregnant rats treated with 2.5-5 times the maximum human dose of hydralazine in another study (Pryde et al., 1993). The relevance of these observations to the use of therapeutic doses of hydralazine in human pregnancy is unknown.

Fetal distress may be more common than expected among hypertensive pregnant women treated with hydralazine near term (Spinnato et al., 1986; Derham & Robinson, 1990; Kirshon et al., 1991).

Transient neonatal thrombocytopenia has been noted in three infants born to women treated chronically with hydralazine for hypertension during the third trimester of pregnancy (Widerlov et al., 1980). Thrombocytopenia is a rare but recognized adverse effect of hydralazine therapy in adults.

Risk Related to Breast-feeding

Hydralazine is excreted in breast milk in low concentrations. The amount of hydralazine that the nursing infant would be expected to ingest is approximately 1% of the lowest neonatal dose of hydralazine, based on data from a single patient (Liedholm et al., 1982).* No adverse effects of maternal hydralazine therapy were observed in the infant.

The American Academy of Pediatrics regards hydralazine to be safe to use during breast-feeding (Committee on Drugs, American Academy of Pediatrics, 1994).

Key References

Committee on Drugs, American Academy of Pediatrics: The transfer of drugs and other chemicals into human milk. Pediatrics 93(1):137-150, 1994.

Danielsson BRG, Reiland S, Rundqvist E, Danielson M: Digital defects induced by vasodilating agents: Relationship to reduction in uteroplacental blood flow. Teratology 40:351-358, 1989.

*This calculation is based on the following assumptions: maternal dose of hydralazine: 150 mg/d; milk concentration of hydralazine: 0.149-0.155 mcg/mL; milk intake by the nursing infant: 150 mL/kg/d; estimated dose of hydralazine ingested by the nursing infant: 0.022-0.023 mg/kg/d; lowest neonatal dose of hydralazine: 2 mg/kg/d.

Derham RJ, Robinson J: Severe preeclampsia: Is vasodilation therapy with hydralazine dangerous for the preterm fetus? Am J Perinatol 7(3):239-244, 1990.

Heinonen OP, Slone D, Shapiro S: *Birth Defects and Drugs in Pregnancy.* Littleton, Mass.: John Wright-PSG, 1977, p 441.

Kirshon B, Wasserstrum N, Cotton DB: Should continuous hydralazine infusions be utilized in severe pregnancy-induced hypertension? Am J Perinatol 8(3):206-208, 1991.

Liedholm H, Wahlin-Boll E, Hanson A, et al.: Transplacental passage and breast milk concentrations of hydralazine. Eur J Clin Pharmacol 21:417-419, 1982.

Pryde PG, Abel EL, Hannigan J, et al.: Effects of hydralazine on pregnant rats and their fetuses. Am J Obstet Gynecol 169:1027-1031, 1993.

Spinnato JA, Sibai BM, Anderson GD: Fetal distress after hydralazine therapy for severe pregnancy-induced hypertension. South Med J 79:559-562, 1986.

USP DI: Hydralazine. In: *USP DI (USP Dispensing Information), Volume 1. Drug Information for the Health Care Professional,* 15th ed. Rockville, Md.: The US Pharmacopeial Convention, 1995, p 1478.

Widerlov E, Karlman I, Storsater J: Hydralazine-induced neonatal thrombocytopenia. N Engl J Med 303:1235, 1980.

HYDROCHLOROTHIAZIDE
(Aprozide®, Esidrix®, Urozide®)

Hydrochlorothiazide is a widely used oral diuretic. It is most often employed in the treatment of edema, hypertension, and heart failure. The usual dose is 12.5-50 mg/d, with doses up to 200 mg/d.

Teratogenic Risk

*Magnitude of teratogenic
risk to child born after
exposure during gestation:*   *Unlikely*

*Quality and quantity of data
on which risk estimate is based:*   *Fair*

305

Therapeutic doses of hydrochlorothiazide are unlikely to pose a substantial teratogenic risk, but the data are insufficient to state that there is no risk.

Neonatal thrombocytopenia has been observed after maternal use of hydrochlorothiazide late in pregnancy (see below).

No increase in the frequency of congenital anomalies was seen among the infants of 107 women treated with hydrochlorothiazide during the first four lunar months of pregnancy in one epidemiological study or among the infants of between 50 and 99 women treated during the first trimester in another study (Heinonen et al., 1977; Jick et al., 1981). Similarly, the frequency of congenital anomalies was no greater than expected among the children of 7575 women treated with hydrochlorothiazide anytime during pregnancy in one study or the children of 506 women treated during the second half of gestation in another investigation (Kraus et al., 1966; Heinonen et al., 1977).

Studies in mice and rats suggest that treatment of pregnant women with hydrochlorothiazide in usual therapeutic doses is unlikely to increase the children's risk of malformations greatly (Maren & Ellison, 1972; George et al., 1984).

Neonatal thrombocytopenia has been observed after maternal use of hydrochlorothiazide and similar diuretics late in pregnancy (Rodriguez et al., 1964). The risk of this problem is unknown but must be small because symptomatic thrombocytopenia was not observed in any of the infants of 506 women treated with hydrochlorothiazide late in pregnancy in the series reported by Kraus et al. (1966).

Risk Related to Breast-feeding

Hydrochlorothiazide is excreted in the breast milk. The amount of hydrochlorothiazide that the nursing infant would be expected to ingest is between <1-2% of the lowest infant dose, based on data from a single patient (Miller et al., 1982).*

Suppression of lactation has been described for other thiazide diuretics (Healy, 1961), but not for hydrochlorothiazide. The American Academy of Pediatrics regards hydrochlorothiazide to be safe to use

*This calculation is based on the following assumptions: maternal dose of hydrochlorothiazide: 50 mg/d; milk concentration of hydrochlorothiazide: 0.05-0.11 mcg/mL; milk intake by the nursing infant: 150 mL/kg/d; estimated dose of hydrochlorothiazide ingested by the nursing infant: 0.007-0.02 mg/kg/d; lowest infant dose of hydrochlorothiazide: 1 mg/kg/d.

while breast-feeding (Committee on Drugs, American Academy of Pediatrics, 1994).

Key References

Committee on Drugs, American Academy of Pediatrics: The transfer of drugs and other chemicals into human milk. Pediatrics 93(1):137-150, 1994.

George JD, Tyl RW, Price CJ, et al.: Teratologic evaluation of hydrochlorothiazide (CAS No. 58-93-5) administered to CD-1 mice on gestational days 6 through 15--Final study report. NTIS (National Technical Information Service) Report/PB 85-103570, 1984.

Healy M: Suppressing lactation with oral diuretics. Lancet 1:1353, 1961.

Heinonen OP, Slone D, Shapiro S: *Birth Defects and Drugs in Pregnancy*. Littleton, Mass.: John Wright-PSG, 1977, pp 372-373, 441.

Jick H, Holmes LB, Hunter JR, et al.: First-trimester drug use and congenital disorders. JAMA 246:343-346, 1981.

Kraus GW, Marchese JR, Yen SSC: Prophylactic use of hydrochlorothiazide in pregnancy. JAMA 198:1150-1154, 1966.

Maren TH, Ellison AC: The teratological effect of certain thiadiazoles related to acetazolamide, with a note on sulfanilamide and thiazide diuretics. Johns Hopkins Med J 130:95-104, 1972.

Miller ME, Cohn RD, Burghart PH: Hydrochlorothiazide disposition in a mother and her breast-fed infant. J Pediatr 101:789-791, 1982.

Rodriguez SU, Leikin SL, Hiller MC: Neonatal thrombocytopenia associated with ante-partum administration of thiazide drugs. N Engl J Med 270:881-884, 1964.

HYDROCODEINE See Dihydrocodeine

HYDROCORTISONE
(A-Hydrocort®, Cortef®, Cortisol®)

Hydrocortisone, the primary glucocorticoid produced by the adrenal cortex, is a potent anti-inflammatory and immunosuppressive agent. It is also used in replacement therapy of adrenal insufficiency. Hydrocortisone is given orally in doses of 20-240 mg/d and rectally in doses of 90-180 mg/d; much larger doses are sometimes given parenterally in acutely ill patients. Hydrocortisone is also given by articular or soft tissue injection and in ophthalmic, otic and topical preparations, from which systemic absorption may occur.

Teratogenic Risk

Magnitude of teratogenic
risk to child born after
exposure during gestation: *Unlikely*

Quality and quantity of data
on which risk estimate is based: *Poor to fair*

Therapeutic doses of hydrocortisone are unlikely to pose a substantial teratogenic risk, but the data are insufficient to state that there is no risk.

The frequency of congenital anomalies was no greater than expected among the children of 21 women treated with hydrocortisone during the first four lunar months of pregnancy or the children of 74 women who were treated with this agent anytime during pregnancy in one study (Heinonen et al., 1977).

Hydrocortisone administration to pregnant mice and hamsters in doses, respectively, greater than 4 and 250 times those used clinically regularly produces cleft palate in the offspring (Roberts & Hendrickx, 1987; Teramoto et al., 1991; Abbott et al., 1992). Polycystic kidney disease was induced among the offspring of pregnant mice treated with 420 times the human therapeutic dose of hydrocortisone (Crocker & Ogborn, 1991). Behavioral alterations have been observed among the offspring of rats treated during pregnancy with 17 times the human dose of hydrocortisone (Fujii et al., 1993). The relevance of these observations to therapeutic use of hydrocortisone in human pregnancy is unknown.

Hydrocortisone has been used to treat women in premature labor to promote pulmonary maturation in their infants (Roberts & Morrison, 1991).

Please see agent summary on prednisone/prednisolone for information on a related agent that has been more thoroughly studied.

Risk Related to Breast-feeding

No information regarding the distribution of hydrocortisone in breast milk has been published.

Key References

Abbott BD, Harris MW, Birnbaum LS: Comparisons of the effects of TCDD and hydrocortisone on growth factor expression provide insight into their interaction in the embryonic mouse palate. Teratology 45(1):35-53, 1992.

Crocker JFS, Ogborn MR: Glucocorticoid teratogenesis in the developing nephron. Teratology 43(6):571-574, 1991.

Fujii T, Horinaka M, Hata M: Functional effects of glucocorticoid exposure during fetal life. Prog Neuropsychopharmacol Biol Psychiatry 17(2):279-293, 1993.

Heinonen OP, Slone D, Shapiro S: *Birth Defects and Drugs in Pregnancy*. Littleton, Mass.: John Wright-PSG, 1977, pp 389, 391, 443.

Roberts LG, Hendrickx AG: Hydrocortisone-induced embryotoxicity and embryonic drug disposition in H-2 congenic mice. J Craniofac Genet Dev Biol 7:341-356, 1987.

Roberts WE, Morrison JC: Pharmacologic induction of fetal lung maturity. Clin Obstet Gynecol 34(2):319-327, 1991.

Teramoto S, Hatakenaka N, Shirasu Y: Effects of the A^y gene on susceptibility to hydrocortisone fetotoxicity and teratogenicity in mice. Teratology 44(1):101-106, 1991.

HYDROXYZINE
(Atarax®, Hy-PAM®, Vistaril®)

Hydroxyzine is a piperazine antihistaminic agent. It is used as an anxiolytic, sedative, antipuritic, and antiemetic drug. Hydroxyzine is administered orally or intramuscularly in doses of 25-200 mg/d, and exceptionally, at doses up to 400 mg.

Teratogenic Risk

Magnitude of teratogenic
risk to child born after
exposure during gestation: *Unlikely*

Quality and quantity of data
on which risk estimate is based: *Poor to Fair*

Therapeutic doses of hydroxyzine are unlikely to pose a substantial teratogenic risk, but the data are insufficient to state that there is no risk.

The frequency of congenital anomalies was no greater than expected among the infants of 50 women treated with hydroxyzine during the first four lunar months of pregnancy or among the infants of 187 women so treated anytime during pregnancy in one epidemiological study (Heinonen et al., 1977). The frequency of congenital anomalies was no greater than expected among 74 infants born to mothers who took hydroxyzine during the first two months of pregnancy in a trial of treatment for gestational nausea and vomiting (Erez et al., 1971). No increase in malformations was observed among 35 infants born to women who had taken hydroxyzine during the first trimester of pregnancy in another series (Einarson et al., 1993).

The frequencies of fetal death and craniofacial and skeletal malformations were increased among the offspring of rats treated with 8-25, but not 3-6 times the dose of hydroxyzine used in humans (King & Howell, 1966; Giurgea & Puigdevall, 1968). The relevance of this finding to the therapeutic use of hydroxyzine in human pregnancy is unknown.

Risk Related to Breast-feeding

No information regarding the distribution of hydroxyzine in breast milk has been published.

Key References

Einarson A, Spizziri D, Berkovich M, et al.: Prospective study of hydroxyzine use in pregnancy. Reprod Toxicol 7:640, 1993.

Erez S, Schifrin BS, Dirim O: Double-blind evaluation of hydroxyzine as an antiemetic in pregnancy. J Reprod Med 7:35-37, 1971.

Giurgia M, Puigdevall J: Maternal and foetal toxicity of some diphenylmethane piperazine derivatives. Proc Eur Soc Study Drug Toxic 9:134-143, 1968.

Heinonen OP, Slone D, Shapiro S: *Birth Defects and Drugs in Pregnancy.* Littleton, Mass.: John Wright-PSG, 1977, pp 335-337, 438.

King CTG, Howell J: Teratogenic effect of buclizine and hydroxyzine in the rat and chlorcyclizine in the mouse. Am J Obstet Gynecol 95:109-111, 1966.

HYGROTON® *See* Chlorthalidone

HYOSCYAMINE
(Anaspaz®, Cystospaz®, Levsin®)

Hyoscyamine is an anticholinergic agent that is used to treat gastrointestinal disorders and bronchial asthma. Hyoscyamine may be given orally, sublingually, or parenterally; the usual dose is 0.125-3 mg/d.

Teratogenic Risk

Magnitude of teratogenic risk to child born after exposure during gestation:	*None*
Quality and quantity of data on which risk estimate is based:	*Fair*

The frequencies of congenital anomalies, of major malformations, and of minor anomalies were no greater than expected among the children of 322 women treated with hyoscyamine during the first four lunar months of pregnancy in one epidemiological study (Heinonen et al., 1977). The frequency of congenital anomalies was not increased among the infants of 1067 women treated anytime during pregnancy in this investigation.

No teratology studies of hyoscyamine in experimental animals have been published.

Risk Related to Breast-feeding

Hyoscyamine is excreted into breast milk (USP DI, 1995), although this has not been quantitated in published reports.

Key References

Heinonen OP, Slone D, Shapiro S: *Birth Defects and Drugs in Pregnancy.* Littleton, Mass.: John Wright-PSG, 1977, pp 346-347, 439.

USP DI: Anticholinergics/Antispasmodics. In: *USP DI (USP Dispensing Information), Volume 1. Drug Information for the Health Care Professional,* 15th ed. Rockville, Md.: The US Pharmacopeial Convention, 1995, p 211.

HY-PAM® *See* Hydroxyzine

HYZYD® *See* Isoniazid

IBUPROFEN
(Advil®, Motrin®, Nuprin®)

Ibuprofen is an oral nonsteroidal anti-inflammatory agent that has analgesic and antipyretic actions. It is used in a dose of 1200-3200 mg/d to treat arthritis, dysmenorrhea, and mild to moderate pain syndromes.

Teratogenic Risk

Magnitude of teratogenic risk to child born after exposure during gestation:	*Unlikely*
Quality and quantity of data on which risk estimate is based:	*Poor to fair*

Therapeutic doses of ibuprofen are unlikely to pose a substantial teratogenic risk, but the data are insufficient to state that there is no risk.

The frequency of congenital anomalies was no greater than expected among 51 infants whose mothers took ibuprofen during the first trimester of pregnancy in one epidemiological study (Aselton et al., 1985). The frequency and nature of anomalies was not unusual among the children of a small group of women who took ibuprofen at various times and at various doses during their pregnancies and whose experience was voluntarily reported to one manufacturer (Barry et al., 1984). No association with maternal ibuprofen use during the first trimester of pregnancy was seen among 76 infants with gastroschisis or 416 infants with a heterogeneous group of congenital anomalies suspected of having a vascular etiology (Werler et al., 1992).

Studies in mice, rats, and rabbits suggest that treatment of pregnant women with ibuprofen in usual therapeutic doses is unlikely to increase the children's risk of malformations greatly (Adams et al., 1969; Ono et al., 1982, 1984a, b; Randall et al., 1991).

Ibuprofen is an inhibitor of prostaglandin synthesis. This class of drugs has been used therapeutically to produce closure of the ductus arteriosus and consequent changes in cardiovascular and pulmonary function in newborns with patent ductus arteriosus. One case in which constriction of the ductus arteriosus was observed in the fetus of a woman who was taking ibuprofen in large doses during the second and early third trimester of pregnancy has been reported, but this case was complicated by several other factors so that a causal inference is difficult (Baker et al., 1993).

The development of oligohydramnios has been associated with maternal ibuprofen treatment to arrest premature labor (Hendricks et al., 1990; Wiggins & Elliott, 1990).

Risk Related to Breast-feeding

Ibuprofen is excreted into breast milk in negligible amounts (Weibert et al., 1982; Townsend et al., 1984).

The American Academy of Pediatrics considers ibuprofen to be safe to use during breast-feeding (Committee on Drugs, American Academy of Pediatrics, 1994).

Key References

Adams SS, Bough RG, Cliffe EE, et al.: Absorption, distribution and toxicity of ibuprofen. Toxicol Appl Pharmacol 15:310-330, 1969.

Aselton P, Jick H, Milunsky A, et al.: First-trimester drug use and congenital disorders. Obstet Gynecol 65:451-455, 1985.

Baker ER, Eberhardt H, Brown ZA: "Stuck twin" syndrome associated with congenital cytomegalovirus infection. Am J Perinatol 10:(1):81-83, 1993.

Barry WS, Meinzinger MM, Howse CR: Ibuprofen overdose and exposure in utero: Results from a postmarketing voluntary reporting system. Am J Med 77(1A):35-39, 1984.

Committee on Drugs, American Academy of Pediatrics: The transfer of drugs and other chemicals into human milk. Pediatrics 93:137-150, 1994.

Hendricks SK, Smith JR, Moore DE, Brown ZA: Oligohydramnios associated with prostaglandin synthetase inhibitors in preterm labour. Br J Obstet Gynaecol 97:312-316, 1990.

Ono M, Hagihara K, Nagase M, Asami K: [Reproductive study of ibuprofen administered in rectum. 4. Organogenesis administration in rabbits.] Kiso To Rinsho 18:569-574, 1984a.

Ono M, Hoshida F, Nagase M, Asami K: Reproductive studies of ibuprofen by rectal administration. 2. Teratogenicity study in rats. Oyo Yakuri 24:531-538, 1982.

Ono M, Sakakibara H, Kodama M, et al.: [Reproductive study of ibuprofen administered in rectum. 5. Administration during organogenesis in rats.] Kiso To Rinsho 18:537-547, 1984b.

Randall CL, Becker HC, Anton RF: Effect of ibuprofen on alcohol-induced teratogenesis in mice. Alcohol Clin Exp Res 15(4):673-677, 1991.

Townsend RJ, Benedetti TJ, Erickson S, et al.: Excretion of ibuprofen into breast milk. Am J Obstet Gynecol 149:184-186, 1984.

Weibert RT, Townsend RJ, Kaiser DG, et al.: Lack of ibuprofen secretion into human milk. Clin Pharm 1:457-458, 1982.

Werler MM, Mitchell AA, Shapiro S: First trimester maternal medication use in relation to gastroschisis. Teratology 45:361-367, 1992.

Wiggins DA, Elliott JP: Oligohydramnios in each sac of a triplet gestation caused by Motrin® - fulfilling Koch's postulates. Am J Obstet Gynecol 162:460-461, 1990.

IMIGRAN® *See* Sumatriptan

IMIPRAMINE
(Norfranil®, Tipramine®, Tofranil®)

Imipramine is a tricyclic antidepressant given orally or parenterally in doses of 75-300 mg/d.

Teratogenic Risk

*Magnitude of teratogenic
risk to child born after
exposure during gestation:*   *Unlikely*

Quality and quantity of data
on which risk estimate is based: *Poor to fair*

Therapeutic doses of imipramine are unlikely to pose a substantial teratogenic risk, but the data are insufficient to state that there is no risk.

Available studies of congenital anomalies among children born to women who used imipramine during the first trimester of pregnancy include too few cases to permit firm conclusions to be drawn (Scanlon, 1969; Banister et al., 1972; Crombie et al., 1972; Kuenssberg & Knox, 1972; Rachelefsky et al., 1972; Idanpaan-Heikkila & Saxen, 1973; Heinonen et al., 1977). None of these investigations includes more than 20 exposed pregnancies, but there is no indication of a major teratogenic effect. The suggestion, based on anecdotal observations, that maternal use of imipramine during pregnancy is associated with limb reduction defects in infants is probably incorrect (Morrow, 1972).

No malformations were observed among the offspring of 17 bonnet monkeys treated during pregnancy with imipramine in doses 7-70 times those used in humans (Hendrickx, 1975). Growth retardation and vertebral anomalies were observed among the offspring of a few rhesus monkeys treated during pregnancy with 4-5 times the human dose of imipramine (Wilson, 1974). Increased frequencies of central nervous system and other malformations were found among the offspring of mice, rabbits, and hamsters treated during pregnancy with imipramine in doses 31, 10, and 9-28 times those used in humans (Harper et al., 1965; Guram et al., 1980; Jurand, 1980). Behavioral and developmental alterations have been reported among the offspring of rats treated with 1-5 times the usual human dose of imipramine during pregnancy (Coyle et al., 1975; Jason et al., 1981; Ali et al., 1986). The relevance of these observations to the therapeutic use of imipramine in human pregnancy is unknown.

Transient abnormalities of neonatal respiratory, circulatory, and neurological adaptation have been reported in three infants whose mothers took imipramine during pregnancy (Eggermont et al., 1972).

Risk Related to Breast-feeding

Imipramine and its active metabolite, desipramine, are excreted in the breast milk. The amount of imipramine and desipramine that the nursing infant would be expected to ingest is <1% of the equivalent lowest pediatric dose of imipramine, based on data obtained from a single patient (Sovner & Orsulak, 1979).* No physical or behavioral changes attributable to imipramine were observed in this infant.

Although no adverse effects in nursing infants have been documented, the American Academy of Pediatrics regards imipramine to be a concern when used in breast-feeding women because of its potential to alter central nervous system functioning (Committee on Drugs, American Academy of Pediatrics, 1994).

Key References

Ali SF, Buelke-Sam J, Newport GD, Slikker W: Early neurobehavioral and neurochemical alterations in rats prenatally exposed to imipramine. Neurotoxicology 7:365-380, 1986.

Banister P, Dafoe C, Smith ESO, Miller J: Possible teratogenicity of tricyclic antidepressants. Lancet 1:838-839, 1972.

Committee on Drugs, American Academy of Pediatrics: The transfer of drugs and other chemicals into human milk. Pediatrics 93(1):137-150, 1994.

Coyle IR: Changes in developing behavior following prenatal administration of imipramine. Pharmacol Biochem Behav 3:799-807, 1975.

Crombie DL, Pinsent RJFH, Fleming D: Imipramine in pregnancy. Br Med J 1:745, 1972.

Eggermont E, Raveschot J, Deneve V, Casteels-Van Daele M: The adverse influence of imipramine on the adaptation of the newborn infant to extrauterine life. Acta Paediatr Belg 26:197-204, 1972.

Guram MK, Gill TS, Geber WF: Teratogenicity of imipramine and amitriptyline in fetal hamsters. Res Commun Psychol Psychiatr Behav 5:275-282, 1980.

Harper KH, Palmer AK, Davies RE: Effect of imipramine upon the pregnancy of laboratory animals. Arzneimittelforsch 15:1218-1221, 1965.

Heinonen OP, Slone D, Shapiro S: *Birth Defects and Drugs in Pregnancy.* Littleton, Mass.: John Wright-PSG, 1977, p 336.

Hendrickx AG: Teratologic evaluation of imipramine hydrochloride in bonnet (*Macaca radiata*) and rhesus monkeys (*Macaca mulatta*). Teratology 11:219-222, 1975.

*This calculation is based on the following assumptions: maternal dose of imipramine: 200 mg/d; milk concentration of imipramine and desipramine: 0.004-0.029 mcg/mL and 0.017-0.035 mcg/mL; milk intake by the nursing infant: 150 mL/kg/d; estimated dose of both imipramine and desipramine ingested by the nursing infant: 0.004-0.01 mg/kg/d; lowest pediatric dose of imipramine: 1 mg/kg/d.

Idanpaan-Heikkila J, Saxen L: Possible teratogenicity of imipramine/chloropyramine. Lancet 2:282-284, 1973.

Jason KM, Cooper TB, Friedman E: Prenatal exposure to imipramine alters early behavioral development and β-adrenergic receptors in rats. J Pharmacol Exp Ther 217:461-466, 1981.

Jurand A: Malformations of the central nervous system induced by neurotropic drugs in mouse embryos. Dev Growth Differ 22:61-78, 1980.

Kuenssberg EV, Knox JDE: Imipramine in pregnancy. Br Med J 2:292, 1972.

Morrow AW: Imipramine and congenital abnormalities. NZ Med J 75:228-229, 1972.

Rachelefsky GS, Flynt JW, Ebbin AJ, Wilson MG: Possible teratogenicity of tricyclic antidepressants. Lancet 1:838, 1972.

Scanlon FJ: Use of antidepressant drugs during the first trimester. Med J Aust 2:1077, 1969.

Sovner R, Orsulak PJ: Excretion of imipramine and desipramine in human breast milk. Am J Psychiatry 136(4A):451-452, 1979.

Wilson JG: Teratologic causation in man and its evaluation in non-human primates. Excerpta Med Int Congr Ser 310:191-203, 1974.

IMITREX® *See* Sumatriptan

IMURAN® *See* Azathioprine

INDERAL® *See* Propranolol

INDOCID® *See* Indomethacin

INDOCIN® *See* Indomethacin

INDOMETHACIN
(Indocid®, Indocin®)

Indomethacin is a prostaglandin synthetase inhibitor that is used as an analgesic, anti-inflammatory, and antipyretic agent. Indomethacin has also been used to arrest premature labor and to treat polyhydramnios. It is usually given orally in doses of 50-200 mg/d.

Teratogenic Risk

Magnitude of teratogenic
risk to child born after
exposure during gestation:
    Malformations: *None to minimal*
    Premature closure of the
    ductus arteriosus: *Small to moderate*

Quality and quantity of data
on which risk estimate is based:
    Malformations: *Poor to fair*
    Premature closure of the
    ductus arteriosus: *Fair to good*

Maternal treatment with indomethacin late in pregnancy may be associated with the development of fetal anuria, oligohydramnios, premature closure of the ductus arteriosus, and consequent problems in perinatal adaptation (see below).

Necrotizing enterocolitis occurs with increased frequency among low-birth-weight infants born to women who were treated with indomethacin shortly before delivery (see below).

The frequency of malformations was no greater than expected among the children of 50 women who had been treated with indomethacin during the first trimester of pregnancy in one epidemiological study (Aselton et al., 1985).

Indomethacin may cause premature closure of the ductus arteriosus and persistent pulmonary hypertension (Besinger et al., 1991; Bivins et al., 1993; Van den Veyver & Moise, 1993; Marpeau et al., 1994). Indomethacin is used to induce closure of the ductus in premature infants (Douidar et al., 1988; Yu, 1993), and similar pharmacologic mechanisms are presumed to operate prenatally. Constriction of the fetal ductus arteriosus and associated tricuspid regurgitation have been demonstrated by fetal echocardiography in women treated with indomethacin in the third trimester of pregnancy (Bivins et al., 1993; Eronen, 1993; Moise, 1993a). The risk of such fetal hemodynamic alterations is greater after about 32 weeks gestation than before (Eronen, 1993; Moise, 1993a).

Several perinatal deaths have been reported in the infants of women treated with indomethacin just prior to delivery (Marpeau et al., 1994), but the occurrence of such events did not appear to be much greater than expected in studies involving 30-880 pregnancies in which the mother was treated with indomethacin to prevent preterm labor (Baerts et al., 1990; Gerson et al., 1990; Bivins et al., 1993; Morales & Madhav, 1993; Marpeau et al., 1994).

The frequency of intracranial hemorrhages was increased among 57 very low-birth-weight infants born to women who had been treated with indomethacin shortly before delivery in comparison to matched control infants in one study (Norton et al., 1993). In another study, hypoxic-ischemic cerebral lesions were more severe, but not more common, among small premature infants whose mothers had received indomethacin tocolysis (Baerts et al., 1990).

Fetal urinary output and amniotic fluid volume are decreased in women who are treated with indomethacin in the second or third trimester of pregnancy (Hendricks et al., 1990; Kirshon et al., 1990, 1991; Wiggins & Elliott, 1990; Bivins et al., 1993). Oligohydramnios may occur as a result. The effect is usually reversible when therapy is stopped, but persistent renal dysfunction has been observed in infants born to women treated with indomethacin late in pregnancy (Buderus et al., 1993; Gloor et al., 1993; Norton et al., 1993; Marpeau et al., 1994; van der Heijden et al., 1994). Maternal indomethacin treatment has been used to decrease polyhydramnios (Mohen et al., 1992; Carmona et al., 1993; Moise, 1993b).

Necrotizing enterocolitis occurs with increased frequency among low-birth-weight neonates delivered shortly after their mothers were treated with indomethacin to arrest premature labor (Norton et al., 1993; Major et al., 1994). Uterine contractions can be reduced and parturition delayed by indomethacin treatment of women with premature labor in the late second or third trimester of pregnancy (Wallenburg & Bremer, 1992; Bivins et al., 1993; Morales & Madhav, 1993; Ven den Veyver & Moise, 1993).

Increased frequencies of fetal death and malformations have been observed in some studies when pregnant mice or rats were treated with indomethacin in doses similar to or a few times greater than those used in humans (Gavin et al., 1974; Persaud & Moore, 1974; Persaud, 1975; Gupta & Goldman, 1986). In other studies, no increase in the frequency of malformations was seen among the offspring of mice or rats treated during pregnancy with indomethacin in doses many times larger than those used in humans (Kalter, 1973; Klein et al., 1981; Randall et al., 1987; Kondoh et al., 1989).

Risk Related to Breast-feeding

Indomethacin is excreted into breast milk. The amount of indomethacin that the nursing infant would be expected to ingest is <1-6% of the lowest pediatric dose, based on data obtained from 16 lactating women (Lebedevs et al., 1991).*

The amount of indomethacin found in the serum of seven infants of women who were being treated with indomethacin during lactation was 0-5% of the therapeutic serum concentration of indomethacin.[†]

Generalized seizures occurred in the nursing infant of a woman who was being treated with indomethacin (Eeg-Oloffson et al., 1978). The infant recovered when indomethacin was discontinued in the mother. No causal inference can be made on the basis of this anecdotal report.

The American Academy of Pediatrics considers indomethacin to be safe to use during breast-feeding (Committee on Drugs, American Academy of Pediatrics, 1994).

Key References

Aselton P, Jick H, Milunsky A, et al.: First-trimester drug use and congenital disorders. Obstet Gynecol 65:451-455, 1985.

Baerts W, Fetter WPF, Hop WCJ, et al.: Cerebral lesions in preterm infants after tocolytic indomethacin. Dev Med Child Neurol 32:910-918, 1990. [Erratum: Dev Med Child Neurol 32(11):1032, 1990.]

Besinger RE, Niebyl JR, Keyes WG, Johnson TRB: Randomized comparative trial of indomethacin and ritodrine for the long-term suppression of preterm labor. Am J Obstet Gynecol 164:981-988, 1991.

Bivins HA Jr, Newman RB, Fyfe DA, et al.: Randomized trial of oral indomethacin and terbutaline sulfate for the long-term suppression of pre-term labor. Am J Obstet Gynecol 169:1065-1070, 1993.

Buderus S, Thomas B, Fahnenstich H, Kowalewski S: Renal failure in two preterm infants: Toxic effect of prenatal maternal indomethacin treatment? Br J Obstet Gynaecol 100:97-98, 1993.

---

*This calculation is based on the following assumptions: maternal dose of indomethacin: 75-300 mg; milk concentrations of indomethacin: <0.002-0.111 mcg/mL; milk intake by the nursing infant: 150 mL/kg/d; estimated dose of indomethacin ingested by the nursing infant: <0.003-0.017 mg/kg/d; lowest pediatric dose of indomethacin: 0.3 mg/kg/d.

†Infant serum level of indomethacin: 0.047 mcg/mL; lowest therapeutic serum level of indomethacin in adults: 1 mcg/mL.

Carmona F, Martinez-Roman S, Mortera C, et al.: Efficacy and safety of indomethacin therapy for polyhydramnios. Eur J Obstet Gynecol Reprod Biol 52:175-180, 1993.

Committee on Drugs, American Academy of Pediatrics: The transfer of drugs and other chemicals into human milk. Pediatrics 93(1):137-150, 1994.

Douidar SM, Richardson J, Snodgrass WR: Role of indomethacin in ductus closure: An update evaluation. Dev Pharmacol Ther 11:196-212, 1988.

Eeg-Oloffson O, Malmros I, Elwin CE, Steen B: Convulsions in a breast-fed infant after maternal indomethacin. Lancet 2:215, 1978.

Eronen M: The hemodynamic effects of antenatal indomethacin and a beta-sympathomimetic agent on the fetus and the newborn: A randomized study. Pediatr Res 33:615-619, 1993.

Gavin MA, Fernandez-Tejerina JCD, De Las Heras MFM, Maeso EV: [Effects of an inhibitor of prostaglandins biosynthesis (indomethacin) on the rat implantation.] Reproduccion 1:177-183, 1974.

Gerson A, Abbasi S, Johnson A, et al.: Safety and efficacy of long-term tocolysis with indomethacin. Am J Perinatol 7:71-74, 1990.

Gloor JM, Muchant DG, Norling LL: Prenatal maternal indomethacin use resulting in prolonged neonatal renal insufficiency. J Perinatol 13(6):425-427, 1993.

Gupta C, Goldman A: The arachidonic acid cascade is involved in the masculinizing action of testosterone on embryonic external genitalia in mice. Proc Natl Acad Sci USA 83:4346-4349, 1986.

Hendricks SK, Smith JR, Moore DE, Brown ZA: Oligohydramnios associated with prostaglandin synthetase inhibitors in preterm labour. Br J Obstet Gynaecol 97:312-316, 1990.

Kalter H: Nonteratogenicity of indomethacin in mice. Teratology 7:A-19, 1973.

Kirshon B, Mari G, Moise KJ Jr: Indomethacin therapy in the treatment of symptomatic polyhydramnios. Obstet Gynecol 75:202-205, 1990.

Kirshon B, Moise KJ Jr, Mari G, Willis R: Long-term indomethacin therapy decreases fetal urine output and results in oligohydramnios. Am J Perinatol 8(2):86-88, 1991.

Klein KL, Scott WJ, Clark KE, Wilson JG: Indomethacin--Placental transfer, cytotoxicity, and teratology in the rat. Am J Obstet Gynecol 141:448-452, 1981.

Kondoh S, Okada F, Goto K, et al.: [Reproduction study of indometacin farnesil (II)--Teratogenicity study in rats by oral administration.] Yakuri To Chiryo 17:63-85, 1989.

Lebedevs T, Wojnar-Horton RE, Yapp P, et al.: Excretion of indomethacin in breast milk. Br J Clin Pharmacol 32:751-754, 1991.

Major CA, Lewis DF, Harding JA, et al.: Tocolysis with indomethacin increases the incidence of necrotizing enterocolitis in the low-birth-weight neonate. Am J Obstet Gynecol 170:102-106, 1994.

Marpeau L, Bouillie J, Barrat J, Milliez J: Obstetrical advantages and perinatal risks of indomethacin: A report of 818 cases. Fetal Diagn Ther 9:110-115, 1994.

Mohen D, Newnham JP, D'Orsogna L: Indomethacin for the treatment of polyhydramnios: A case of constriction of the ductus arteriosus. Aust NZ J Obstet Gynaecol 32(3):243-246, 1992.

Moise KJ Jr: Effect of advancing gestational age on the frequency of fetal ductal constriction in association with maternal indomethacin use. Am J Obstet Gynecol 168:1350-1353, 1993a.

Moise KJ Jr: Polyhydramnios: Problems and treatment. Semin Perinatol 17(3):197-209, 1993b.

Morales WJK, Madhav H: Efficacy and safety of indomethacin compared with magnesium sulfate in the management of preterm labor: A randomized study. Am J Obstet Gynecol 169:97-102, 1993.

Norton ME, Merrill J, Cooper BAB, et al.: Neonatal complications after the administration of indomethacin for preterm labor. N Engl J Med 329:1602-1607, 1993.

Persaud TVN: Prolongation of pregnancy and abnormal fetal development in rats treated with indomethacin. IRCS Med Sci Libr Compend 3:300, 1975.

Persaud TVN, Moore KL: Inhibitors of prostaglandin synthesis during pregnancy. Anat Anz 136:349-353, 1974.

Randall CL, Anton RF, Becker HC: Effect of indomethacin on alcohol-induced morphological anomalies in mice. Life Sci 41:361-369, 1987.

Van den Veyver IB, Moise KJ Jr: Prostaglandin synthetase inhibitors in pregnancy. Obstet Gynecol Surv 48:493-502, 1993.

van der Heijden AJ, Carlus C, Narcy F, et al.: Persistent anuria, neonatal death, and renal microcystic lesions after prenatal exposure to indomethacin. Am J Obstet Gynecol 171:617-623, 1994.

Wallenburg HCS, Bremer HA: Principles and applications of manipulation of prostaglandin synthesis in pregnancy. Baillieres Clin Obstet Gynaecol 6(4):859-891, 1992.

Wiggins DA, Elliott JP: Oligohydramnios in each sac of a triplet gestation caused by Motrin®--fulfilling Koch's postulates. Am J Obstet Gynecol 162:460-461, 1990.

Yu VYH: Patent ductus arteriosus in the preterm infant. Early Hum Dev 35:1-14, 1993.

INFLUENZA VIRUS VACCINE
(Flu-Immune®, Fluogen®, Fluzone®)

Conventional influenza vaccine consists of whole or fractionated inactivated (i.e., killed) influenza virus that is administered by injection (Anonymous, 1993). An attenuated live influenza virus vaccine has been used by intranasal administration.

Teratogenic Risk

*Magnitude of teratogenic
risk to child born after
exposure during gestation:*   *None*

*Quality and quantity of data
on which risk estimate is based:*   *Fair*

This rating is for inactivated influenza virus vaccine. Live influenza virus vaccine is not currently in use in the US.
The formulation of influenza virus vaccine varies each year.
Since influenza is not known to be teratogenic and the vaccine used is inactivated, the risk of congenital anomalies in children is unlikely to be affected by maternal immunization with influenza vaccine during pregnancy.

The frequencies of congenital anomalies in general, of major malformations, of minor anomalies, and of principal classes of malformations were no greater than expected among the children of 650 women who were immunized with influenza virus vaccine during the first four lunar months of pregnancy in one epidemiological study (Heinonen et al., 1977). The frequency of congenital anomalies was not increased among the children of 2283 women who had been given influenza virus vaccine anytime during pregnancy in this study. The frequency of congenital anomalies was no greater than expected among the infants of 39 women immunized with inactivated influenza virus vaccine during the first trimester of pregnancy or among the infants of 56 or 135 infants immunized with such vaccine during the last two trimesters in other studies (Sumaya & Gibbs, 1979; Deinard & Ogburn, 1981).

No animal teratology studies of inactivated influenza vaccine have been published.

Risk Related to Breast-feeding

No information regarding the distribution of inactivated influenza vaccine in breast milk has been published. The Advisory Committee on Immunization Practices regards maternal immunization with inactivated influenza vaccine during breast-feeding to be safe for both the mother and her infant (ACIP, 1994).

Key References

ACIP: General recommendations on immunization. Recommendations of the Advisory Committee on Immunization Practices (ACIP). MMWR 43(RR-1):1-38, 1994.

Anonymous: Prevention and Control of Influenza: Part I, Vaccines. Recommendations of the Advisory Committee on Immunization Practices (ACIP). MMWR 42:1-14, 1993.

Deinard AS, Ogburn P: A/NJ/8/76 influenza vaccination program: Effects on maternal health and pregnancy outcome. Am J Obstet Gynecol 140:240-245, 1981.

Heinonen OP, Slone D, Shapiro S: *Birth Defects and Drugs in Pregnancy*. Littleton, Mass.: John Wright-PSG, 1977, pp 314-316, 318-319, 436, 474, 488.

Sumaya CV, Gibbs RS: Immunization of pregnant women with influenza A/New Jersey/76 virus vaccine: Reactogenicity and immunogenicity in mother and infant. J Infect Dis 140(2):141-146, 1979.

INSULIN
(Humulin®, Novolin®, Velosulin®)

Insulin is a protein hormone produced by the pancreatic β cells. Insulin regulates glucose metabolism and is involved in many other metabolic processes in the body. Insulin is administered parenterally in the treatment of diabetes mellitus. The dosage varies greatly, depending on each indvidual patient's needs.

Teratogenic Risk

*Magnitude of teratogenic
risk to child born after
exposure during gestation:*   *Unlikely*

*Quality and quantity of data
on which risk estimate is based:*   *Fair*

Therapeutic doses of insulin are unlikely to pose a substantial teratogenic risk, but the data are insufficient to state that there is no risk.

Many epidemiological studies have established that the risk of congenital anomalies is increased two- to four-fold or more among the children of insulin-dependent diabetic women receiving conventional insulin treatment (Reece & Hobbins, 1986; Becerra et al., 1990; Ramos-Arroyo et al., 1992; Hawthorne et al., 1994). Central nervous system, cardiovascular, renal, and skeletal malformations are the most frequent congenital anomalies among these children (Becerra et al., 1990; Ramos-Arroyo et al., 1992; Martinez-Frias, 1994). Since many metabolic alterations occur among insulin-dependent diabetics, and since diabetics who require insulin differ greatly from those who do not, neither pregnancies in normal women nor pregnancies in diabetic women who do not require insulin treatment can be used as a control to distinguish the effects of maternal insulin therapy from the effects of the underlying illness on embryogenesis in diabetic mothers. Recent evidence suggesting that congenital anomalies can be reduced by improved control of maternal diabetes very early in pregnancy is consistent with the interpretation that the increased risk of malformations among infants of diabetic mothers is largely a manifestation of the disease itself and not of its treatment with insulin (Gregory et al., 1992; Kitzmiller et al., 1993; Miller, 1994; Rosenn et al., 1994, 1995).

A high incidence of fetal death and congenital anomalies has been observed among the children of women treated in the first trimester of pregnancy with insulin-induced hypoglycemic coma for psychiatric illness (Impastato et al., 1964). This treatment produces an adverse metabolic reaction in the mother that may pose a substantial risk to the embryo.

Although central nervous system, skeletal, and other malformations can be produced among the offspring of mice, rats, and rabbits treated with insulin during pregnancy (Buchanan et al., 1986; Eriksson et al., 1989; Tanigawa et al., 1991), such treatment also causes major alterations of maternal metabolic homeostasis. Thus, it is uncertain whether the teratogenic effects are due to insulin per se, to maternal metabolic derangement, or both. The observation that insulin treatment decreases the frequency of malformations among the offspring of diabetic rats and among mouse embryos cultured in diabetic rat serum suggests that maternal metabolic derangement is largely responsible for the teratogenic effects associated with the insulin treatment (Sadler & Horton, 1983; Wilson et al., 1985; Eriksson et al., 1987).

Risk Related to Breast-feeding

Insulin is destroyed in the gastrointestinal tract when administered orally (Atchinson et al., 1989; Reynolds et al., 1993) and therefore would not be expected to be absorbed intact by the nursing infant of a treated woman regardless of the amount transferred in milk (Catz & Giacoia, 1972). However, inadequate or excessive insulin treatment of diabetic mothers inhibits milk production (Benz, 1992).

Key References

Atchinson JA, Grizzle WE, Pillion DJ: Colonic absorption of insulin: An in vitro and in vivo evaluation. J Pharmacol Exper Ther 248:567-572, 1989.

Becerra JE, Khoury MJ, Cordero JF, Erickson JD: Diabetes mellitus during pregnancy and the risks for specific birth defects: A population based case-control study. Pediatrics 85:1-9, 1990.

Benz J: The galactopharmacopedia. Antidiabetic agents and lactation. J Hum Lact 8(1):27-28, 1992.

Buchanan TA, Schemmer JK, Freinkel N: Embryotoxic effects of brief maternal insulin-hypoglycemia during organogenesis in the rat. J Clin Invest 78:643-649, 1986.

Catz CS, Giacoia GP: Drugs and breast milk. Pediatr Clin North Am 19(1):151-166, 1972.

Eriksson RSM, Thunberg L, Eriksson UJ: Effects of interrupted insulin treatment on fetal outcome of pregnant diabetic rats. Diabetes 38:764-772, 1989.

Eriksson UJ, Karlsson M-G, Styrud J: Mechanisms of congenital malformations in diabetic pregnancy. Biol Neonate 51:113-118, 1987.

Gregory R, Scott AR, Mohajer M, Tattersall RB: Diabetic pregnancy 1977-1990: Have we reached a plateau? J R Coll Physicians Lond 26(2):162-166, 1992.

Hawthorne G, Snodgrass A, Tunbridge M: Outcome of diabetic pregnancy and glucose intolerance in pregnancy: An audit of fetal loss in Newcastle General Hospital 1977-1990. Diabetes Res Clin Prac 25:183-190, 1994.

Impastato DJ, Gabriel AR, Lardaro HH: Electric and insulin shock therapy during pregnancy. Dis Nerv Syst 25:542-546, 1964.

Kitzmiller JL: Sweet success with diabetes--The development of insulin therapy and glycemic control for pregnancy. Diabetes Care 16(3):107-121, 1993.

Martinez-Frias ML: Epidemiological analysis of outcomes of pregnancy in diabetic mothers: Identification of the most characteristic and most frequent congenital anomalies. Am J Med Genet 51:108-113, 1994.

Miller EH: Metabolic management of diabetes in pregnancy. Semin Perinatol 18(5):414-431, 1994.

Ramos-Arroyo MA, Rodriguez-Pinilla E, Cordero JF: Maternal diabetes: The risk for specific birth defects. Eur J Epidemiol 8(4):503-508, 1992.

Reece EA, Hobbins JC: Diabetic embryopathy: Pathogenesis, prenatal diagnosis and prevention. Obstet Gynecol Surv 41(6):325-335, 1986.

Reynolds JEF, Parfitt K, Parsons AV, Sweetman SC (eds): *Martindale: The Extra Pharmacopoeia*, 30th ed. London: The Pharmaceutical Press, 1993, p 285.

Rosenn B, Miodovnik M, Combs CA, et al.: Glycemic thresholds for spontaneous abortion and congenital malformations in insulin-dependent diabetes mellitus. Obstet Gynecol 84:515-520, 1994.

Rosenn BM, Miodovnik M, Holcberg G, et al.: Hypoglycemia: The price of intensive insulin therapy for pregnant women with insulin-dependent diabetes mellitus. Obstet Gynecol 85:417-422, 1995.

Sadler TW, Horton WE: Effects of maternal diabetes on early embryogenesis. The role of insulin and insulin therapy. Diabetes 32:1070-1074, 1983.

Tanigawa K, Kawaguchi M, Tanaka O, Kato Y: Skeletal malformations in rat offspring: Long-term effect of maternal insulin-induced hypoglycemia during organogenesis. Diabetes 40:1114-1121, 1991.

Wilson GN, Howe M, Stover JM: Delayed developmental sequences in rodent diabetic embryopathy. Pediatr Res 19(12):1337-1339, 1985.

IRON
(Ferrous Fumurate, Ferrous Gluconate, Ferrous Sulfate)

Iron is an essential element of the diet. The body's iron requirements increase dramatically in pregnancy, and supplementation is often necessary to prevent development of anemia. The US recommended dietary allowance in pregnancy is 30 mg of elemental iron per day (NRC, 1989). Iron is usually given orally; therapeutic doses range from 150-2600 mg/d, depending on the preparation and the severity of the anemia being treated. Iron is also given parenterally in smaller doses.

Teratogenic Risk

*Magnitude of teratogenic
risk to child born after
exposure during gestation:*   *None*

*Quality and quantity of data
on which risk estimate is based:*   *Poor to fair*

This assessment refers to the risk associated with maternal use of iron in therapeutic doses. The risk may be greater in cases in which the mother has taken a toxic overdose of iron.

The frequency of congenital anomalies was no higher than expected among the children of 66 women treated with parenteral iron during the first four lunar months of pregnancy or among 1864 women who received such treatment anytime during pregnancy in one epidemiological study (Heinonen et al., 1977). No difference in the frequency of congenital anomalies was observed between the infants of 1336 women who received supplemental iron routinely in the second and third trimester of pregnancy and the infants of a similar number of women who received iron only if they were anemic (Hemminki & Rimpela, 1991). The perinatal mortality was significantly higher in pregnancies of the routinely supplemented women, but this did not appear to be related to the treatment.

A decreased risk was found with maternal use of iron supplements during pregnancy in studies of 166 young children with primitive neuroectodermal brain tumors and of 155 young children with astrocytomas of the brain (Bunin et al., 1993, 1994).

In one series of 66 pregnancies in which the mother took an iron overdose, only one of 59 liveborn infants had a major malformation (McElhatton et al., 1991, 1993). The mother had taken the iron overdose after the first trimester in this case. About half of the exposures produced maternal serum iron levels in the moderate to severely toxic range; just four overdoses in this series occurred in the first trimester. No abnormalities have been reported in other infants born to women who ingested toxic doses of iron during pregnancy (Blanc et al., 1984; Olenmark et al., 1987; Tenenbein, 1989; Lacoste et al., 1992; Turk et al., 1993). A few spontaneous abortions have been reported among such women, and a direct or indirect toxic effect of the iron overdose is possible in these cases (Strom et al., 1976; McElhatton et al., 1991).

Animal teratology studies using iron have produced inconsistent results. No increase in the frequency of malformations was observed in the offspring of mice or rats treated during pregnancy in doses 1-100 times those used therapeutically in humans (Flodh et al., 1977; Tadokoro et al., 1979). No teratogenic effect was observed among the offspring of rats or rabbits treated during pregnancy with iron protein succinylate in doses of 100-900 mg/kg/d (Forster, 1993). In contrast, malformations have been observed in the offspring of rabbits treated with maternally toxic doses of iron during pregnancy (Flodh et al., 1977). Malformations were also observed in the offspring of treated mice in another investigation in which neither dose nor maternal toxicity was adequately measured (Kuchta, 1982). In both investigations, the most frequently observed fetal anomalies involved the central nervous system and skeleton. The relevance of these observations to the therapeutic use of iron in human pregnancy is unknown.

Risk Related to Breast-feeding

Iron is a normal constituent of breast milk and is present in low concentrations. The concentration of iron in breast milk does not correlate with maternal iron status or increase with maternal supplementation (Vuori et al., 1980; Lonnerdal, 1986; Arnaud et al., 1993). No adverse effects of maternal iron supplementation on the nursing infant have been reported.

Key References

Arnaud J, Prual A, Preziosi P, et al.: Effect of iron supplementation during pregnancy on trace element (Cu, Se, Zn) concentrations in serum and breast milk from Nigerien Women. Ann Nutr Metab 37:262-271, 1993.

Blanc P, Hryhorczuk D, Danel I: Deferoxamine treatment of acute iron intoxication in pregnancy. Obstet Gynecol 64(3):12S-14S, 1984.

Bunin GR, Kuijten RR, Boesel CP, et al.: Maternal diet and risk of astrocytic glioma in children: A report from the Childrens Cancer Group (United States and Canada). Cancer Causes Control 5:177-187, 1994.

Bunin GR, Kuijten RR, Buckley JD, et al.: Relation between maternal diet and subsequent primitive neuroectodermal brain tumors in young children. N Engl J Med 329:536-541, 1993.

Flodh H, Magnusson G, Malmfors T: Teratological, peri- and postnatal studies on Ferastral®, an iron-poly (sorbitol-gluconic acid) complex. Scand J Haematol (Suppl) 32:69-83, 1977.

Forster R: Iron protein succinylate: Preclinical safety assessment. Int J Clin Pharmacol Ther Toxicol 31(2):53-60, 1993.

Heinonen OP, Slone D, Shapiro S: *Birth Defects and Drugs in Pregnancy*. Littleton, Mass.: John Wright-PSG, 1977, pp 402, 444.

Hemminki E, Rimpela U: A randomized comparison of routine versus selective iron supplementation during pregnancy. J Am Coll Nutr 10(1):3-10, 1991.

Kuchta B: Experiments and ultrastructural investigations on the mouse embryo during early teratogen-sensitive stages. Acta Anat 113:218-225, 1982.

Lacoste H, Goyert GL, Goldman LS, et al.: Acute iron intoxication in pregnancy: Case report and review of the literature. Obstet Gynecol 80:500-501, 1992.

Lonnerdal LB: Effect of maternal iron status on iron in human milk. In: Hamosh M, Goldman AS (eds). *Human Lactation. 2. Maternal and Environmental Factors*. New York: Plenum Press, 1986.

McElhatton PR, Roberts JC, Sullivan FM: The consequences of iron overdose and its treatment with desferrioxamine in pregnancy. Hum Exp Toxicol 10:251-259, 1991.

McElhatton PR, Sullivan FM, Volans GN: Outcome of pregnancy following deliberate iron overdose by the mother. Hum Exp Toxicol 12(6):579, 1993.

NRC (National Research Council): *Recommended Dietary Allowances, 10th ed. Report of the Subcommittee on the Tenth Edition of the RDAs, Food and Nutrition Board, Commission on Life Sciences*. Washington, DC: National Academy Press, 1989, p 262.

Olenmark M, Biber B, Dottori O, Rybo G: Fatal iron intoxication in late pregnancy. Clin Toxicol 25(4):347-359, 1987.

Strom RL, Schiller P, Seeds AE, Bensel RT: Fatal iron poisoning in a pregnant female. Case report. Minn Med 59:483-489, 1976.

Tadokoro T, Miyaji T, Okumura M: Teratogenicity studies of slow-Fe in mice and rats. Oyo Yakuri (Pharmacometrics) 17:483-495, 1979.

Tenenbein M: Iron overdose during pregnancy. Vet Hum Toxicol 31(4):346, 1989.

Turk J, Aks S, Ampuero F, Hryhorczuk DO: Successful therapy of iron intoxication in pregnancy with intravenous deferoxamine and whole bowel irrigation. Vet Hum Toxicol 35(5):441-444, 1993.

Vuori E, Makinen SM, Kara R, et al.: The effects of the dietary intakes of copper, iron manganese and zinc on the trace element content of milk. Am J Clin Nutr 33:227-231, 1980.

ISONIAZID
(Hyzyd®, Isotamine®, Nydrazid®)

Isoniazid is a hydrazine derivative used to treat tuberculosis. Isoniazid is given orally or parenterally; the usual dose is 300 mg/d.

Teratogenic Risk

Magnitude of teratogenic risk to child born after exposure during gestation:	*Minimal*
Quality and quantity of data on which risk estimate is based:	*Poor to fair*

Prophylactic administration of pyridoxine is recommended for pregnant women on isoniazid therapy to prevent fetal neurotoxicity (see below).

The frequency of congenital anomalies was not significantly increased among the children of 85 women treated with isoniazid during the first four lunar months of pregnancy or the children of 146 women treated with this drug anytime during gestation in one epidemiological study (Heinonen et al., 1977). In another study, congenital anomalies were more frequent than expected among the children of 42 women treated with isoniazid and other medications during the first trimester of pregnancy, but there was no specificity to the kind of anomalies observed (Varpela, 1964). Several other investigations of congenital anomalies among infants born to women treated with antituberculous drugs during pregnancy have been reported (Warkany, 1979; Snider et al., 1980), but these studies are difficult to interpret because many patients are treated with more than one drug and individual agents are usually not considered separately. Moreover, the time and duration of therapy during pregnancy is variable and often incompletely documented, and underascertainment of congenital anomalies among the control infants seems likely. In general, however, no association between congenital anomalies and maternal use of isoniazid during pregnancy was apparent in these studies.

At least seven children with mental retardation, seizures, or other evidence of central nervous system dysfunction whose mothers took isoniazid and other antituberculous agents at various times during pregnancy have been reported (Varpela, 1964; Monnet et al., 1967). Available data are inadequate to determine whether or not this association is causal, but these reports are of concern because neurotoxicity is a recognized side-effect of isoniazid therapy in adults. Prophylactic administration of 50 mg/d of pyridoxine to pregnant women who are receiving isoniazid therapy has been recommended to prevent this complication (American Thoracic Society, 1986; Medchill & Gillum, 1989).

A study of 11,169 children with cancer showed no apparent association with maternal isoniazid treatment during the mothers' pregnancies (Sanders & Draper, 1979), but very few of the mothers in either group took isoniazid. In another investigation, no neoplasms were found among 660 one- to 13-year-old children born to women treated with isoniazid for various periods during their pregnancies (Hammond et al., 1967).

No increase in the frequency of malformations was observed among the offspring of mice treated with isoniazid during pregnancy in doses as high as 60 times those used in humans (Kalter, 1972; Menon & Bhide, 1980). No teratogenic effect was seen among the offspring of rabbits treated with isoniazid during pregnancy in doses equivalent to those used clinically, but in rats such treatment did increase the frequency of skeletal anomalies (Dluzniewski & Gastol-Lewinska, 1971).

An increased frequency of pulmonary adenocarcinomas has been observed among the offspring of mice treated with about 30 times the usual human dose of isoniazid during pregnancy and lactation (Menon & Bhide, 1983). The relevance of this observation to the therapeutic use of isoniazid in human pregnancy is uncertain.

Risk Related to Breast-feeding

Isoniazid and its active metabolite, acetylisoniazid, are excreted in the breast milk. The amount of isoniazid and acetylisoniazid that the nursing infant would be expected to ingest is equivalent to 9-31% of the lowest prophylactic dose of isoniazid (Vorherr, 1974; Berlin & Lee, 1979).*

The American Academy of Pediatrics regards isoniazid to be safe to use while breast-feeding (Committee on Drugs, American Academy of Pediatrics, 1994). Peripheral neuropathy is a common side effect of isoniazid therapy in adults (USP DI, 1995). Although this side effect occurs less often in children, breast-fed infants whose mothers are taking large doses of isoniazid should be monitored for signs of central nervous system toxicity.

Key References

American Thoracic Society: Treatment of tuberculosis and tuberculosis infection in adults and children. Am Rev Respir Dis 134:355-363, 1986.

Berlin CM Jr, Lee C: Isoniazid and acetylisoniazid disposition in human milk. Fed Proc 38:426, 1979.

Committee on Drugs, American Academy of Pediatrics: The transfer of drugs and other chemicals into human milk. Pediatrics 93(1):137-150, 1994.

Dluzniewski A, Gastol-Lewinska L: The search for teratogenic activity of some tuberculostatic drugs. Diss Pharm Pharmacol 23(4):383-392, 1971.

Hammond EC, Selikoff IJ, Robitzek EH: Isoniazid therapy in relation to later occurrence of cancer in adults and in infants. Br Med J 2:792-795, 1967.

Heinonen OP, Slone D, Shapiro S: *Birth Defects and Drugs in Pregnancy.* Littleton, Mass.: John Wright-PSG, 1977, pp 298-299, 302, 313, 435.

*This calculation is based on the following assumptions: maternal dose: 300 mg; milk concentrations of isoniazid and acetylisoniazid: 6-16.6 mcg/mL and 3.76 mcg/mL, respectively; milk intake by the nursing infant: 150 mL/kg/d; estimated dose of both isoniazid and acetylisoniazid ingested by the nursing infant, assuming 100% bioavailability, and similar activity and molecular weights: 0.9-3.1 mg/kg/d; lowest prophylactic dose of isoniazid in children: 10 mg/kg/d.

Kalter H: Nonteratogenicity of isoniazid in mice. Teratology 5:259, 1972.

Medchill MT, Gillum M: Diagnosis and management of tuberculosis during pregnancy. Obstet Gynecol Surv 44:81-84, 1989.

Menon MM, Bhide SV: Perinatal carcinogenicity of isoniazid (INH) in Swiss Mice. J Cancer Res Clin Oncol 105:258-261, 1983.

Menon MM, Bhide SV: Transplacental, biological and metabolic effects of isoniazid (INH) in Swiss mice. Indian J Exp Biol 18:1104-1106, 1980.

Monnet P, Kalb JC, Pujol M: [Harmful effects of isoniazid on the fetus and infants.] Lyon Med 218:431-455, 1967.

Sanders BM, Draper GJ: Childhood cancer and drugs in pregnancy. Br Med J 1:717-718, 1979.

Snider DE Jr, Layde PM, Johnson MW, Lyle MA: Treatment of tuberculosis during pregnancy. Am Rev Respir Dis 122:65-79, 1980.

USP DI: Isoniazid. In: *USP DI (USP Dispensing Information), Volume 1. Drug Information for the Health Care Professional,* 15th ed. Rockville, Md.: The US Pharmacopeial Convention, 1995, pp 1629-1630.

Varpela E: On the effect exerted by the first-line tuberculosis medicines on the foetus. Acta Tuberc Scand 35:53-69, 1964.

Vorherr H: Drug excretion in breast milk. Postgrad Med 56(4):97-104, 1974.

Warkany J: Antituberculous drugs. Teratology 20:133-138, 1979.

ISOPROTERENOL
(Aerolone®, Isuprel®, Vapo-Iso®)

Isoproterenol is a sympathomimetic agent that stimulates β-adrenergic receptors. It is widely used in the treatment of asthma and cardiac dysfunction. Isoproterenol is given in sublingual doses of 15-60 mg/d. Smaller doses are used by inhalation and parenterally.

Teratogenic Risk

*Magnitude of teratogenic
risk to child born after
exposure during gestation:*   Unlikely

*Quality and quantity of data
on which risk estimate is based:*   Poor to fair

Therapeutic doses of isoproterenol are unlikely to pose a substantial teratogenic risk, but the data are insufficient to state that there is no risk.

The frequency of congenital anomalies was no greater than expected among the children of 31 women treated with isoproterenol during the first four lunar months of pregnancy in one epidemiological study (Heinonen et al., 1977).

No teratogenic effect was observed among the offspring of rats or rabbits treated with isoproterenol by inhalation in doses 5-15 times those used in humans (Vogin et al., 1970). Similarly, the frequency of malformations was not increased among the offspring of pregnant rats injected intraperitoneally with 6-22 times the maximal human oral dose of isoproterenol or of pregnant rabbits fed 4-14 times the maximal human dose (Hollingsworth et al., 1971; Jones-Price et al., 1982). In contrast, the frequency of central nervous system and other malformations was increased among the offspring of pregnant hamsters given isoproterenol in single subcutaneous injections 1250-8700 times those used in humans (Geber, 1969). Increased frequencies of congenital anomalies have also been reported among the offspring of pregnant mice given single isoproterenol injections about 720 times those used subcutaneously in humans (Sullivan & Robson, 1965). The relevance of these observations to the therapeutic use of isoproterenol in human pregnancy is unknown.

Alterations in heart rate and blood pressure have been observed near term in the fetuses of rhesus monkeys given intravenous infusions of 2.5-20 times the usual human dose of isoproterenol (Myers et al., 1978).

Risk Related to Breast-feeding

No information regarding the distribution of isoproterenol in breast milk has been published.

Key References

Geber WF: Comparative teratogenicity of isoproterenol and trypan blue in the fetal hamster. Proc Soc Exp Biol Med 130:1168-1170, 1969.

Heinonen OP, Slone D, Shapiro S: *Birth Defects and Drugs in Pregnancy.* Littleton, Mass.: John Wright-PSG, 1977, pp 346-347.

Hollingsworth RL, Scott WJ Jr, Woodard MW, Woodard G: Fetal rabbit ductus arteriosus assessed in a teratological study on isoproterenol and metaproterenol. Toxicol Appl Pharmacol 18:231-234, 1971

Jones-Price C, Ledoux TA, Reel JR, et al.: Teratologic evaluation of isoproterenol hydrochloride (CAS No. 51-30-9) in CD rats. NTIS (National Technical Information Service) Report/PB83-153007, 1982.

Myers RE, Joelsson I, Adamsons K: The effects of isoproterenol on fetal oxygenation. Acta Obstet Gynecol Scand 57:317-322, 1978.

Sullivan FM, Robson JM: Discussion. In: Robson JM, Sullivan FM, Smith RL (eds). *Embryopathic Activity of Drugs*. Boston, Mass.: Little Brown and Co., 1965, pp 110-115.

Vogin EE, Goldhamer RE, Scheimberg J, Carson S: Teratology studies in rats and rabbits exposed to an isoproterenol aerosol. Toxicol Appl Pharmacol 16:374-381, 1970.

ISOPTIN® *See* Verapamil

ISOTAMINE® *See* Isoniazid

ISOTRETINOIN
(Accutane®)

Isotretinoin (13-cis-retinoic acid) is a vitamin A congener used in the treatment of cystic acne and other dermatologic diseases. The usual oral dose is 0.5-2 mg/kg/d, although doses up to 8 mg/kg/d are sometimes employed. Topical preparations usually contain 0.05% isotretinoin.

Teratogenic Risk

Magnitude of teratogenic risk to child born after exposure during gestation:	*High*
Quality and quantity of data on which risk estimate is based:	*Excellent*

This risk is for oral treatment during embryogenesis.

A very uncommon but strikingly similar pattern of anomalies has been observed in more than 80 children born to women who took oral isotretinoin during early pregnancy (Lammer et al., 1985; Rosa et al., 1986; Teratology Society, 1991). Characteristic features of this embryopathy include central nervous system (CNS) malformations, microtia/anotia, micrognathia, cleft palate, cardiac and great vessel defects, thymic abnormalities, and eye anomalies. Limb reduction defects may occasionally occur (Rizzo et al., 1991). Among 115 continuing pregnancies in women treated with oral isotretinoin that were voluntarily reported to the manufacturer before the outcome was known, 18% ended in spontaneous abortion (Dai et al., 1992). Twenty-eight percent of the 94 liveborn infants, almost all of whose mothers had taken isotretinoin during the first trimester, had at least one major malformation. Typical malformations occurred in children born to women who took various dosages of isotretinoin within the usual therapeutic range and in women who were treated for less than one week in the first trimester of pregnancy (Chen et al., 1990; Dai et al., 1992). In a follow-up study of 31 five-year-old children born to women who had been treated with oral isotretinoin during the first 60 days after conception, 47% performed in the subnormal range on standard intelligence tests (Adams, 1990; Adams et al., 1991; Adams & Lammer, 1992, 1993). Of the 12 children in this study who had major malformations, six (including four with major CNS anomalies) had IQ <70, four (including one with major CNS anomalies) had IQ 70-85, and two had IQ >85. Six of 19 children with no major malformations had IQ 70-85; the others had IQ >85.

The frequency of congenital anomalies does not appear to be increased among the children of women who discontinue oral isotretinoin therapy *prior to conception* (Dai et al., 1989). This finding is consistent with the ten- to 12-hour average serum half-life of isotretinoin.

Systemic isotretinoin treatment during pregnancy produces a similar spectrum of malformations in experimental animals. Teratogenic effects have been reported in monkeys, rabbits, hamsters, mice, and rats after administration of isotretinoin to pregnant females in doses several to many times greater than those used clinically (Hummler et al., 1990; Teratology Society, 1991; Korte et al., 1993; Eckhoff et al., 1994).

Risk Related to Breast-feeding

No information regarding the excretion of isotretinoin in breast milk has been published. However, because it is a retinoid with high lipid solubility, isotretinoin is likely to be present in the milk of treated women.

Key References

Adams J: High incidence of intellectual deficits in 5 year old children exposed to isotretinoin "in utero". Teratology 41(5):614, 1990.

Adams J, Lammer EJ: Neurobehavioral teratology of isotretinoin. Reprod Toxicol 7:175-177, 1993.

Adams J, Lammer EJ: Relationship between dysmorphology and neuro-psychological function in children exposed to isotretinoin "in utero." In: Fujii T, Boer GJ (eds). *Functional Neuroteratology of Short-Term Exposure to Drugs.* Tokyo: Teikyo University Press, 1992, pp 159-170.

Adams J, Lammer EJ, Holmes LB: A syndrome of cognitive dysfunctions following human embryonic exposure to isotretinoin. Teratology 43(5):497, 1991.

Chen DT, Jacobson MM, Kuntzman RG: Experience with the retinoids in human pregnancy. In: Volans GN (ed). *Basic Science in Toxicology (International Congress of Toxicology),* 5th ed. London: Francis Taylor Publishing Co., 1990, pp 473-482.

Dai WS, Hsu M-A, Itri LM: Safety of pregnancy after discontinuation of isotretinoin. Arch Dermatol 125:362-365, 1989.

Dai WS, LaBraico JM, Stern RS: Epidemiology of isotretinoin exposure during pregnancy. J Am Acad Dermatol 26:599-606, 1992.

Eckhoff C, Chari S, Kromka M, et al.: Teratogenicity and transplacental pharmacokinetics of 13-cis-retinoic acid in rabbits. Toxicol Appl Pharmacol 125:34-41, 1994.

Hummler H, Korte R, Hendrickx AG: Induction of malformations in the cynomolgus monkey with 13-cis retinoic acid. Teratology 42:263-272, 1990.

Korte R, Hummler H, Hendrickx AG: Importance of early exposure to 13-cis retinoic acid to induce teratogenicity in the cynomolgus monkey. Teratology 47:37-45, 1993.

Lammer EJ, Chen DT, Hoar RM, et al.: Retinoic acid embryopathy. N Engl J Med 313:837-841, 1985.

Rizzo R, Lammer EJ, Parano E, et al.: Limb reduction defects in humans associated with prenatal isotretinoin exposure. Teratology 44:599-604, 1991.

Rosa FW, Wilk AL, Kelsey FO: Teratogen update: Vitamin A congeners. Teratology 33:355-364, 1986.

Teratology Society: Recommendations for isotretinoin use in women of childbearing potential. Teratology 44:1-6, 1991.

ISUPREL® *See* Isoproterenol

K-10® *See* Potassium Chloride

KABIKINASE® *See* Streptokinase

KAOCHLOR-10® *See* Potassium Chloride

KEFUROX® *See* Cefuroxime

KEFLEX® *See* Cephalexin

KENACORT® *See* Triamcinolone

KETOCONAZOLE
(Nizoral®)

Ketoconazole is given orally in a dose of 200-1000 mg/d to treat systemic fungal infections. Topical ketoconazole is used to treat cutaneous mycoses and seborrhea. Systemic absorption of ketoconazole from the skin is very poor, although some absorption may occur from the vagina. Ketoconazole blocks the activity of several enzymes involved in synthesis of adrenal steroid hormones and is also used for symptomatic treatment of Cushing's syndrome. For this purpose, oral doses as great as 1200 mg/d may be given.

Teratogenic Risk

Magnitude of teratogenic
risk to child born after
exposure during gestation:
  Topical use: *Undetermined*
  Systemic use: *Undetermined*

Quality and quantity of data
on which risk estimate is based:
  Topical use: *None*
  Systemic use: *Very poor*

A small risk cannot be excluded, but there is no indication that the risk of congenital anomalies in children of women treated with topical ketoconazole during pregnancy is likely to be great.

Because ketoconazole interferes with steroid hormonogenesis, systemic maternal treatment with this drug early in pregnancy may affect genital development in male fetuses (Amado et al., 1990).

No epidemiological studies of congenital anomalies in infants born to women who took ketoconazole during pregnancy have been reported. No adverse effect was noted in a female infant whose mother was treated with ketoconazole during the last five weeks of pregnancy for Cushing's syndrome (Amado et al., 1990).

The frequencies of fetal death and anomalies were increased among the offspring of rats treated during pregnancy with 2-4 times the human dose of ketoconazole (Nishikawa et al., 1984; Buttar et al., 1989). Ventricular septal defect and cleft palate were among the most frequently observed anomalies. Increased frequencies of fetal death were also seen among the offspring of pregnant mice and rabbits treated with 1-2 and 1-4 times the human therapeutic dose of ketoconazole (Nishikawa et al., 1984; Buttar et al., 1989).

Risk Related to Breast-feeding

No information regarding the distribution of ketoconazole in breast milk has been published; however, it is unlikely that topical application of ketoconazole would produce breast milk levels large enough to affect the nursing infant (USP DI, 1995).

Key References

Amado JA, Pesquera C, Gonzalez EM, et al.: Successful treatment with ketoconazole of Cushing's syndrome in pregnancy. Postgrad Med J 66:221-223, 1990.

Buttar HS, Moffatt JH, Bura C: Pregnancy outcome in ketoconazole treated rats and mice. Teratology 39(5):444, 1989.

Nishikawa S, Hara T, Miyazaki H, Ohguro Y: Reproduction studies of KW-1414 in rats and rabbits. Kiso To Rinsho (Clin Rep) 18:1433-1448, 1984.

USP DI: Ketoconazole. In: *USP DI (USP Dispensing Information), Volume 1. Drug Information for the Health Care Professional,* 15th ed. Rockville, Md.: The US Pharmacopeial Convention, 1995, p 1650.

KETOROLAC
(Toradol®)

Ketorolac is a prostaglandin synthetase inhibitor that is used as an anti-inflammatory and analgesic agent. Ketorolac may be administered orally, parenterally, or as an ophthalmic preparation. The usual oral dose is 10-40 mg/d; doses as high as 120-150 mg/d are sometimes used parenterally. Systemic absorption of the ophthalmic preparation is negligible.

Teratogenic Risk

*Magnitude of teratogenic
risk to child born after
exposure during gestation:*   *Undetermined*

*Quality and quantity of data
on which risk estimate is based:*   *Very poor*

A small risk cannot be excluded, but a greatly increased risk of congenital anomalies is unlikely in the children of women treated with ophthalmic ketorolac preparations during pregnancy.

Because ketorolac is a prostaglandin synthetase inhibitor, maternal treatment with this drug late in pregnancy may cause premature closure of the fetal ductus arteriosus. This effect has not been studied directly with ketorolac.

No epidemiological studies of congenital anomalies among the children of women treated with ketorolac during pregnancy have been reported.

Decreased platelet aggregation, a recognized side-effect of ketorolac therapy, was observed in cord blood following administration of ketorolac to a pregnant woman during labor (Greer et al., 1988). No adverse effect was observed clinically among the infants of 40 women who were treated with ketorolac during labor in a controlled therapeutic trial (Walker et al., 1992).

Unpublished studies in rats and rabbits are said to suggest that treatment of pregnant women with ketorolac in usual therapeutic doses is unlikely to increase the children's risk of malformations greatly (USP DI, 1995).

Please see agent summary on indomethacin for information on a similar drug that has been more thoroughly studied.

Risk Related to Breast-feeding

Ketorolac is excreted into breast milk in very low concentrations. The amount of ketorolac that the nursing infant would be expected to ingest is <1% of the lowest weight-adjusted therapeutic dose of ketorolac, based on data from ten lactating women (Wischnik et al., 1989).*

The American Academy of Pediatrics regards ketorolac to be safe to use while breast-feeding (Committee on Drugs, American Academy of Pediatrics, 1994).

Key References

Committee on Drugs, American Academy of Pediatrics: The transfer of drugs and other chemicals into human milk. Pediatrics 93(1):137-150, 1994.

Greer LA, Johnston J, Tulloch I, Walker JJ: Effect of maternal ketorolac administration on platelet function in the newborn. Eur J Obstet Gynecol Reprod Biol 29:257-260, 1988.

USP DI: Ketorolac. In: *USP DI (USP Dispensing Information), Volume 1. Drug Information for the Health Care Professional*, 15th

---

*This calculation is based on the following assumptions: maternal dose of ketorolac: 40 mg/d; milk concentration of ketorolac: 0.005-0.008 mcg/mL; milk intake by the nursing infant: 150 mL/kg/d; estimated dose of ketorolac ingested by the nursing infant: 0.0007-0.001 mg/kg/d; lowest therapeutic dose of ketorolac in adults: 0.31 mg/kg/d.

ed. Rockville, Md.: The US Pharmacopeial Convention, 1995, pp 1651-1657.

Walker JJ, Johnston J, Fairlie FM, et al.: A comparative study of intramuscular ketorolac and pethidine in labour pain. Eur J Obstet Gynecol Reprod Biol 46:87-94, 1992.

Wischnik A, Manth SM, Lloyd J, et al.: The excretion of ketorolac tromethamine into breast milk after multiple oral dosing. Eur J Clin Pharmacol 36:521-524, 1989.

KLONOPIN® *See* Clonazepam

KOROSTATIN® *See* Nystatin

LANOXICAPS® *See* Digoxin

LANOXIN® *See* Digoxin

LARIAM® *See* Mefloquine

LASIX® *See* Furosemide

LEDERCORT® *See* Triamcinolone

LEUPROLIDE
(Lupron®, Procrin®)

Leuprolide is a synthetic peptide analog of luteinizing hormone-releasing hormone. Leuprolide is given intramuscularly as a depot injection (usually 3.75 mg per dose) to treat endometriosis. Leuprolide has also been used subcutaneously as part of a regimen for pharmacological stimulation of ovulation. The intramuscular depot formulation is released slowly with 85-100% absorption in four weeks (AHFS Drug Information, 1991). In contrast, the subcutaneous preparation of leuprolide is rapidly absorbed and eliminated from the plasma.

Teratogenic Risk

Magnitude of teratogenic
risk to child born after
exposure during gestation: Undetermined

Quality and quantity of data
on which risk estimate is based: Very poor

A small risk cannot be excluded, but a high risk of congenital anomalies in the children of women treated with leuprolide during pregnancy is unlikely. This rating is for malformations and excludes the risk of deformations associated with multifetal pregnancies.

Multifetal pregnancies may be especially frequent in women who conceive after ovulation stimulation with leuprolide and gonadotropin (see below).

No epidemiological studies of congenital anomalies among infants born to women treated with leuprolide during pregnancy have been reported. No congenital anomalies were seen among 15 liveborn infants delivered to women who had been treated with subcutaneous leuprolide for ovulation induction (Wilshire et al., 1993; Young et al., 1993). These series also included seven spontaneous pregnancy losses and one therapeutic abortion for trisomy 18 in the fetus.

Multifetal pregnancies may be even more frequent in women who conceive after ovulation has been stimulated with leuprolide and gonadotropin than after other methods of ovulation stimulation (Jansen et al., 1990).

Fetal death and growth retardation were observed with increased frequency among the offspring of rats and rabbits treated during pregnancy with leuprolide in doses similar to or smaller than those used in humans (Ooshima et al., 1990a, b; USP DI, 1995). In unpublished studies, the frequency of major fetal anomalies is said to have been increased among the offspring of pregnant rabbits treated with leuprolide in doses similar to or greater than those used in humans (USP DI, 1995). No increase in the frequency of malformations was observed among the offspring of either rats or rabbits in other studies using the same doses (Ooshima et al., 1990a, b; USP DI, 1995). The relevance of these observations to the use of leuprolide in human pregnancy is uncertain.

Risk Related to Breast-feeding

No information regarding the distribution of leuprolide in breast milk has been published.

Key References

AHFS Drug Information--91. Bethesda, Md.: Board of Directors of the Amer Society of Hospital Pharmacists, 1991, pp 568-574.

Jansen RPS, Anderson JC, Birrell WSR, et al.: Outpatient gamete intrafallopian transfer: A clinical analysis of 710 cases. Med J Aust 153:182-188, 1990.

Ooshima Y, Nakamura H, Negishi R, et al.: [Teratological study of TAP-144-SR in rabbits.] Yakuri To Chiryo (Suppl) 18(3):S633-639, 1990b.

Ooshima Y, Negishi R, Yoshida T, et al.: [Teratological study of TAP-144-SR in rats.] Yakuri To Chiryo (Suppl) 18(3):S609-S623, 1990a.

USP DI: Leuprolide. In: *USP DI (USP Dispensing Information), Volume 1. Drug Information for the Health Care Professional,* 15th ed. Rockville, Md.: The US Pharmacopeial Convention, 1995, p 1708.

Wilshire GB, Emmi AM, Gagliardi CC, Weiss G: Gonadotropin-releasing hormone agonist administration in early human pregnancy is associated with normal outcomes. Fertil Steril 60(6):980-983, 1993.

Young DC, Snabes MC, Poindexter AN III: GnRH agonist exposure during the first trimester of pregnancy. Obstet Gynecol 81:587-589, 1993.

LEVOTHROID® *See Levothyroxine*

LEVOTHYROXINE
(Eltroxin®, Levothroid®, Syroxine®)

Levothyroxine (T4), a thyroid hormone, is used to treat goiter and thyroid deficiency states. Levothyroxine is usually given orally in a dose of 12.5-200 mcg/d. It may also be given parenterally for severe myxedema in doses as high as 500 mcg/d.

Teratogenic Risk

Magnitude of teratogenic
risk to child born after
exposure during gestation: *None*

Quality and quantity of data
on which risk estimate is based: *Fair*

The frequencies of congenital anomalies, major malformations, minor anomalies, and major classes of anomalies were not increased among 537 children of women treated with levothyroxine or thyroid extract during the first four lunar months of pregnancy in one epidemiological study (Heinonen et al., 1977). The frequency of congenital anomalies was no greater than expected among 1605 children of women treated with levothyroxine or thyroid extract anytime during pregnancy in this study.

Studies in rats and mice suggest that treatment of pregnant women with levothyroxine in usual therapeutic doses is unlikely to increase the children's risk of malformations greatly (Baksi, 1978; Lamb et al., 1986). The offspring of pregnant rats treated with levothyroxine in doses more than 25 times those used in humans often had cataracts, permanent impairment of hypothalamo-pituitary-thyroid function, and fetal or neonatal death (Giroud & de Rothschild, 1951; Lammers et al., 1978; Porterfield, 1985). The relevance, if any, of these findings with thyrotoxic doses to the therapeutic use of levothyroxine during human pregnancy is unknown.

In humans, direct fetal treatment with levothyroxine late in pregnancy has been used for fetal hypothyroidism and goiter (Davidson et al., 1991; Noia et al., 1992). Intra-amniotic instillation of levothyroxine has also been used to induce fetal lung maturity prior to premature delivery in the third trimester of pregnancy (Romaguera et al., 1990; Roberts & Morrison, 1991; Barkai et al., 1992). Such therapy does not appear to have any adverse effect on the child (Barkai et al., 1988).

Risk Related to Breast-feeding

Levothyroxine is normally present in breast milk in small amounts. Concentrations of levothyroxine measured in breast milk have varied widely across studies, primarily because of differences in techniques used (Jansson et al., 1983). No data regarding the effects of maternal supplementation with levothyroxine on the nursing infant have been published.

Key References

Baksi SN: Effect of dichlorvos on embryonal and fetal development in thyroparathyroidectomized, thyroxine-treated and euthyroid rats. Toxicol Lett 2:213-216, 1978.

Barkai G, Reichman B, Lusky A, et al.: The effect of thyroxine and corticosteroids upon amniotic fluid fluorescence polarization: A randomized controlled study. J Perinat Med 20:459-464, 1992.

Barkai G, Zarfin Y, Ben-Harari M, et al.: In utero thyroxine therapy for the induction of fetal lung maturity: Long term effects. J Perinat Med 16:145-148, 1988.

Davidson KM, Richards DS, Schatz DA, Fisher DA: Successful in utero treatment of fetal goiter and hypothyroidism. N Engl J Med 324:543-546, 1991.

Giroud A, de Rothschild B: [Effects of thyroxine on the fetal eye.] C R Soc Biol 145:525-526, 1951.

Heinonen OP, Slone D, Shapiro S: *Birth Defects and Drugs in Pregnancy.* Littleton, Mass.: John Wright-PSG, 1977, pp 397-398, 443.

Jansson L, Ivarsson S, Larsson I, Ekman R: Tri-iodothyronine and thyroxine in human milk. Acta Paediatr Scand 72:703-705, 1983.

Lamb JC IV, Harris MW, McKinney JD, et al.: Effects of thyroid hormones on the induction of cleft palate by 2,3,7,8-tetrachlorodibenzo-p-dioxin (TCDD) in C57BL/6N mice. Toxicol Appl Pharmacol 84(1):115-124, 1986.

Lammers M, von zur Muhlen A, Dohler U: Prenatal thyroxine treatment causes permanent impairment of hypothalamopituitary-thyroid function in rats. Acta Endocrinol (Copenh) Suppl 215:73-74, 1978.

Noia G, De Santis M, Tocci A, et al.: Early prenatal diagnosis and therapy of fetal hypothyroid goiter. Fetal Diagn Ther 7:138-143, 1992.

Porterfield SP: Prenatal exposure of the fetal rat to excessive L-thyroxine or 3,5-dimethyl-3'-isopropyl-thyronine produces persistent changes in the thyroid control system. Horm Metab Res 17:655-659, 1985.

Roberts WE, Morrison JC: Pharmacologic induction of fetal lung maturity. Clin Obstet Gynecol 34(2):319-327, 1991.

Romaguera J, Zorrilla C, de la Vega A, et al.: Responsiveness of L-S ratio of the amniotic fluid to intra-amniotic administration of thyroxine--role of fetal age.   Acta Obstet Gynecol Scand 69:119-122, 1990.

LEVSIN® *See* Hyoscyamine

LIBRITABS® *See* Chlordiazepoxide

LIBRIUM® *See* Chlordiazepoxide

LIDEX® *See* Fluocinonide

LIDOCAINE
(Dulcaine®, LidoPen®, Xylocaine®)

Lidocaine is a local anesthetic of the amide class that is widely used by injection and topical application.   Lidocaine is also used intravenously to treat cardiac arrhythmia's.   The parenteral dose may be as great as 300 mg/hr.   Systemic absorption of topical or locally administered lidocaine occurs.

Teratogenic Risk

Magnitude of teratogenic
risk to child born fate
exposure during gestation:
    Local or topical administration: *None*
    Intravenous administration: *Undetermined*

Quality and quantity of data
on which risk estimate is based:
    Local or topical administration: *Fair*
    Intravenous administration: *Poor*

The frequencies of congenital anomalies in general, of major malformations, of minor anomalies, and of major classes of congenital anomalies were not increased among the children of 293 women who received lidocaine as a local anesthetic during the first four lunar months of pregnancy in one epidemiological study (Heinonen et al., 1977).   The frequency of congenital anomalies was no greater than expected among children born to 947 women who received lidocaine as a local anesthetic anytime during pregnancy in this study. No epidemiological investigations of congenital anomalies among children born to women treated with intravenous lidocaine during pregnancy have been reported.

No teratogenic effect was observed among the offspring of rats treated continuously during pregnancy with lidocaine in doses 1-5 times those given by parenterally in humans (Fujinaga & Mazze, 1986). In another study, no teratogenic effect was noted among the offspring of rats treated with single daily doses of lidocaine that were similar in magnitude to the total daily parenteral dose used in humans (Ramazzotto et al., 1985). Increased frequencies of dilatation of the fourth ventricle and other central nervous system anomalies were observed among embryos of pregnant mice given single injections of lidocaine 50-70% as great as the daily parental dose in humans, but these examinations were performed before embryogenesis was completed and the anomalies may not have resulted in malformations at birth (Martin & Jurand, 1992). Alterations of neonatal behavior have been noted among the offspring of pregnant rats treated with single injections of lidocaine that are 1-2 times those used on an hourly basis in humans (Smith et al., 1986), but the effect on behavior later in life was variable (Teiling et al., 1987; Smith et al., 1989). The relevance of these observations to the use of lidocaine in human pregnancy is uncertain.

Transient alterations of perinatal cardiopulmonary adaptation have been reported after maternal local or regional anesthesia with lidocaine, but serious changes appear to be uncommon (Bratteby, 1981; Abboud et al., 1982; Kileff et al., 1982; Guay et al., 1992) except when inadvertent direct injection of drug into the fetus occurs during delivery (Kim et al., 1979; De Praeter et al., 1991). Alterations of brain stem auditory evoked responses have been observed in neonates born to women who had received regional anesthesia with lidocaine during delivery (Diaz et al., 1988; Bozynski et al., 1989).

Risk Related to Breast-feeding

Lidocaine is excreted in the breast milk in low concentrations. Based on data from a single patient, the amount of lidocaine systemically absorbed by the nursing infant following local administration of a single dose to a woman for a dental procedure is <1% of the lowest pediatric dose (Lebedevs et al. 1993).*

In a second case, the amount of lidocaine that would be ingested by the nursing infant following maternal intravenous treatment with lidocaine for seven hours for ventricular dysrthythmia is <1% of the lowest pediatric dose (Zeisler et al., 1986).[†]

The American Academy of Pediatrics regards lidocaine to be safe to use while breast-feeding (Committee on Drugs, American Academy of Pediatrics, 1994).

Key References

Abboud TK, Khoo SS, Miller F, et al.: Maternal, fetal, and neonatal responses after epidural anesthesia with bupivacaine, 2-chloroprocaine, or lidocaine. Anesth Analg 61:638-644, 1982.

Bozynski MEA, Schumacher RE, Deschner LS, Kileny P: Effect of prenatal lignocaine on auditory brain stem evoked response. Arch Dis Child 64:934-938, 1989.

Bratteby LE: Effects on the infant of obstetric regional analgesia. J Perinat Med 9(Suppl 1):54-56, 1981.

Committee on Drugs, American Academy of Pediatrics: The transfer of drugs and other chemicals into human milk. Pediatrics 93(1):137-150, 1994.

De Praeter C, Vanhaesebrouck P, De Praeter N, et al.: Episiotomy and neonatal lidocaine intoxication. Eur J Pediatr 150:685-686, 1991.

Diaz M, Graff M, Hiatt M, et al.: Prenatal lidocaine and the auditory evoked responses in term infants. Am J Dis Child 142:160-161, 1988.

Fujinaga M, Mazze RI: Reproductive and teratogenic effects of lidocaine in Sprague-Dawley rats. Anesthesiology 65:626-632, 1986.

Guay J, Gaudreault P, Boulanger A, et al.: Lidocaine hydrocarbonate and lidocaine hydrochloride for cesarean section: Transplacental passage and neonatal effects. Acta Anaesthesiol Scand 36:722-727, 1992.

*This calculation is based on the following assumptions: maternal dose: 20 mg of lidocaine for a dental procedure; milk concentration of lidocaine: 0.044-0.066 mcg/mL; milk intake by the nursing infant: 150 mL/kg/d; estimated dose of lidocaine ingested by the nursing infant, assuming 35% absorption following oral administration: 0.002-0.003 mg/kg/d; lowest pediatric antiarrhythmic dose of lidocaine: 15.4 mg/kg.

†This calculation is based on the following assumptions: maternal dose of lidocaine: 15.4 mg/kg/d; milk concentration of lidocaine: 0.8 mcg/mL; estimated dose of lidocaine ingested by the nursing infant, assuming 35% absorption following oral administration: 0.04 mg/kg/d; lowest pediatric antiarrhythmic dose of lidocaine: 15.4 mg/kg/d.

Heinonen OP, Slone D, Shapiro S: *Birth Defects and Drugs in Pregnancy.* Littleton, Mass.: John Wright-PSG, 1977, pp 358, 360, 477, 493.

Kileff M, James FM III, Dewan D, et al.: Neonatal neurobehavioral responses after epidural anesthesia for cesarean section with lidocaine and bupivacaine. Anesthesiology 57(3)Suppl:A403, 1982.

Kim WY, Pomerance JJ, Miller AA: Lidocaine intoxication in a newborn following local anesthesia for episiotomy. Pediatrics 64:643-645, 1979.

Lebedevs TH, Wojnar-Horton RE, Yapp P, et al.: Excretion of lignocaine and its metabolite monoethylglycinexylidide in breast milk following its use in a dental procedure. A case report. J Clin Periodontal 20:606-608, 1993.

Martin LVH, Jurand A: The absence of teratogenic effects of some analgesics used in anaesthesia. Additional evidence from a mouse model. Anaesthesia 47:473-476, 1992.

Ramazzotto LJ, Curro FA, Paterson JA, et al.: Toxicological assessment of lidocaine in the pregnant rat. J Dent Res 164:1214-1217, 1985.

Rey E, Radvani-Bouvet, Bodiou MF, et al.: Intravenous lidocaine in the treatment of convulsions in the neonatal period: Monitoring plasma levels. Ther Drug Monitor 12:316-320, 1990.

Smith RF, Kurkjian MF, Mattran KM, Kurtz SL: Behavioral effects of prenatal exposure to lidocaine in the rat: Effects of dosage and of gestational age at administration. Neurotoxicol Teratol 11:395-403, 1989.

Smith RF, Wharton GG, Kurtz SL, et al.: Behavioral effects of mid-pregnancy administration of lidocaine and mepivacaine in the rat. Neurobehav Toxicol Teratol 8:61-68, 1986.

Teiling AKY, Mohammed AK, Minor BG, et al.: Lack of effects of prenatal exposure to lidocaine on development of behavior in rats. Anesth Analg 66:533-541, 1987.

Zeisler JA, Gaarder TD, De Mesquita SA: Lidocaine excretion in breast milk. Drug Intell Clin Pharm 20(9):691-693, 1986.

LIDOPEN® *See* Lidocaine

LIQUAEMIN® *See* Heparin

LISINOPRIL
(Prinivil®, Zestril®)

Lisinopril is an angiotensin-converting enzyme (ACE) inhibitor that is given orally to treat hypertension. The drug is also used as a vasodilator in the treatment of congestive heart failure. Lisinopril is given orally in doses of 1.25-80 mg/d.

Teratogenic Risk

Magnitude of teratogenic
risk to child born after
exposure during gestation
    First trimester use: *None to minimal*
    Use later in pregnancy: *Moderate*

Quality and quantity of data
on which risk estimate is based
    First trimester use: *Poor to fair*
    Use later in pregnancy: *Fair to good*

There is a substantial risk of oligohydramnios and fetal distress or death in hypertensive women treated with lisinopril in the latter part of pregnancy. The effect appears to be related to the pharmacological action of this drug on the fetus (see below).

The risk associated with maternal use of lisinopril during the second or third trimester of pregnancy increases with the duration of treatment.

One malformed infant was observed in a series of 12 born to women given lisinopril or another ACE inhibitor during the first trimester of pregnancy (Piper et al., 1992). This child, whose mother had been treated with a different ACE inhibitor during the first and second trimesters, had an occipital encephalocele.

One case has been reported in which hypocalvaria, an unusual underdevelopment of the skull bones, occurred in the infant of a woman who had been treated with lisinopril throughout pregnancy (Barr & Cohen, 1991; Pryde et al., 1993). Six infants with similar unusual skull defects have been observed after maternal treatment throughout pregnancy with other ACE inhibitors (Duminy & Berger, 1981; Rothberg & Lorenz, 1984; Mehta & Modi, 1989; Cunniff et al.,

1990; Barr & Cohen, 1991; Pryde et al., 1993; Shotan et al., 1994). Renal tubular dysplasia has been observed among infants who died in the neonatal period with anuria after maternal treatment during pregnancy with lisinopril or another ACE inhibitor (Cunniff et al., 1990; Pryde et al., 1993).

Oligohydramnios, fetal growth retardation and neonatal renal failure, hypotension, pulmonary hypoplasia, joint contractures, and death have been repeatedly observed after maternal treatment with lisinopril or related drugs during pregnancy (Hulton et al., 1990; Barr & Cohen, 1991; Hanssens et al., 1991; Rosa & Bosco, 1991; Bhatt-Mehta & Deluga, 1993; Pryde et al., 1993; Shotan et al., 1994). One infant among 15 in one series born to women treated with lisinopril or other ACE inhibitors during the second or third trimester of pregnancy had oligohydramnios and neonatal hypotension and anuria (Piper et al., 1992). It is important to note that these effects do not appear to reflect abnormal embryogenesis but rather a pharmacologic response of the fetus to lisinopril during the second half of gestation (Beckman & Brent, 1990; Brent & Beckman, 1991; Martin et al., 1992).

Studies in mice, rats, and rabbits suggest that treatment of pregnant women with lisinopril in usual therapeutic doses early in pregnancy is unlikely to increase the children's risk of malformations greatly (Bagdon et al., 1993a, b).

Please see agent summary on captopril for information on a related agent that has been more thoroughly studied.

Risk Related to Breast-feeding

No information regarding the distribution of lisinopril in breast milk has been published.

Key References

Bagdon WJ, Clark RL, Minsker DH, et al.: Developmental toxicity studies of lisinopril in mice and rabbits. Yakuri To Chiryo 21(7):87-94, 1993b.

Bagdon WJ, Clark RL, Minsker DH, et al.: Reproductive and developmental toxicity studies of lisinopril in rats. Yakuri To Chiryo 21(7):67-85, 1993a.

Barr M Jr, Cohen MM Jr: ACE inhibitor fetopathy and hypocalvaria: The kidney-skull connection. Teratology 44:485-495, 1991.

Beckman DA, Brent RL: Teratogenesis: Alcohol, angiotensin-converting-enzyme inhibitors, and cocaine. Curr Opin Obstet Gynecol 2:236-245, 1990.

Bhatt-Mehta V, Deluga KS: Fetal exposure to lisinopril: Neonatal manifestations and management. Pharmacotherapy 13(5):515-518, 1993.

Brent RL, Beckman DA: Angiotensin-converting enzyme inhibitors, an embryopathic class of drugs with unique properties: Information for clinical teratology counselors. Teratology 43:543-546, 1991.

Cunniff C, Jones KL, Phillipson J, et al.: Oligohydramnios sequence and renal tubular malformation associated with maternal enalapril use. Am J Obstet Gynecol 162:187-189, 1990.

Duminy PC, Burger P du T: Fetal abnormality associated with the use of captopril during pregnancy. S Afr Med J 60:805, 1981.

Hanssens M, Keirse MJNC, Vankelecom F, Van Assche FA: Fetal and neonatal effects of treatment with angiotensin-converting enzyme inhibitors in pregnancy. Obstet Gynecol 78(1):128-135, 1991.

Hulton SA, Thomson PD, Cooper PA, Rothberg AD: Angiotensin-converting enzyme inhibitors in pregnancy may result in neonatal renal failure. S Afr Med J 78:673-676, 1990.

Martin RA, Jones KL, Mendoza A, et al.: Effect of ACE inhibition on the fetal kidney: Decreased renal blood flow. Teratology 46:317-321, 1992.

Mehta N, Modi N: ACE inhibitors in pregnancy. Lancet 2:96-97, 1989.

Piper JM, Ray WA, Rosa FW: Pregnancy outcome following exposure to angiotensin-converting enzyme inhibitors. Obstet Gynecol 80:429-432, 1992.

Pryde PG, Nugent CE, Barr M Jr, et al.: Angiotensin-converting enzyme inhibitor fetopathy. J Am Soc Nephrol 3:1575-1582, 1993.

Rosa F, Bosco L: Infant renal failure with maternal ACE inhibition. Am J Obstet Gynecol 164:273, 1991.

Rothberg AD, Lorenz R: Can captopril cause fetal and noenatal renal failure? Pediatr Pharmacol 4:189-192, 1984.

Shotan A, Widerhorn J, Hurst A, Elkayam U: Risks of angiotensin-converting enzyme inhibition during pregnancy: Experimental and clinical evidence, potential mechanisms, and recommendations for use. Am J Med 96(5):451-456, 1994.

LITHANE® *See* Lithium

LITHIUM
(Carbolith®, Eskalith®, Lithane®)

Lithium carbonate and some other lithium salts are used for the prevention and treatment of affective mental illness. Lithium is usually given orally in doses of 300-2400 mg/d. Serum lithium levels of 0.8-1.2 mEq/L are considered to be therapeutic in acute bipolar disorder.

Teratogenic Risk

Magnitude of teratogenic risk to child born after exposure during gestation: *Small*

Quality and quantity of data on which risk estimate is based: *Fair to good*

Fetal echocardiography should be offered to pregnant women who have been treated with lithium early in pregnancy (see below).

An association has been observed between maternal treatment with lithium carbonate during pregnancy and the occurrence of cardiovascular malformations, especially Ebstein's anomaly, in children (Elia et al., 1987; Thiels, 1987; Warkany, 1988; Cohen et al., 1994). Eighteen (8%) of 225 infants voluntarily reported to an international registry because they had been born to mothers treated with lithium salts during the first trimester of pregnancy had serious congenital cardiovascular anomalies (Weinstein, 1980). Six of the affected infants (2.7% of the total) had Ebstein's anomaly, a malformation that occurs with an expected incidence of only about 1/20,000. Noncardiovascular malformations occurred in seven (3.1%) of the 225 infants, a frequency not much different from that expected. Because these cases were voluntarily reported and because no appropriate control data are available, it is not possible to use this registry to estimate the risk of congenital anomalies in children of women who take lithium during early pregnancy.

Controlled epidemiological studies indicate that this risk is likely to be small. No instance of maternal lithium use during pregnancy was observed in studies of 59, 40, or 34 children with Ebstein's anomaly or of 44 children with tricuspid atresia (Kallen, 1988; Edmonds & Oakley, 1990; Zalzstein et al., 1990; Cohen et al., 1994).

355

The frequency of congenital anomalies was no greater than expected among 105 liveborn infants whose mothers had taken lithium during the first trimester of pregnancy in another study (Jacobson et al., 1992). There was a total of 138 pregnancies with known outcome in this series; one fetus with Ebstein's anomaly was diagnosed prenatally. The occurrence of this rare malformation in so small a series of patients is remarkable (Ferner & Smith, 1992; Cohen et al., 1994).

In a study of children born to women with manic-depressive illness, 59 infants were delivered by mothers who took lithium salts early in pregnancy (Kallen & Tanberg, 1983). Eleven (19%) of these infants had congenital anomalies and four (7%) had congenital heart disease. None had Ebstein's anomaly. The frequencies of congenital anomalies and of heart defects were significantly greater than among the children of manic-depressive women who had not been treated with lithium during pregnancy.

Prenatal diagnosis by fetal echocardiography is recommended for women who have been treated with lithium early in pregnancy (Allan et al., 1982; Long & Willis, 1984; Cohen et al., 1994).

Associations between maternal lithium treatment during pregnancy and both premature delivery and higher than expected birth weight have been observed (Jacobson et al., 1992; Troyer et al., 1993).

No differences were found between 60 children born of pregnancies in which the mother took lithium and their unexposed siblings in a postal survey of physical and mental developmental problems five or more years after birth (Schou, 1976).

Increased frequencies of cleft palate and fetal loss have been observed among the offspring of mice treated during pregnancy with lithium carbonate in doses that produce blood levels within the human therapeutic range (Szabo, 1970; Smithberg & Dixit, 1982). No teratogenic effect was noted among pregnant rats or rabbits treated with lithium carbonate in doses calculated to produce serum levels within the human therapeutic range (Gralla & McIlhenny, 1972). In another investigation, increased frequencies of eye and ear anomalies were observed in the offspring of pregnant rats given lithium chloride in doses that caused maternal toxicity but produced blood levels below the human therapeutic range (Wright et al., 1971).

Several other animal teratology studies have been done with lithium salts, but these investigations do not include measurements of serum levels and are therefore more difficult to interpret. Most involve treatment with lithium salts in doses one to several times those used in humans, and many of the studies are complicated by maternal toxicity. The results have been inconsistent (Jurand, 1988).

Lithium toxicity may occur in infants born to women who are receiving treatment with lithium salts near term. The abnormalities, which resemble those seen in adults with lithium toxicity, include neurological, cardiac, and hepatic dysfunction (Arnon et al., 1981; Filtenborg, 1982; Morrell et al., 1983). Manifestations of fetal lithium toxicity such as polyhydramnios and goiter may be apparent prenatally in some cases (Arnon et al., 1981; Krause et al., 1990). Fetal or neonatal lithium toxicity may develop when maternal blood lithium levels are within the therapeutic range (Filtenborg, 1982; Krause et al., 1990).

Premature delivery and large for gestational age infants may occur more frequently than expected among the pregnancies of women who are treated with lithium (Troyer et al., 1993).

Risk Related to Breast-feeding

Lithium is excreted in the breast milk. Based on data from nine lactating women, the amount of lithium that the nursing infant would be expected to ingest is approximately 5-30% of the lowest therapeutic dose on a weight-adjusted basis (Schou & Amdisen, 1973; Sykes et al., 1976).*

Serum levels of lithium in seven infants whose mothers were treated with lithium while breast-feeding were within the range of therapeutic serum concentrations of lithium (Schou & Amdisen, 1973; Sykes et al., 1976).[†]

Cyanosis, lethargy, and EKG abnormalities were observed in a nursing infant whose mother received lithium while breast-feeding (Tunnessen & Hertz, 1972). The infant's serum level of lithium was within the serum therapeutic range. No other adverse effects of lithium have been reported in nursing infants.

Because reported serum levels in infants have been found to approach therapeutic levels, the American Academy of Pediatrics regards maternal treatment with lithium to be contraindicated during breast-feeding (Committee on Drugs, American Academy of Pediatrics, 1994).

---

*This calculation is based on the following assumptions: maternal dose of lithium: 400-800 mg/d; milk concentration of lithium: 4.5-28 mcg/mL; milk intake by the nursing infant: 150 mL/kg/d; estimated dose of lithium ingested by the nursing infant: 0.7-4.5 mg/kg/d; lowest therapeutic dose of lithium in children: 15 mg/kg/d.

[†]This calculation is based on the following assumptions: infant serum levels of lithium: 3.7-22.5 mcg/mL; therapeutic serum concentrations of lithium in adults: 15-37 mcg/mL.

Key References

Allan LD, Desai G, Tynan MJ: Prenatal echocardiographic screening for Ebstein's anomaly for mothers on lithium therapy. Lancet 2:875-876, 1982.

Arnon RG, Marin-Garcia J, Peeden JN: Tricuspid valve regurgitation and lithium carbonate toxicity in a newborn infant. Am J Dis Child 135:941-943, 1981.

Cohen LS, Friedman JM, Jefferson JW, et al.: A reevaluation of risk of in utero exposure to lithium. JAMA 271:146-150, 1994.

Committee on Drugs, American Academy of Pediatrics: The transfer of drugs and other chemicals into human milk. Pediatrics 93(1):137-150, 1994.

Edmonds LD, Oakley GP: Ebstein's anomaly and maternal lithium exposure during pregnancy. Teratology 41:551-552, 1990.

Elia J, Katz IR, Simpson GM: Teratogenicity of psychotherapeutic medications. Psychopharmacol Bull 23(4):531-586, 1987.

Ferner RE, Smith JM: Lithium and pregnancy. Lancet 339(8797): 869, 1992.

Filtenborg JA: Persistent pulmonary hypertension after lithium intoxication in the newborn. Eur J Pediatr 138:321-323, 1982.

Gralla EJ, McIlhenny HM: Studies in pregnant rats, rabbits and monkeys with lithium carbonate. Toxicol Appl Pharmacol 21:428-433, 1972.

Jacobson SJ, Jones K, Johnson K, et al.: Prospective multicentre study of pregnancy outcome after lithium exposure during first trimester. Lancet 339:530-533, 1992.

Jurand A: Teratogenic activity of lithium carbonate: An experimental update. Teratology 38:101-111, 1988.

Kallen B: Comments on teratogen update: Lithium. Teratology 38:597, 1988.

Kallen B, Tanberg A: Lithium and pregnancy. A cohort study on manic-depressive women. Acta Psychiatr Scand 68:134-139, 1983.

Krause S, Ebbesen F, Lange AP: Polyhydramnios with maternal lithium treatment. Obstet Gynecol 75:504-506, 1990.

Long WA, Willis PW IV: Maternal lithium and neonatal Ebstein's anomaly: Evaluation with cross-sectional echocardiography. Am J Perinatol 1(2):182-184, 1984.

Morrell P, Sutherland GR, Buamah PK, et al.: Lithium toxicity in a neonate. Arch Dis Child 58:539-541, 1983.

Schou M: What happened later to the lithium babies? A follow-up study of children born without malformations. Acta Psychiatr Scand 54:193-197, 1976.

Schou M, Amdisen A. Lithium and pregnancy. III. Lithium ingestion by children breast-fed by women on lithium treatment. Br Med J 2:138, 1973.

Sykes PA, Quarrie J, Alexander FW: Lithium carbonate and breast-feeding. Br Med J 2:1299, 1976.

Smithberg M, Dixit PK: Teratogenic effects of lithium in mice. Teratology 26:239-246, 1982.

Szabo KT: Teratogenic effect of lithium carbonate in the foetal mouse. Nature 225:73-75, 1970.

Thiels C: Pharmacotherapy of psychiatric disorder in pregnancy and during breastfeeding: A review. Pharmacopsychiatry 20:133-146, 1987.

Troyer WA, Pereira GR, Lannon RA, et al.: Association of maternal lithium exposure and premature delivery. J Perinatol 13(2):123-127, 1993.

Tunnessen WW Jr, Hertz CG: Toxic effects of lithium in newborn infants: A commentary. J Pediatr 81:804-807, 1972.

Warkany J: Teratogen update: Lithium. Teratology 38:593-596, 1988.

Weinstein MR: Lithium treatment of women during pregnancy and in the post-delivery period. In: Johnson FN (ed). *Handbook of Lithium Therapy*. Baltimore, Md.: University Park Press, 1980, pp 421-429.

Wright TL, Hoffman LH, Davies J: Teratogenic effects of lithium in rats. Teratology 4:151-156, 1971.

Zalzstein E, Koren G, Einarson T, et al.: A case-control study on the association between first trimester exposure to lithium and Ebstein's anomaly. Am J Cardiol 65:817-818, 1990.

LOMOCOT® *See* Diphenoxylate

LOMOTIL® *See* Diphenoxylate

LORAZEPAM
(Alzapam®, Ativan®)

Lorazepam is a benzodiazepine tranquilizer. It is given orally in doses of 2-10 mg/d or parenterally in doses of 2.5-4 mg/d.

Teratogenic Risk

*Magnitude of teratogenic
risk to child born after
exposure during gestation:*   Undetermined

*Quality and quantity of data
on which risk estimate is based:*   Poor

Maternal lorazepam treatment late in pregnancy has been associated with problems in neonatal adaptation (see below).

No epidemiological studies of congenital anomalies in infants whose mothers were treated with lorazepam during pregnancy have been reported.

The frequency of malformations was not increased among the offspring of pregnant mice or rats treated orally with 2-20 times the human dose of lorazepam (Esaki et al., 1975). In another study, no "gross dysmorphism" was seen, but decreased weight and increased activity were observed among the offspring of mice treated with 10 times the maximum human dose of lorazepam during pregnancy (Chesley et al., 1991). Cleft palate occurred with increased frequency among the offspring of mice injected with 400 times the maximum human parenteral dose of lorazepam during pregnancy (Jurand & Martin, 1994). The relevance of these observations to therapeutic use of lorazepam in human pregnancy is unknown.

Neonatal hypotonia and feeding difficulties have been reported in infants born to women treated with lorazepam late in pregnancy (Whitelaw et al., 1981; McAuley et al., 1982; Sanchis et al., 1991). In one study, maternal intravenous lorazepam treatment for hypertension was associated with low Apgar scores, hypothermia, poor feeding, and need for assisted ventilation in the neonates (Whitelaw et al., 1981). Preterm infants appear to be especially susceptible to these adverse effects of lorazepam.

Please see agent summary on diazepam for information on a related agent that has been more thoroughly studied.

Risk Related to Breast-feeding

Lorazepam is excreted in breast milk in low concentrations. Based on data from four lactating women, the amount of lorazepam that the nursing infant would be expected to ingest is approximately 4% of the lowest therapeutic dose on a weight-adjusted basis (Summerfield & Nielsen, 1985).*

Because of its potential to affect neurobehavioral development, the American Academy of Pediatrics regards lorazepam to be a drug of special concern when given to breast-feeding mothers over a long period of time. However, no adverse effects in nursing infants have thus far been reported (Committee on Drugs, American Academy of Pediatrics, 1994).

Key References

Chesley S, Lumpkin M, Schatzki A, et al.: Prenatal exposure to benzodiazepine--I. Prenatal exposure to lorazepam in mice alters open-field activity and GABAA receptor function. Neuropharmacology 30(1):53-58, 1991.

Committee on Drugs, American Academy of Pediatrics: The transfer of drugs and other chemicals into human milk. Pediatrics 93(1):137-150, 1994.

Esaki K, Tanioka Y, Tsukada M, Izumiyama K: Teratogenicity of lorazepam (WY-4036) in mice and rats. CIEA Preclin Rep 1:25-34, 1975.

Jurand A, Martin LVH: Cleft palate and open eyelids inducing activity of lorazepam and the effect of flumazenil, the benzodiazepine antagonist. Pharmacol Toxicol 74:228-235, 1994.

McAuley DM, O'Neill MP, Moore J, Dundee JW: Lorazepam premedication for labour. Br J Obstet Gynaecol 89:149-154, 1982.

Sanchis A, Rosique D, Catala J: Adverse effects of maternal lorazepam on neonates. DICP Ann Pharmacother 25(10):1137-1138, 1991.

*This calculation is based on the following assumptions: maternal dose of lorazepam: 3.5 mg; milk concentration of lorazepam: 0.008-0.009 mcg/mL; milk intake by the nursing infant: 150 mL/kg/d; estimated dose of lorazepam ingested by the nursing infant: 0.001 mg/kg/d; lowest therapeutic dose of lorazepam in adults: 0.03 mg/kg/d.

Summerfield RJ, Nielsen MS: Excretion of lorazepam into breast milk. Br J Anaesth 57:1042-1043, 1985.

Whitelaw AGL, Cummings AJ, McFadyen IR: Effect of maternal lorazepam on the neonate. Br Med J 282:1106-1108, 1981.

LOTRIMIN® *See* Clotrimazole

LOVASTATIN
(Mevacor®, Mevinolin)

Lovastatin is a fungal product used in the treatment of hypercholesterolemia. Lovostatin is given orally in doses of 20-80 mg/d.

Teratogenic Risk

*Magnitude of teratogenic
risk to child born after
exposure during gestation:*   *Undetermined*

*Quality and quantity of data
on which risk estimate is based:*   *Very poor*

A small risk cannot be excluded, but a high risk of congenital anomalies in the children of women treated with lovastatin during pregnancy is unlikely.

No epidemiological studies of congenital anomalies among infants born to women treated with lovastatin during pregnancy have been reported. A child with limb and vertebral malformations compatible with the VATER association whose mother took lovastatin early in pregnancy has been described (Ghidini et al., 1992). No causal inference can be made on the basis of this single anecdotal observation.

An increased frequency of gastroschisis was observed among the offspring of rats treated during pregnancy with lovastatin in a dose 500 times that used in humans; no teratogenic effect was observed at doses 5-50 times those used clinically (Minsker et al., 1983). The relevance of this observation to the therapeutic use of lovastatin in human pregnancy is unknown.

Risk Related to Breast-feeding

No information regarding the distribution of lovastatin in breast milk has been published.

Key References

Ghidini A, Sicherer S, Willner J: Congenital abnormalities (VATER) in baby born to mothers using lovastatin. Lancet 339:1416-1417, 1992.

Minsker DH, MacDonald JS, Robertson RT, Bokelman DL: Mevalonate supplementation in pregnant rats suppresses the teratogenicity of mevinolinic acid, an inhibitor of 3-hydroxy-3-methylglutaryl-coenzyme A reductase. Teratology 28:449-456, 1983.

LUDIOMIL® *See* Maprotiline

LUMINA® *See* Phenobarbital

LUPRON® *See* Leuprolide

LUTEONORM® *See* Ethynodiol Diacetate

LYDERM® *See* Fluocinonide

MACRODANTIN® *See* Nitrofurantoin

MAGNESIUM HYDROXIDE
(Milk of Magnesia)

Magnesium hydroxide is an inorganic salt that is administered orally as an antacid or laxative. Magnesium hydroxide is a component of many over-the-counter antacid preparations, which often contain calcium carbonate, aluminum hydroxide, and/or simethicone as well. About 10% of the magnesium in a dose of magnesium hydroxide is absorbed through the intestine. The amount of magnesium hydroxide in various preparations varies greatly, but doses as great as 7200 mg/d may be taken by some patients.

Teratogenic Risk

*Magnitude of teratogenic
risk to child born after
exposure during gestation:*   *Undetermined*

*Quality and quantity of data
on which risk estimate is based:*   *Very poor*

A small risk cannot be excluded, but a greatly increased risk of congenital anomalies in the children of women treated with magnesium hydroxide during pregnancy is very unlikely.

No epidemiological studies of congenital anomalies among the children of women who took magnesium hydroxide during early pregnancy have been reported. No adverse effect was noted among 27 infants of women who took magnesium hydroxide during the third trimester in a therapeutic trial for pregnancy-induced hypertension (Rudnicki et al., 1991).

No animal teratology studies of magnesium hydroxide have been published.

Risk Related to Breast-feeding

No information regarding the distribution of magnesium hydroxide in breast milk has been published.

Key References

Rudnicki M, Frolich A, Rasmussen WF, McNair P: The effect of magnesium on maternal blood pressure in pregnancy-induced hypertension. A randomized double-blind placebo-controlled trial. Acta Obstet Gynecol Scand 70:445-450, 1991.

MAPROTILINE
(Ludiomil®)

Maprotiline is a tetracyclic antidepressant with sedative action. It is given orally in doses of 25-225 mg/d.

Teratogenic Risk

Magnitude of teratogenic risk to child born after exposure during gestation:	*Undetermined*
Quality and quantity of data on which risk estimate is based:	*Very poor*

No epidemiological studies of congenital anomalies in infants born to women treated with maprotiline during pregnancy have been published.

Studies in mice, rats, and rabbits suggest that treatment of pregnant women with maprotiline in usual therapeutic doses is unlikely to increase the children's risk of malformations greatly (Esaki et al., 1976; Hirooka et al., 1978).

Please see agent summary on amitriptyline for information on a related drug.

Risk Related to Breast-feeding

Maprotiline is excreted in breast milk in concentrations similar to those in maternal serum (Lloyd, 1977). The amount of maprotiline that the nursing infant would be expected to ingest is approximately 4-8% of the lowest therapeutic dose on a weight-adjusted basis (Lloyd, 1977; Reiss, 1980).*

Key References

Esaki K, Tanioka Y, Tsukada M, Izumiyama K: Teratogenicity of maprotiline tested by oral administration in mice and rats. Jitchuken Zenrinsho Kenkyuho 2:69-77, 1976.

Hirooka T, Morimoto K, Tadokoro T, et al.: Teratogenicity test on maprotiline (CIBA 34, 276-Ba) in rabbits. Oyo Yakuri (Pharmacometrics) 15:555-565, 1978.

Lloyd AH: Practical considerations in the use of maprotiline (Ludiomil®) in general practice. J Int Med Res 5(Suppl 4):122-138, 1977.

*This calculation is based on the following assumptions: maternal dose of maprotiline: 100-150 mg/d; milk concentration of maprotiline: 0.1-0.2 mcg/mL; milk intake by the nursing infant: 150 mL/kg/d; estimated dose of maprotiline ingested by the nursing infant: 0.015-0.03 mg/kg/d; lowest therapeutic dose of maprotiline in adults: 0.39 mg/kg/d.

Reiss W: The relevance of blood level determinations during the evaluation of maprotiline in man. In: Murphy JE (ed). *Research and Clinical Investigation in Depression.* Northampton, England: Cambridge Medical Publications, 1980, pp 19-38.

MARCAINE® *See* Bupivacaine

MARIJUANA
(Hash, Pot, Weed)

Marijuana is widely used as a "recreational" drug. It is usually smoked or eaten. The active ingredient is Δ^9-tetrahydrocannabinol (THC). Marijuana is used medically in treatment of glaucoma and as an antiemetic during cancer chemotherapy at doses ranging 5-120 mg/d.

Teratogenic Risk

*Magnitude of teratogenic
risk to child born after
exposure during gestation:*   *Unlikely*

*Quality and quantity of data
on which risk estimate is based:*   *Fair to good*

Occasional maternal "recreational" use of marijuana in conventional amounts is unlikely to pose a substantially increased risk of malformations in the offspring, but the data are insufficient to state that there is no risk.

Behavioral alterations have been observed among the infants of women who smoked marijuana during pregnancy in some studies (see below).

Most published epidemiological studies of infants of women who smoked marijuana during pregnancy are compromised by poor or absent information on the magnitude, duration, and gestational timing of exposures (Day & Richardson, 1991; Zuckerman & Frank, 1992; Richardson, 1993). Moreover, many of these studies may be confounded by correlated factors such as alcohol and tobacco use, race, and socioeconomic status among the mothers.

The frequency of major malformations was no greater than expected among the children of 1246 women who smoked marijuana while pregnant (Linn et al., 1983). A similar result was obtained when only the children of 137 women who smoked marijuana daily were considered. In three other studies, the frequency of congenital anomalies was no greater than expected among 392, 331, or 417 infants of women who reported marijuana use during pregnancy (Gibson et al., 1983; Zuckerman et al., 1989; Witter & Niebyl, 1990). Five infants with intrauterine growth retardation and minor dysmorphic features have been reported whose mothers smoked marijuana daily during pregnancy (Qazi et al., 1985). The prevalence of this exposure in the general population and the nonspecificity of the anomalies in the infants preclude any causal inference. The frequency of minor physical anomalies was no greater than expected among the children of women who smoked marijuana during pregnancy in other studies (Zuckerman et al., 1989; Day et al., 1991, 1992; Astley et al., 1992).

Decreased birth weight and length do not appear to be associated with maternal marijuana smoking during pregnancy in most well-controlled studies when the effects of confounding variables are eliminated (Behnke & Eyler, 1993; Fried, 1993; Richardson et al., 1993). No association with marijuana use during pregnancy was observed among the mothers of either 567 chromosomally normal or 393 chromosomally abnormal spontaneous abortuses (Kline et al., 1991).

Behavioral abnormalities have been observed among the infants of women who used marijuana during pregnancy in some studies but not others (Parker et al., 1990; Fried, 1991, 1993; Dalterio & Fried, 1992; Dreher et al., 1994). Neurobehavioral alterations have also been found among older children who had been born to mothers who used marijuana during pregnancy in some studies (Fried & Watkinson, 1990; Fried, 1991; Fried et al., 1992b), but postnatal environmental conditions appear to exert increasingly important effects on these assessments as children grow older (O'Connell & Fried, 1991; Fried et al., 1992a).

Many teratologic studies of marijuana and THC have been performed in rats, mice, hamsters, and rabbits (Abel, 1985b; Schardein, 1985; Dalterio & Fried, 1992). Various anomalies have been reported among the offspring of animals treated during pregnancy with marijuana in doses many times greater than those usually encountered in humans. Most animal teratology studies of marijuana have been negative, however, especially if dosing is more comparable to the human situation in magnitude and route. Fetal growth retardation and embryo or fetal mortality are frequently seen at high doses. These effects may be more marked in pregnant animals treated with both marijuana and alcohol concomitantly (Abel, 1985a; Abel & Dintcheff, 1986). People often use this combination of agents together, and there is some evidence that intrauterine growth retardation occurs more commonly in human pregnancies exposed to both substances than in pregnancies exposed to either alone (Hingson et al., 1982).

Risk Related to Breast-feeding

Marijuana and its metabolites, 11-hydroxy-tetrahydrocannabinol and 9-carboxy-tetrahydrocannabinol, are excreted in breast milk. Based on data from two mothers who smoked one and seven marijuana pipes per day, the nursing infant would be expected to ingest 3-17% of the lowest pharmacologically-active dose of canabinoids on a weight-adjusted basis (Perez-Reyes & Wall, 1982).* No adverse effects were observed in either of the nursing infants.

Nursing infants of women who smoked marijuana daily were found to have significantly decreased motor development at one year of age in one study (Astley & Little, 1990) but not in another (Tennes et al., 1985). No significant difference in growth or other aspects of mental development was observed in infants of mothers who smoked marijuana during lactation compared to nursed infants whose mothers did not smoke marijuana in either study.

The American Academy of Pediatrics regards marijuana use to be contraindicated in breast-feeding mothers because it can be detrimental to the health of both the mother and her nursing infant (Committee on Drugs, American Academy of Pediatrics, 1994).

Key References

Abel EL: Alcohol enhancement of marijuana-induced fetotoxicity. Teratology 31:35-40, 1985a.

Abel EL: Effects of prenatal exposure to cannabinoids. NIDA Res Monogr Ser 59:20-35, 1985b.

---

*This calculation is based on the following assumptions: milk concentration of marijuana: 0.06-0.34 mcg/mL; milk intake by the nursing infant: 150 mL/kg/d; estimated dose of marijuana ingested by the nursing infant: 0.01-0.05 mg/kg/d; lowest pharmacologically-active dose of marijuana in children: 0.3 mg/kg/d.

Abel EL, Dintcheff BA: Increased marihuana-induced fetotoxicity by a low dose of concomitant alcohol administration. J Stud Alcohol 47:440-443, 1986.

Astley SJ, Clarren SK, Little RE, et al.: Analysis of facial shape in children gestationally exposed to marijuana, alcohol, and/or cocaine. Pediatrics 89:67-77, 1992.

Astley SJ, Little RE: Maternal marijuana use during lactation and infant development at one year. Neurotoxicol Teratol 12:161-168, 1990.

Behnke M, Eyler FD: The consequences of prenatal substance use for the developing fetus, newborn, and young child. Int J Addict 28(13):1341-1391, 1993.

Committee on Drugs, American Academy of Pediatrics: The transfer of drugs and other chemicals into human milk. Pediatrics 93(1):137-150, 1994.

Dalterio SL, Fried PA: The effects of marijuana use on offspring. In: Sonderegger TB (ed). *Perinatal Substance Abuse: Research Findings and Clinical Implications*. Baltimore, Md.: Johns Hopkins University Press, 1992, pp 161-183.

Day N, Cornelius M, Goldschmidt L, et al.: The effects of prenatal tobacco and marijuana use on offspring growth from birth through 3 years of age. Neurotoxicol Teratol 14(6):407-414, 1992.

Day N, Sambamoorthi U, Taylor P, et al.: Prenatal marijuana use and neonatal outcome. Neurotoxicol Teratol 13(3):329-334, 1991.

Day NL, Richardson GA: Prenatal marijuana use: Epidemiology, methodologic issues, and infant outcome. Clin Perinatol 18(1):77-92, 1991.

Dreher MC, Nugent K, Hudgins R: Prenatal marijuana exposure and neonatal outcomes in Jamaica: An ethnographic study. Pediatrics 93:254-260, 1994.

Fried PA: Marijuana use during pregnancy: Consequences for the offspring. Semin Perinatol 15(4):280-287, 1991.

Fried PA: Prenatal exposure to tobacco and marijuana: Effects during pregnancy, infancy, and early childhood. Clin Obstet Gynecol 36(2):319-337, 1993.

Fried PA, O'Connell CM, Watkinson B: 60- and 72-month follow-up of children prenatally exposed to marijuana, cigarettes, and alcohol: Cognitive and language assessment. J Dev Behav Pediatr 13:383-391, 1992a.

Fried PA, Watkinson B: 36-and 48-month neurobehavioral follow-up of children prenatally exposed to marijuana, cigarettes, and alcohol. J Dev Behav Pediatr 11:49-58, 1990.

Fried PA, Watkinson B, Gray R: A follow-up study of attentional behavior in 6-year-old children exposed prenatally to marihuana, cigarettes, and alcohol. Neurotoxicol Teratol 14(5):299-311, 1992b.

Gibson GT, Baghurst PA, Colley DP: Maternal alcohol, tobacco and cannabis consumption and the outcome of pregnancy. Aust NZ J Obstet Gynaecol 23:15-19, 1983.

Hingson R, Alpert JJ, Day N, et al.: Effects of maternal drinking and marijuana use on fetal growth and development. Pediatrics 70:539-546, 1982.

Kline J, Hutzler M, Levin B, et al.: Marijuana and spontaneous abortion of known karyotype. Paediatr Perinat Epidemiol 5:320-332, 1991.

Linn S, Schoenbaum SC, Monson RR, et al.: The association of marijuana use with outcome of pregnancy. Am J Public Health 73:1161-1164, 1983.

O'Connell CM, Fried PA: Prenatal exposure to cannabis: A preliminary report of postnatal consequences in school-age children. Neurotoxicol Teratol 13(6):631-639, 1991.

Parker S, Zuckerman B, Bauchner H, et al.: Jitteriness in full-term neonates: Prevalence and correlates. Pediatrics 85(1):17-23, 1990.

Perez-Reyes M, Wall ME: Presence of a Δ^9-tetrahydrocannabinol in human milk. N Engl J Med 307:819-820, 1982.

Qazi QH, Mariano E, Milman DH, et al.: Abnormalities in offspring associated with prenatal marihuana exposure. Dev Pharmacol Ther 8:141-148, 1985.

Richardson GA, Day NL, McGauhey PJ: The impact of prenatal marijuana and cocaine use on the infant and child. Clin Obstet Gynecol 36(2):302-318, 1993.

Schardein JL: Chemically Induced Birth Defects. New York: Marcel Dekker, 1985, pp 774-775.

Tennes K, Avitable N, Blackard C, et al.: Marijuana: Prenatal and postnatal exposure in the human. Natl Inst Drug Abuse Res Monogr Ser 59:48-60, 1985.

Witter FR, Niebyl JR: Marijuana use in pregnancy and pregnancy outcome. Am J Perinatol 7(1):36-38, 1990.

Zuckerman B, Frank DA: Prenatal cocaine and marijuana exposure: Research and clinical implications. In: Zagon IS, Slotkin TA (eds). Maternal Substance Abuse and the Developing Nervous System. San Diego, Calif.: Academic Press, 1992, pp 125-153.

Zuckerman B, Frank DA, Hingson R, et al.: Effects of maternal marijuana and cocaine use on fetal growth. N Engl J Med 320:762-768, 1989.

MAX-CARO® *See* Beta-Carotene

MAZEPINE® *See* Carbamazepine

MEASLES VACCINE, LIVE
(Attenuvax®)

Live measles vaccine contains living attenuated measles virus. It is administered subcutaneously to elicit immunity to measles (rubeola).

Teratogenic Risk

Magnitude of teratogenic
risk to child born after
exposure during gestation: *Unlikely*

Quality and quantity of data
which risk estimate is based: *Poor*

Immunization with live measles vaccine is unlikely to pose a substantial teratogenic risk, but the data are insufficient to state that there is no risk.

No malformations were observed among the children of 37 women immunized with live measles vaccine during the first four lunar months of pregnancy in one epidemiological study (Heinonen et al., 1977).

No animal teratology studies of live measles vaccine have been published.

Risk Related to Breast-feeding

No information regarding the distribution of live measles vaccine in breast milk has been published. The Advisory Committee on Immunization Practices considers live measles vaccine to be safe to administer during breast-feeding for both mother and infant (ACIP, 1994).

Key References

ACIP: General recommendations on immunization. Recommendations of the Advisory Committee on Immunization Practices (ACIP). MMWR 43(RR-1):1-38, 1994.

Heinonen OP, Slone E, Shapiro S: *Birth Defects and Drugs in Pregnancy.* Littleton, Mass.: John Wright-PSG, 1977, pp 315-316.

MECLIZINE
(Antivert®, Bonamine®,D-Vert®)

Meclizine is an antihistamine used primarily as an antiemetic. Meclizine is given orally in doses of 25-100 mg/d.

Teratogenic Risk

*Magnitude of teratogenic
risk to child born after
exposure during gestation:*   *Unlikely*

*Quality and quantity of data
on which risk estimate is based:*   *Good*

Therapeutic doses of meclizine are unlikely to pose a substantial teratogenic risk, but the data are insufficient to state that there is no risk.

The frequencies of congenital anomalies in general, of major malformations, and of minor anomalies were no greater than expected among the children of 1014 women who took meclizine during the first four lunar months of pregnancy in one epidemiological study (Heinonen et al., 1977). A weak association was seen between maternal use of meclizine in the first four lunar months of pregnancy and congenital anomalies of the ear or eye among these infants, but the biological significance of this association is uncertain. Studies such as this one that include multiple comparisons between maternal drug exposures and various birth defect outcomes are expected to show occasional associations with nominal statistical significance purely by chance. Congenital anomalies were no more frequent than expected among children of 1463 women who used meclizine anytime during pregnancy in this study (Heinonen et al., 1977).

The frequency of congenital anomalies was no greater than expected among the children of 613 women treated with meclizine during the first trimester of pregnancy in another study (Milkovich & van den Berg, 1976). In three studies involving, respectively, 266, 175, and 836 infants with various malformations, the frequency of maternal use of meclizine during the first trimester of pregnancy was no greater than expected (Mellin, 1964; Nelson & Forfar, 1971; Greenberg et al., 1977).

No teratogenic effect was observed among the offspring of 14 macaque monkeys treated with 10 times the usual human dose of meclizine during early pregnancy (Wilson & Gavan, 1967; Courtney & Valerio, 1968). In rats, a variety of craniofacial and skeletal malformations were induced in the offspring by maternal treatment with meclizine in doses more than 175 times greater than those used clinically, but not usually in doses 25-125 those used in humans (King, 1963). The relevance, if any, of these observations to therapeutic use of meclizine by pregnant women is unknown.

Risk Related to Breast-feeding

No information regarding the distribution of meclizine in breast milk has been published.

Key References

Courtney KD, Valerio DA: Teratology in the *Macaca mulatta*. Teratology 1:163-172, 1968.

Greenberg G, Inman WHW, Weatherall JAC, et al.:   Maternal drug histories and congenital abnormalities.   Br Med J 2:853-856, 1977.

Heinonen OP, Slone D, Shapiro S: *Birth Defects and Drugs in Pregnancy*.   Littleton, Mass.:   John Wright-PSG, 1977, pp 323-324, 437.

King CTG: Teratogenic effects of meclizine hydrochloride on the rat.   Science 141:353-355, 1963.

Mellin GW: Drugs in the first trimester of pregnancy and the fetal life of *Homo sapiens*.   Am J Obstet Gynecol 90:1169-1180, 1964.

Milkovich L, van den Berg BJ: An evaluation of the teratogenicity of certain antinauseant drugs.   Am J Obstet Gynecol 125:244-248, 1976.

Nelson MM, Forfar JO: Associations between drugs administrered during pregnancy and congenital abnormalities of the fetus. Br Med J 1:523-527, 1971.

Wilson JG, Gavan JA: Congenital malformations in nonhuman primates: Spontaneous and experimentally induced. Anat Rec 158:99-109, 1967.

MECLOFENAMATE
(Meclomen®)

Meclofenamate is a nonsteroidal anti-inflammatory agent that has analgesic and antipyretic actions. It is used to treat rheumatic disorders. Meclofenamate is given orally in doses of 200-400 mg/d.

Teratogenic Risk

Magnitude of teratogenic risk to child born after exposure during gestation:	*Undetermined*
Quality and quantity of data on which risk estimate is based:	*Very poor*

No epidemiological studies of malformations in the infants of women treated with meclofenamate during pregnancy have been reported.

The frequency of malformations was not increased among the offspring of pregnant rats treated with 0.4-2.5 times the maximal human dose of meclofenamate (Schardein et al., 1969; Patrere et al., 1985). No teratogenic effect was observed among the offspring of rabbits treated with meclofenamate during pregnancy in a dose 0.4 times that used in humans (Schardein et al., 1969).

Please see agent summary on indomethacin for information on a related agent that has been more thoroughly studied.

Risk Related to Breast-feeding

Meclofenamate is excreted into breast milk in trace amounts (USP DI, 1995); however, the effects of maternal exposure to meclofenamate on the nursing infant are unknown.

Key References

Patrere JA, Humphrey RR, Anderson JA, et al.: Studies on reproduction in rats with meclofenamate sodium, a nonsteroidal anti-inflammatory agent. Fundam Appl Toxicol 5:665-671, 1985.

Schardein JL, Blatz AT, Woosley ET, Kaump DH: Reproduction studies on sodium meclofenamate in comparison to aspirin and phenylbutazone. Toxicol Appl Pharmacol 15:46-55, 1969.

USP DI: Nonsteroidal anti-inflammatory drugs. In: *USP DI (USP Dispensing Information), Volume 1. Drug Information for the Health Care Professional*, 15th ed. Rockville, Md.: The US Pharmacopeial Convention, 1995, p 2002.

MECLOMEN® *See* Meclofenamate

MEDIHALER-ERGOTAMINE
See Ergotamine

MEDROL® *See* Methylprednisolone

MEDRONE® *See* Methylprednisolone

MEDROXYPROGESTERONE
(Depo-Provera®, MPA, Provera®)

Medroxyprogesterone is a long-acting synthetic progestin that is used orally in doses of 5-10 mg/d to treat menstrual disorders. An injectable form of medroxyprogesterone is given intramuscularly in a dose of 150 mg every three months as a contraceptive and in a dose of 400-1000 mg/wk to treat cancer.

Teratogenic Risk

*Magnitude of teratogenic
risk to child born after
exposure during gestation:*   *Unlikely*

*Quality and quantity of data
on which risk estimate is based:*   *Fair to good*

Therapeutic doses of medroxyprogesterone are unlikely to pose a substantial teratogenic risk, but the data are insufficient to state that there is no risk.

A minimal risk for virilization of the genitalia in a female fetus appears to exist with maternal use of large doses of this agent during pregnancy. Assessment of this risk is based primarily on studies involving use of progestational hormones at doses much greater than those used for contraception (Schardein, 1993).

The frequency of congenital anomalies was slightly increased among the children of 130 women treated with medroxyprogesterone during the first four lunar months of pregnancy in one epidemiological study, but a causal association seems unlikely because the increase was due entirely to a difference in the frequency of mild anomalies that had nonuniform rates at participating institutions (Heinonen et al., 1977).

The frequency of congenital anomalies among the infants of 217 women treated with medroxyprogesterone anytime during pregnancy was no greater than expected in this study. Congenital anomalies were seen with a frequency no greater than expected among 366 infants whose mothers were treated with medroxyprogesterone during the first trimester of pregnancy for recurrent or threatened abortion (Yovich et al., 1988). In another study, the frequency of polysyndactyly and of chromosomal abnormalities was increased among the children of 1229 women who had used medroxyprogesterone as an injectable contraceptive at some time prior to or during pregnancy, but these associations were not seen if only the 724 women who had received an injection of medroxyprogesterone within six months of conception were considered (Pardthaisong et al., 1988).

Ambiguity of the external genitalia has been reported among both sons and daughters of women who were treated with high-dose medroxyprogesterone to prevent miscarriage during pregnancy, but genital abnormalities among these infants are uncommon (Yovich et al., 1988; Schardein, 1993).

Increased frequencies of perinatal death and low birth weight were observed in a study of 1431 infants whose mothers had received depot medroxyprogesterone injections for contraception around the time of conception (Gray & Pardthaisong, 1991; Pardthaisong & Gray, 1991). Substantial differences existed between the exposed and control groups in this study, however, and these differences may account for the associations observed. No major adverse effects on growth or pubertal development were found among the exposed children up to 17 years of age (Pardthaisong et al., 1992). Similarly, no alteration of growth, general health, sexual maturation, or sexually dimorphic behavior was found among 74 teenage boys or 98 teenage girls who had been exposed to medroxyprogesterone in utero in another study (Jaffe et al., 1989, 1990).

Most studies in baboons, cynomologus monkeys, rats, and mice suggest that women who become pregnant despite injection of medroxyprogesterone as a contraceptive are unlikely to be at a greatly increased risk of having children with nongenital congenital anomalies (Andrew & Staples, 1977; Tarara, 1984; Prahalada et al., 1985a, b; Carbone et al., 1990). In other studies, increased frequencies of cleft palate and other malformations were observed among the offspring of pregnant rats or rabbits treated with medroxyprogesterone in doses respectively 2-300 or 1-10 times the human contraceptive dose during pregnancy (Andrew & Staples, 1977; Eibs et al., 1982). The relevance of these observations to the risk of malformations among the children of women treated with medroxyprogesterone during pregnancy is unknown.

Genital ambiguity has been observed among the offspring of baboons, cynomolgus monkeys, guinea pigs, and rats treated during pregnancy with medroxyprogesterone in doses greater than those used in humans (Lerner et al., 1962; Foote et al., 1968; Kawashima et al., 1977; Prahalada et al., 1985a, b).

Risk Related to Breast-feeding

Medroxyprogesterone is excreted in breast milk in low concentrations. The amount of medroxyprogesterone that the nursing infant would be expected to ingest is between 0.1-1.5% of the lowest therapeutic dose of medroxyprogesterone on a weight-adjusted basis (Saxena et al., 1977; Koetsawang et al., 1982).*

Milk volume and duration of lactation have been found to be increased in breast-feeding mothers receiving medroxyprogesterone (Toddywalla et al., 1977; Hull, 1981; Jimenez et al., 1984; Zacharias et al., 1986). No adverse effects of medroxyprogesterone on the long-term growth and development of nursed infants have been found (WHO, 1988, 1994a, b; Pardthaisong et al., 1992).

*This calculation is based on the following assumptions: maternal dose of medroxyprogesterone: 150 mg; milk concentration of medroxyprogesterone: 0.0004-0.008 mcg/mL; milk intake by the nursing infant: 150 mL/kg/d; estimated dose of medroxyprogesterone ingested by the nursing infant: 0.00006-0.0012 mg/kg/d; lowest therapeutic dose of medroxyprogesterone in adults: 0.08 mg/kg/d.

Both the American Academy of Pediatrics (Committee on Drugs, American Academy of Pediatrics, 1994) and the WHO Working Group on Drugs and Human Lactation (1988) regard medroxyprogesterone to be safe to use while breast-feeding.

Key References

Andrew FD, Staples RE: Prenatal toxicity of medroxyprogesterone acetate in rabbits, rats, and mice. Teratology 15:25-32, 1977.

Carbone JP, Figurska K, Buck S, Brent RL: Effect of gestational sex steroid exposure on limb development and endochondral ossification in the pregnant C57B1/6J mouse I. Medroxyprogesterone acetate. Teratology 42(2):121-130, 1990.

Committee on Drugs, American Academy of Pediatrics: The transfer of drugs and other chemicals into human milk. Pediatrics 93(1):137-150, 1994.

Eibs HG, Spielmann H, Hagele M: Teratogenic effects of cyproterone acetate and medroxyprogesterone treatment during the pre- and postimplantation period of mouse embryos. I. Teratology 25:27-36, 1982.

Foote WD, Foote WC, Foote LH: Influence of certain natural and synthetic steroids on genital development in guinea pigs. Fertil Steril 19:606-615, 1968.

Gray RH, Pardthaisong T: In utero exposure to steroid contraceptives and survival during infancy. Am J Epidemiol 134(8):804-811, 1991.

Heinonen OP, Slone D, Shapiro S: *Birth Defects and Drugs in Pregnancy*. Littleton, Mass.: John Wright-PSG, 1977, pp 389-391, 443.

Hull VJ: The effects of hormonal contraceptives on lactation: Current findings, methodological considerations, and future priorities. Stud Fam Plan 12:156-163, 1981.

Jaffe B, Shye D, Harlap S, et al.: Aggression, physical activity levels and sex role identity in teenagers exposed in utero to MPA. Contraception 40:351-363, 1989.

Jaffe B, Shye D, Harlap S, et al.: Health, growth and sexual development of teenagers exposed in utero to medroxyprogesterone acetate. Paediatr Perinat Epidemiol 4(2):184-195, 1990.

Jimenez J, Ochoa, Soler MP, Portales P: Long-term follow-up of children breast-fed by mothers receiving depot-medroxyprogesterone acetate. Contraception 30:523-533, 1984.

Kawashima K, Nakaura S, Nagao S, et al.: Virilizing activities of various steroids in female rat fetuses. Endocrinol Jpn 24:77-81, 1977.

Koetsawang S, Nukulkarn P, Fotherby K, et al.: Transfer of contraception steroids in milk of women using long-acting gestagens. Contraception 25:321-331, 1982.

Lerner LJ, DePhillipo M, Yiacas E, et al.: Comparison of the acetophenone derivative of 16α, 17α-dihydroxyprogesterone with other progestational steroids for masculinization of the rat fetus. Endocrinology 71:448-451, 1962.

Pardthaisong T, Gray RH: In utero exposure to steroid contraceptives and outcome of pregnancy. Am J Epidemiol 134(8):795-803, 1991.

Pardthaisong T, Gray RH, McDaniel EB, et al.: Steroid contraceptive use and pregnancy outcome. Teratology 38:51-58, 1988.

Pardthaisong T, Yenchit C, Gray R: The long-term growth and development of children exposed to Depo-Provera® during pregnancy or lactation. Contraception 45(4):313-324, 1992.

Prahalada S, Carroad E, Cukierski M, Hendrickx AG: Embryotoxicity of a single dose of medroxyprogesterone acetate (MPA) and maternal serum MPA concentrations in cynomolgus monkey (Macaca fascicularis). Teratology 32:421-432, 1985a.

Prahalada S, Carroad E, Hendrickx AG: Embryotoxicity and maternal serum concentrations of medroxyprogesterone acetate (MPA) in baboons (Papio cynocephalus). Contraception 32:497-515, 1985b.

Saxena BN, Shrimanker K, Grudzinskas JG: Levels of contraceptive steroids in breast milk and plasma of lactating women. Contraception 16(6):605-613, 1977.

Schardein JL: Chemically Induced Birth Defects. New York: Marcel Dekker, 1993, pp 284-301.

Tarara R: The effect of medroxyprogesterone acetate (Depo-Provera®) on prenatal development in the baboon (Papio anubis): Preliminary study. Teratology 30:181-185, 1984.

Toddywalla VS, Joshi L, Virkar K: Effect of contraceptive steroids on human lactation. Am J Obstet Gynecol 127:245-249, 1977.

WHO Working Group on Drugs and Human Lactation. In: Bennet PN (ed): Drugs and Human Lactation. Amsterdam: Elsevier, 1988, pp 168-169.

WHO (World Health Organization Task Force on Oral Contraceptives, Special Programme of Research, Development, and Research Training in Human Reproduction): Effects of hormonal contraceptives on breast milk composition and infant growth. Stud Fam Plan 19(6):361-369, 1988.

WHO (World Health Organization Task Force on Oral Contraceptives, Special Programme of Research, Development, and Research Training in Human Reproduction): Progestogen-only contraceptives during lactation: I. Infant growth. Contraception 50:35-53, 1994a.

WHO (World Health Organization Task Force on Oral Contraceptives, Special Programme of Research, Development, and Research Training in Human Reproduction): Progestogen-only contraceptives during lactation: II. Infant development. Contraception 50:55-68, 1994b.

Yovich JL, Turner SR, Draper R: Medroxyprogesterone acetate therapy in early pregnancy has no apparent fetal effects. Teratology 38:135-144, 1988.

Zacharias S, Aguilera E, Assenzo JR, Zanartu J: Effects of hormonal and nonhormonal contraceptives on lactation and incidence of pregnancy. Contraception 33(3):203-213, 1986.

MEFLOQUINE
(Lariam®)

Mefloquine, a quincline-methanol compound, is given orally for prophylaxis and treatment of malaria (Palmer et al., 1993). The usual prophylactic dose is 250 mg once a week; 1250 mg is usually given as a single dose for treatment.

Teratogenic Risk

Magnitude of teratogenic
risk to child born after
exposure during gestation:
    Therapeutic doses: *None to minimal*
    Prophylactic doses: *Unlikely*

Quality and quantity of data
on which risk estimate is based:
    Therapeutic doses: *Poor to fair*
    Prophylactic doses: *Fair*

Prophylactic doses of mefloquine are unlikely to pose a substantial teratogenic risk, but the data are insufficient to state that there is no risk.

This drug is chemically related to quinine which has been associated with deafness and possibly other congenital anomalies in children born after high-dose maternal treatment during pregnancy.

The half-life for elimination of mefloquine from the body averages 12 days in patients with malaria and 18 days in healthy individuals (Palmer et al., 1993). Possible effects of treatment prior to or immediately after conception should be considered.

Untreated malaria poses a substantial risk to fetal survival.

Six fetal anomalies were observed in 66 pregnancies of women who were treated with mefloquine in one series (Anonymous, 1991), but no consistent malformation or pattern of anomalies was seen. Among 45 infants born to women treated with mefloquine early in pregnancy and reported to the manufacturer prior to delivery, there were four with congenital anomalies (Bricaire et al., 1991). One child had hydrocephalus, another congenital heart disease, a third fetal growth retardation, and the fourth congenital toxoplasmosis (which is clearly unrelated). Three infants with congenital anomalies were born to 85 women who were treated with mefloquine at various times during pregnancy in a controlled therapeutic trial (Harinasuta et al., 1990). None of these anomalies was thought to be related to the medication. The frequency of congenital anomalies was not increased among 157 infants of women given mefloquine prophylaxis after 20 weeks of pregnancy in another controlled therapeutic trial (Nosten et al., 1994). No adverse effect of the maternal treatment was found on the growth or development of these children up to two years of age. Growth and development were normal up to two years of age in the children of 20 women who received mefloquine prophylaxis during the third trimester of pregnancy in an earlier series by these authors (Nosten et al., 1990).

Unpublished studies are said to have shown an increased frequency of malformations among the offspring of rats, mice, and rabbits treated during pregnancy with mefloquine in doses respectively 6, 6, and 5 times those used therapeutically in humans (Palmer et al., 1993; USP DI, 1995). Soft tissue and skeletal anomalies were seen most often in rats and cleft palate was most common in mice. Fetal death is said to have occurred with increased frequency among pregnant rats and rabbits treated respectively with 1-3 or 10 times the human therapeutic dose of mefloquine. These studies cannot be fully evaluated because they are unpublished, and the relevance of the findings to therapeutic or prophylactic use of mefloquine in human pregnancy is unknown.

Risk Related to Breast-feeding

Mefloquine is excreted in the breast milk. Based on data from two lactating women, the amount of mefloquine that the nursing infant would be expected to ingest is <1% of the lowest therapeutic dose or approximately 1% of the lowest weekly prophylactic dose, on a weight-adjusted basis (Edstein et al., 1988).*

Using calculations based on the area under the milk concentration-time curve, the authors in this study estimated that the average amount of mefloquine ingested by the nursing infant over a period of 56 days is 3% of the lowest prophylactic dose in children.

Mefloquine has a median elimination rate of 20 days (USP DI, 1995), and therefore accumulation of mefloquine in infant serum is possible with chronic exposures.

Key References

Anonymous: Mefloquine--a new antimalarial. Drug Ther Bull 29:51-52, 1991.

Bricaire PF, Salmon D, Danis M, Gentilini M: [Antimalarials and pregnancy.] Bull Soc Pathol Exot 84:721-738, 1991.

Edstein MD, Veenendaal JR, Hyslop R: Excretion of mefloquine in human breast milk. Chemotherapy 34:165-169, 1988.

Harinasuta T, Kietinum S, Somlaw SB, et al.: A clinical trial of mefloquine on multi-resistant falciparum malaria in pregnant women in Thailand. Bull Soc Fr Parasitol 8(Suppl 1):429, 1990.

Nosten F, Karbwang J, White NJ, et al.: Mefloquine antimalarial prophylaxis in pregnancy: Dose finding and pharmacokinetic study. Br J Clin Pharmacol 30:79-85, 1990.

Nosten F, ter Kuile F, Maelankiri, T, et al.: Mefloquine prophylaxis prevents malaria during pregnancy: A double-blind placebo-controlled study. J Infect Dis 169:595-603, 1994.

Palmer KJ, Holliday SM, Brogden RN: Mefloquine. A review of its antimalarial activity, pharmacokinetic properties and therapeutic efficacy. Drugs 45(3):430-475, 1993.

*This calculation is based on the following assumptions: maternal dose of mefloquine: single bolus of 250 mg; milk concentration of mefloquine: 0.032-0.053 mcg/mL; milk intake by the nursing infant: 150 mL/kg/d; estimated dose of mefloquine ingested by the nursing infant: 0.005-0.008 mg/kg/d or 0.034-0.056 mg/kg per week; lowest therapeutic dose in children: 15 mg/kg/d; lowest prophylactic dose in children: 4.6 mg/kg/wk.

USP DI: Mefloquine. In: *USP DI (USP Dispensing Information), Volume 1. Drug Information for the Health Care Professional*, 15th ed. Rockville, Md.: The US Pharmacopeial Convention, 1995, p 1792.

MEGACE® *See* Megestrol

MEGESTROL
(Megace®, Pallace®)

Megestrol is a progestational agent used in the treatment of breast and uterine cancer. Megestrol is given orally in doses of 40-320 mg/d, with doses up to 1200 mg/d.

Teratogenic Risk

*Magnitude of teratogenic
risk to child born after
exposure during gestation:*   *Undetermined*

*Quality and quantity of data
on which risk estimate is based:*   *Very poor*

A small risk cannot be excluded, but a high risk of congenital anomalies in the children of women treated with megestrol during pregnancy is unlikely.

A minimal risk for virilization of the genitalia in female fetuses may exist with maternal use of megestrol in large doses during pregnancy (Katz et al., 1985).

No epidemiological studies of congenital anomalies among infants born to women treated with megestrol during pregnancy have been reported.

Virilization of the external genitalia was observed among the female offspring of rats treated during pregnancy with megestrol in doses six times those used in humans (Kawashima et al., 1977).

Please see agent summary on medroxyprogesterone for information on a related drug that has been more thoroughly studied.

Risk Related to Breast-feeding

Megestrol is excreted in the breast milk. Based on data from five lactating mothers who took a combination oral contraceptive containing megestrol, the amount of megestrol that the nursing infant would be expected to ingest is between <1-5% of the lowest contraceptive dose on a weight-adjusted basis (Nilsson et al., 1977).* No adverse effects of megestrol on the nursing infants were noted.

The American Academy of Pediatrics regards oral contraceptives to be safe to use while breast-feeding (Committee on Drugs, American Academy of Pediatrics, 1994).

Key References

Committee on Drugs, American Academy of Pediatrics: The transfer of drugs and other chemicals into human milk. Pediatrics 93(1):137-150, 1994.

Katz Z, Lancet M, Skornik J, et al.: Teratogenicity of progestogens given during the first trimester of pregnancy. Obstet Gynecol 65:775-780, 1985.

Kawashima K, Nakaura S, Nagao S, et al.: Virilizing activities of various steroids in female rat fetuses. Endocrinol Jpn 24(1):77-81, 1977.

Nilsson S, Nygren K-G, Johansson EDB: Megestrol acetate concentrations in plasma and milk during administration of an oral contraceptive containing 4 mg megestrol acetate to nursing women. Contraception 16:615-624, 1977.

*This calculation is based on the following assumptions: maternal dose of megestrol: 4 mg/d; milk concentration of megestrol: 0.001-0.02 mcg/mL; milk intake by the nursing infant: 150 mL/kg/d; estimated dose of megestrol ingested by the nursing infant: 0.0001-0.003 mg/kg/d; lowest oral contraceptive dose in adults: 0.06 mg/kg/d.

MELLARIL® See Thioridazine

MEPERIDINE
(Demerol®)

Meperidine is a widely used synthetic narcotic analgesic. It is given orally or parenterally, usually in a dose of 100 mg every three to four hours. Doses as high as 150 mg every three hours are sometimes used.

Teratogenic Risk

*Magnitude of teratogenic
risk to child born after
exposure during gestation:*   *Unlikely*

*Quality and quantity of data
on which risk estimate is based:*   *Fair*

> *Therapeutic doses of meperidine are unlikely to pose a substantial teratogenic risk, but the data are insufficient to state that there is no risk.*
> *Respiratory depression and behavioral alterations occur with increased frequency among infants born within a few hours of maternal treatment with meperidine.*

The frequency of congenital anomalies was no greater than expected among the infants of 268 women who were treated with meperidine during the first four lunar months of pregnancy or the infants of 1100 women who were treated with the drug anytime during pregnancy in one epidemiological study (Heinonen et al., 1977). No association was observed between maternal use of meperidine during the first trimester of pregnancy and congenital anomalies in more than 50 infants in another study (Jick et al., 1981).

An increase in the frequency of central nervous system and other anomalies was observed in the offspring of pregnant hamsters treated with meperidine in doses 8-29 times those used in humans but not in the offspring of pregnant mice treated with even larger doses (Geber & Schramm, 1975; Martin & Jurand, 1992). The relevance of these observations to the clinical use of meperidine in human pregnancy is unknown.

Maternal treatment with meperidine within a few hours of delivery may cause transient respiratory depression in newborn infants (Goldsmith & Starrett, 1991; Hamza et al., 1992; Clyburn & Rosen, 1993). Behavioral alterations have also been observed among such infants in the newborn period (Belsey et al., 1981; Busacca et al., 1982; Hodgkinson et al., 1982; Goldsmith & Starrett, 1991), but no physical or psychological deficit was apparent at age five to ten years in one series of 70 children born to mothers treated with meperidine shortly before birth (Buck, 1975).

Risk Related to Breast-feeding

Meperidine is excreted in the breast milk in low concentrations. The amount of meperidine that the nursing infant would be expected to receive is <2.5% of the lowest therapeutic dose in infants (Vorherr, 1974).*

Key References

Belsey EM, Rosenblatt DB, Lieberman BA, et al.: The influence of maternal analgesia on neonatal behaviour: I. Pethidine. Br J Obstet Gynaecol 88:398-406, 1981.

Buck C: Drugs in pregnancy. Can Med Assoc J 112:1285, 1975.

Busacca M, Gementi P, Gambini E, et al.: Neonatal effects of the administration of meperidine and promethazine to the mother in labor. Double blind study. J Perinat Med 10:48-53, 1982.

Clyburn PA, Rosen M: The effects of opioid and inhalation analgesia on the newborn. In: *The Effects on the Baby of Maternal Analgesia and Anaesthesia*, 1993, pp 169-190.

Geber WF, Schramm LC: Congenital malformations of the central nervous system produced by narcotic analgesics in the hamster. Am J Obstet Gynecol 123:705-713, 1975.

Goldsmith JP Strait AL: The neonatal effects of anesthetic agents and techniques. In: Diaz JH (ed). *Perinatal Anesthesia and Critical Care*. Philadelphia, Pa.: WB Saunders Company, 1991, pp 242-262.

Hamza J, Benlabed M, Orhant E, et al.: Neonatal pattern of breathing during active and quiet sleep after maternal administration of meperidine. Pediatr Res 32:412-416, 1992.

Heinonen OP, Slone D, Shapiro S: *Birth Defects and Drugs in Pregnancy*. Littleton, Mass.: John Wright-PSG, 1977, pp 287, 288, 434, 471, 484.

Hodgkinson R, Husain FJ: The duration of effect of maternally administered meperidine on neonatal neurobehavior. Anesthesiology 56(1):51-52, 1982.

*This calculation is based on the following assumptions: maternal dose: unspecified; milk concentration of meperidine: <0.001 mg/mL; milk intake by the nursing infant: 150 mL/kg/d; estimated dose of meperidine ingested by the nursing infant: 0.15 mg/kg/d; lowest therapeutic dose of meperidine in infants: 6 mg/kg/d.

Jick H, Holmes LB, Hunter JR, et al.: First-trimester drug use and congenital disorders. JAMA 246:343-346, 1981.

Martin LVH, Jurand A: The absence of teratogenic effects of some analgesics used in anaesthesia. Anaesthesia 47:473-476, 1992.

Vorherr H: Drug excretion in breast milk. Postgrad Med 56(4):97-104, 1974.

MEPROLONE® *See* Methylprednisolone

MERUVAX® *See* Rubella Vaccine

MESTRANOL

Mestranol is an estrogenic agent that is widely used, generally in combination with a progestin, in oral contraception and in treatment of menstrual disorders. The usual oral dose of mestranol is 50-100 mcg/d for contraception.

Teratogenic Risk

Magnitude of teratogenic risk to child born after exposure during gestation:	*None*
Quality and quantity of data on which risk estimate is based:	*Fair*

The frequency of congenital anomalies was no greater than expected among the infants of 179 women who had taken mestranol during the first four lunar months of pregnancy or of 206 women who had taken this drug anytime in pregnancy in one epidemiological study (Heinonen et al., 1977).

Studies in mice, rats, and rabbits suggest that treatment of pregnant women with mestranol in usual therapeutic or contraceptive doses is unlikely to increase the children's risk of malformations greatly (Takano et al., 1966; Saunders & Elton, 1967). Fetal loss occurred with increased frequency in pregnant mice and rats treated with mestranol in doses 100 or more times those used in humans.

Increased aggressive behavior was observed among the male (but not the female) offspring of mice treated during pregnancy with mestranol combined with norethynodrel (a progestin) in a dose about 50 times greater than that used in human contraception (Abbatiello & Scudder, 1970). Decreased serum testosterone concentrations were found in adult male rats born to mothers that had been treated with 50 times the human dose of mestranol in another study (Varma & Bloch, 1987). The clinical relevance of these observations is unknown.

Risk Related to Breast-feeding

No information regarding the distribution of mestranol in breast milk has been published. Combination oral contraceptives containing usual doses of mestranol were found to reduce milk intake by nursing infants in some studies (Kaern, 1967; Kora, 1969; Miller & Hughes, 1970; Borglin & Sandholm, 1971), but not in others (Semm, 1966; Kamal et al., 1969, 1970). The effect of oral contraceptives on milk intake by nursing infants may be minimized if treatment with oral contraceptives is not initiated until lactation is well-established (Committee on Drugs, American Academy of Pediatrics, 1981).

The American Academy of Pediatrics regards oral contraceptives to be safe to take while breast-feeding (Committee on Drugs, American Academy of Pediatrics, 1994).

Key References

Abbatiello E, Scudder CL: The effect of norethynodrel with mestranol treatment of pregnant mice on the isolation-induced aggression of their male offspring. Int J Fertil 15:182-189, 1970.

Borglin N, Sandholm L: Effect of oral contraceptives on lactation. Fertil Steril 22:39-41, 1971.

Committee on Drugs, American Academy of Pediatrics: Breast-feeding and contraception. Pediatrics 68:138-140, 1981.

Committee on Drugs, American Academy of Pediatrics: The transfer of drugs and other chemicals into human milk. Pediatrics 93(1):137-150, 1994.

Heinonen OP, Slone D, Shapiro S: *Birth Defects and Drugs in Pregnancy.* Littleton, Mass.: John Wright-PSG, 1977, pp 389-391, 443.

Kaern T: Effect of an oral contraceptive immediately postpartum on inhibition of lactation. Br Med J 3:644-645, 1967.

Kamal I, Hefnawi F, Ghoneim M, et al.: Clinical, biochemical, and experimental studies on lactation. II. Clinical effects of gestagens on lactation. Am J Obstet Gynecol 105:324-334, 1969.

Kamal I, Hefnawi F, Ghoneim M, et al.: Clinical, biochemical, and experimental studies on lactation. V. Clinical effects of steroids on the initiation of lactation. Am J Obstet Gynecol 108:655-658, 1970.

Kora SJ: Effect of oral contraceptives on lactation. Fertil Steril 20:419-423, 1969.

Miller GH, Hughes LR: Lactation and genital involution effects of a new low-dose oral contraceptive on breast-feeding mothers and their infants. Obstet Gynecol 35:44-50, 1970.

Saunders FJ, Elton RL: Effects of ethynodiol diacetate and mestranol in rats and rabbits, on conception, on the outcome of pregnancy and on the offspring. Toxicol Appl Pharmacol 11:229-244, 1967.

Semm K: Social and medical aspects of oral contraception. *International Congress Series No. 130.* Princeton, NJ: Excerpta Medica Foundation, 1966, pp 98-100.

Takano K, Yamamura H, Suzuki M, et al.: Teratogenic effect of chlormadinone acetate in mice and rabbits. Proc Soc Exp Biol Med 121:455-457, 1966.

Varma SK, Bloch E: Effects of prenatal administration of mestranol and two progestins on testosterone synthesis and reproductive tract development in male rats. Acta Endocrinol (Copenh) 116:193-199, 1987.

METAMUCIL® *See* Psyllium

METAPREL® *See* Metaproterenol

METAPROTERENOL
(Alupent®, Metaprel®, Prometa®)

Metaproterenol is a β_2 selective adrenergic receptor blocking agent. It is used in treatment of bronchospasm and in management of premature labor. The usual oral dose is 60-80 mg/d; metaproterenol is also given by inhalation in smaller doses.

Teratogenic Risk

*Magnitude of teratogenic
risk to child born after
exposure during gestation:*   *Undetermined*

No epidemiological studies of congenital anomalies among the children of women treated with metaproterenol during pregnancy have been reported.

No increase in the frequency of malformations was apparent among the offspring of 12 rhesus monkeys treated with about 3 times the usual human dose of metaproterenol during pregnancy (Banerjee & Woodard, 1971). The frequency of malformations was no greater than expected among the offspring of rabbits given 2-25 times the usual human dose of metaproterenol during pregnancy (Hollingsworth et al., 1971; Matsuo et al., 1982). An increased frequency of cleft palate was observed among the offspring of mice treated during pregnancy with 25-250 but not 2.5 times the usual human dose of metaproterenol (Iida et al., 1988). Increased fetal death and maternal cardiotoxicity occurred at the highest dose. The relevance of these observations to therapeutic use of metaproterenol in human pregnancy is unknown.

Risk Related to Breast-feeding

No information regarding the distribution of metaproterenol in breast milk has been published.

Key References

Banerjee BN, Woodard G: Teratologic evaluation of metaproterenol in the rhesus monkey (*Macaca mulatta*). Toxicol Appl Pharmacol 20:562-564, 1971.

Hollingsworth RL, Scott WJ Jr, Woodard MW, Woodard G: Fetal rabbit ductus arteriosus assessed in a teratological study on isoproterenol and metaproterenol. Toxicol Appl Pharmacol 18:231-234, 1971.

Iida H, Kast A, Tsunenari Y, Asakura M: Corticosterone induction of cleft palate in mice dosed with orciprenaline sulfate. Teratology 38:15-27, 1988.

Matsuo A, Kast A, Tsunenari Y: Teratology study with orciprenaline sulfate in rabbits. Arzneimittelforsch 32:808-810, 1982.

METHAMPEX® *See* Methamphetamine

METHAMPHETAMINE
(Desoxyn®, Methampex®)

Methamphetamine is a sympathomimetic agent and a potent central nervous system stimulant. It is used to promote weight loss and in the treatment of narcolepsy and childhood hyperkinetic states. Methamphetamine is a popular "recreational drug." It is also used illicitly to "cut" or dilute other drugs. The oral therapeutic dose of methamphetamine is 5-25 mg/d.

Teratogenic Risk

*Magnitude of teratogenic
risk to child born after
exposure during gestation:*
    Therapeutic use: *Unlikely*
    Abuse: *Small*

*Quality and quantity of data
on which risk estimate is based:*
    Therapeutic use: *Poor to fair*
    Abuse: *Fair*

Therapeutic use of methamphetamine is unlikely to pose a substantial teratogenic risk, but the data are insufficient to state that there is no risk.

The frequency of congenital anomalies was no greater than expected among the children of 89 women treated with methamphetamine during the first four lunar months of pregnancy or among the infants of 320 women treated anytime during pregnancy in one epidemiological study (Heinonen et al., 1977). In a study of 52 infants born to women who abused methamphetamine intravenously throughout pregnancy, the frequency of congenital anomalies was no greater than expected, but birth weight, length, and head circumference were decreased (Little et al., 1988). Abnormal echoencephalograms with evidence of intracranial hemorrhage were observed in nine of 24 infants of mothers who abused methamphetamine during pregnancy in another investigation (Dixon & Bejar, 1989).

No malformations were found among the offspring of five macaque monkeys treated during pregnancy with methamphetamine in doses similar to those used in humans (Courtney & Valerio, 1968). Increased frequencies of fetal death, growth retardation, and brain and eye malformations were observed among the offspring of rabbits and mice treated during pregnancy with methamphetamine in doses respectively 2 and 16-42 times those used clinically (Kasirsky & Tansy, 1971; Yamamoto et al., 1992). High frequencies of anophthalmia were seen among the offspring of pregnant rats treated with 200 times the human therapeutic dose of methamphetamine (Vorhees & Acuff-Smith, 1990; Acuff-Smith et al., 1992). Persistently decreased weight and long-lasting behavioral alterations were noted in the offspring of rats treated during pregnancy with methamphetamine in doses 4 or more times those used clinically (Cho et al., 1991; Acuff-Smith et al., 1992; Weissman & Caldecott-Hazard, 1993). The relevance of these observations to the risks associated with therapeutic or "recreational" use of methamphetamine in human pregnancy is unknown.

Please see agent summary on dextroamphetamine for information on a related agent that has been more thoroughly studied.

Risk Related to Breast-feeding

No information regarding the distribution of methamphetamine in breast milk has been published. Since amphetamines are potential drugs of abuse, the American Academy of Pediatrics regards amphetamines to be contraindicated during breast-feeding even though no adverse effects on the nursing infant have been reported (Committee on Drugs, American Academy of Pediatrics, 1994).

Key References

Acuff-Smith KD, George M, Lorens SA, Vorhees CV: Preliminary evidence for methamphetamine-induced behavioral and ocular effects in rat offspring following exposure during early organogenesis. Psychopharmacology 109:255-263, 1992.

Cho D-H, Lyu H-M, Lee H-B, et al.: Behavioral teratogenicity of methamphetamine. J Toxicol Sci 16(Suppl 1):37-49, 1991.

Committee on Drugs, American Academy of Pediatrics: The transfer of drugs and other chemicals into human milk. Pediatrics 93(1):137-150, 1994.

Courtney KD, Valerio DA: Teratology in the *Macaca mulatta*. Teratology 1:163-172, 1968.

Dixon SD, Bejar R: Echoencephalographic findings in neonates associated with maternal cocaine and methamphetamine use: Incidence and clinical correlates. J Pediatr 115:770-778, 1989.

Heinonen OP, Slone D, Shapiro S: *Birth Defects and Drugs in Pregnancy.* Littleton, Mass.: John Wright-PSG, 1977, pp 346-347, 439.

Kasirsky G, Tansy MF: Teratogenic effects of methamphetamine in mice and rabbits. Teratology 4:131-134, 1971.

Little BB, Snell LM, Gilstrap LC III: Methamphetamine abuse during pregnancy: Outcome and fetal effects. Obstet Gynecol 72(4):541-544, 1988.

Vorhees CV, Acuff-Smith KD: Prenatal methamphetamine-induced anophthalmia in rats. Neurotoxicol Teratol 12:409, 1990.

Weissman AD, Caldecott-Hazard S: In utero methamphetamine effects: I. Behavior and monoamine uptake sites in adult offspring. Synapse 13:241-250, 1993.

Yamamoto Y, Yamamoto K, Fukui Y, Kurishita A: Teratogenic effects of methamphetamine in mice. Nippon Hoigaku Zasshi [Jpn J Legal Med] 46(2):126-131, 1992.

METHANOXANOL® *See* Sulfamethoxazole

METHOTREXATE
(Amethopterin, Folex®, Mexate®)

Methotrexate is a folic acid antagonist. It is used in the treatment of neoplastic and rheumatic diseases. Methotrexate is administered orally and parenterally. The dose given in one day varies from 5 mg to as much as 22,500 mg in cancer therapy and from 5-25 mg in rheumatic disease.

Teratogenic Risk

Magnitude of teratogenic risk to child born after exposure during gestation:	*Moderate to high*
Quality and quantity of data on which risk estimate is based:	*Fair to good*

Features of methotrexate embryopathy have occurred in an infant whose mother took as little as 12.5 mg of methotrexate a week during the first trimester of pregnancy, but the teratogenic risk is probably higher with higher doses.

The effect on the fetus of maternal treatment with methotrexate during the second or third trimester of pregnancy is unknown.

At least four children with a very uncommon and characteristic pattern of congenital anomalies have been born to women treated with methotrexate during the first trimester of pregnancy (Milunsky et al., 1968; Powell & Ekert, 1971; Diniz et al., 1978; Sosa Munoz et al., 1983). These children exhibited abnormal head shape, large fontanelles, craniosynostosis, ocular hypertelorism, and skeletal defects. The pattern of anomalies is strikingly similar to that seen in children born to women who took aminopterin, a closely-related agent, early in pregnancy (Warkany, 1978). The frequency of malformations among infants of women treated with methotrexate during pregnancy does not appear to be extremely high and is probably dose-related (Kozlowski et al., 1990; Aviles et al., 1991; Feldkamp & Carey, 1993; Donnenfeld et al., 1994; Wiebe & Sipila, 1994). Most infants of women treated with low-dose methotrexate during pregnancy appear normal at birth.

The rate of miscarriage is high among women who were treated with methotrexate early in pregnancy (Kozlowski et al., 1990; Donnenfeld et al., 1994). Methotrexate has been used as an abortifacient and in the treatment of ectopic pregnancy (Stovall et al., 1991; Pansky et al., 1989, 1993; Creinin & Darney, 1993; Wiebe, 1994).

No increase in the incidence of congenital anomalies was apparent in the children of over 375 women who had been treated with methotrexate for neoplasia prior to becoming pregnant (van Thiel et al., 1970; Rustin et al., 1984; Hsieh et al., 1985; Green et al., 1991).

Fetal death occurs with increased frequency in pregnant monkeys, mice, rats, cats, and rabbits treated with methotrexate in doses equivalent to or greater than those used in humans (Skalko & Gold, 1974; Khera, 1976; Jordan et al., 1977; Wilson et al., 1979; DeSesso & Goeringer, 1991, 1992). Increased frequencies of malformations were observed among the offspring of mice, rats, and rabbits treated during pregnancy with methotrexate in doses equivalent to or greater than those used in humans (Skalko & Gold, 1974; Jordan et al., 1977; Darab et al., 1987). Cleft palate and limb malformations were the anomalies observed most often.

Risk Related to Breast-feeding

Methotrexate is excreted in the breast milk in very low concentrations. The amount of methotrexate that the nursing infant would be expected to ingest is <1% of the lowest antineoplastic dose for infants (Johns et al., 1972).*

Methotrexate is considered to be contraindicated during breast-feeding by the American Academy of Pediatrics because of possible adverse effects, such as immune suppression, carcinogenicity, or mutagenicity in the nursing infant (Committee on Drugs, American Academy of Pediatrics, 1994).

Key References

Aviles A, Diaz-Macqueo JC, Talavera A, et al.: Growth and development of children of mothers treated with chemotherapy during pregnancy: Current status of 43 children. Am J Hematol 36:243-248, 1991.

Committee on Drugs, American Academy of Pediatrics: The transfer of drugs and other chemicals into human milk. Pediatrics 93(1):137-150, 1994.

Creinin MD, Darney PD: Methotrexate and misoprostol for early abortion. Contraception 48:339-348, 1993.

Darab DJ, Minkoff R, Sciote J, Sulik KK: Pathogenesis of median facial clefts in mice treated with methotrexate. Teratology 36:77-88, 1987.

DeSesso JM, Goeringer GC: Amelioration by leucovorin of methotrexate developmental toxicity of rabbits. Teratology 43:201-215, 1991.

DeSesso JM, Goeringer GC: Methotrexate-induced developmental toxicity in rabbits is ameliorated by 1-(p-tosyl)-3,4,4-trimethylimidazolidine, a functional analog for tetrahydrofolate-mediated one-carbon transfer. Teratology 45:271-283, 1992.

Diniz EMA, Corradini HB, Ramos JLA, Brock R: [The effects of methotrexate on the developing fetus.] Rev Hosp Clin Fac Med Sao Paulo 33:286-290, 1978.

*This calculation is based on the following assumptions: maternal dose of methotrexate: 22.5 mg/d; milk concentration of methotrexate: 0.003 mcg/mL; milk intake by the nursing infant: 150 mL/kg/d; estimated dose of methotrexate ingested by the nursing infant: 0.0004 mg/kg/d; lowest antineoplastic dose of methotrexate for infants: 1.5 mg/kg/d.

Donnenfeld AE, Pastuszak A, Noah JS, et al.: Methotrexate exposure prior to and during pregnancy. Teratology 49:79-81, 1994.

Feldkamp M, Carey JC: Clinical teratology counseling and consultation case report: Low dose methotrexate exposure in the early weeks of pregnancy. Teratology 47:533-539, 1993.

Green DM, Zevon MA, Lowrie G, et al.: Congenital anomalies in children of patients who received chemotherapy for cancer in childhood and adolescence. N Engl J Med 325:141-146, 1991.

Hsieh F-J, Chen T-CG, Cheng Y-T, et al.: The outcome of pregnancy after chemotherapy for gestational trophoblastic disease. Biol Res Pregnancy Perinatol 6(4):177-180, 1985.

Johns DG, Rutherford LD, Leighton PC, Vogel CL: Secretion of methotrexate into human milk. Am J Obstet Gynecol 112:978-980, 1972.

Jordan RL, Wilson JG, Schumacher HJ: Embryotoxicity of the folate antagonist methotrexate in rats and rabbits. Teratology 15:73-80, 1977.

Khera KS: Teratogenicity studies with methotrexate, aminopterin, and acetylsalicylic acid in domestic cats. Teratology 14:21-28, 1976.

Kozlowski RD, Steinbrunner JV, MacKenzie AH, et al.: Outcome of first-trimester exposure to low-dose methotrexate in eight patients with rheumatic disease. Am J Med 88(6):589-592, 1990.

Milunsky A, Graef JW, Gaynor MF Jr: Methotrexate-induced congenital malformations. J Pediatr 72:790-795, 1968.

Pansky M, Bukovsky I, Golan A, et al.: Local methotrexate injection: A nonsurgical treatment of ectopic pregnancy. Am J Obstet Gynecol 161:393-396, 1989.

Pansky M, Bukovsky J, Golan A, et al.: Reproductive outcome after laparoscopic local methotrexate injection for tubal pregnancy. Fertil Steril 60:85-87, 1993.

Powell HR, Ekert H: Methotrexate-induced congenital malformations. Med J Aust 2:1076-1077, 1971.

Rustin GJS, Booth M, Dent J, et al.: Pregnancy after cytotoxic chemotherapy for gestational trophoblastic tumours. Br Med J 288:103-106, 1984.

Skalko RG, Gold MP: Teratogenicity of methotrexate in mice. Teratology 9:159-164, 1974.

Sosa Munoz JL, Perez Santana MT, Sosa Sanchez R, Labardini JR: [Acute leukemia and pregnancy.] Rev Invest Clin (Mex) 35:55-58, 1983.

Stovall TG, Ling FW, Gray LA, et al.: Methotrexate treatment of unruptured ectopic pregnancy. A report of 100 cases. Obstet Gynecol 77:749-753, 1991.

van Thiel DH, Ross GT, Lipsett MB: Pregnancies after chemotherapy of trophoblastic neoplasms. Science 169:1326-1327, 1970.

Warkany J: Aminopterin and methotrexate: Folic acid deficiency. Teratology 17:353-358, 1978.

Wiebe ER: Methotrexate and misoprostol used in abortions. Can Med Assoc J 150(9):1381-1382, 1994.

Wiebe VJ, Sipila PEH: Pharmacology of antineoplastic agents in pregnancy. Crit Rev Oncol Hematol 16:75-112, 1994.

Wilson JG, Scott WJ, Ritter EJ, Fradkin R: Comparative distribution and embryotoxicity of methotrexate in pregnant rats and rhesus monkeys. Teratology 19:71-80, 1979.

METHYCLOTHIAZIDE
(Aquatensen®, Enduron®)

Methyclothiazide is a thiazide diuretic. It is given orally in doses of 2.5-10 mg/d to treat edema and hypertension.

Teratogenic Risk

Magnitude of teratogenic risk to child born after exposure during gestation:	*Minimal*
Quality and quantity of data on which risk estimate is based:	*Poor to fair*

The frequency of patent ductus arteriosus appeared higher than expected among the children of 942 women who took methyclothiazide anytime during pregnancy in one epidemiological study (Heinonen et al., 1977). Only three of these women were treated during the first four lunar months of gestation. Studies such as this one that include multiple comparisons between maternal drug exposures and various birth defect outcomes are expected to show occasional associations with nominal statistical significance purely by chance.

Unpublished studies in rats and rabbits are said to suggest that treatment of pregnant women with methyclothiazide in usual therapeutic doses is unlikely to increase the children's risk of malformations greatly (USP DI, 1995).

Neonatal thrombocytopenic purpura was observed in one infant whose mother was treated with methyclothiazide during pregnancy (Rodriguez et al., 1964). Thrombocytopenia has also been reported among the newborn infants of women treated during pregnancy with other thiazide diuretics, but it appears to be very uncommon under such circumstances (Finnerty & Assali, 1964).

Please see agent summary on chlorothiazide for information on a closely related drug that has been more thoroughly studied.

Risk Related to Breast-feeding

No information regarding the distribution of methyclothiazide in breast milk has been published.

Key References

Finnerty FA, Assali NS: Thiazide and neonatal thrombocytopenia. N Engl J Med 271:160-161, 1964.

Heinonen OP, Slone D, Shapiro S: *Birth Defects and Drugs in Pregnancy.* Littleton, Mass.: John Wright-PSG, 1977, pp 372, 495.

Rodriguez SU, Leikin SL, Hiller MC: Neonatal thrombocytopenia associated with ante-partum administration of thiazide drugs. N Engl J Med 270:881-884, 1964.

USP DI: Methyclothiazide. In: *USP DI (USP Dispensing Information), Volume 1. Drug Information for the Health Care Professional,* 15th ed. Rockville, Md.: The US Pharmacopeial Convention, 1995, p 1161.

METHYLDOPA
(Aldomet®, Dopamet®, Novomedopa®)

Methyldopa is an antihypertensive agent that is administered orally or parenterally. The usual dose is 500-2000 mg/d, although doses as large as 3000 mg/d are sometimes employed.

Teratogenic Risk

*Magnitude of teratogenic
risk to child born after
exposure during gestation:*   Undetermined

*Quality and quantity of data
on which risk estimate is based:*   Poor

A small risk cannot be excluded, but a greatly increased risk of congenital anomalies in children of women treated with methyldopa during pregnancy is unlikely.

No epidemiological studies of malformations in children born to women treated with methyldopa early in pregnancy have been reported.

No consistent adverse effect has been observed among children born to women treated with methyldopa late in pregnancy (Cockburn et al., 1982; Fidler et al., 1983). In one well-controlled study involving about 100 children born to women treated with methyldopa during pregnancy, a small but statistically significant decrease in head circumference was observed at birth and four years of age among males whose mothers' treatment had begun between 16 and 20 weeks gestation (Redman et al., 1976; Moar et al., 1978; Ounsted et al., 1980). This effect was not seen in the boys at 7.5 years of age, was not seen in girls, was not associated with any functional deficits, and was not observed in independent studies (Moar et al., 1978; Ounsted et al., 1980; Cockburn et al., 1982; Fidler et al., 1983).

Transient neonatal tremor, irritability, and mildly decreased systolic blood pressure have been noted in infants of mothers treated chronically with methyldopa late in pregnancy (Whitelaw, 1981; Bodis et al., 1982; Sulyok et al., 1991). No clinically significant problems have been associated with these findings, however.

Studies in mice, rats, and rabbits suggest that treatment of pregnant women with methyldopa in usual therapeutic doses is unlikely to increase the children's risk of malformations greatly (Peck et al., 1965).

Risk Related to Breast-feeding

Methyldopa is excreted in the breast milk in low concentrations. Based on data from four lactating women, the amount of methyldopa that the nursing infant would be expected to ingest is between 0.1-1.6%

of the lowest therapeutic dose on a weight-adjusted basis (Jones & Cummings, 1978).*

Both the American Academy of Pediatrics (Committee on Drugs, American Academy of Pediatrics, 1994) and the WHO Working Group on Drugs and Human Lactation (1988) regard methyldopa to be safe to use while breast-feeding.

Key References

Bodis J, Sulyok E, Ertl T, et al.: Methyldopa in pregnancy hypertension and the newborn. Lancet 2:498-499, 1982.

Cockburn J, Moar VA, Ounsted M, Redman CWG: Final report of study on hypertension during pregnancy: The effects of specific treatment on the growth and development of the children. Lancet 2:647-648, 1982.

Committee on Drugs, American Academy of Pediatrics: The transfer of drugs and other chemicals into human milk. Pediatrics 93(1):137-150, 1994.

Fidler J, Smith V, Fayers P, De Swiet M: Randomised controlled comparative study of methyldopa and oxprenolol in treatment of hypertension in pregnancy. Br Med J 286:1927-1930, 1983.

Jones HMR, Cummings AJ: A study of the transfer of α-methyldopa to the human foetus and newborn infant. Br J Clin Pharmacol 6:432-434, 1978.

Moar VA, Jefferies MA, Mutch LMM, et al.: Neonatal head circumference and the treatment of maternal hypertension. Br J Obstet Gynaecol 85:933-937, 1978.

Ounsted MK, Moar VA, Good FJ, Redman CWG: Hypertension during pregnancy with and without specific treatment; the development of the children at the age of four years. Br J Obstet Gynaecol 87:19-24, 1980.

Peck HM, Mattis PA, Zawoiski EJ: The evaluation of drugs for their effects on reproduction and fetal development. Excerpta Med Int Congr Serv 85:19-29, 1965.

Redman CWG, Beilin LJ, Bonnar J, Ounsted MK: Fetal outcome in trial of antihypertensive treatment in pregnancy. Lancet 2:753-756, 1976.

*This calculation is based on the following assumptions: maternal dose of methyldopa: 750-2000 mg/d; milk concentration of free and conjugated methyldopa: <0.1-0.2 and >0.1-0.9 mcg/mL, respectively; milk intake by the nursing infant: 150 mL/kg/d; estimated dose of methyldopa ingested by the nursing infant: 0.01-0.16 mg/kg/d; lowest therapeutic dose of methyldopa in children: 10 mg/kg/d.

Sulyok E, Bodis J, Hartman G, Ertl T: Neonatal effects of methyldopa therapy in pregnancy hypertension. Acta Paediatr Hung 31(1):53-63, 1991.

Whitelaw A: Maternal methyldopa treatment and neonatal blood pressure. Br Med J 283:471, 1981.

WHO Working Group on Drugs and Human Lactation. In: Bennet PN (ed). *Drugs and Human Lactation*. Amsterdam: Elsevier, 1988, p 114.

METHYLMORPHINE PHOSPHATE
See Codeine

METHYLPREDNISOLONE
(Medrol®, Medrone®, Meprolone®)

Methylprednisolone is a synthetic glucocorticoid used for its anti-inflammatory and immunosuppressive properties. The usual oral dose of methylprednisolone is 4-48 mg/d, but higher doses are used in the treatment of multiple sclerosis. Parenteral doses vary greatly and may be as large as 180 mg/kg/d (9000 mg/d in a 110 pound woman) in very serious acute illnesses.

Teratogenic Risk

*Magnitude of teratogenic
risk to child born after
exposure during gestation:*   *Unlikely*

*Quality and quantity of data
on which risk estimate is based:*   *Very poor*

Conventional oral doses of methylprednisolone during pregnancy are unlikely to pose a substantial teratogenic risk, but the data are insufficient to state that there is no risk.

The risk associated with use of very large doses of methylprednisolone in pregnancy is unknown.

No epidemiological studies of congenital anomalies in infants born to women treated with methylprednisolone during pregnancy have been reported.

An increased frequency of cleft palate was observed among the offspring of mice treated during pregnancy with methylprednisolone in doses similar to those used orally in humans (Walker, 1971). An increased frequency of cardiovascular defects and decreased body weight were observed in one study among the offspring of pregnant rats treated with methylprednisolone in a dose that was similar to that used orally in humans but was toxic to the rat dams (Kageyama et al., 1991). High frequencies of fetal death and a variety of central nervous system and skeletal anomalies were reported in the offspring of pregnant rabbits treated with methylprednisolone in doses less than those used in humans (Walker, 1967; Langhoff et al., 1979). The relevance of these findings to the risk of malformations in human infants born to mothers treated with methylprednisolone in pregnancy is unknown.

Please see agent summary on prednisone/prednisolone for information on a closely related drug that has been more thoroughly studied.

Risk Related to Breast-feeding

Methylprednisolone is excreted in the breast milk in low concentrations. Based on data from a single patient, the amount of methylprednisolone that the nursing infant would be expected to ingest is <1% of the lowest therapeutic dose of methylprednisolone on a weight-adjusted basis (Coulam et al., 1982).*

Breast milk concentration of IgA in this study was similar to IgA concentrations in the breast milk of women not taking immunosuppressive medications. The nursing infant had normal blood counts, no increase in infections, and above-average growth. Similar normal outcomes were observed in two breast-fed infants whose mothers were treated with methylprednisolone during lactation in another report (Grekas et al., 1984).

Key References

Coulam CB, Moyer TP, Jiang N-S, Zincke H: Breast-feeding after renal transplantation. Transplant Proc 14:605-609, 1982.

*This calculation is based on the following assumptions: maternal dose of methylprednisolone: 6 mg/d; milk concentration of methylprednisolone: 0.001-0.007 mcg/mL; milk intake by the nursing infant: 150 mL/kg/d; estimated dose of methylprednisolone ingested by the nursing infant: 0.0001-0.001 mg/kg/d; lowest therapeutic dose of methylprednisolone in children: 0.12 mg/kg/d.

Grekas DM, Vasiliou SS, Lazarides AN: Immunosuppressive therapy and breast-feeding after renal transplantation. Nephron 37:68, 1984.

Kageyama A, Kato K, Urabe K, et al.: [Toxicity study of methylprednisolone aceponate (ZK 91 588) (V)--Teratogenicity study in rats.] Yakuri To Chiryo 19(8):91-106, 1991.

Langhoff LM, Rudiger HF, Hoar RM: Teratology of methylprednisolone acetate (Depo-Medrol®) in rabbits. Anat Rec 193:598, 1979.

Walker BE: Induction of cleft palate in rabbits by several glucocorticoids. Proc Soc Exp Biol Med 125:1281-1284, 1967.

Walker BE: Induction of cleft palate in rats with antiinflammatory drugs. Teratology 4:39-42, 1971.

METICORTEN® *See* Prednisone/Prednisolone

METOCLOPRAMIDE
(Clopra®, Emex®)

Metoclopramide is used to treat disorders of gastrointestinal motility and as an antiemetic. Metoclopramide is given orally or parenterally. The usual dose is 5-60 mg/d, but larger doses are sometimes given when metoclopromide is used as an adjunct to cancer chemotherapy.

Teratogenic Risk

*Magnitude of teratogenic
risk to child born after
exposure during gestation:*　　　　　　　*Unlikely*

*Quality and quantity of data
on which risk estimate is based:*　　　　　*Poor to fair*

Therapeutic doses of metoclopramide are unlikely to pose a substantial teratogenic risk, but the data are insufficient to state that there is no risk.

No malformations were observed among the children of about 25 women treated with metoclopramide during the first trimester of pregnancy in one study (Sidhu & Lean, 1970).

Studies in mice, rats, and rabbits suggest that treatment of pregnant women with metoclopramide in usual therapeutic doses is unlikely to increase the children's risk of malformations greatly (Watanabe et al., 1968).

No adverse effects of metoclopramide therapy were observed among infants whose mothers were given the drug just before cesarean delivery in randomized clinical trials involving 21 and 31 treated women, respectively (Lussos et al., 1992; Orr et al., 1993).

Risk Related to Breast-feeding

Metoclopramide is excreted in the breast milk. The amount of metoclopramide that the nursing infant would be expected to ingest is between <1-5% of the therapeutic dose on a weight-adjusted basis (Lewis et al., 1980; Kauppila et al., 1983).*

Serum levels of metoclopramide in five nursing infants of mothers who were being treated with this drug were 0-17% of the lowest therapeutic serum level in adults (Kauppila et al., 1983).[†]

Metoclopramide treatment has been used to improve lactation in mothers with faltering milk production (Guzman et al., 1979; Gupta & Gupta, 1985; Kauppila et al., 1985; Ehrenkranz & Ackerman, 1986). No adverse effect of metoclopramide on the nursing infants was found in these studies.

The American Academy of Pediatrics states that maternal metoclopramide treatment during breast-feeding could be of concern because of possible antidopaminergic effects on the infant. The American Academy of Pediatrics therefore recommends that serum concentrations of metoclopramide be measured in nursing infants whenever possible (Committee on Drugs, American Academy of Pediatrics, 1994).

Key References

Committee on Drugs, American Academy of Pediatrics: The transfer of drugs and other chemicals into human milk. Pediatrics 93(1):137-150, 1994.

*This calculation is based on the following assumptions: maternal dose of metoclopramide: 10-30 mg; milk concentration of metoclopramide: 0.02-0.16 mcg/mL; milk intake by the nursing infant: 150 mL/kg/d; estimated dose of metoclopramide ingested by the nursing infant: 0.003-0.02 mg/kg/d; therapeutic dose of metoclopramide in children: 0.5 mg/kg/d.

[†]Infant serum levels of metoclopromide: 0-0.03 mcg/mL; lowest therapeutic serum level of metoclopramide in adults: 0.12 mcg/mL.

Ehrenkranz RA, Ackerman BA: Metoclopramide effect on faltering milk production by mothers of premature infants. Pediatrics 78:614-620, 1986.

Gupta AP, Gupta PK: Metoclopramide as a lactogogue. Clin Pediatr 24:269-272, 1985.

Guzman V, Toscano G, Canales ES, Zarate A: Improvement of defective lactation by using oral metoclopramide. Acta Obstet Gynecol Scand 58:53-55, 1979.

Kauppila A, Anunti P, Kivinen S, et al.: Metoclopramide and breast feeding: Efficacy and anterior pituitary responses of the mother and the child. Eur J Obstet Gynecol Reprod Biol 19:19-22, 1985.

Kauppila A, Arvela P, Koivisto M, et al.: Metoclopramide and breast feeding: Transfer into milk and the newborn. Eur J Clin Pharmacol 25:819-823, 1983.

Lewis PJ, Devenish C, Kahn C: Controlled trial of metoclopramide in the initiation of breast feeding. Br J Clin Pharmacol 9:217-219, 1980.

Lussos SA, Bader AM, Thornhill ML, Datta S: The antiemetic efficacy and safety of prophylactic metoclopramide for elective cesarean delivery during spinal anesthesia. Reg Anesth 17(3):126-130, 1992.

Orr DA, Bill KM, Gillon KRW, et al.: Effects of omeprazole, with and without metoclopramide, in elective obstetric anaesthesia. Anaesthesia 48(2):114-119, 1993.

Sidhu MS, Lean TH: The use of metoclopramide (Maxolon®) in hyperemesis gravidarum. Proc Obstet Gynaecol Soc Singapore 1:43-46, 1970.

Watanabe N, Iwanami K, Nakahara N: Teratogenicity of metoclopramide. Yukagaku Kenkyu (Jpn J Pharmacy Chem) 39:92-106, 1968.

METOLAZONE
(Diulo®, Mykrox®, Zaroxolyn®)

Metolazone is a diuretic used to treat hypertension and edema. Metolazone is given orally in doses of 0.5-20 mg/d.

Teratogenic Risk

*Magnitude of teratogenic
risk to child born after
exposure during gestation:*   *Undetermined*

No epidemiological studies of congenital anomalies in infants born to women who took metolazone during pregnancy have been reported.

Studies in mice, rats, and rabbits suggest that treatment of pregnant women with metolazone in usual therapeutic doses is unlikely to increase the children's risk of malformations greatly (Nakajima et al., 1978a, b; USP DI, 1995).

No adverse effects attributable to metolazone were noted in babies born to 35 women treated with this drug in the third trimester for pregnancy-induced hypertension in one study (Duffy et al., 1972).

Risk Related to Breast-feeding

No information regarding the distribution of metolazone in breast milk has been published.

Key References

Duffy GJ, O'Dwyer WF, Martin F: The effects of a new diuretic (Metolazone) on pre-eclamptic toxaemia of pregnancy. J Ir Med Assoc 65:615-619, 1972.

Nakajima T, Ishisaka K, Taylor P, Matsuda S: Effects of metolazone on the reproduction function of rats. 2. Teratogenicity test. Clin Rep 12:3394-3406, 1978a.

Nakajima T, Ishisaka K, Taylor P, Matsuda S: Effects of metolazone on reproduction of rabbits. Teratogenicity test. Clin Rep 12:3417-3421, 1978b.

USP DI: Diuretics, thiazide. In: *USP DI (USP Dispensing Information), Volume 1. Drug Information for the Health Care Professional*, 15th ed. Rockville, Md.: The US Pharmacopeial Convention, 1995, pp 1160-1161.

METOPROLOL
(Lopressor®)

Metoprolol is a β-adrenergic receptor blocking agent used in the treatment of hypertension, angina, and cardiac arrythmias. The oral dosage varies from 50-450 mg/d. Metoprolol is also given intravenously in much smaller doses in the therapy of acute myocardial infarction.

Teratogenic Risk

*Magnitude of teratogenic
risk to child born after
exposure during gestation:*   *Undetermined*

*Quality and quantity of data
on which risk estimate is based:*   *Poor*

A small risk cannot be excluded, but there is no indication that the risk of congenital anomalies in the children of women treated with metoprolol during pregnancy is likely to be great.

No epidemiological studies of congenital anomalies among infants born to women treated with metoprolol during pregnancy have been reported.

Studies in rats and rabbits suggest that treatment of pregnant women with metoprolol in usual therapeutic doses is unlikely to increase the children's risk of malformations greatly (Bodin et al., 1975).

Kaaja et al. (1992) found a higher rate of neonatal death among 19 very low birth weight infants of women who had been treated for hypertension late in pregnancy with a β-blocker than among similar infants whose mothers were treated with other antihypertensive agents. Most of the women in the β-blocker group took metoprolol in this study. In another series of 184 infants born to women with hypertension who were treated with metoprolol and other agents after the first trimester, the only adverse effect noted was mild fetal growth retardation; this may have been due to the maternal hypertension rather than to its treatment (Sandstrom, 1982). No adverse effect of maternal metoprolol therapy was found among infants of women treated for hypertension during the second and third trimesters of pregnancy in controlled therapeutic trials involving 15, 50, and 69 treated women, respectively (Hogstedt et al., 1985; Oumachigui et al., 1992; Jannet et al., 1994). No significant differences in birth weight, head circumference, or neonatal complications were observed among 69 infants born to women treated with metoprolol for hypertension during the second and third trimesters of pregnancy when compared to control infants in another study.

407

Please see agent summary on propranolol for information on a closely related drug that has been more thoroughly studied.

Risk Related to Breast feeding

Metoprolol is excreted in breast milk. The amount of metoprolol that the nursing infant would be expected to ingest is between <1-17% of the lowest therapeutic dose on a weight-adjusted basis (Sandstrom & Regardh, 1980; Lindeberg et al., 1984).*

The highest concentration of metoprolol measured in the serum of eight nursing infants whose mothers were treated with metoprolol while breast-feeding was within the therapeutic range (Lindeberg et al., 1984).[†]

Although no adverse effects were observed in the infants reported in the above studies, symptoms of β-adrenergic blockade have been described in breast-fed infants whose mothers were treated with other beta-adrenergic blocking agents (USP DI, 1995). Breast-fed infants of women who are being treated with metoprolol should therefore be monitored for such symptoms of β-adrenergic blockade as bradycardia, hypotension, and respiratory distress.

Both the American Academy of Pediatrics (Committee on Drugs, American Academy of Pediatrics, 1994) and the WHO Working Group on Drugs and Human Lactation (1988) regard metoprolol to be safe to use while breast-feeding.

Key References

Bodin NO, Flodh H, Magnusson G, et al.: Toxicological studies on metoprolol. Acta Pharmacol Toxicol 36(Suppl V):96-103, 1975.

Committee on Drugs, American Academy of Pediatrics: The transfer of drugs and other chemicals into human milk. Pediatrics 93(1):137-150, 1994.

Hogstedt S, Lindeberg S, Axelsson O, et al.: A prospective controlled trial of metoprolol-hydralazine treatment in hypertension during pregnancy. Acta Obstet Gynecol Scand 64:505-510, 1985.

*This calculation is based on the following assumptions: maternal dose of metoprolol: 100-200 mg/d; milk concentration of metoprolol: 0.0014-1.73 mcg/mL; milk intake by the nursing infant: 150 mL/kg/d; estimated dose of metoprolol ingested by the nursing infant: 0.00021-0.26 mg/kg/d; lowest therapeutic dose of metoprolol in adults: 1.56 mg/kg/d.

†Infant serum levels of metoprolol: 0.0014-0.114 mcg/mL; range of therapeutic serum levels of metoprolol in adults: 0.008-0.144 mcg/mL.

Jannet D, Carbonne B Sebban E, Milliez J: Nicardipine versus metoprolol in the treatment of hypertension during pregnancy: A randomized comparative trial. Obstet Gynecol 84:354-359, 1994.

Kaaja R, Hiilesmaa V, Holma K, Jarvenpaa A-L: Maternal antihypertensive therapy with beta-blockers associated with poor outcome in very-low birthweight infants. Int J Gynaecol Obstet 38:195-199, 1992.

Lindeberg S, Sandstrom B, Lundborg P, Regardh C-G: Disposition of the adrenergic blocker metoprolol in the late-pregnant woman, the amniotic fluid, the cord blood and the neonate. Acta Obstet Gynecol Scand 118 (Suppl):61-64, 1984.

Oumachigui A, Verghese M, Balachander J: A comparative evaluation of metoprolol and methyldopa in the management of pregnancy induced hypertension. Indian Heart J 44(1):39-41, 1992.

Sandstrom B: Adrenergic β-receptor blockers in hypertension of pregnancy. Clin Exp Hypertens [B] B1:127-141, 1982.

Sandstrom B, Regardh C-G: Metoprolol excretion into breast milk. Br J Clin Pharmacol 9:518-519, 1980.

USP DI: β-adrenergic blocking agents. In: *USP DI (USP Dispensing Information), Volume 1. Drug Information for the Health Care Professional*, 15th ed. Rockville, Md.: The US Pharmacopeial Convention, 1995, p 494.

WHO Working Group on Drugs and Human Lactation. In: Bennet PN (ed). *Drugs and Human Lactation*. Amsterdam: Elsevier, 1988, pp 331-332.

METOSYN® *See* Fluocinonide

METROGEL® *See* Metronidazole

METRONIDAZOLE
(Flagyl®, MetroGel®)

Metronidazole is an imidazole that is widely used in the treatment of vaginal trichomonal and bacterial infections. Substantial absorption may occur from the vaginal preparations that are used for this purpose; such preparations usually provide 75-1000 mg/d of metronidazole. Metronidazole is also given orally or intravenously in doses of 1500-4000 mg/d to treat amebiasis and other parasitic and anaerobic bacterial infections. Topical metronidazole is used to treat acne, but absorption through the skin is minimal.

Teratogenic Risk

*Magnitude of teratogenic
risk to child born after
exposure during gestation:*   *None*

*Quality and quantity of data
on which risk estimate is based:*   *Good*

This rating is for vaginal use of metronidazole. The risk associated with systemic administration of metronidazole during pregnancy is unknown.

The frequency of maternal treatment with metronidazole during the first four lunar months of pregnancy was no greater than expected among 4264 spontaneous abortions or among 6564 infants with various birth defects, 984 infants with cardiovascular defects, 122 infants with oral clefts, or 56 infants with spina bifida in a large epidemiological study (Rosa et al., 1987). The frequencies of major congenital anomalies and of specific categories of congenital anomalies were no greater than expected among the infants of 718 women for whom metronidazole was prescribed in the first trimester of pregnancy in another study (Piper et al., 1993). Similarly, no significant increase in the frequency of congenital anomalies was seen among the children of more than 200 women, 62 women, or 31 women treated with metronidazole during the first trimester of pregnancy in three other epidemiological investigations (Heinonen et al., 1977; Morgan 1978; Jick et al., 1981; Aselton et al., 1985).

Most studies in mice, rats, guinea pigs, and rabbits suggest that treatment of pregnant women with metronidazole in usual therapeutic doses is unlikely to increase the children's risk of malformations greatly (Bost, 1977; Roe, 1985; Dobias et al., 1994). However, other studies have found an increased frequency of fetal anomalies among the offspring of pregnant mice, rats, and guinea pigs treated with metronidazole in doses equivalent to those used in humans (Ivanov, 1969; Giknis & Damjanov, 1983). The relevance of these observations to metronidazole therapy in human pregnancy is unknown.

Metronidazole is mutagenic in bacterial systems, but the drug has not been found to cause gene mutations or chromosomal damage in most studies in mammals (Goldman, 1980; Roe, 1983, 1985; Drinkwater, 1987; Dobias et al., 1994).

Risk Related to Breast-feeding

Metronidazole and its metabolite, hydroxymetronidazole, are excreted in the breast milk. Based on data from 27 lactating mothers given metronidazole in divided doses, the amount of metronidazole and hydroxymetronidazole that the nursing infant would be expected to ingest is equivalent to 2-18% of the lowest therapeutic dose on a weight-adjusted basis (Heisterberg & Branebjerg, 1983; Passmore et al., 1988).* Following maternal administration of a single small dose or a single large dose of metronidazole, the amount of metronidazole that the nursing infant would be expected to ingest is between 1-8% or 3.5-45.8%, respectively, of the lowest weight-adjusted therapeutic dose (Gray et al., 1961; Erickson et al., 1981).†

Serum levels of both metronidazole and hydroxymetronidazole in nursing infants following maternal administration of metronidazole were between <1.2-140% of the lowest therapeutic serum level in adults (Gray et al., 1960; Heisterberg & Branebjerg, 1983: Passmore et al., 1988).‡ Higher infant serum levels occurred with higher and more frequent maternal doses of metronidazole. No adverse effects that could be attributed to metronidazole were observed in the nursing infants in any of these studies.

Although no adverse effects in nursing infants have been reported, the American Academy of Pediatrics recommends that women discontinue breast-feeding for 12-24 hours following administration of a single high dose of metronidazole (Committee on Drugs, American Academy of Pediatrics, 1994).

*This calculation is based on the following assumptions: maternal dose of metronidazole: 600 or 1200 mg/d in divided doses; milk concentration of metronidazole and hydroxymetronidazole: 1.6-16 mcg/mL and 1.1-6.3 mcg/mL, respectively; milk intake by the nursing infant: 150 mL/kg/d; estimated dose of both metronidazole and hydroxymetronidazole ingested by the nursing infant, assuming hydroxymetronidazole has similar bioavailability and molecular weight, and 30% of the activity of metronidazole: 0.29-2.68 mg/kg/d; lowest therapeutic dose of metronidazole in children: 15 mg/kg/d.

†This calculation is based on the following assumptions: maternal doses of metronidazole: 200 mg (low) or 2000 mg (high); milk concentration of metronidazole following low and high maternal doses: 1.0-7.7 mcg/mL and 3.5-45.8 mcg/mL, respectively; estimated doses of metronidazole ingested by the nursing infant following low and high maternal doses: 0.15-1.2 mg/kg/d and 0.52-6.9 mg/kg/d, respectively.

‡This calculation is based on the following assumptions: Infant serum levels of metronidazole and hydroxymetronidazole, assuming hydroxymetronidazole has similar bioavailability and molecular weight, and 30% of the activity of metronidazole: <0.05-5.6 mcg/mL; lowest therapeutic serum level of metronidazole in adults: 4 mcg/mL.

Key References

Aselton P, Jick H, Milunsky A, et al.: First-trimester drug use and congenital disorders. Obstet Gynecol 65:451-455, 1985.

Bost RG: Metronidazole: Toxicology and teratology. In: Finegold SM (ed). *Metronidazole: Proceedings of the International Metronidazole Conference, 1976.* New York: Excerpta Medica, 1977, pp 112-118.

Committee on Drugs, American Academy of Pediatrics: The transfer of drugs and other chemicals into human milk. Pediatrics 93(1):137-150, 1994.

Dobias L, Cerna M, Rossner P, Sram R: Genotoxicity and carcinogenicity of metronidazole. Mutat Res 317:177-194, 1994.

Drinkwater P: Metronidazole. Aust NZ J Obstet Gynaecol 27:228-230, 1987.

Erickson SH, Oppenheim GL, Smith GH: Metronidazole in breast milk. Obstet Gynecol 57(1):48-50, 1981.

Giknis MLA, Damjanov I: The transplacental effects of ethanol and metronidazole in Swiss Webster mice. Toxicol Lett 19:37-42, 1983.

Goldman P: Metronidazole. N Engl J Med 303:1212-1218, 1980.

Gray MS, Kane PO, Squires S: Further observations on metronidazole (Flagyl®. Br J Vener Dis 37:278, 1961.

Heinonen OP, Slone D, Shapiro S: *Birth Defects and Drugs in Pregnancy.* Littleton, Mass.: John Wright-PSG, 1977, pp 298-299, 302.

Heisterberg L, Branebjerg PE: Blood and milk concentrations of metronidazole in mothers and infants. J Perinat Med 11:114-120, 1983.

Ivanov I: [The effect of the preparation "trichomonacid" on the pregnancy of experimental animals.] Akush Ginekol (Sofiia) 8:241-244, 1969.

Jick H, Holmes LB, Hunter JR, et al.: First-trimester drug use and congenital disorders. JAMA 246:343-346, 1981.

Morgan I: Metronidazole treatment in pregnancy. Int J Gynaecol Obstet 15:501-502, 1978.

Passmore CM, McElnay JC, Rainey EA, D'Arcy PF: Metronidazole excretion in human milk and its effect on the suckling neonate. Br J Clin Pharmacol 26:45-51, 1988.

Piper JM, Mitchel EF, Ray WA: Prenatal use of metronidazole and birth defects: No association. Obstet Gynecol 82:348-352, 1993.

Roe FJC: Safety of nitroimidazoles. Scand J Infect Dis (Suppl 46):72-81, 1985.

Roe FJC: Toxicologic evaluation of metronidazole with particular reference to carcinogenic, mutagenic, and teratogenic potential. Surgery 93:158-164, 1983.

Rosa FW, Baum C, Shaw M: Pregnancy outcomes after first-trimester vaginitis drug therapy. Obstet Gynecol 69:751-755, 1987.

MEVACOR® *See* Lovastatin

MEVINOLIN® *See* Lovastatin

MEXATE® *See* Methotrexate

MICATIN 3® *See* Miconazole

MICONAZOLE
(Micatin 3®, Monistat®)

Miconazole is an imidazole antifungal agent. It is used intravenously in doses of 200-4800 mg/d to treat severe systemic mycotic infections. Local preparations of miconazole for oral, vaginal, and topical use are poorly absorbed.

Teratogenic Risk

Magnitude of teratogenic
risk to child born after
exposure during gestation:
    Systemic: *Undetermined*
    Topical: *Unlikely*

Quality and quantity of data
on which risk estimate is based:
    Systemic: *Poor*
    Topical: *Fair to good*

Topical use of miconazole in usual amounts during pregnancy is unlikely to pose a substantial teratogenic risk, but the data are insufficient to state that there is no risk.

The frequency of congenital anomalies was not increased among 360 infants of women treated during the first trimester of pregnancy with miconazole in one epidemiological study (Jick et al., 1981). In another study, Rosa et al. (1987) observed no association with maternal use of vaginal miconazole during the first trimester of pregnancy among 6564 infants with congenital anomalies, 122 infants with oral clefts, 984 infants with congenital cardiovascular defects, or 56 infants with spina bifida. Similarly, the rate of congenital anomalies did not appear unusual among the children of 43 women treated with miconazole vaginal cream in the first trimester or the infants of 248 women treated later in pregnancy in another investigation (McNellis et al., 1977). No epidemiological studies of congenital anomalies among infants born to women treated with systemic miconazole during pregnancy have been reported.

A study of vaginal miconazole use and spontaneous abortion based on Medicare records (Rosa et al., 1987) is difficult to interpret because of uncertainty regarding the exposures.

The frequency of malformations was not increased among the offspring of rats or rabbits treated with 1-2.5 times the systemic human dose of miconazole during pregnancy (Ito et al., 1976a, b). Increased fetal loss occurred in both species at the high dose which was also toxic to the mother.

Risk Related to Breast-feeding

No information regarding the distribution of miconazole in breast milk has been published.

Key References

Ito C, Shibutani Y, Inoue K, et al.: Toxicological studies of miconazole. II. Teratological studies of miconazole in rats. Iyakuhin Kenkyu 7:367-376, 1976a.

Ito C, Shibutani Y, Taya K, et al.: Toxicological studies of miconazole. III. Teratological studies of miconazole in rabbits. Iyakuhin Kenkyu 7:377-381, 1976b.

Jick H, Holmes LB, Hunter JR, et al.: First-trimester drug use and congenital disorders. JAMA 246:343-346, 1981.

McNellis D, McLeod M, Lawson J, Pasquale SA: Treatment of vulvovaginal candidiasis in pregnancy. Obstet Gynecol 50:674-678, 1977.

Rosa FW, Baum C, Shaw M: Pregnancy outcomes after first-trimester vaginitis drug therapy. Obstet Gynecol 69(5):751-755, 1987.

MICRONOR® *See* Norethindrone

MICROSULFON® *See* Sulfadiazine

MIDAMOR® *See* Amiloride

MILK OF MAGNESIA *See* Magnesium Hydroxide

MILLAZINE® *See* Thioridazine

MINIPRESS® *See* Prazosin

MINOCIN® *See* Minocycline

MINOCRIN® *See* Aminacrine

MINOCYCLINE
(Minocin®, Ultramycin®, Vectrin®)

Minocycline is a broad-spectrum antibiotic agent that is chemically related to tetracycline. Minocycline is given orally, usually in a dose of 200 mg/d, or intravenously in doses of 200-400 mg/d.

Teratogenic Risk

Magnitude of teratogenic risk to child born after exposure during gestation: Undetermined

Quality and quantity of data on which risk estimate is based: Very poor

No epidemiological studies of congenital anomalies in children born to women who were treated with minocycline during pregnancy have been published.

No teratogenic effect was apparent among the offspring of pregnant macaque monkeys given 1-4 times the usual human dose of minocycline during pregnancy (Jackson et al., 1975).

Tetracycline causes staining of the primary dentition in fetuses exposed during the second or third trimesters of pregnancy (*please see tetracycline agent summary*); it is not known whether or not minocycline produces similar problems.

Risk Related to Breast-feeding

No information regarding the distribution of minocycline in breast milk has been published. As with other tetracyclines, dental staining or inhibition of bone growth associated with ingestion of minocycline through the breast milk is a theoretical possibility with chronic use (USP DI, 1995), but these effects have not been documented in humans.

Key References

Jackson BA, Rodwell DE, Kanegis LA, Noble JF: Effect of maternally administered minocycline on embryonic and fetal development in the rhesus monkey (*Macaca mulatta*). Toxicol Appl Pharmacol 33:156, 1975.

USP DI: Tetracyclines. In: *USP DI (USP Dispensing Information), Volume 1. Drug Information for the Health Care Professional*, 15th ed. Rockville, Md.: The US Pharmacopeial Convention, 1995, p 2634.

MODAMIDE® *See* Amiloride

MONACRIN® *See* Aminacrine

MONISTAT® *See* Miconazole

MONODOX® *See* Doxycycline

MORPHINE
(Morphitec®, Roxanol®, Statex®)

Morphine is a narcotic analgesic. It is used as a pain reliever, particularly in the treatment of myocardial infarction and cardiac failure. Morphine is also used as an antitussive. The usual dose of morphine is 60-450 mg/d when given orally, 30-120 mg/d when given parenterally, and 40-180 mg/d when given rectally.

Teratogenic Risk

Magnitude of teratogenic
risk to child born after
exposure during gestation:
Congenital anomalies:	*Unlikely*
Neonatal neurobehavioral effects:	*Moderate*

Quality and quantity of data
on which risk estimate is based:
Congenital anomalies:	*Fair to good*
Neonatal neurobehavioral effects:	*Fair to good*

The risk of congenital anomalies is unlikely to be substantially increased among the children of women who are treated with therapeutic doses of morphine, but the data are insufficient to state that there is no risk.

Neonatal withdrawal symptoms often occur among infants born to women who regularly use morphine during pregnancy.

The frequency of congenital anomalies was no greater than expected among the children of 70 women who were treated with morphine during the first four lunar months of pregnancy or among the children of 448 women treated with this drug anytime during pregnancy in one epidemiological study (Heinonen et al., 1977).

No malformations were observed in the infant of a woman who attempted suicide by taking an overdose of morphine and other medication during the first trimester of pregnancy (Czeizel et al., 1988).

The frequency of malformations was no greater than expected among the offspring of mice or rats treated during pregnancy with morphine in doses 2-17 times those used clinically (Yamamoto et al.,

1972; Fujinaga & Mazze, 1988), but fetal growth retardation and increased frequencies of central nervous system and other anomalies were seen among the offspring of pregnant mice and hamsters treated respectively with doses 40-200 and 15-130 times those used in humans (Harpel & Gautieri, 1968; Geber & Schramm, 1975; Geber, 1977; Gupta et al., 1990). Fetal growth retardation was also seen among the offspring of pregnant rabbits or rats treated with morphine at 20-40 or 5-60 times the human dose (Raye et al., 1977; Zagon & McLaughlin, 1977; Eriksson & Ronnback, 1989). Increased rates of fetal and neonatal death were observed after treatment of pregnant rats with morphine in doses 5 or more times those used in humans (Fujinaga & Mazze, 1988; Eriksson & Ronnback, 1989). Long-lasting alterations of central nervous system development and function have been observed among the offspring of mice, rats, and hamsters treated with large doses of morphine during pregnancy (Johnston et al., 1992, 1994; Vathy & Katay, 1992; Zagon & McLaughlin, 1992; Koyuncuoglu & Aricioglu, 1993; Ramsey et al., 1993; Vathy et al., 1994, 1995).

Neonatal withdrawal symptoms similar to those seen in the infants of heroin addicts have been observed in the infants of morphine-addicted women (Perlstein, 1947; Cobrinik et al., 1959; Levy & Spino, 1993). These symptoms include tremors, irritability, sneezing, diarrhea, vomiting, and occasionally seizures.

Risk Related to Breast-feeding

Morphine is excreted in the breast milk. Based on data from eight lactating women, the amount of morphine that the nursing infant would be expected to ingest is between <1-10% of the lowest therapeutic dose of morphine, on a weight-adjusted basis (Terwilliger & Hatcher, 1934; Feilberg et al., 1989; Robieux et al., 1990).*

The serum level of morphine measured in one infant was 15% of the average analgesic serum level of morphine in infants (Olkkola et al., 1988; Robieux et al., 1990).[†] No signs of withdrawal or other adverse effects of morphine were observed in the nursing infant.

*This calculation is based on the following assumptions: maternal dose of morphine: 4-5 mg epidurally, 5-10 mg intravenously or intramuscularly, 20 mg orally; milk concentration of morphine: 0.002-0.5 mcg/mL; milk intake by the nursing infant: 150 mL/kg/d; estimated dose of morphine by the nursing infant: 0.0003-0.075 mg/kg/d; lowest therapeutic dose of morphine in adults: 0.75 mg/kg/d.

†Infant serum level of morphine: 0.004 mcg/mL; average analgesic serum level of morphine in infants: 0.026 mcg/mL.

The American Academy of Pediatrics regards therapeutic use of morphine to be safe while breast-feeding (Committee on Drugs, American Academy of Pediatrics, 1994).

Key References

Cobrinik RW, Hood RT Jr, Chusid E: The effect of maternal narcotic addiction on the newborn infant. Pediatrics 24:288-304, 1959.

Committee on Drugs, American Academy of Pediatrics: The transfer of drugs and other chemicals into human milk. Pediatrics 93(1):137-150, 1994.

Czeizel A, Szentesi I, Szekeres I, et al.: A study of adverse effects on the progeny after intoxication during pregnancy. Arch Toxicol 62:1-7, 1988.

Eriksson PS, Ronnback L: Effects of prenatal morphine treatment of rats on mortality, bodyweight and analgesic response in the offspring. Drug Alcohol Depend 24:187-194, 1989.

Feilberg VL, Rosenborg D, Christensen CB, Mogensen JV: Excretion of morphine in human breast milk. Acta Anaesthesiol Scand 33:426-428, 1989.

Fujinaga M, Mazze RI: Teratogenic and postnatal developmental studies of morphine in Sprague-Dawley rats. Teratology 38:401-410, 1988.

Geber WF: Effects of central nervous system active and nonactive drugs on the fetal central nervous system. Neurotoxicology 1:585-593, 1977.

Geber WF, Schramm LC: Congenital malformations of the central nervous system produced by narcotic analgesics in the hamster. Am J Obstet Gynecol 123:705-713, 1975.

Gupta U, Gautieri RF, Lemke PM: Influence of aminophylline on the teratogenic potential of morphine in mice. Res Commun Subst Abuse 11(3):105-121, 1990.

Harpel HS Jr, Gautieri RF: Morphine-induced fetal malformations. I. Exencephaly and axial skeletal fusions. J Pharm Sci 57:1590-1597, 1968.

Heinonen OP, Slone D, Shapiro S: *Birth Defects and Drugs in Pregnancy*. Littleton, Mass.: John Wright-PSG, 1977, pp 287-288, 434, 484.

Johnston HM, Payne AP, Gilmore DP: Effect of exposure to morphine throughout gestation on feminine and masculine adult sexual behaviour in golden hamsters. J Reprod Fertil 100:173-176, 1994.

Johnston HM, Payne AP, Gilmore DP: Perinatal exposure to morphine affects adult sexual behavior of the male golden hamster. Pharmacol Biochem Behav 42(1):41-44, 1992.

Koyuncuoglu H, Aricioglu F: Prenatal exposure to morphine or naloxone intensifies morphine dependence at maturity. Pharmacol Biochem Behav 44(4):939-941, 1993.

Levy M, Spino M: Neonatal withdrawal syndrome: Associated drugs and pharmacologic management. Pharmacotherapy 13(3):202-211, 1993.

Olkkola KT, Maunuskela EL, Korpela R, Rosenberg PH: Kinetics and dynamics of postoperative intravenous morphine in children. Clin Pharmacol Ther 44:128-136, 1988.

Perlstein MA: Congenital morphinism. JAMA 10:633, 1947.

Ramsey NF, Niesink RJM, Van Ree JM: Prenatal exposure to morphine enhances cocaine and heroin self-administration in drug-naive rats. Drug Alcohol Depend 33:41-51, 1993.

Raye JR, Dubin JW, Blechner JN: Fetal growth retardation following maternal morphine administration: Nutritional or drug effect? Biol Neonate 32:222-228, 1977.

Robieux I, Koren G, Vandenbergh H, Schneiderman J: Morphine excretion in breast milk and resultant exposure of a nursing infant. Clin Toxicol 28(3):365-370, 1990.

Terwilliger WG, Hatcher RA: The elimination of morphine and quinine in human milk. Surg Gynecol Obstet 58:823-826, 1934.

Vathy I, Katay L: Effects of prenatal morphine on adult sexual behavior and brain catecholamines in rats. Dev Brain Res 68(1):125-131, 1992.

Vathy I, Rimanoczy A, Eaton RC, Katay L: Modulation of catecholamine turnover rate in brain regions of rats exposed prenatally to morphine. Brain Res 662:209-215, 1994.

Vathy I, Rimanoczy A, Eaton RC, Katay L: Sex dimorphic alterations in postnatal brain catecholamines after gestational morphine. Brain Res Bull 36(2):185-193, 1995.

Yamamoto H, Kuchii M, Hayano T, Nishino H: [A study on teratogenicity of both CG-315 and morphine in mice and rats.] Oyo Yakuri (Pharmacometrics) 6:1055-1069, 1972.

Zagon IS, McLaughlin PJ: Effects of chronic morphine administration on pregnant rats and their offspring. Pharmacology 15:302-310, 1977.

Zagon IS, McLaughlin PJ: Maternal exposure to opioids and the developing nervous system: Laboratory findings. In: Zagon IS, Slotkin TA (eds). *Maternal Substance Abuse and the Developing Nervous System.* San Diego, Calif.: Academic Press, 1992, pp 241-282.

MORPHITEC® *See* Morphine

MOTRIN® *See* Ibuprofen

MPA *See* Medroxyprogesterone

MUMPSVAX® *See* Mumps Virus Vaccine

MUMPS VIRUS VACCINE
(Mumpsvax®)

Mumps virus vaccine is a live attenuated virus vaccine that is used for immunization against mumps.

Teratogenic Risk

*Magnitude of teratogenic
risk to child born after
exposure during gestation:*   *Undetermined*

*Quality and quantity of data
on which risk estimate is based:*   *None*

A small risk cannot be excluded, but a high risk of congenital anomalies in the children of women immunized with mumps virus vaccine during pregnancy is unlikely.

No epidemiological studies of congenital anomalies in infants born to women who were inoculated with mumps virus vaccine during pregnancy have been reported.

No animal teratology studies of mumps virus vaccine have been published.

Risk Related to Breast-feeding

No information regarding the distribution of mumps virus vaccine in breast milk has been published. Live vaccinations are safe to administer during breast-feeding for both mother and infant (ACIP, 1994).

Key References

ACIP: General recommendations on immunization. Recommendations of the Advisory Committee on Immunization Practices (ACIP). MMWR 43(RR-1):1-38, 1994.

MYAMBUTOL® *See* Ethambutol

MYCELEX CREAM® *See* Clotrimazole

MYCIFRADIN® *See* Neomycin

MYCIGUENT® *See* Neomycin

MYCOSTATIN® *See* Nystatin

MYDFRIN® *See* Phenylephrine

MYKROX® *See* Metolazone

NADOLOL
(Corgard®, Solgol®)

Nadolol is a β-adrenergic receptor-blocking agent used in the treatment of hypertension and angina pectoris. Nadolol is given orally in doses of 20-320 mg/d.

Teratogenic Risk

*Magnitude of teratogenic
risk to child born after
exposure during gestation:*   *Undetermined*

No epidemiological studies of congenital anomalies among infants born to women treated with nadolol during pregnancy have been reported.

The frequency of malformations was no greater than expected among the offspring of rats, hamsters, or rabbits treated during pregnancy with nadolol in doses, respectively, 8-156, 16-47, and 4-47 times those used in humans (Sibley et al., 1978; Saegusa et al., 1983; Stevens et al., 1984). Fetal growth retardation was observed among the rats and fetal death among the rabbits at the higher doses. The relevance of these observations to therapeutic use of nadolol in human pregnancy is uncertain.

One infant with cardiorespiratory depression, hypoglycemia, and growth retardation whose mother was treated with nadolol throughout pregnancy has been reported (Fox et al., 1985). Similar neonatal effects have been observed among infants whose mothers were treated with propranolol during pregnancy.

Please see agent summary on propranolol for information on this closely related agent that has been more thoroughly studied.

Risk Related to Breast-feeding

Nadolol is excreted in the breast milk. The amount of nadolol that the nursing infant would be expected to ingest is between 1-11% of the lowest weight-adjusted therapeutic dose, based on data from thirteen lactating women (Devlin et al., 1981).*

The American Academy of Pediatrics regards nadolol to be safe to use while breast-feeding (Committee on Drugs, American Academy of Pediatrics, 1994).

Key References

Committee on Drugs, American Academy of Pediatrics: The transfer of drugs and other chemicals into human milk. Pediatrics 93(1):137-150, 1994.

*This calculation is based on the following assumptions: maternal dose of nadolol: 20-80 mg/d; milk concentration of nadolol: <0.05-0.44 mcg/mL; milk intake by the nursing infant: 150 mL/kg/d; estimated dose of nadolol ingested by the nursing infant: 0.007-0.07 mg/kg/d; lowest therapeutic dose of nadolol in adults: 0.62 mg/kg/d.

Devlin RG, Duchin KL, Fleiss PM: Nadolol in human serum and breast milk. Br J Clin Pharmac 12:393-396, 1981.

Fox RE, Marx C, Stark AR: Neonatal effects of maternal nadolol therapy. Am J Obstet Gynecol 152:1045-1046, 1985.

Saegusa T, Suzuki T, Narama I: [Reproduction studies of nadolol a new beta-adrenergic blocking agent.] Yakuri To Chiryo 11:5119-5138, 1983.

Sibley PL, Keim GR, Murphy BF, et al.: Preclinical toxicologic evaluation of nadolol, a new beta-adrenergic antagonist. Toxicol Appl Pharmacol 44:379-389, 1978.

Stevens AC, Keysser CH, Kulesza JS, et al.: Preclinical safety evaluations of the nadolol/bendroflumethiazide combination in mice, rats and dogs. Fundam Appl Toxicol 4:360-369, 1984.

NADOPEN V® *See* Penicillin

NALCROM® *See* Cromolyn

NALFON® *See* Fenoprofen

NALICIDIN® *See* Nalidixic Acid

NALIDIXIC ACID
(Nalicidin®, NegGram®, Uropan®)

Nalidixic acid is an antibacterial agent of the 4-quinolone class. It is given orally in doses of 2000-4000 mg/d to treat urinary tract infections.

Teratogenic Risk

Magnitude of teratogenic
risk to child born after
exposure during gestation: *Unlikely*

Quality and quantity of data
on which risk estimate is based: *Poor to fair*

Therapeutic doses of nalidixic acid are unlikely to pose a substantial teratogenic risk, but the data are insufficient to state that there is no risk.

No controlled epidemiological studies of congenital anomalies among infants born to women treated with nalidixic acid during pregnancy have been reported. No adverse effects were noted among the children of 63 women treated with nalidixic acid during pregnancy in one clinical series (Murray, 1981). Treatment occurred during the first trimester in six of these cases, and during the second or third trimester in 57.

The frequency of congenital anomalies was no greater than expected among the offspring of rabbits treated during pregnancy with nalidixic acid in doses <1-10 times those used in humans; fetal growth retardation and fetal death were seen with the highest dose (Pagnini et al., 1971; Sato & Kobayashi, 1980). No increase in the frequency of congenital anomalies was observed among the offspring of pregnant rats treated with <1 to almost 4 times the usual human dose of nalidixic acid (Pagnini et al., 1971; Sato et al., 1980). Stillbirth and neonatal death were unusually frequent at the highest dose. The relevance of these observations to therapeutic use of nalidixic acid in human pregnancy is unknown.

Risk Related to Breast-feeding

Nalidixic acid is excreted in the breast milk in low concentrations. Based on data from 13 lactating women, the amount of nalidixic acid that the nursing infant would be expected to receive is <1% of the lowest pediatric maintenance dose (Traeger & Peiker, 1980).*

Hemolytic anemia has been described in one infant whose mother was treated with large doses of nalidixic acid (Belton & Jones, 1965). The infant recovered following blood transfusion and termination of breast-feeding. No causal inference can be made on the basis of this single anecdotal report.

The American Academy of Pediatrics regards nalidixic acid to be safe to use while breast-feeding (Committee on Drugs, American Academy of Pediatrics, 1994).

*This calculation is based on the following assumptions: maternal dose of nalidixic acid: 2 g; milk concentration of nalidixic acid: 0.3-1.1 mcg/mL; milk intake by the nursing infant: 150 mL/kg/d; estimated dose of nalidixic acid by the nursing infant: 0.04-0.16 mg/kg/d; lowest pediatric maintenance dose of nalidixic acid: 33 mg/kg/d.

Key References

Belton EM, Jones RV: Hemolytic anaemia due to nalidixic acid. Lancet 2:691, 1965.

Committee on Drugs, American Academy of Pediatrics: The transfer of drugs and other chemicals into human milk. Pediatrics 93(1):137-150, 1994.

Murray EDS: Nalidixic acid in pregnancy. Br Med J 282:224, 1981.

Pagnini G, Pelagalli GV, Di Carlo F: Effect of nalidixic acid on the chick embryo and on pregnancy and embryonic development in rabbits and rats. Atti Soc Ital Sci Vet 25:137-140, 1971.

Sato T, Kaneko Y, Saegusa T, Kobayashi F: Reproduction studies of cinoxacin in rats. Chemotherapy 28(Suppl 4):484-507, 1980.

Sato T, Kobayashi F: Teratological study on cinoxacin in rabbits. Chemotherapy 28(Suppl 4):508-515, 1980.

Traeger A, Peiker G: Excretion of nalidixic acid via mother's milk. Arch Toxicol (Suppl 4):388-390, 1980.

NAPROSYN® *See Naproxen*

NAPROXEN
(Anaprox®, Apranax®, Naprosyn®)

Naproxen is a nonsteroidal anti-inflammatory agent with analgesic and antipyretic actions. It is used orally in the treatment of dysmenorrhea, arthritis, and other painful conditions. The usual dose is 500-1000 mg/d, although sometimes higher doses (up to 1650 mg/d) are used for short periods or lower doses are used chronically. Similar doses have also been administered rectally.

Teratogenic Risk

*Magnitude of teratogenic
risk to child born after
exposure during gestation:*   *Undetermined*

*Quality and quantity of data
on which risk estimate is based:*   *Poor*

A small risk cannot be excluded, but there is no indication that the risk of congenital anomalies in the children of women treated with naproxen during pregnancy is likely to be great.
Maternal use of naproxen just before delivery may be associated with abnormalities of neonatal cardiovascular adaptation (see below).

There are no published epidemiological studies of congenital anomalies among children of women treated with naproxen during pregnancy.

Increased frequencies of cleft palate were observed among the offspring of pregnant mice treated with naproxen in doses similar to those used in humans in one study (Montenegro & Palomino, 1990) but not in another (Kuramoto et al., 1973). The clinical relevance of this observation is uncertain.

Increased frequencies of fetal death have been observed in pregnant mice and rabbits treated with naproxen in doses similar to those used in humans (Hallesy et al., 1973; Montenegro & Palomino, 1990).

Persistent pulmonary hypertension and premature closure of the ductus arteriosus have been reported in infants whose mothers took naproxen just before delivery (Wilkinson et al., 1979, Wilkinson, 1980). This observation is consistent with the fact that naproxen is a prostaglandin inhibitor, a class of drugs that has been used therapeutically to produce closure of the ductus arteriosus in infants. Naproxen and pharmacologically related drugs appear capable of delaying labor when given to women late in pregnancy (Csapo et al., 1974; Grella & Zanor, 1978).

Please see agent summary on indomethacin for information on a related agent that has been more thoroughly studied.

Risk Related to Breast-feeding

Naproxen is excreted into breast milk in small amounts (Brogden et al., 1975; Jamali & Stevens, 1983). The amount of naproxen that the nursing infant would be expected to ingest is between 2-7% of the lowest pediatric dose, based on data obtained from a single patient (Jamali & Stevens, 1983).*

*This calculation is based on the following assumptions: maternal dose of naproxen: 500-750 mg/d; milk concentration of naproxen: 0.7-2.4 mcg/mL; milk intake by the nursing infant: 150 mL/kg/d; estimated dose of naproxen ingested by the nursing infant: 0.1-0.36 mg/kg/d; lowest pediatric dose of naproxen: 5 mg/kg/d.

Both the American Academy of Pediatrics (Committee on Drugs, American Academy of Pediatrics, 1994) and the WHO Working Group on Drugs and Human Lactation (1988) consider naproxen to be safe to use during breast-feeding.

Key References

Brogden RN, Pinder RM, Sawyer PR, et al.: Naproxen: A review of its pharmacological properties and therapeutic efficacy and use. Drugs 9:326-363, 1975.

Committee on Drugs, American Academy of Pediatrics: The transfer of drugs and other chemicals into human milk. Pediatrics 93:137-150, 1994.

Csapo AI, Henzl MR, Kaihola HL, et al.: Suppression of uterine activity and abortion by inhibition of prostaglandin synthesis. Prostaglandins 7:39-47, 1974.

Grella P, Zanor P: Premature labor and indomethacin. Prostaglandins 16:1007-1017, 1978.

Hallesy DW, Shott LD, Hill R: Comparative toxicology of naproxen. Scand J Rheumatol (Suppl 2):20-28, 1973.

Jamali F, Stevens DRS: Naproxen excretion in breast milk and its uptake by the infant. Drug Intell Clin Pharm 17:910-911, 1983.

Kuramoto M, Ishimura Y, Daikoku S, Hashimoto T: Studies on teratogenicity of naproxen on mice and rats. Shikoku Igaku Zasshi 29:465-470, 1973.

Montenegro MA, Palomino H: Induction of cleft palate in mice by inhibitors of prostaglandin synthesis. J Craniofac Genet Dev Biol 10:83-94, 1990.

WHO Working Group on Human Lactation. In: Bennet PN (ed). *Drugs and Human Lactation.* Amsterdam: Elsevier, 1988, pp 299-300.

Wilkinson AR: Naproxen levels in preterm infants after maternal treatment. Lancet 2:591-592, 1980.

Wilkinson AR, Aynsley-Green A, Mitchell MD: Persistent pulmonary hypertension and abnormal prostaglandin E levels in preterm infants after maternal treatment with naproxen. Arch Dis Child 54:942-945, 1979.

NASALIDE® *See* Flunisolide

NAVANE® *See* Thiothixene

NEGGRAM® *See* Nalidixic Acid

NELULEN® *See* Ethynodiol Diacetate

NEMASOL SODIUM® *See* Aminosalicylic Acid

NEOMYCIN
(Mycifradin®, Myciguent®)

Neomycin is a broad-spectrum antibiotic used locally in a variety of infections. Some absorption may occur from topical and systemic preparations. An oral preparation, which is poorly absorbed, is used to kill bowel flora in preparation for surgery or in treatment of hepatic coma.

Teratogenic Risk

*Magnitude of teratogenic
risk to child born after
exposure during gestation:*   *None*

*Quality and quantity of data
on which risk estimate is based:*   *Poor to fair*

The frequency of congenital anomalies was not increased among the children of 30 women treated with neomycin during the first four lunar months of pregnancy in one epidemiological study (Heinonen et al., 1977).

The frequency of malformations was not increased among the offspring of pregnant mice given drinking water containing 4 g/L of neomycin (Skalko & Gold, 1974). No teratogenic effect was observed among the offspring of pregnant rats given twice the human dose of neomycin orally (Takeno & Sakai, 1991). Decreased hearing was seen among the offspring of pregnant rats given intramuscular injections of neomycin in a dose similar to that used orally in humans (Kameyama et al., 1982). The relevance of this observation to the oral or local use of neomycin in human pregnancy is unknown.

Risk Related to Breast-feeding

No information regarding the distribution of neomycin in breast milk has been published.

Key References

Heinonen OP, Slone D, Shapiro S: *Birth Defects and Drugs in Pregnancy.* Littleton, Mass.: John Wright-PSG, 1977, p 297.

Kameyama T, Nabeshima T, Itoh J: Measurement of an auditory impairment induced by prenatal administration of aminoglycosides using a shuttle box method. Folia Pharmacol Jpn 80:525-535, 1982.

Skalko RG, Gold MP: Teratogenicity of methotrexate in mice. Teratology 9:159-164, 1974.

Takeno S, Sakai T: Involvement of the intestinal microflora in nitrazepam-induced teratogenicity in rats and its relationship to nitroreduction. Teratology 44:209-214, 1991.

NEORESPIN® *See* Ephedrine

NEO-SYNEPHRINE® *See* Phenylephrine

NEOTIGASONE® *See* Acitretin

NIACIN
(Nicobid®, Nicotinic Acid, Vitamin B₃)

Niacin is a vitamin of the B complex that occurs naturally in many foods. The recommended dietary allowance is 17 mg/d in pregnancy. Niacin is given in larger amounts to treat deficiency and hyperlipidemia. Therapeutic doses range from 100-6000 mg/d orally or 50-500 mg/d parenterally.

Teratogenic Risk

*Magnitude of teratogenic
risk to child born after
exposure during gestation:*   *Undetermined*

*Quality and quantity of data
on which risk estimate is based:*   *None*

> *A small risk cannot be excluded, but there is no indication that the risk of congenital anomalies in the children of women who take therapeutic doses of niacin during pregnancy is likely to be great.*

No epidemiological studies of congenital anomalies in infants born to women who took niacin in pharmacologic doses during pregnancy have been reported.

No studies of the teratogenicity of therapeutic or greater doses of niacin in mammals have been published.

Risk Related to Breast-feeding

Niacin is a normal constituent of breast milk and is present in low concentrations (Schanler & Prestridge, 1991). Progressive supplementation for eight months with niacin at doses up to 60 mg/d in lactating women who had low dietary intakes of niacin (2.4 mg/d) steadily increased the niacin content of breast milk (Deodhar et al., 1964). However, this increased content of niacin would not be expected to produce levels of niacin in the nursing infant that exceeded the RDA for infants.*

Key References

Deodhar AD, Rajalkashmi R, Ramakrishnan CV: Studies on human lactation. Part III. Effect of dietary vitamin supplementation on vitamin contents of breast milk. Acta Paediatr 53:42-48, 1964.

Schanler RJ, Prestridge LL: Neonatal vitamin metabolism--water soluble. In: Cowett RM (ed). *Principles of Perinatal-Neonatal Metabolism.* New York: Springer-Verlag, 1991, pp 559-582.

*RDA of niacin for infants: 5 mg.

NICOBID® *See* Niacin

NICOTINIC ACID *See* Niacin

NIFEDICOR® *See* Nifedipine

NIFEDIPINE
(Adalat®, Nifedicor®, Procardia®)

Nifedipine is a calcium channel-blocking agent used as a vasodilator in the treatment of hypertension and angina pectoris (Childress & Katz, 1994). Nifedipine has also been used to arrest premature labor. The drug is administered orally in doses of 30-60 mg/d; doses as high as 180 mg/d are sometimes used.

Teratogenic Risk

Magnitude of teratogenic risk to child born after exposure during gestation:	*Undetermined*
Quality and quantity of data on which risk estimate is based:	*Poor*

The frequency of congenital anomalies was not significantly increased among 57 infants of women who had been treated with nifedipine or another calcium channel-blocking agent during the first trimester of pregnancy in one series (Magee et al., 1994). No adverse effects related to maternal treatment with nifedipine in the second or third trimester of pregnancy were observed among infants born in clinical trials and series in which the mothers were treated for preterm labor of pregnancy-induced hypertension (Read & Wellby, 1986; Ferguson et al., 1990; Meyer et al., 1990; Bracero et al., 1991; Fenakel et al., 1991; Murray et al., 1992; Sibai et al., 1992; Glock & Morales, 1993; Roy & Pan, 1993; Smith & Woodland, 1993; Childress & Katz, 1994). Each of these studies included 20-99 treated pregnancies.

Severe maternal hypotension and fetal distress have been reported in a woman who was treated with sublingual nifedipine for pregnancy-induced hypertension (Impey, 1993).

Increased frequencies of fetal death, growth retardation, and skeletal and cardiovascular malformations have been seen among the offspring of rats treated with nifedipine during pregnancy in doses 4-62 times those used in humans (Fukunishi et al., 1980; Yoshida et al., 1988; Furuhashi et al., 1991; Komai et al., 1991; Richichi & Vasilenko, 1992). Cardiac failure was observed among the offspring of pregnant rats treated just prior to delivery with <1-4 times the human dose of nifedipine (Momma & Takao, 1989). Distal digital hypoplasia occurred with increased frequency among the offspring of rabbits treated with 3.5-14 times the human therapeutic dose of nifedipine during pregnancy (Danielsson et al., 1989). The relevance of these observations to the treatment of pregnant women with therapeutic doses of nifedipine is unknown.

Risk Related to Breast-feeding

Nifedipine is excreted in breast milk in low concentrations. The amount of nifedipine that the nursing infant would be expected to receive is between <1-3% of the lowest pediatric dose (Ehrenkranz, et al. 1989; Penny & Lewis, 1989; Manninen & Juhakoski, 1991).*

The American Academy of Pediatrics regards nifedipine to be safe to use while breast-feeding (Committee on Drugs, American Academy of Pediatrics, 1994).

Key References

Bracero LA, Leikin E, Kirshenbaum N, Tejani N: Comparison of nifedipine and ritodrine for the treatment of preterm labor. Am J Perinatol 8(6):365-369, 1991.

Childress CH, Katz VL: Nifedipine and its indications in obstetrics and gynecology. Obstet Gynecol 83:616-624, 1994.

Committee on Drugs, American Academy of Pediatrics: The transfer of drugs and other chemicals into human milk. Pediatrics 93(1):137-150, 1994.

Danielsson BRG, Reiland S, Rundqvist E, Danielson M: Digital defects induced by vasodilating agents: Relationship to reduction in uteroplacental blood flow. Teratology 40:351-358, 1989.

Ehrenkranz RA, Ackerman BA, Hulse JD: Nifedipine transfer into human milk. J Pediatr 114:478-480, 1989.

Fenakel K, Fenakel G, Appelman ZVI, et al.: Nifedipine in the treatment of severe preeclampsia. Obstet Gynecol 77:331-337, 1991.

Ferguson JE II, Dyson DC, Schutz T, Stevenson DK: A comparison of tocolysis with nifedipine or ritodrine: Analysis of efficacy and maternal, fetal, and neonatal outcome. Am J Obstet Gynecol 163:105-111, 1990.

*This calculation is based on the following assumptions: maternal dose of nifedipine: 30-90 mg/d; milk concentration of nifedipine: 0.001-0.053 mcg/mL; milk intake by the nursing infant: 150 mL/kg/d; estimated dose of nifedipine ingested by the nursing infant: 0.001-0.008 mg/kg/d; lowest pediatric dose of nifedipine: 0.25 mg/kg/d.

Fukunishi K, Yokoi Y, Yoshida H, Nose T: [Effects of nifedipine on rat fetuses]. Med Consult New Remed [Shinryo To Shinyakie] 17:2245-2256, 1980.

Furuhashi N, Tsujiei M, Kimura H, Yajima A: Effects of nifedipine on normotensive rat placental blood flow, placental weight and fetal weight. Gynecol Obstet Invest 32:1-3, 1991.

Glock JL, Morales WJ: Efficacy and safety of nifedipine versus magnesium sulfate in the management of preterm labor: A randomized study. Am J Obstet Gynecol 169:960-964, 1993.

Impey L: Severe hypotension and fetal distress following sublingual administration of nifedipine to a patient with severe pregnancy induced hypertension at 33 weeks. Br J Obstet Gynaecol 100:959-961, 1993.

Komai Y, Ito I, Ishimura K, et al.: [Reproduction study of S-1230: Teratogenicity study in rats by oral administration]. Yakuri To Chiryo 19(7):95-121, 1991.

Magee LA, Conover B, Schick B, et al.: Exposure to calcium channel blockers in human pregnancy. A prospective, controlled, multicentre cohort study. Teratology 49(5):372, 1994.

Manninen Ak, Juhakoski A: Nifedipine concentrations in maternal and umbilical serum, amniotic fluid, breast milk and urine of mothers and offspring. Int J Clin Pharm Res 11(5):231-236, 1991.

Meyer WR, Randall HW, Graves WL: Nifedipine versus ritodrine for suppressing preterm labor. J Reprod Med 35:649-653, 1990.

Momma K, Takao A: Fetal cardiovascular effects of nifedipine in rats. Pediatr Res 26(5):442-447, 1989.

Murray C, Haverkamp AD, Orleans M, et al.: Nifedipine for treatment of preterm labor: A historic prospective study. Am J Obstet Gynecol 167:52-56, 1992.

Penny WJ, Lewis MJ: Nifedipine is excreted in human milk. Eur J Clin Pharmacol 36:427-428, 1989.

Read MD, Wellby DE: The use of a calcium antagonist (nifedipine) to suppress preterm labour. Br J Obstet Gynaecol 93:933-937, 1986.

Richichi J, Vasilenko P: The effects of nifedipine on pregnancy outcome and morphology of the placenta, uterus, and cervix during late pregnancy in the rat. Am J Obstet Gynecol 167:797-803, 1992.

Roy UK, Pan S: Use of calcium antagonist (nifedipine) in premature labour. J Indian Med Assoc 91:8-10, 1993.

Sibai BM, Barton JR, Akl S, et al.: A randomized prospective comparison of nifedipine and bed rest versus bed rest alone in the management of preeclampsia remote from term. Am J Obstet Gynecol 167:879-884, 1992.

Smith CS, Woodland MB: Clinical comparison of oral nifedipine and subcutaneous terbutaline for initial tocolysis. Am J Perinatol 10:280-284, 1993.

Yoshida T, Kanamori S, Hasegawa Y: Hyperphalangeal bones induced in rat pups by maternal treatment with nifedipine. Toxicol Lett 40:127-132, 1988.

NILSTAT® *See* Nystatin

NITROFAN® *See* Nitrofurantoin

NITROFURANTOIN
(Furadantin®, Macrodantin®, Nitrofan®)

Nitrofurantoin is an antimicrobial agent used frequently in prophylaxis and treatment of urinary tract infections. Nitrofurantoin is given orally in doses of 50-600 mg/d.

Teratogenic Risk

Magnitude of teratogenic risk to child born after exposure during gestation:	*Unlikely*
Quality and quantity of data on which risk estimate is based:	*Poor to fair*

Therapeutic doses of nitrofurantoin are unlikely to pose a substantial teratogenic risk, but the data are insufficient to state that there is no risk.

The frequency of congenital anomalies was no greater than expected among the children of 83 woman who took nitrofurantoin during the first four lunar months of pregnancy or the children of 590 women who took this drug anytime during pregnancy in one epidemiological study (Heinonen et al., 1977).

The frequency of malformations was not increased among the offspring of pregnant rats and rabbits given 2-6 times the usual human dose of nitrofurantoin (Prytherch et al., 1984). The frequency of malformations was slightly but significantly increased among the offspring of mice given nitrofurantoin during pregnancy in doses about 50 times greater than those used clinically (Nomura et al., 1976). The relevance of this finding to the therapeutic use of nitrofurantoin in human pregnancy is unknown.

Risk Related to Breast-feeding

Nitrofurantoin is excreted in the breast milk in low concentrations. The amount of nitrofurantoin that the nursing infant would be expected to ingest is between <1-6% of the lowest therapeutic dose for infants (Varsano, 1973; Pons et al., 1990).*

The American Academy of Pediatrics regards nitrofurantoin to be safe to use while breast-feeding (Committee on Drugs, American Academy of Pediatrics, 1994).

Key References

Committee on Drugs, American Academy of Pediatrics: The transfer of drugs and other chemicals into human milk. Pediatrics 93(1):137-150, 1994.

Heinonen OP, Slone D, Shapiro S: *Birth Defects and Drugs in Pregnancy.* Littleton, Mass.: John Wright-PSG, 1977, pp 435, 486.

Nomura T, Kimura S, Isa Y, et al.: Teratogenic effects of some antimicrobial agents on mouse embryo. Teratology 14:250, 1976.

Pons G, Rey E, Richard M-O, et al.: Nitrofurantoin excretion in human milk. Dev Pharmacol Ther 14:148-152, 1990.

Prytherch JP, Sutton ML, Denine EP: General reproduction, peri-natal-postnatal, and teratology studies of nitrofurantoin macrocrystals in rats and rabbits. J Toxicol Environ Health 13:811-823, 1984.

Varsano I, Fischl J, Shochet SB: The excretion of orally ingested nitrofurantoin in human milk. J Pediatr 82:886-887, 1973.

*This calculation is based on the following assumptions: maternal dose of nitrofurantoin: 100-400 mg/d; milk concentration of nitrofurantoin: <0.2-1.2 mcg/mL; milk intake by the nursing infant: 150 mL/kg/d; estimated dose of nitrofurantoin by the nursing infant: <0.03-0.18 mg/kg/d; lowest therapeutic dose of nitrofurantoin in infants: 3 mg/kg/d.

NIZORAL® *See* Ketoconazole

NODOZ® *See* Caffeine

NOLVADEX® *See Tamoxifen*

NONOXYNOLS
(Delfen®, Gynol II®, Ortho-Creme®)

The nonoxynols are a series of nonionic surfactants of various chain lengths. Nonoxynol 9, 10, and 11 are used as vaginal spermicides. Nonoxynol 4, 15, and 30 are used as solubilizing and emulsifying agents.

Teratogenic Risk

Magnitude of teratogenic risk to child born after exposure during gestation:	*None*
Quality and quantity of data on which risk estimate is based:	*Good*

The frequency of malformations was no greater than expected among the infants of 1355 women who used nonoxynol-containing vaginal contraceptives before the last menstrual period preceding their pregnancy or among the infants of 943 women who used such contraceptives after their last menstrual period (Mills et al., 1982). Similarly, no increase in the frequency of malformations was observed among the children of 342 women who used vaginal contraceptives containing nonoxynol 9 early in pregnancy in another epidemiological study (Heinonen et al., 1977). Negative findings have also been reported in five large cohort studies in which data for nonoxynol were included with those for other spermicides (Huggins et al., 1982; Polednak et al., 1982; Linn et al., 1983; Harlap et al., 1985; Strobino et al., 1988).

No association was observed with maternal use of spermicides containing nonoxynol around the time of conception or in the first trimester of pregnancy among infants with a variety of anomalies including 264 with Down syndrome, 396 with hypospadias, 146 with limb reduction defects, and 115 with neoplasms (Louik et al., 1987). Similarly, no association was found with maternal use of various vaginal spermicides around the time of conception in large studies involving cases with stillbirth, chromosomal abnormalities, limb reduction defects, or a variety of other congenital anomalies (Cordero & Layde, 1981; Bracken & Vita, 1983; Porter et al., 1986; Warburton et al., 1987; Adams et al., 1989).

Jick et al. (1981) reported that the frequency of a heterogenous group of anomalies (especially limb reduction defects, neoplasms, chromosomal abnormalities, and hypospadias) was greater than expected among the offspring of 763 women who had obtained a vaginal spermicide (nonoxynol 9 in about 20%) within ten months of becoming pregnant. This study has serious methodological limitations (Cordero & Layde, 1981; Bracken, 1985; Watkins, 1986) and is not supported by the findings in other investigations (Anonymous, 1986; Einarson et al., 1990).

The frequency of malformations was not increased among the offspring of pregnant rats administered nonoxynol 9 vaginally in doses 2 and 20 times those used in humans (Abrutyn et al., 1982). Similarly, no teratogenic effect was observed among the offspring of pregnant rats given nonoxynol 9 orally or parenterally in a dose 25 times those used vaginally in humans (Meyer et al., 1988). Increased frequencies of skeletal variants were observed among the offspring of rats treated orally or parenterally with 125-250 times the human vaginal dose, but such doses were toxic to the mothers. Embryonic loss occurred with increased frequency among rats given 25 times the human dose of nonoxynol 9 intravaginally early in pregnancy (Tryphonas & Buttar, 1986). The relevance of these observations to the vaginal use of nonoxynol-containing spermacides by pregnant women is uncertain.

Risk Related to Breast-feeding

No information regarding the distribution of nonoxynols in breast milk has been published.

Key References

Abrutyn D, McKenzie BE, Nadaskay N: Teratology study of intravaginally administered nonoxynol-9-containing contraceptive cream in rats. Fertil Steril 37:113-117, 1982.

Adams MM, Mulinare J, Dooley K: Risk factors for conotruncal cardiac defects in Atlanta. J Am Coll Cardiol 14:432-442, 1989.

Anonymous: Data do not support association between spermicides, birth defects. FDA Drug Bull 16:21, 1986.

Bracken MB: Spermicidal contraceptives and poor reproductive outcomes: The epidemiologic evidence against an association. Am J Obstet Gynecol 151(5):552-556, 1985.

Bracken MB, Vita K: Frequency of non-hormonal contraception around conception and association with congenital malformations in offspring. Am J Epidemiol 117(3):281-291, 1983.

Cordero JF, Layde PM: Vaginal spermicides, chromosome abnormalities and limb reduction defects. Am J Hum Genet 33:74A, 1981.

Einarson TR, Koren G, Mattice D, Schechter-Tsafriri O: Maternal spermicide use and adverse reproductive outcome: A meta-analysis. Am J Obstet Gynecol 162:655-660, 1990.

Harlap S, Shiono PH, Ramcharan S: Congenital abnormalities in the offspring of women who used oral and other contraceptives around the time of conception. Int J Fertil 30(2):39-47, 1985.

Heinonen OP, Slone D, Shapiro S: *Birth Defects and Drugs in Pregnancy.* Littleton, Mass.: John Wright-PSG, 1977, p 392.

Huggins G, Vessey M, Flavel R, et al.: Vaginal spermicides and outcome of pregnancy: Findings in a large cohort study. Contraception 25:219-230, 1982.

Jick H, Walker AM, Rothman KJ, et al.: Vaginal spermicides and congenital disorders. JAMA 245:1329-1332, 1981.

Linn S, Schoenbaum SC, Monson RR, et al.: Lack of association between contraceptive usage and congenital malformations in offspring. Am J Obstet Gynecol 147:923-928, 1983.

Louik C, Mitchell AA, Werler MM, et al.: Maternal exposure to spermicides in relation to certain birth defects. N Engl J Med 317:474-478, 1987.

Meyer O, Andersen PH, Hansen EV, Larsen JC: Teratogenicity and in vitro mutagenicity studies on nonoxynol-9 and -30. Pharmacol Toxicol 62:236-238, 1988.

Mills JL, Harley EE, Reed GF, Berendes HW: Are spermicides teratogenic? JAMA 248:2148-2151, 1982.

Polednak AP, Janerich DT, Glebatis DM: Birth weight and birth defects in relation to maternal spermicide use. Teratology 26:27-38, 1982.

Porter JB, Hunter-Mitchell J, Jick H, Walker AM: Drugs and stillbirth. Am J Public Health 76(12):1428-1431, 1986.

Strobino B, Kline J, Warburton D: Spermicide use and pregnancy outcome. Am J Public Health 78(3):260-263, 1988.

Tryphonas L, Buttar HS: Effects of the spermicide nonoxynol-9 on the pregnant uterus and the conceptus of rat. Toxicology 39:177-186, 1986.

Warburton D, Neugut RH, Lustenberger A, et al.: Lack of association between spermicide use and trisomy. N Engl J Med 317(8):478-482, 1987.

Watkins RN: Vaginal spermicides and congenital disorders: The validity of a study. JAMA 256(22):3095, 1986.

NORETHINDRONE
(Micronor®, Norlutin®, Nor-Q.D.®)

Norethindrone is a synthetic progestin that is used as an oral contraceptive (when formulated with an estrogenic compound) and in treatment of menstrual disorders. The dose used to treat endometriosis (up to 15 mg/d) is much greater than that currently used in oral contraceptives (0.4-2.5 mg/d).

Teratogenic Risk

Magnitude of teratogenic risk to child born after exposure during gestation:	
Nongenital congenital anomalies:	*None*
Virilization of female fetus with large doses (used to treat endometriosis):	*Small*
Virilization of female fetus with small doses (used in oral contraceptives):	*None*
Quality and quantity of data on which risk estimate is based:	
Nongenital congenital anomalies:	*Fair*
Virilization of female fetus with large doses (used to treat endometriosis):	*Fair*
Virilization of female fetus with small doses (used in oral contraceptives):	*Fair*

Maternal use of large doses of norethindrone during pregnancy has been associated with the occurrence of masculinization of the external genitalia in female infants (Schardein, 1980, 1993). The genital anomalies observed include various degrees of clitoral hypertrophy with or without labioscrotal fusion (Wilkins et al., 1958; Overzier, 1963). Internal genitalia and pubertal development are not affected. Labioscrotal fusion is associated with exposure between the seventh and thirteenth week of gestation, but clitoral hypertrophy can develop with exposure at this time or later in pregnancy. The frequency of genital virilization among daughters of women who took norethindrone during pregnancy in doses similiar to or greater than those used to treat endometriosis was 13% and 19% in clinical series of 39 and 82 female infants, respectively (Jacobson, 1968; Beischer et al., 1992).

The overall frequency of congenital anomalies was not significantly greater than expected among the children of 132 women who took norethindrone during the first four lunar months of pregnancy or of 148 women who took this drug anytime in pregnancy in a large epidemiological study (Heinonen et al., 1977). In another study, maternal use of norethindrone during pregnancy was not significantly increased among 171 children with various congenital anomalies (Spira et al., 1972). Similarly, the frequency of hormonal pregnancy tests using norethindrone and ethinyl estradiol (an estrogenic agent) during the second month of pregnancy was not increased among the mothers of 194 infants with major malformations or 551 infants with minor congenital anomalies (Kullander & Kallen, 1976).

Masculinization of the genitalia of female offspring can be induced in several species of experimental animals by treatment of the mother with norethindrone in high doses during pregnancy (Hendrickx et al., 1983; Schardein, 1993).

Studies in nonhuman primates, mice, and rabbits suggest that treatment of pregnant women with norethindrone in usual therapeutic or contraceptive doses is unlikely to increase the children's risk of nongenital congenital anomalies greatly (Takano et al., 1966; Hendrickx et al., 1987; Harada et al., 1991a, b).

Risk Related to Breast-feeding

Norethindrone is excreted in breast milk. The amount of nore-thindrone that the nursing infant would be expected to ingest is <1-24% of the lowest weight-adjusted dose used for oral contraception

(Toddywalla et al., 1980; Koetsawang et al., 1982; Fotherby et al., 1983; Betrabet et al., 1987).*

Norethindrone concentrations ranging from 0.07-0.42 ng/mL were measured in the serum of 15 breast-fed infants whose mothers took an oral contraceptive containing norethindrone (Betrabet et al., 1987). These levels of norethindrone were between 4-25% of those found in the maternal serum. In another study, no norethindrone was found in the serum of breast-fed infants whose mothers had been given an intramuscular injection of norethindrone (Melis et al., 1981).

Maternal use of norethindrone as a contraceptive during lactation had no adverse effects on growth or development of infants followed up to one year of age (WHO, 1994a, b).

The American Academy of Pediatrics regards oral contraceptives to be safe to use while breast-feeding (Committee on Drugs, American Academy of Pediatrics, 1994).

Key References

Beischer NA, Cookson T, Sheedy M, Wein P: Norethisterone and gestational diabetes. Aust NZ J Obstet Gynaecol 32(3):233-238, 1992.

Betrabet SS, Shikary ZK, Toddywalla VS: Transfer of norethisterone (NET) and levonorgestrel (LNG) from a single tablet into the infant's circulation through the mother's milk. Contraception 35(6):517-522, 1987.

Committee on Drugs, American Academy of Pediatrics: The transfer of drugs and other chemicals into human milk. Pediatrics 93(1):137-150, 1994.

Fotherby K, Towobola O, Muggeridge J, Elder MG: Norethisterone levels in maternal serum and milk after intramuscular injection of norethisterone oenanthate as a contraceptive. Contraception 28:405-411, 1983.

Harada S, Takayama S, Miyazaki Y, et al.: [Teratogenicity study of oral contraceptives DT-5061 and DT-5062 (1/35) in rabbits.] Yakuri To Chiryo 19(Suppl 4):233-249, 1991a.

*This calculation is based on the following assumptions: maternal dose of norethindrone: 200 mg (intramuscular) or 3 mg (oral); milk concentration of norethindrone: <0.5-8 ng/mL; milk intake by the nursing infant: 150 mL/kg/d; estimated dose of norethindrone ingested by the nursing infant: 0.007-1.2 mcg/kg/d; lowest oral contraceptive dose in adults: 0.005 mg/kg/d.

Harada S, Takayama S, Shibano T, et al.: [Teratogenicity study of oral contraceptives DT-5061 and DT-5062 (1/35) in rats.] Yakuri To Chiryo 19(Suppl 4):197-231, 1991b.

Heinonen OP, Slone D, Shapiro S: *Birth Defects and Drugs in Pregnancy.* Littleton, Mass.: John Wright-PSG, 1977, pp 389-391, 443.

Hendrickx AG, Binkerd PE, Rowland JM: Developmental toxicity and nonhuman primates. Interspecies comparisons. Issues Rev Teratol 1:149-180, 1983.

Hendrickx AG, Korte R, Leuschner F, et al.: Embryotoxicity of sex steroidal hormone combinations in nonhuman primates: I. Norethisterone acetate + ethinylestradiol and progesterone + estradiol benzoate (*Macaca mulatta, Macaca fascicularis,* and *Papio cynocephalus*). Teratology 35:119-127, 1987.

Jacobson BD: Hazards of norethindrone therapy during pregnancy. Am J Obstet Gynecol 84:962-968, 1968.

Koetsawang S, Nukulkarn P, Fotherby K, et al.: Transfer of contraceptive steroids in milk of women using long-acting gestagens. Contraception 25:321-331, 1982.

Kullander S, Kallen B: A prospective study of drugs and pregnancy. 3. Hormones. Acta Obstet Gynecol Scand 55:221-224, 1976.

Melis GB, Strigini F, Fruzzetti F, et al.: Norethisterone enanthate as an injectable contraceptive in puerperal and non-puerperal women. Contraception 23:77-88, 1981.

Overzier C: Induced pseudo-hermaphroditism. In: *Intersexuality.* New York, Academic Press, 1963, pp 387-401.

Schardein JL: *Chemically Induced Birth Defects,* 2nd ed. New York: Marcel Dekker, 1993, pp 284-301.

Schardein JL: Congenital abnormalities and hormones during pregnancy: A clinical review. Teratology 22:251-270, 1980.

Spira N, Goujard J, Huel G, Rumeau-Rouquette C: [Investigation into the teratogenic action of sex hormones first results of an epidemiologic survey involving 20,000 women.] Rev Med 41:2683-2694, 1972.

Takano K, Yamamura H, Suzuki M, Nishimura H: Teratogenic effect of chlormadione acetate in mice and rabbits. Proc Soc Exp Biol Med 121:455-457, 1966.

Toddywalla VS, Mehta S, Virkar KD, Saxena BN: Release of 19-nor-testosterone type of contraceptive steroids through different drug delivery systems into serum and breast milk of lactating women. Contraception 21:217-223, 1980.

WHO (World Health Organization Task Force on Oral Contraceptives, Special Programme of Research, Development, and Research Training in Human Reproduction): Progestogen-only contraceptives during lactation: I. Infant growth. Contraception 50:35-53, 1994a.

WHO (World Health Organization Task Force on Oral Contraceptives, Special Programme of Research, Development, and Research Training in Human Reproduction): Progestogen-only contraceptives during lactation: II. Infant development. Contraception 50:55-68, 1994b.

Wilkins L, Jones HW, Holman GH et al.: Masculinization of the female fetus associated with administration of oral and intramuscular progestins during gestation: Non-adrenal female pseudohermaphrodism. J Clin Endocrinol Metab 18:559-585, 1958.

NORFRANIL® *See* Imipramine

NORGESTREL
(Follistrel®, Norplant®, Ovrette®)

Norgestrel is a synthetic progestin that is used alone or in combination with an estrogenic compound as an oral contraceptive and in treatment of menstrual disorders. The usual dose is 75-150 mcg/d, but doses as large as 2000 mcg/d are given when norgestrel is used as a postcoital contraceptive.

Teratogenic Risk

*Magnitude of teratogenic
risk to child born after
exposure during gestation:*   *Unlikely*

*Quality and quantity of data
on which risk estimate is based:*   *Poor to fair*

Contraceptive doses of norgestrel are unlikely to pose a substantial teratogenic risk, but the data are insufficient to state that there is no risk.

A minimal risk for virilization of the genitalia in a female fetus may exist with maternal use of large doses of norgestrel during pregnancy. This assessment is based primarily on studies involving use of progestational hormones at doses much greater than those

No epidemiological studies of congenital anomalies in infants born to women who took norgestrel specifically during pregnancy have been reported. Extensive epidemiological data are available regarding the frequency of malformations in infants of women who took oral contraceptives early in pregnancy, but the findings are inconsistent (Smitthels, 1981; Wilson & Brent, 1981; Schardein, 1994). If the risk of congenital anomalies in children of women who took oral contraceptives early in pregnancy is increased, this increase is small compared to the background risk of birth defects in the general population.

Studies in mice and rabbits suggest that maternal use of conventional oral contraceptives containing norgestrel during pregnancy is unlikely to increase the children's risk of malformations greatly (Heinecke & Kohler, 1983; Klaus, 1983)

Risk Related to Breast-feeding

Norgestrel is excreted in the breast milk. The amount of norgestrel that the nursing infant would ingest is between <1.5-32% of the lowest dose used for oral contraception (Nilsson et al., 1977; Toddywalla et al., 1980).[*]

Serum levels of norgestrel in three infants whose mothers used a norgestrel-only contraceptive while breast-feeding were between 0-38% of the lowest therapeutic serum level for oral contraception (Nilsson et al., 1977).[†]

No adverse effects of norgestrel use were found on milk volume in lactating women or on the growth or psychomotor development of their infants (WHO, 1984; 1988; Moggia et al., 1991; Shaaban, 1991).

Breast enlargement was described in one 18-month-old infant whose mother had been on norgestrel for three months (Madhavapeddi & Ramachandran, 1985). The enlargement disappeared six months after termination of breast-feeding. Nevertheless, gynecomastia has not

[*]This calculation is based on the following assumptions: maternal dose of norgestrel: 30-250 mcg/d; milk concentration of norgestrel: 0.00005-0.001 mcg/mL; milk intake by the nursing infant: 150 mL/kg/d; estimated dose of norgestrel ingested by the nursing infant: 0.007-0.15 mcg/kg/d; lowest oral contraceptive dose of norgestrel in adults: 0.47 mcg/kg/d.

[†]Lowest serum level of norgestrel in adults: 0.29 ng/mL.

been consistently observed in other reports (Committee on Drugs, American Academy of Pediatrics, 1981).

The American Academy of Pediatrics regards combination oral contraceptives to be safe to use while breast-feeding (Committee on Drugs, American Academy of Pediatrics, 1994).

Key References

Committee on Drugs, American Academy of Pediatrics: Breast-feeding and contraception. Pediatrics 68(1):138-140, 1981.

Committee on Drugs, American Academy of Pediatrics: The transfer of drugs and other chemicals into human milk. Pediatrics 93(1):137-150, 1994.

Heinecke H, Kohler D: Prenatal toxic effects of STS 557. II. Investigation in rabbits--preliminary results. Exp Clin Endocrinol 81:206-209, 1983.

Klaus S: Prenatal toxic effects of STS 557. I. Investigations in mice. Exp Clin Endocrinol 81:197-205, 1983.

Madhavapeddi R, Ramachandran P: Side effects of oral contraceptive use in lactating women--enlargement of breast in a breast-fed child. Contraception 32(5):437-443, 1985.

Moggia AV, Harris GS, Dunson TR, et al.: A comparative study of a progestin-only oral contraceptive versus non-hormonal methods in lactating women in Buenos Aires, Argentina. Contraception 44(1):31-43, 1991.

Nilsson S, Nygren K-G, Johansson EDB: d-Norgestrel concentrations in maternal plasma, milk, and child plasma during administration of oral contraceptives to nursing women. Am J Obstet Gynecol 129:178-184, 1977.

Smithells RW: Oral contraceptive, and birth defects. Dev Med Child Neurol 23:369-372, 1981.

Shaaban MM: Contraception with progestogens and progesterone during lactation. J Steroid Biochem Mol Biol 40(4-6):705-710, 1991.

Toddywalla VS, Mehta S, Virkar KD, Saxena BN: Release of 19-nor-testosterone type of contraceptive steroids through different drug delivery systems into serum and breast milk of lactating women. Contraception 21(3):217-222, 1980.

WHO (World Health Organization Special Programme of Research, Development and Research Training in Human Reproduction. Task force on oral contraceptives): Effects of hormonal contraceptives on milk volume and infant growth. Contraception 30(6):505-522, 1984.

WHO (World Health Organization Task Force on Oral Contraceptives, Special Programme of Research, Development, and Research Training in Human Reproduction): Effects of hormonal contraceptives on breast milk composition and infant growth. Stud Fam Plan 19(6):361-369, 1988.

Wilson JG, Brent RL: Are female sex hormones teratogenic? Am J Obstet Gynecol 141:567-580, 1981.

NORLUTIN® *See* Norethindrone

NORPACE® *See* Disopyramide

NORPLANT® *See* Norgestrel

NOR-QD® *See* Norethindrone

NORTRIPTYLINE
(Aventyl®, Pamelor®)

Nortriptyline is a tricyclic antidepressant that is administered orally in doses of 75-150 mg/d.

Teratogenic Risk

Magnitude of teratogenic risk to child born after exposure during gestation:	*Undetermined*
Quality and quantity of data on which risk estimate is based:	*None*

No epidemiological studies of congenital anomalies among the infants of women treated with nortriptyline during pregnancy have been reported.

No animal teratology studies of nortriptyline have been published.

Urinary retention, a recognized complication of nortriptyline therapy in adults, has been reported in the newborn infant of a woman who took this drug throughout pregnancy (Shearer et al., 1972). *Please see agent summary on amitriptyline for information on a closely related drug that has been studied.*

Risk Related to Breast-feeding

Nortriptyline is excreted in breast milk in low concentrations. The amount of nortriptyline that the nursing infant would be expected to ingest is approximately 1-6% of the lowest weight-adjusted therapeutic dose, based on data from a single patient (Matheson & Skjaeraasen, 1988).*

No measurable levels of nortriptyline were found in infant serum following maternal administration of nortriptyline in three studies (Erickson et al., 1979; Wisner & Perel, 1991; Altshuler et al., 1995); however, low concentrations of its metabolite, 10-hydroxynortriptyline, were found in the plasma of two infants in one small series (Wisner & Perel, 1991). No adverse effects were observed in the nursing infants.

The American Academy of Pediatrics states that nortriptyline may be a concern for the nursing infant when taken by the mother while breast-feeding because of its potential effect on central nervous system function (Committee on Drugs, American Academy of Pediatrics, 1994).

Key References

Altshuler LL, Burt VK, McMullen M, Hendrick V: Breastfeeding and sertraline: A 24-hour analysis. J Clin Psychiatry 56:243-245, 1995.

Committee on Drugs, American Academy of Pediatrics: The transfer of drugs and other chemicals into human milk. Pediatrics 93(1):137-150, 1994.

Erickson ST, Smither GH, Heidrich F: Tricyclics and breast feeding. Am J Psychiatry 136:11, 1979.

*This calculation is based on the following assumptions: maternal dose of nortriptyline: 75-125 mg/d; milk concentration of nortriptyline: 0.09-0.4 mcg/mL; milk intake by the nursing infant: 150 mL/kg/d; estimated dose of nortriptyline ingested by the nursing infant: 0.013-0.06 mg/kg/d; lowest therapeutic dose of nortriptyline in children: 1 mg/kg/d.

Matheson L, Skjaeraasen J: Milk concentrations of flupenthixol, nortriptyline and zuclopenthixol and between-breast differences in two patients. Eur J Clin Pharmacol 35:217-220, 1988.

Shearer WT, Schreiner RL, Marshall RE: Urinary retention in a neonate secondary to maternal ingestion of nortriptyline. J Pediatr 81(3):570-572, 1972.

Wisner KL, Perel JM: Serum nortriptyline levels in nursing mothers and their infants. Am J Psychiatry 148:1234-1236, 1991.

NOVACIMETINE® *See* Cimetidine

NOVOBUTAMIDE® *See* Tolbutamide

NOVO-FOLACID® *See* Folic Acid

NOVOLIN® *See* Insulin

NOVOMEDOP® *See* Methyldopa

NOVO-PIROCAM® *See* Piroxicam

NOVOSPIRATON® *See* Spironolactone

NOVOSTREP® *See* Streptomycin

NU-PIROX® *See* Piroxicam

NUPRIN® *See* Ibuprofen

NYDRAZID® *See* Isoniazid

NYSTATIN
(Korostatin®, Mycostatin®, Nilstat®)

Nystatin is a polyene antibiotic used in local treatment of candidiasis and other fungal infections. Nystatin is poorly absorbed from the gastrointestinal tract and is not absorbed through the skin or mucous membranes when applied locally.

Teratogenic Risk

Magnitude of teratogenic risk to child born after exposure during gestation:	*None*
Quality and quantity of data on which risk estimate is based:	*Fair to good*

The frequencies of malformations in general, of major malformations, and of minor malformations were no greater than expected among infants born to 142 women treated with nystatin during the first four lunar months of pregnancy in one epidemiological study (Heinonen et al., 1977). The frequency of congenital anomalies was not increased among the children of 230 women treated with nystatin anytime during pregnancy in this study. In two separate cohorts of another epidemiological investigation, malformations were no more frequent than expected among children born to a total of 401 women treated with nystatin during the first trimester of gestation (Jick et al., 1981; Aselton et al., 1985). No association was found between maternal vaginal nystatin use during the first trimester of pregnancy and congenital anomalies among 66 children in a third study (Rosa et al., 1987).

Studies in rats suggest that treatment of pregnant women with nystatin in usual therapeutic doses is unlikely to increase the children's risk of malformations greatly (Slonitskaya & Mikhailets, 1975).

Risk Related to Breast-feeding

No information regarding the distribution of nystatin in breast milk has been published.

Key References

Aselton P, Jick H, Milunsky A, et al.: First-trimester drug use and congenital disorders. Obstet Gynecol 65:451-455, 1985.
Heinonen OP, Slone D, Shapiro S: *Birth Defects and Drugs in Pregnancy.* Littleton, Mass.: John Wright-PSG, 1977, pp 305, 435.

Jick H, Holmes LB, Hunter JR, et al.: First-trimester drug use and congenital disorders. JAMA 246:343-346, 1981.

Rosa FW, Baum C, Shaw M: Pregnancy outcomes after first-trimester vaginitis drug therapy. Obstet Gynecol 69:751-755, 1987.

Slonitskaya NM, Mikhailets GA: [Study of nystatin and mycoheptin effect on intrauterine development of rat fetus.] Antibiotiki 20:45-47, 1975.

OMNIPEN® *See* Ampicillin

OPTIMINE® *See* Azatadine

ORAJEL® *See* Benzocaine

ORAMIDE® *See* Tolbutamide

ORASONE® *See* Prednisone/Prednisolone

ORINASE® *See* Tolbutamide

ORTHO-CREME® *See* Nonoxynols

OVRETTE® *See* Norgestrel

OXAZEPAM
(Alopam®, Durazepam®, Praxiten®)

Oxazepam is a benzodiazepine tranquilizer. It is administered orally in the treatment of anxiety, as a sedative, and as a preoperative medication. The usual dose is 30-120 mg/d.

Teratogenic Risk

Magnitude of teratogenic
risk to child born after
exposure during gestation: *Undetermined*

No epidemiological studies of malformations in infants born to women who took oxazepam during pregnancy have been reported. The suggestion that there exists a "benzodiazepine embryofetopathy" comprised of typical facial features, neurological dysfunction, and other anomalies (Laegreid et al., 1987, 1989, 1990, 1992) is not generally accepted.

The frequency of malformations was not increased among the offspring of rabbits or rats treated during pregnancy with oxazepam in doses respectively 10-21 and 42 times those used in humans (Owen et al., 1970; Saito et al., 1984). Increased frequencies of craniofacial, central nervous system and eye malformations were observed among the offspring of mice treated with 312-833 times the human dose of oxazepam (Simon et al., 1992). Behavioral alterations were noted among the offspring of mice treated during pregnancy with 4-42 times the usual human dose of oxazepam (Laviola et al., 1991a, b, 1992a, b; Bignami et al., 1992; Ricceri et al., 1994). The relevance of these observations to therapeutic use of oxazepam in human pregnancy is uncertain.

Oxazepam is a major metabolite of diazepam.

Please see agent summary on diazepam for information on a more thoroughly studied benzodiazepine tranquilizer.

Risk Related to Breast-feeding

Oxazepam is excreted in the breast milk in very low concentrations. The amount of oxazepam that the nursing infant would be expected to ingest is <1% of the lowest weight-adjusted therapeutic dose, based on data from a single patient (Dusci et al., 1990).*

Key References

Bignami G, Alleva E, Chiarotti F, Laviola G: Selective changes in mouse behavioral development after prenatal benzodiazepine exposure:

*This calculation is based on the following assumptions: maternal dose: 30 mg of oxazepam and 80 mg of diazepam per day; milk concentration of oxazepam: 0.008-0.03 mcg/mL; milk intake by the nursing infant: 150 mL/kg/d; estimated dose of oxazepam by the nursing infant: 0.001-0.004 mg/kg/d; lowest therapeutic dose of oxazepam in adults: 0.47 mg/kg/d.

A progress report. Prog Neuropsychopharmacol Biol Psychiatry 16:587-604, 1992.

Dusci LJ, Good SM, Hall RW, Ilett KF: Excretion of diazepam and its metabolites in human milk during withdrawal from combination high dose diazepam and oxazepam. Br J Clin Pharmacol 29:123-126, 1990.

Laegreid L, Hagberg G, Lundberg A: Neurodevelopment in late infancy after prenatal exposure to benzodiazepines--A prospective study. Neuropediatrics 23:60-67, 1992.

Laegreid L, Olegard R, Conradi N, et al.: Congenital malformations and maternal consumption of benzodiazepines. A case-control study. Dev Med Child Neurol 32:432-441, 1990.

Laegreid L, Olegard R, Wahlstrom J, Conradi N: Abrnomalities in children exposed to benzodiazepines in utero. Lancet 1:108-109, 1987.

Laegreid L, Olegard R, Wahlstrom J, Conradi N: Teratogenic effects of benzodiazepine use during pregnancy. J Pediatr 114:126-131, 1989.

Laviola G, Bignami G, Alleva E: Interacting effects of oxazepam in late pregnancy and fostering procedure on mouse maternal behavior. Neurosci Biobehav Rev 15:501-504, 1991b.

Laviola G, Chiarotti F, Alleva E: Development of GABAergic modulation of mouse locomotor activity and pain sensitivity after prenatal benzodiazepine exposure. Neurotoxicol Teratol 14(1):1-5, 1992a.

Laviola G, de Acetis L, Bignami G, Alleva E: Prenatal oxazepam enhances mouse maternal aggression in the offspring, without modifying acute chlordiazepoxide effects. Neurotoxicol Teratol 13:75-81, 1991a.

Laviola G, Pick CG, Yanai J, Alleva E: Eight-arm maze performance, neophobia, and hippocampal cholinergic alterations after prenatal oxazepam in mice. Brain Res Bull 29(5):609-616, 1992b.

Owen G, Smith THF, Agersborg HPK Jr: Toxicity of some benzodiazepine compounds with CNS activity. Toxicol Appl Pharmacol 16:556-570, 1970.

Ricceri L, Calamandrei G, Alleva E: Prenatal oxazepam affects passive avoidance performance of preweaning mice. Brain Res Bull 33(3):267-271, 1994.

Saito H, Kobayashi H, Takeno S, Sakai T: Fetal toxicity of benzodiazepines in rats. Res Commun Chem Pathol Pharmacol 46:437-447, 1984.

Simon AR, Rogers JM, Sulik KK: Benzodiazepine-induced craniofacial malformations in C57BL/6J mice. Teratology 45(5):479, 1992.

OXYCODONE
(Roxicodone®, Supeudol®)

Oxycodone is a narcotic analgesic that is given orally in doses of 20-40 mg/d or rectally in doses of 30-160 mg/d.

Teratogenic Risk

Magnitude of teratogenic risk to child born after exposure during gestation:	*Undetermined*
Quality and quantity of data on which risk estimate is based:	*Poor*

A small risk cannot be excluded, but there is no indication that the risk of congenital anomalies in the children of women treated with oxycodone during pregnancy is likely to be great.
Possible effects on perinatal adaptation are discussed below.

The frequency of maternal exposure to oxycodone during the first trimester of pregnancy was not significantly greater than expected among 1370 infants with malformations in one study, but only five exposed cases were included in this investigation (Bracken & Holford, 1981).

Teratogenicity studies of oxycodone in experimental animals have not been published.

Neonatal withdrawal symptoms and respiratory depression are regularly observed following chronic maternal treatment late in pregnancy with chemically related narcotics (*please see agent summary for codeine.*) These complications have not been reported with oxycodone but probably can occur.

Please see agent summary on codeine for information on a related agent.

Risk Related to Breast-feeding

Oxycodone is excreted in the breast milk. The amount of oxycodone that the nursing infant would be expected to ingest is between <1-10% of the lowest weight-adjusted therapeutic dose, based on data from six lactating women (Marx et al., 1986).* No adverse effects of oxycodone on the nursing infants were noted in this study.

Key References

Bracken MB, Holford TR: Exposure to prescribed drugs in pregnancy and association with congenital malformations. Obstet Gynecol 58:336-344, 1981.
Marx CM, Pucino F, Carlson JD, et al.: Oxycodone excretion in human milk in the puerperium. Drug Intell Clin Pharm 20(6):474, 1986.

*This calculation is based on the following assumptions: milk concentration of oxycodone: <0.005-0.226 mcg/mL; milk intake by the nursing infant: 150 mL/kg/d; estimated dose of oxycodone ingested by the nursing infant: <0.001-0.03 mg/kg/d; lowest therapeutic dose of oxycodone in adults: 0.31 mg/kg/d.

OXYMETHOLONE
(Anadrol®, Anapolon®)

Oxymetholone is an anabolic and androgenic steroid that is used in the treatment of anemia. Oxymetholone is given orally in doses of 1-5 mg/kg/d (50-250 mg/d for a 110 pound woman).

Teratogenic Risk

Magnitude of teratogenic
risk to child born after
exposure during gestation: *Undetermined*

Quality and quantity of data
on which risk estimate is based: *Very poor*

Because it is an androgen, oxymetholone would be expected to have the capacity to cause virilization of the external genitalia of female fetuses exposed during pregnancy.

No epidemiological studies of congenital anomalies among the infants of women treated with oxymetholone during pregnancy have been reported.

Embryonic loss frequently occurred after injection of about 4 times the usual human dose of oxymetholone to rats in early pregnancy (Naqvi & Warren, 1971).

Please see agent summary on testosterone for information on a related agent that has been more thoroughly studied.

Risk Related to Breast-feeding

No information regarding the distribution of oxymetholone in breast milk has been published.

Key References

Naqvi RH, Warren JC: Interceptives: Drugs interrupting pregnancy after implantation. Steroids 18:731-739, 1971.

PALLACE® *See* Megestrol

PAMELOR® *See* Nortriptyline

PANMYCIN® *See* Tetracycline

PANWARFIN® *See* Warfarin

PARAFLEX® *See* Chlorzoxazone

PARAFON FORTE DSC® *See* Chlorzoxazone

PARLODEL® *See* Bromocriptine

PAROXETINE
(Paxil®)

Paroxetine, an inhibitor of neuronal serotonin reuptake, is used to treat depression. Paroxetine is given orally in a dose of 20-50 mg/d.

Teratogenic Risk

Magnitude of teratogenic risk to child born after exposure during gestation:	*Undetermined*
Quality and quantity of data on which risk estimate is based:	*Very poor*

No epidemiological studies of congenital anomalies among the children of women treated with paroxetine during pregnancy have been published.

Studies in rats and rabbits suggest that treatment of pregnant women with paroxetine in usual therapeutic doses is unlikely to increase the children's risk of malformations greatly (Baldwin et al., 1989).

Risk Related to Breast-feeding

Paroxetine is excreted in breast milk in concentrations similar to those found in the maternal plasma (USP DI, 1995). The effects of maternal exposure to paroxetine on the nursing infant are unknown.

Key References

Baldwin JA, Davidson EJ, Pritchard AL, Ridings JE: The reproductive toxicology of paroxetine. Acta Psychiatr Scand 80(Suppl 350):37-39, 1989.

USP DI: Paroxetine. In: *USP DI (USP Dispensing Information), Volume 1. Drug Information for the Health Care Professional*, 15th ed. Rockville, Md.: The US Pharmacopeial Convention, 1995, p 2138.

PAS® *See* Aminosalicylic Acid

PAXIL® *See* Paroxetine

PCP *See* Phencyclidine

PEDIACARE® *See* Pseudoephedrine

PENICILLIN
(Ayercillin®, Betapen-VK®, Nadopen V®)

Penicillin is an antibiotic that is given orally in doses of 800,000-2,000,000 units/d. Similar doses are usually employed parenterally, although doses as high as 80,000,000 units/d may be given in some serious infections such a bacterial endocarditis.

Teratogenic Risk

*Magnitude of teratogenic
risk to child born after
exposure during gestation:*   *None*

*Quality and quantity of data
on which risk estimate is based:*   *Good*

Available data deal with the use of penicillin in usual therapeutic doses. No information is available on the effects of exposure to exceptionally large doses as may be used to treat bacterial endocarditis.

The frequencies of congenital anomalies in general and of major classes of malformations were no greater than expected among the children of 3546 women who had been treated with penicillin or its derivatives during the first four lunar months of pregnancy or the children of 7171 women so treated anytime during gestation in one epidemiological study (Heinonen et al., 1977). The frequency of congenital anomalies was no greater than expected among the infants of a total of 646 women who had been treated with penicillin during the first trimester of pregnancy in two cohorts of another investigation (Jick et al., 1981; Aselton et al., 1985). In a study of 194 infants with major malformations, the frequency of first-trimester penicillin use was no greater than expected (Kullander & Kallen, 1976).

No teratogenic effect was observed among the offspring of rabbits treated during pregnancy with penicillin in doses similar to those used in humans (Brown et al., 1968).

Risk Related to Breast-feeding

Penicillin is excreted in the breast milk in very low concentrations. The amount of penicillin that the nursing infant would be expected to receive is less than 1% of the lowest weight-adjusted therapeutic dose, based on data from 11 lacatating women (Greene et al., 1946).*

Key References

Aselton P, Jick H, Milunsky A, et al.: First-trimester drug use and congenital disorders. Obstet Gynecol 65(4):451-455, 1985.

Brown DM, Harper KH, Palmer AK, Tesh SA: Effect of antibiotics upon pregnancy in the rabbit. Toxicol Appl Pharmacol 12:295, 1968.

Greene HJ, Burkhart B, Hobby GL: Excretion of penicillin in human milk following parturition. Am J Obstet Gynecol 57:732-733, 1946.

Heinonen OP, Slone D, Shapiro S: *Birth Defects and Drugs in Pregnancy.* Littleton, Mass.: John Wright-PSG, 1977, pp 312, 435.

Jick H, Holmes LB, Hunter JR, et al.: First-trimester drug use and congenital disorders. JAMA 246:343-346, 1981.

Kullander S, Kallen B: A prospective study of drugs and pregnancy. 4. Miscellaneous drugs. Acta Obstet Gynecol Scand 55:287-295, 1976.

*This calculation is based on the following assumptions: maternal dose of penicillin: 60-240 mg/d; milk concentration of penicillin: 0.004-0.036 mcg/mL; milk intake by the nursing infant: 150 mL/kg/d; estimated dose of penicillin ingested by the nursing infant: 0.0006-0.005 mg/kg/d; lowest therapeutic dose of penicillin in children: 25 mg/kg/d.

PEPCID® *See* Famotidine

PEPTO-BISMOL® *See* Bismuth Subsalicylate

PEPTOL® *See* Cimetidine

PERIDOL® *See* Haloperidol

PERSANTINE® *See* Dipyridamole

PHENAZODINE® *See* Phenazopyridine

PHENAZOPYRIDINE
(Baridium®, Phenazodine®, Pyridium®)

Phenazopyridine is used to relieve urinary tract pain and irritability in cystitis and urethritis. Phenazopyridine is given orally, usually in a dose of 600 mg/d.

Teratogenic Risk

Magnitude of teratogenic risk to child born after exposure during gestation: *None*

Quality and quantity of data on which risk estimate is based: *Fair to good*

The frequencies of congenital anomalies in general, of major malformations, and of minor anomalies were no greater than expected among the children of 219 women who used phenazopyridine during the first four lunar months or the children of 1109 women who used this medication anytime during pregnancy in one epidemiological study (Heinonen et al., 1977). In another study, the frequency of malformations in infants born to more than 300 women who used phenazopyridine during the first trimester of pregnancy was no greater than expected (Jick et al., 1981; Aselton et al., 1985).

No animal teratology studies of phenazopyridine have been published.

Risk Related to Breast-feeding

No information regarding the distribution of phenazopyridine in breast milk has been published.

Key References

Aselton P, Jick H, Milunsky A, et al.: First-trimester drug use and congenital disorders. Obstet Gynecol 65:451-455, 1985.
Heinonen OP, Slone D, Shapiro S: *Birth Defects and Drugs in Pregnancy*. Littleton, Mass.: John Wright-PSG, 1977, pp 308, 486.
Jick H, Holmes LB, Hunter JR, et al: First-trimester drug use and congenital disorders. JAMA 246:343-346, 1981.

PHENCYCLIDINE
(Angel Dust, PCP)

Phencyclidine is widely used as a "recreational" drug. It was formerly employed as a human and veterinary anesthetic. Phencyclidine may be taken orally, injected intravenously, or smoked. Central nervous system effects resembling ethanol intoxication are seen with doses of 1-5 mg; excitation, confusion, and ataxia with 5-10 mg; and prolonged coma, seizures, and death with doses of 20 mg or more.

Teratogenic Risk

*Magnitude of teratogenic
risk to child born after
exposure during gestation:*   *Minimal*

*Quality and quantity of data
on which risk estimate is based:*   *Poor to fair*

Neurobehavioral alterations have been observed in infants of women who abused phencyclidine during pregnancy (see below), but it is not known if persistent drug-related effects occur.

No malformations were noted in series of 94 and 37 infants of women who abused phencyclidine at some time during pregnancy (Golden et al., 1987; Tabor et al., 1990). No "special physical characteristics" were observed among 83 infants of mothers who abused phencyclidine regularly during pregnancy in another series (Rahbar et al., 1993). Two of 57 infants whose mothers abused phencyclidine during pregnancy looked "morphologically unusual" in yet another series, but no consistent pattern of congenital anomalies was found (Wachsman et al., 1989). One of these children exhibited severe developmental delay. No direct relationship of these abnormalities to the maternal use of phencyclidine during gestation has been established.

Alterations of neonatal neurological function and behavior have frequently been observed among the children of women who abused phencyclidine during pregnancy (Chasnoff et al., 1983; Golden et al., 1987; Wachsman et al., 1989; Tabor et al., 1990; Harry & Howard, 1992; Rahbar et al., 1993). The abnormalities seen include symptoms resembling narcotic withdrawal (jitteriness, abnormal suck, irritability) as well as alterations of tone, abnormal eye movements, sudden outbursts of agitation, and rapid changes in the level of consciousness. Lower than expected weight, length, and head circumference have also been noted among these infants (Wachsman et al., 1989). Various mild behavioral and developmental abnormalities have been found among preschool children whose mothers abused phencyclidine during pregnancy (Harry & Howard, 1992). It is difficult to know if these findings are due to an effect of the phencyclidine or to other socioeconomic or biological factors associated with children of women who abuse drugs during pregnancy.

An increased frequency of limb and cranial defects occurred in the offspring of pregnant rats given phencyclidine in doses 25-30 times those used in humans (Jordan et al., 1978). Teratogenic effects were observed in mice at doses of phencyclidine that were toxic to the mothers (120 times the usual human dose) but not at lower doses (5-100 times the usual human dose) (Goodwin et al., 1980; Marks et al., 1980; Nicholas & Schreiber, 1983). Behavioral abnormalities occur among the offspring of mice and rats treated with phencyclidine during pregnancy in doses 10-20 times those used by humans (Goodwin et al., 1980; Nicholas & Schreiber, 1983; Nabeshima et al., 1987, 1988; Yanai et al., 1992). The relevance of these observations to the risk of maternal abuse of smaller doses of phencyclidine in human pregnancy is unknown.

Risk Related to Breast-feeding

No information regarding the distribution of phencyclidine in breast milk has been published. Although no adverse effects on the nursing infant have been reported, the American Academy of Pediatrics regards phencyclidine to be contraindicated during breast-feeding because of its potential for abuse (Committee on Drugs, American Academy of Pediatrics, 1994).

Key References

Chasnoff IJ, Burns WJ, Hatcher RP, et al.: Phencyclidine: Effects on the fetus and neonate. Dev Pharmacol Ther 6:404-408, 1983.

Committee on Drugs, American Academy of Pediatrics: The transfer of drugs and other chemicals into human milk. Pediatrics 93(1):137-150, 1994.

Golden NL, Kuhnert BR, Sokol RJ, et al.: Neonatal manifestations of maternal phencyclidine exposure. J Perinat Med 15:185-191, 1987.

Goodwin PJ, Perez VJ, Eatwell JC, et al.: Phencyclidine: Effects of chronic administration in the female mouse on gestation, maternal behavior, and the neonates. Psychopharmacology 69:63-67, 1980.

Harry GJ, Howard J: Phencyclidine: Experimental studies in animals and long-term developmental effects on humans. In: Sonderegger TB (ed). *Perinatal Substance Abuse: Research Findings and Clinical Implications.* Baltimore, Md: The Johns Hopkins University Press, 1992. pp 254-278.

Jordan RL, Young TR, Harry GJ: Teratology of phencyclidine in rats: Preliminary studies. Teratology 17:40A, 1978.

Marks TA, Worthy WC, Staples RE: Teratogenic potential of phencyclidine in the mouse. Teratology 21:241-246, 1980.

Nabeshima T, Hiramatsu M, Yamaguchi K, et al.: Effects of prenatal administration of phencyclidine on the learning and memory processes of rat offspring. J Pharmacobio-Dyn 11:816-823, 1988.

Nabeshima T, Yamaguchi K, Hiramatsu M, et al.: Effects of prenatal and perinatal administration of phencyclidine on the behavioral development of rat offspring. Pharmacol Biochem Behav 28:411-418, 1987.

Nicholas JM, Schreiber EC: Phencyclidine exposure and the developing mouse: Behavioral teratological implications. Teratology 28:319-326, 1983.

Rahbar F, Fomufod A, White D, Westney LS: Impact of intrauterine exposure to phencyclidine (PCP) and cocaine on neonates. J Natl Med Assoc 85:349-352, 1993.

Tabor BL, Smith-Wallace T, Yonekura ML: Perinatal outcome associated with PCP versus cocaine use. Am J Drug Alcohol Abuse 16(3 & 4):337-348, 1990.

Wachsman L, Schuetz S, Chan LS, et al.: What happens to babies exposed to phencyclidine (PCP) in utero? Am J Drug Alcohol Abuse 15(10):31-39, 1989.

Yanai J, Avraham Y, Levy S, et al.: Alterations in septohippocampal cholinergic innervations and related behaviors after early exposure to heroin and phencyclidine. Dev Brain Res 69(2):207-214, 1992.

PHENERGAN® *See* Promethazine

PHENOBARBITAL
(Barbita®, Luminal®, Solfoton®)

Phenobarbital is a barbiturate used as a hypnotic, sedative, and anticonvulsant. Phenobarbital is given orally in doses of 30-320 mg/d or parenterally in doses of 30-600 mg/d.

Teratogenic Risk

Magnitude of teratogenic risk to child born after exposure during gestation:	*Minimal to small*
Quality and quantity of data on which risk estimate is based:	*Fair to good*

This assessment is for chronic treatment with phenobarbital in usual therapeutic doses. The risk of teratogenic effects may be greater with a toxic overdose of phenobarbital in pregnancy.

The risk of congenital anomalies is unlikely to be increased in an infant because of maternal treatment during pregnancy with a single or occasional therapeutic dose of phenobarbital.

The frequencies of congenital anomalies in general, of major malformations, of minor anomalies, and of major classes of congenital anomalies were no greater than expected among the children of 1415 women treated with phenobarbital during the first four lunar months of pregnancy in one epidemiological study (Heinonen et al., 1977). There was no increase in the frequency of congenital anomalies among the children of 8037 women treated with phenobarbital anytime during pregnancy in this study.

Several epidemiological studies in which phenobarbital was taken for maternal epilepsy have demonstrated a higher-than-expected frequency of malformations, especially facial clefts and congenital heart disease, among the children (Greenberg et al., 1977; Rothman et al., 1979; Nakane et al., 1980; Robert et al., 1986; Dansky & Finnell,

1991; Waters et al., 1994). One interpretation of the data is that the increased risk of malformations seen in some studies may be due to teratogenic effects of factors associated with the mother's seizure disorder rather than to a specific effect of phenobarbital (Kelly, 1984).

The frequency of congenital anomalies among 250 infants born to epileptic women treated with phenobarbital monotherapy was no greater than that in infants of epileptic women treated with other anticonvulsant monotherapy in a multinational European collaborative study (Bertollini et al., 1987). The risk of congenital anomalies appears to be greater among infants whose mothers were treated with phenobarbital and phenytoin (and/or other anticonvulsants) during pregnancy than among infants of mothers treated with phenobarbital alone (Dansky & Finnell, 1991; Dravet et al., 1992; Lindhout et al., 1992; Tanganelli & Regesta, 1992).

A characteristic pattern of minor dysmorphic features has been observed in children born to women treated with anticonvulsant drugs during pregnancy. The features of this "fetal anticonvulsant syndrome" include nail hypoplasia and midface hypoplasia, depressed nasal bridge, epicanthal folds, and ocular hypertelorism (**please see agent summary on phenytoin for further discussion**). A similar pattern of minor anomalies has been reported in children of epileptic women who were treated only with phenobarbital during pregnancy (Thakker et al., 1991; Jones et al, 1992; Koch et al., 1992).

A small but statistically significant decrease in the birth weight and head circumference was observed among 55 infants born to epileptic women treated with phenobarbital when compared with the infants of nonepileptic women in one study, but a similar effect on head circumference was seen among the infants of epileptic women who were untreated (Mastroiacovo et al., 1988). Smaller than expected head circumferences were seen among six- to 13-year-old children whose mothers had been treated during pregnancy with phenobarbital for a seizure disorder in another study (van der Pol et al., 1991).

The adjusted intelligence quotient at age four years was no different in children exposed to phenobarbital during gestation than in unexposed children in one large epidemiological study (Shapiro et al., 1976). Poor performance in arithmetic and spelling and short attention span were seen more frequently than expected among six- to 13-year-old children whose mothers had been treated with phenobarbital during pregnancy for a seizure disorder in another study (van der Pol et al., 1991). The relative contribution of anticonvulsant drug exposure, maternal seizures during pregnancy, genetic factors, and psychosocial influences on developmental differences that have been observed in children of women treated with anticonvulsants during pregnancy is uncertain (Gaily et al., 1990; Fisher & Vorhees, 1992).

In a follow-up study of children born to women who had participated in a controlled trial of third-trimester phenobarbital therapy for prevention of neonatal jaundice, boys born to women in the treatment group were taller, had smaller testicular volumes, and scored higher on standardized intelligence tests as adolescents (Yaffe & Dorn, 1990). It is not clear whether the associations observed are due to the treatment or to other differences between the treated and untreated groups.

None of three children in one series whose mothers took phenobarbital overdoses in the first trimester of pregnancy had congenital anomalies (Czeizel et al., 1984, 1988). Four of 18 children born to women who had taken overdoses of phenobarbital during the second or third trimester of pregnancy had congenital anomalies (Czeizel et al., 1984, 1988). The problems differed among the affected children and may not be attributable to the phenobarbital.

In animal studies, increased frequencies of cleft palate, cardiovascular malformations, and other congenital anomalies have been observed among the offspring of pregnant mice or rats treated with many times the usual human dose of phenobarbital (Finnell & Dansky, 1991). An increase in the frequency of congenital anomalies was observed among the offspring of mice treated chronically with 8-33 times the human dose of phenobarbital in one study; although the doses used in this investigation were large, they produced blood levels that were near or within the human therapeutic range (Finnell et al., 1987a, b). Some of the affected mice had facial features reminiscent of the "fetal anticonvulsant syndrome" seen among the children of epileptic women treated with phenobarbital during pregnancy.

Chronic maternal use of phenobarbital late in pregnancy has been associated with transient neonatal sedation or withdrawal symptoms in the infants (Koch et al., 1985). Features include hyperactivity, irritability, and tremors.

Maternal treatment with phenobarbital shortly before delivery has been used to prevent intraventricular hemorrhage in premature infants (Kaempf et al., 1990; Paneth & Pinto-Martin, 1991; Barnes & Thompson, 1993).

Risk Related to Breast-feeding

Phenobarbital is excreted in the breast milk. The amount of phenobarbital that the nursing infant would be expected to ingest is between 2.3-163% of the lowest therapeutic dose (Horning et al., 1975; Kaneko et al., 1979).*

Knott et al. (1987) describe a case of withdrawal symptoms in the infant of a woman who took phenobarbital chronically for a seizure disorder following abrupt termination of breast-feeding at seven months. Prior to that time, the infant's saliva level of phenobarbital had been found to approach the therapeutic range of phenobarbital for adults. The infant's withdrawal symptoms resolved following treatment with phenobarbital and gradual withdrawal of the drug over a period of nine months.

The American Academy of Pediatrics lists phenobarbital as a drug that should be used with caution during breast-feeding (Committee on Drugs, American Academy of Pediatrics, 1994).

Key References

Barnes ER, Thompson DF: Antenatal phenobarbital to prevent or minimize intraventricular hemorrhage in the low-birthweight neonate. Ann Pharmacother 27:49-52, 1993.

Bertollini R, Kallen B, Mastroiacovo P, Robert E: Anticonvulsant drugs in monotherapy. Effect on the fetus. Eur J Epidemiol 3(2):164-171, 1987.

Committee on Drugs, American Academy of Pediatrics: The transfer of drugs and other chemicals into human milk. Pediatrics 93(1):137-150, 1994.

Czeizel A, Szentesi I, Szekeres I, et al.: A study of adverse effects on the progeny after intoxication during pregnancy. Arch Toxicol 62:1-7, 1988.

Czeizel A, Szentesi I, Szekeres I, et al.: Pregnancy outcome and health conditions of offspring of self-poisoned pregnant women. Acta Paediatr Hung 25(3):209-236, 1984.

Dansky LV, Finnell RH: Parental epilepsy, anticonvulsant drugs, and reproductive outcome: Epidemiologic and experimental findings spanning three decades; 2: Human studies. Reprod Toxicol 5(4):301-335, 1991.

*This calculation is based on the following assumptions: milk concentration of phenobarbital: 0.5-33 mcg/mL; milk intake by the nursing infant: 150 mL/kg/d; estimated dose of phenobarbital ingested by the nursing infant: 0.07-4.9 mg/kg/d; lowest therapeutic dose of phenobarbital in neonates: 3 mg/kg/d.

Dravet C, Julian C, Legras C, et al.: Epilepsy, antiepileptic drugs, and malformations in children of women with epilepsy: A French prospective cohort study. Neurology 42(Suppl 5):75-82, 1992.

Finnell RH, Dansky LV: Parental epilepsy, anticonvulsant drugs, and reproductive outcome: Epidemiologic and experimental findings spanning three decades; 1: Animal studies. Reprod Toxicol 5:281-299, 1991.

Finnell RH, Shields HE, Chernoff GF: Variable patterns in anticonvulsant drug-induced malformations in mice: Comparisons of phenytoin and phenobarbital. Teratogenesis Carcinog Mutagen 7:541-549, 1987b.

Finnell RH, Shields HE, Taylor SM, Chernoff GF: Strain differences in phenobarbital-induced teratogenesis in mice. Teratology 35:177-185, 1987a.

Fisher JE, Vorhees CV: Developmental toxicity of antiepileptic drugs: Relationship to postnatal dysfunction. Pharmacol Res 26(3):207-221, 1992.

Gaily E, Kantola-Sorsa E, Granstrom M-L: Specific cognitive dysfunction in children with epileptic mothers. Dev Med Child Neurol 32:403-414, 1990.

Greenberg G, Inman WHW, Weatherall JAC, et al.: Maternal drug histories and congenital abnormalities. Br Med J 2:853-856, 1977.

Heinonen OP, Slone D, Shapiro S: *Birth Defects and Drugs in Pregnancy.* Littleton, Mass.: John Wright-PSG, 1977, p 343.

Horning MG, Stillwell WG, Nowlin J, et al.: Identification and quantification of drugs and drug metabolites in human breast milk using GC-MS-COM methods. Mod Probl Paediatr 15:73-79, 1975.

Jones KL, Johnson KA, Chamber CC: Pregnancy outcome in women treated with phenobarbital monotherapy. Teratology 45:452-453, 1992.

Kaempf JW, Porreco R, Molina R, et al.: Antenatal phenobarbital for the prevention of periventricular and intraventricular hemorrhage: A double-blind, randomized, placebo-controlled, multihospital trial. J Pediatr 117:933-938, 1990.

Kaneko S, Sato T, Suzuki K: The levels of anticonvulsants in breast milk. Br J Clin Pharmacol 7:624-627, 1979.

Kelly TE: Teratogenicity of anticonvulsant drugs. I: Review of the literature. Am J Med Genet 19:413-434, 1984.

Knott C, Reynolds F, Clayden G: Infantile spasms on weaning from breast milk containing anticonvulsants. Lancet 2:272-273, 1987.

Koch S, Gopfert-Geyer I, Hauser I, et al.: Neonatal behaviour disturbances in infants of epileptic women treated during pregnancy. Prog Clin Biol Res 163B:453-461, 1985.

Koch S, Losche G, Jager-Roman E, et al.: Major and minor birth malformations and antiepileptic drugs. Neurology 42(Suppl 5):83-88, 1992.

Lindhout D, Meinardi H, Meijer JWA, Nau H: Antiepileptic drugs and teratogenesis in two consecutive cohorts: Changes in prescription policy paralleled by changes in pattern of malformations. Neurology 42(Suppl 5):94-110, 1992.

Mastroiacovo P, Bertollini R, Licata D: Fetal growth in the offspring of epileptic women: Results of an Italian multicentric cohort study. Acta Neurol Scand 78:110-114, 1988.

Nakane Y, Okuma T, Takahashi R, et al.: Multi-institutional study on the teratogenicity and fetal toxicity of antiepileptic drugs: A report of a collaborative study group in Japan. Epilepsia 21:663-680, 1980.

Paneth N, Pinto-Martin J: The epidemiology of germinal matrix/intraventricular hemorrhage. In: Kiely M (ed). *Reproductive and Perinatal Epidemiology*. Boca Raton, Fla: CRC Press, Inc., 1991, pp 371-399.

Robert E, Lofkvist E, Mauguiere F, Robert JM: Evaluation of drug therapy and teratogenic risk in a Rhone-Alpes District population of pregnant epileptic women. Eur Neurol 25:436-443, 1986.

Rothman KJ, Fyler DC, Goldblatt A, Kreidberg MB: Exogenous hormones and other drug exposures of children with congenital heart disease. Am J Epidemiol 109:433-439, 1979.

Shapiro S, Hartz SC, Siskind V, et al.: Anticonvulsants and parental epilepsy in the development of birth defects. Lancet 1:272-275, 1976.

Tanganelli P, Regesta G: Epilepsy, pregnancy, and major birth anomalies: An Italian prospective, controlled study. Neurology 42(Suppl 5):89-93, 1992.

Thakker JC, Kothari SS, Deshmukh CT, et al.: Hypoplasia of nails and phalanges: A teratogenic manifestation of phenobarbitone. Indian Pediatr 28(1):73-75, 1991.

van der Pol MC, Hadders-Algra M, Huisjes HJ, Touwen BCL: Antiepileptic medication in pregnancy: Late effects on the children's central nervous system development. Am J Obstet Gynecol 164:121-128, 1991.

Waters CH, Belai Y, Gott PS, et al.: Outcomes of pregnancy associated with antiepileptic drugs. Arch Neurol 51:250-253, 1994.

Yaffe SJ, Dorn LD: Effects of prenatal treatment with phenobarbital. Dev Pharmacol Ther 15:215-223, 1990.

PHENYLEPHRINE
(Mydfrin®, Neo-Synephrine®, Sinex®)

Phenylephrine is a sympathomimetic agent used as a nasal decongestant and for temporary relief of glaucoma. Phenylepherine is given orally in doses of 20-100 mg/d for these purposes. It is also used parenterally in single doses of 0.5-10 mg to treat hypotensive states.

Teratogenic Risk

Magnitude of teratogenic risk to child born after exposure during gestation:	*None to minimal*
Quality and quantity of data on which risk estimate is based:	*Fair to good*

Epidemiological studies of congenital anomalies among infants born to women treated with phenylephrine during pregnancy have produced inconsistent results. The frequency of congenital anomalies was slightly higher than expected among the children of 1249 women who used phenylephrine during the first four lunar months of pregnancy in one epidemiological study (Heinonen et al., 1977). This association primarily involved minor anomalies, although "malformations of the eye and ear" as a group occurred more often than expected among the children of treated women. The frequency of congenital anomalies was no greater than expected among 4194 infants whose mothers took phenylephrine anytime in pregnancy. Studies such as this one that include multiple comparisons between maternal drug exposures and various birth defect outcomes are expected to show occasional associations with nominal statistical significance purely by chance. In contrast, the frequency of malformations was no greater than expected among a total of more than 225 infants born to women treated with phenylephrine during the first trimester of pregnancy in another investigation (Jick et al., 1981; Aselton et al., 1985).

In a study of 390 children with congenital heart disease, Rothman et al. (1979) observed a slightly higher than expected rate of maternal use of phenylephrine early in pregnancy. This observation was confirmed in a later and more rigorous study by the same investigators of 298 children with congenital heart disease (Zierler & Rothman, 1985). No association between first-trimester maternal use of phenylephrine and congenital heart disease in the offspring was seen in another study (Heinonen et al., 1977). Interpretation of these investigations is complicated by the fact that phenylephrine is usually used as part of a multi-drug combination in treatment of viral illnesses. The possibility exists that the weak associations observed with maternal phenylephrine use, if real, might be due to another drug or the underlying illness.

Increased frequencies of fetal growth retardation and premature delivery have been reported in the offspring of rabbits treated chronically during gestation with phenylephrine in doses equivalent to those used in humans (Shabanah et al., 1969a, b). Similar doses of phenylephrine, when administered to sheep late in pregnancy, produced acidosis and hypoxemia in the fetuses (Cottle et al., 1982). These effects have not been studied in human pregnancies.

Risk Related to Breast-feeding

No information regarding the distribution of phenylephrine in breast milk has been published.

Key References

Aselton P, Jick H, Milunsky A, et al.: First-trimester drug use and congenital disorders. Obstet Gynecol 65:451-455, 1985.

Cottle MKW, Van Petten GR, van Muyden P: Effects of phenylephrine and sodium salicylate on maternal and fetal cardiovascular indices and blood oxygenation in sheep. Am J Obstet Gynecol 143:170-176, 1982.

Heinonen OP, Slone D, Shapiro S: *Birth Defects and Drugs in Pregnancy*. Littleton, Mass.: John Wright-PSG, 1977, pp 345-347, 439.

Jick H, Holmes LB, Hunter JR, et al.: First-trimester drug use and congenital disorders. JAMA 246:343-346, 1981.

Rothman KJ, Fyler DC, Goldblatt A, Kreidberg MB: Exogenous hormones and other drug exposures of children with congenital heart disease. Am J Epidemiol 109:433-439, 1979.

Shabanah EH, Tricomi V, Suarez JR: Effect of epinephrine on fetal growth and the length of gestation. Surg Gynecol Obstet 129:341-343, 1969a.

Shabanah EH, Tricomi V, Suarez JR: Fetal environment and its influence on fetal development. Surg Gynecol Obstet 129:556-564, 1969b.

Zierler S, Rothman KJ: Congenital heart disease in relation to maternal use of Bendectin and other drugs in early pregnancy. N Engl J Med 313:347-352, 1985.

PHENYLPROPANOLAMINE
(Acutrim®, Dexatrim®, Stay-Trim®)

Phenylpropanolamine is a sympathomimetic agent given for relief of nasal congestion. Phenylpropanolamine has also been used for urinary incontinence and as an anorectic. The drug is given orally in doses of 50-150 mg/d.

Teratogenic Risk

Magnitude of teratogenic risk to child born after exposure during gestation:	*Unlikely*
Quality and quantity of data on which risk estimate is based:	*Fair to good*

Therapeutic doses of phenylpropanolamine are unlikely to pose a substantial teratogenic risk, but the data are insufficient to state that there is no risk.

The frequency of major malformations was not increased among the children of 726 women who took phenylpropanolamine during the first four lunar months of pregnancy in one epidemiological study, but increased frequencies of minor anomalies and of eye and ear defects were observed (Heinonen et al., 1977). Studies such as this one that include multiple comparisons between maternal drug exposures and various birth defect outcomes are expected to show occasional associations with nominal statistical significance purely by chance. The frequency of congenital anomalies was no greater than expected among the infants of 2489 women who took phenylpropanolamine anytime during pregnancy in this investigation. The frequency of malformations was not increased among a total of more than 350 infants born to women who took phenylpropanolamine during the first trimester of pregnancy in two cohorts of another epidemiological study (Jick et al., 1981; Aselton et al., 1985). No significant association was observed with maternal phenylpropanolamine use during the first trimester of pregnancy in a study of 76 children with gastroschisis (Werler et al., 1992).

No animal teratology studies of the phenylpropanolamine have been published.

Risk Related to Breast-feeding

No information regarding the distribution of phenylpropanolamine in breast milk has been published.

Key References

Aselton P, Jick H, Milunsky A, et al.: First-trimester drug use and congenital disorders. Obstet Gynecol 65:451-455, 1985.

Heinonen OP, Slone D, Shapiro S: *Birth Defects and Drugs in Pregnancy*. Littleton, Mass.: John Wright-PSG, 1977, pp 346-347, 349, 351, 439, 477, 491.

Jick H, Holmes LB, Hunter JR, et al.: First-trimester drug use and congenital disorders. JAMA 246:343-346, 1981.

Werler MM, Mitchell AA, Shapiro S: First trimester maternal medication use in relation to gastroschisis. Teratology 45:361-367, 1992. [E]

PHENYTOIN
(Dilantin®)

Phenytoin is an anticonvulsant administered orally or intravenously in the treatment of seizure disorders. Phenytoin is also used to treat digitalis-induced cardiac arrhythmias. The usual oral dosage is 300-600 mg/d; intravenous doses up to 18 mg/kg/d are sometimes used in the treatment of status epilepticus. A serum concentration of 10-20 mcg/mL is considered to be therapeutic in most patients.

Teratogenic Risk

*Magnitude of teratogenic
risk to child born after
exposure during gestation:*   *Small to moderate*

Quality and quantity of data
on which risk estimate is based: *Fair to good*

> *This assessment is based on data for continuous treatment of maternal seizure disorders with phenytoin throughout pregnancy. No data are available on the effects of acute exposure.*

A "fetal hydantoin syndrome," which consists of an unusual and characteristic pattern of anomalies, has been described in about 10% of infants born to epileptic women who took phenytoin during pregnancy (Kelly, 1984; Kelly et al., 1984a; Hanson, 1986). Typical features of this syndrome include apparent ocular hypertelorism, flat nasal bridge, and nail hypoplasia. None of these features is of great clinical importance, but some authors believe that cleft palate, congenital heart disease, microcephaly, developmental delay, and prenatal and postnatal growth retardation also occur as occasional manifestations of fetal hydantoin syndrome (Bracken, 1986; Hanson, 1986; Friis, 1989; Adams et al., 1990). This conclusion is controversial, however. Other authorities believe that most of the anomalies that occur more frequently among the children of epileptic women taking phenytoin during pregnancy than among the children of normal untreated women are due to underlying familial factors or effects of maternal epilepsy per se rather than to the teratogenic action of phenytoin (Kelly, 1984; Kelly et al., 1984a, b; Gaily et al., 1988a, b, 1990; Gaily & Granstrom, 1989, 1992; Kaneko, 1991; Koch et al., 1992). Distal digital hypoplasia is one feature in the children that does appear to be due to maternal phenytoin treatment during pregnancy (Kelly et al., 1984a; D'Souza et al., 1990; Gaily, 1990; Gaily & Granstrom, 1992; Koch et al., 1992).

Although many large epidemiologic studies of the offspring of epileptic women have been published, currently available data are incapable of resolving this controversy because assessment of the effects of phenytoin exposure is confounded by many other factors (Kelly, 1984; Hanson, 1986; Schardein, 1993). Among these confounders are the facts that most women with seizures are treated with some anticonvulsant drug, that many women are treated with more than one anticonvulsant at a time, that women who are not treated or are treated with a single agent probably have milder disease, and that phenytoin exposure rarely occurs in women without seizures.

This much seems clear: The frequency of major malformations among the children of epileptic women treated with phenytoin during pregnancy is about twice as great as the frequency of such anomalies in the general population (Kelly, 1984; Delgado-Escueta & Janz, 1992; Dravet et al.,

1992; Lindhout & Omtzigt, 1992). The risk of malformations in the offspring is probably even greater if the mother requires treatment with other anticonvulsants in addition to phenytoin during pregnancy (Lindhout et al., 1984; Kaneko et al., 1988; Lindhout & Omtzigt, 1992; Tanganelli & Regesta, 1992) or if the mother has previously had a child with features of fetal hydantoin syndrome (Van Dyke et al., 1988). Genetic factors in the fetus may be important in determining whether or not congenital anomalies occur when a pregnant epileptic woman is treated with phenytoin (Buehler et al., 1990).

Full-scale IQs, performance IQs, and Visual Motor Integration Test scores were significantly lower among 20 four- to eight-year-old children whose mothers took phenytoin during pregnancy than among controls (Vanoverloop et al., 1992). None of the children tested in this study was mentally retarded. Global IQ averaged ten points lower than controls in a study of 34 eighteen- to thirty-six-month-old children of mothers who were treated with phenytoin during pregnancy (Scolnik et al., 1994).

Prenatal diagnosis by means of ultrasound examination has been advocated for pregnant epileptic women who are being treated with anticonvulsant medication, but such screening does not appear to be very sensitive for the kinds of anomalies most often seen in the children of these women (Wladimiroff et al., 1988; Delgado-Escueta & Janz, 1992; Lindhout & Omtzigt, 1992).

Phenytoin, in doses producing therapeutic blood levels or in greater doses, is teratogenic in mice, rats, and rabbits (Finnell & Dansky, 1991). Cleft palate, cardiac defects, and skeletal anomalies are the malformations most frequently observed. Frequent embryonic death but no increase in fetal malformations was observed among pregnant rhesus monkeys treated with phenytoin in doses that caused maternal toxicity even though they produced blood levels only 1-2 times those considered to be therapeutic in humans (Hendrie et al., 1990). Behavioral alterations have been demonstrated among the offspring of rats and rhesus monkeys treated during pregnancy with phenytoin in doses that produce blood levels similar to those used therapeutically in humans (Adams et al., 1990).

Exposure to phenytoin during embryogenesis has also been associated with an increased risk of tumor development in humans; neuroblastoma and other neoplasms have been reported in such children with surprisingly high frequency (Lipson & Bale, 1985; Koren et al., 1989; Al-Shammri et al., 1992). Malignancy in childhood is rare, however, and the risk of neoplasia in a child who was exposed to phenytoin during gestation is probably small.

Perinatal and neonatal hemorrhage associated with deficiency of vitamin K-dependent clotting factors has been observed in infants of women treated with phenytoin during pregnancy (Gimovsky & Petrie, 1986; McNinch & Tripp, 1991). Administration of vitamin K to these infants appears to be useful both prophylactically and therapeutically.

Risk Related to Breast-feeding

Phenytoin is excreted into breast milk. The amount of phenytoin that the nursing infant would be expected to ingest is between 1-15% of the lowest therapeutic dose (Kaneko et al., 1979, 1981; Chaplin et al., 1982; Steen et al., 1982).* No adverse effects in the infants were found in these studies.

Serum levels of phenytoin in six infants were found to be between 0-2% of the lowest therapeutic serum level in adults (Steen et al., 1982).[†]

Both the American Academy of Pediatrics (Committee on Drugs, American Academy of Pediatrics, 1994) and the WHO Working Group on Drugs and Human Lactation (1988) regard phenytoin to be safe to use while breast-feeding.

Key References

Adams J, Vorhees CV, Middaugh LD: Developmental neurotoxicity of anticonvulsants: Human and animal evidence on phenytoin. Neurotoxicol Teratol 12:203-214, 1990.

Al-Shammri S, Guberman A, Hsu E: Neuroblastoma and fetal exposure to phenytoin in a child without dysmorphic features. Can J Neurol Sci 19:243-245, 1992.

Bracken MB: Drug use in pregnancy and congenital heart disease in offspring. N Engl J Med 314:1120, 1986.

Buehler BA, Delimont D, van Waes M, Finnell RH: Prenatal prediction of risk of the fetal hydantoin syndrome. N Engl J Med 322:1567-1572, 1990.

Chaplin S, Sanders GL, Smith JM: Drug excretion in human breast milk. Adv Drug React Ac Pois Rev 1:255-287, 1982.

Committee on Drugs, American Academy of Pediatrics: The transfer of drugs and other chemicals into human milk. Pediatrics 93(1):137-150, 1994.

*This calculation is based on the following assumptions: maternal dose of phenytoin: 100-700 mg/d; milk concentration of phenytoin: 0.26-4 mcg/mL; milk intake by the nursing infant: 150 mL/kg/d; estimated dose of phenytoin ingested by the nursing infant: 0.04-0.6 mg/kg/d; lowest therapeutic dose of phenytoin in infants: 4 mg/kg/d.

[†]Infant serum levels of phenytoin: 0.0-0.18 mcg/mL; lowest therapeutic serum level of phenytoin in adults: 10 mcg/mL.

Delgado-Escueta AV, Janz D: Consensus guidelines: Preconception counseling, management, and care of the pregnant woman with epilepsy. Neurology 42(Suppl 5):149-160, 1992.

Dravet C, Julian C, Legras C, et al.: Epilepsy, antiepileptic drugs, and malformations in children of women with epilepsy: A French prospective cohort study. Neurology 42(Suppl 5):75-82, 1992.

D'Souza SW, Robertson IG, Donnai D, Mawer G: Fetal phenytoin exposure, hypoplastic nails and jitteriness. Arch Dis Child 65:320-324, 1990.

Finnell RH, Dansky LV: Parental epilepsy, anticonvulsant drugs, and reproductive outcome: Epidemiologic and experimental findings spanning three decades; 1: Animal studies. Reprod Toxicol 5:281-299, 1991.

Friis ML: Facial clefts and congenital heart defects in children of parents with epilepsy: Genetic and environmental etiologic factors. Acta Neurol Scand 79:433-459, 1989.

Gaily E, Granstrom M-L: A transient retardation of early postnatal growth in drug-exposed children of epileptic mothers. Epilepsy Res 4:147-155, 1989.

Gaily E, Granstrom M-L: Minor anomalies in children of mothers with epilepsy. Neurology 42(Suppl 5):128-131, 1992.

Gaily E, Granstrom M-L, Hiilesmaa V, Bardy A: Minor anomalies in offspring of epileptic mothers. J Pediatr 112:520-529, 1988a.

Gaily E, Kantola-Sorsa E, Granstrom M-L: Intelligence of children of epileptic mothers. J Pediatr 113:677-684, 1988b.

Gaily EK, Granstrom M-L, Hiilesmaa VK, Bardy AH: Head circumference in children of epileptic mothers: Contributions of drug exposure and genetic background. Epilepsy Res 5:217-222, 1990.

Gimovsky ML, Petrie R: Maternal anticonvulsants and fetal hemorrhage. A report of two cases. J Reprod Med 31:61-62, 1986.

Hanson JW: Teratogen update: Fetal hydantoin effects. Teratology 33:349-353, 1986.

Hendrie TA, Rowland JR, Binkerd PE, Hendrickx AG: Developmental toxicity and pharmacokinetics of phenytoin in the rhesus macaque: An interspecies comparison. Reprod Toxicol 4:257-266, 1990.

Kaneko S: Antiepileptic drug therapy and reproductive consequences: Functional and morphologic effects. Reprod Toxicol 5:179-198, 1991.

Kaneko S, Otani K, Fukushima Y, et al.: Teratogenicity of antiepileptic drugs. Analysis of possible risk factors. Epilepsia 29(4):459-467, 1988.

Kaneko S, Sato T, Suzuki K: The levels of anticonvulsants in breast milk. Br J Clin Pharmacol 7:624-629, 1979.

Kaneko S, Suzuki K, Sato T, et al.: The problems of anticonvulsant medication at the neonatal period: Is breast feeding advisable? In: Janz D et al. (eds). Epilepsy, Pregnancy and the Child. New York: Raven Press, 1981, pp 343-347.

Kelly TE: Teratogenicity of anticonvulsant drugs. I: Review of the literature. Am J Med Genet 19:413-434, 1984.

Kelly TE, Edwards P, Rein M, et al.: Teratogenicity of anticonvulsant drugs. II: A prospective study. Am J Med Genet 19:435-443, 1984a.

Kelly TE, Rein M, Edwards P: Teratogenicity of anticonvulsant drugs. IV: The association of clefting and epilepsy. Am J Med Genet 19:451-458, 1984b.

Koch S, Losche G, Jager-Roman E, et al.: Major and minor birth malformations and antiepileptic drugs. Neurology 42(Suppl 5):83-88, 1992.

Koren G, Demitrakoudis D, Weksberg R, et al.: Neuroblastoma after prenatal exposure to phenytoin: Cause and effect? Teratology 40:157-162, 1989.

Lindhout D, Hoppener RJEA, Meinardi H: Teratogenicity of antiepileptic drug combinations with special emphasis on epoxidation (of carbamazepine). Epilepsia 25:77-83, 1984.

Lindhout D, Omtzigt JGC: Pregnancy and the risk of teratogenicity. Epilepsia 33(Suppl 4):S41-S48, 1992.

Lipson A, Bale P: Ependymoblastoma associated with prenatal exposure to diphenylhydantoin and methylphenobarbitone. Cancer 55:1859-1862, 1985.

McNinch AW, Tripp JH: Haemorrhagic disease of the newborn in the British Isles: Two year prospective study. BMJ 303:1105-1109, 1991.

Schardein JL: Chemically Induced Birth Defects. New York: Marcel Dekker, 1993, pp 169-173.

Scolnik D, Nulman I, Rovet J, et al.: Neurodevelopment of children exposed in utero to phenytoin and carbamazepine monotherapy. JAMA 271:767-770, 1994.

Steen B, Rane A, Lonnerholm G, et al.: Phenytoin excretion in human breast milk and plasma levels in nursed infants. Ther Drug Monit 4:331-334, 1982.

Tanganelli P, Regesta G: Epilepsy, pregnancy, and major birth anomalies: An Italian prospective, controlled study. Neurology 42(Suppl 5):89-93, 1992.

Van Dyke DC, Hodge SE, Heide F, Hill LR: Family studies in fetal phenytoin exposure. J Pediatr 113:301-306, 1988.

Vanoverloop D, Schnelll RR, Harvey EA, Holmes LB: The effects of prenatal exposure to phenytoin and other anticonvulsants on intellectual function at 4 to 8 years of age. Neurotoxicol Teratol 14:(5):329-335, 1992.

WHO Working Group on Drugs and Human Lactation. In: Bennet PN (ed). *Drugs and Human Lactation*. Amsterdam: Elsevier, 1988, pp 331-332.

Wladimiroff JW, Stewart PA, Reuss A, et al.: The role of ultrasound in the early diagnosis of fetal structural defects following maternal anticonvulsant therapy. Ultrasound Med Biol 14(8):657-660, 1988.

PILOCAR® *See* Pilocarpine

PILOCARPINE
(Akarpine®, Pilocar®, Salagen®)

Pilocarpine is a muscarinic parasympathomimetic agent. Ophthalmic preparations are used to induce pupillary contraction and to decrease intraocular pressure in glaucoma and retinal detachment.

Teratogenic Risk

Magnitude of teratogenic risk to child born after exposure during gestation:	*Undetermined*
Quality and quantity of data on which risk estimate is based:	*None*

No epidemiological studies of congenital anomalies in infants born to women treated with pilocarpine during pregnancy have been reported.

Behavioral alterations were observed among the offspring of pregnant rats treated parenterally with 5 mg/kg of body weight per day of pilocarpine (Watanabe et al., 1985). The relevance of this observation to the therapeutic use of pilocarpine in human pregnancy is unknown.

Risk Related to Breast-feeding

No information regarding the distribution of pilocarpine in breast milk has been published.

Key References

Watanabe T, Matsuhashi K, Takayama S: Study on the postnatal neurobehavioral development in rats treated prenatally with drugs acting on the autonomic nervous systems. Folia Pharmacol Jpn 85:79-90, 1985.

PIROXICAM
(Feldene®, Novo-Pirocam®, Nu-Pirox®

Piroxicam is a nonsteroidal anti-inflammatory agent with antipyretic action. It is used in the treatment of arthritis and other musculoskeletal disorders. The drug is given orally, usually in a dose of 20 mg/d. Piroxicam is eliminated from the body slowly; the half-life averages about 50 hours.

Teratogenic Risk

*Magnitude of teratogenic
risk to child born after
exposure during gestation:*   *Undetermined*

*Quality and quantity of data
on which risk estimate is based:*   *Poor*

Maternal treatment with piroxicam late in pregnancy may be associated with premature closure of the fetal ductus arteriosus.

There are no published epidemiological studies of congenital anomalies among children of women treated with piroxicam during pregnancy.

Studies in rats and rabbits suggest that treatment of pregnant women with proxicam in usual therapeutic doses is unlikely to increase the children's risk of malformations greatly (Sakai et al., 1980; Perraud et al., 1984).

In rats, piroxicam administered in late pregnancy was found to delay delivery (Powell & Cochrane, 1982). The effect of piroxicam on human parturition has not been studied, but other nonsteroidal anti-inflammatory agents may delay delivery in humans.

Constriction or closure of the ductus arteriosus was observed in fetal rats exposed to 1-10 times the human therapeutic dose of piroxicam late in pregnancy (Momma et al., 1984). Treatment of women late in pregnancy with chemically related nonsteroidal anti-inflammatory agents has been associated with premature closure of the ductus arteriosus in utero and pulmonary hypertension in their infants. *Please see agent summary on indomethacin for more information on this point.*

Risk Related to Breast-feeding

Piroxicam is excreted into breast milk in small quantities. The amount of piroxicam that the nursing infant would be expected to receive is between <1-7.3% of the lowest pediatric dose, based on data from six lactating women (Ostensen, 1983; Ostensen et al., 1988).*

Both the American Academy of Pediatrics (Committee on Drugs, American Academy of Pediatrics, 1994) and the WHO Working Group on Drugs and Human Lactation (1988) consider piroxicam to be safe to use during breast-feeding, although the latter recommend avoidance of breast-feeding if piroxicam is taken for long periods of time.

Key References

Committee on Drugs, American Academy of Pediatrics: The transfer of drugs and other chemicals into the human milk. Pediatrics 93(1):137-150, 1994.

Momma K, Hagiwara H, Konishi T: Constriction of fetal ductus arteriosus by non-steroidal anti-inflammatory drugs: Study of additional 34 drugs. Prostaglandins 28:527-536, 1984.

Ostensen M: Piroxicam in human breast milk. Eur J Clin Pharmacol 25:829-830, 1983.

*This calculation is based on the following assumptions: maternal dose of piroxicam: 20-40 mg/d; milk concentration of piroxicam: 0.027-0.22 mcg/mL; milk intake by the nursing infant: 150 mL/kg/d; estimated dose of piroxicam ingested by the nursing infant: 0.004-0.033 mg/kg/d; lowest pediatric dose of piroxicam: 0.45 mg/kg/d.

Ostensen M, Matheson I, Laufen H: Piroxicam in breast milk after long-term treatment. Eur J Clin Pharmacol 35:567-569, 1988.

Perraud J, Stadler J, Kessedjlan MJ, Monro AM: Reproductive studies with the anti-inflammatory agent, piroxicam: Modification of classical protocols. Toxicology 30:59-63, 1984.

Powell JG, Cochrane RL: The effects of a number of non-steroidal anti-inflammatory compounds on parturition in the rat. Prostaglandins 23:469-488, 1982.

Sakai T, Ohtsuki I, Noguchi Y: [Reproduction studies of piroxicam. Effects of piroxicam on fertility.] Yakuri To Chiryo 8:4655-4671, 1980.

WHO Working Group on Drugs and Human Lactation. In: Bennet PN (ed). *Drugs and Human Lactation*. Amsterdam: Elsevier, 1988, pp 311-312.

POLYCILLIN® *See* Ampicillin

POLYCITRA® *See* Citrate

POLYMOX® *See* Amoxicillin

POLYMYXIN B
(Aerosporin®)

Polymyxin B is a polypeptide antibiotic. It is used topically and in ophthalmic preparations. Polymyxin B may be absorbed after ophthalmic administration, but systemic absorption is minimal after topical use.

Teratogenic Risk

Magnitude of teratogenic risk to child born after exposure during gestation:	*Undetermined*
Quality and quantity of data on which risk estimate is based:	*None*

A small risk cannot be excluded, but a substantial risk of congenital anomalies in the children of women treated locally with polymyxin B during pregnancy is unlikely.

No epidemiological studies of infants born after maternal polymyxin B treatment during pregnancy have been reported.

No adequate teratology studies of polymyxin B in experimental animals have been published.

Risk Related to Breast-feeding

No information regarding the distribution of polymyxin B in breast milk has been published.

Key References

None available.

POT *See* Marijuana

POTASSIUM CHLORIDE
(K-10®, Kaochlor-10®, Slow-K®)

Potassium is an essential element, the concentration of which is closely regulated in body fluids. Potassium chloride is used for replenishment of potassium depletion due to factors such as malnutrition, dehydration, or diuretic therapy. For this purpose potassium chloride is given orally in a dose of 1200-7500 mg (16-100 mEq of potassium) per day. Doses up to 30,000 mg (400 mEq of potassium) per day are sometimes given intravenously for severe depletion. Potassium chloride is also used as a dietary substitute for table salt.

Teratogenic Risk

*Magnitude of teratogenic
risk to child born after
exposure during gestation:*   *None*

*Quality and quantity of data
on which risk estimate is based:*   *Poor*

No epidemiological studies of congenital anomalies in children of women who took large amounts of potassium chloride during pregnancy have been reported.

The frequency of malformations among the offspring of mice treated with 0.6-60 times the usual human dose of potassium chloride during pregnancy was no greater than expected (Anonymous, 1975). Increased rates of fetal death and growth retardation were seen in association with evidence of maternal toxicity when pregnant rats were treated with about 10 times the human therapeutic dose of potassium chloride (Hayasaka et al., 1990).

Direct injection of potassium chloride into the fetal thorax, pericardium, or heart has been used for selective fetocide in multifetal pregnancies or in association with second trimester pregnancy termination (Evans et al., 1990; Wapner et al., 1990; Isada et al., 1992; Berkowitz et al., 1993).

Risk Related to Breast-feeding

Potassium chloride is a natural constituent of human milk (Bates & Prentice, 1994). The effect of maternal supplementation with potassium chloride on the nursing infant is unknown.

Key References

Anonymous: Teratologic evaluation of FDA 73-78, potassium chloride, in mice and rats. NTIS (National Technical Information Service) Report/PB-245 528, 1975.

Bates C, Prentice A: Breast milk as a source of vitamins, essential minerals and trace elements. Pharmacol Ther 62:193-220, 1994.

Berkowitz RL, Lynch L, Lapinsko R, Bergh P: First-trimester transabdominal multifetal pregnancy reduction: A report of two hundred complete cases. Am J Obstet Gynecol 169:17-21, 1993.

Evans MI, May M, Drugan A, et al.: Selective termination. Clinical experience and residual risks. Am J Obstet Gynecol 162(6):1568-1575, 1990.

Hayasaka I, Murakami K, Kato Z, et al.: Preventive effects of maternal electrolyte supplementation on azosemide-induced skeletal malformations in rats. Environ Med 34:61-67, 1990.

Isada NB, Pryde PG, Johnson MP, et al.: Fetal intracardiac potassium chloride injection to avoid the hopeless resuscitation of an abnormal abortus: I. Clinical issues. Obstet Gynecol 80:296-299, 1992.

Wapner RJ, Davis GH, Johnson A, et al.: Selective reduction of multifetal pregnancies. Lancet 335:90-93, 1990.

PRAXITEN® *See* Oxazepam

PRAZENE® *See* Prazepam

PRAZEPAM
(Centrax®, Prazene®)

Prazepam is a benzodiazepine minor tranquilizer used to treat anxiety. Prazepam is given orally in doses of 20-60 mg/d.

Teratogenic Risk

Magnitude of teratogenic risk to child born after exposure during gestation:	*Undetermined*
Quality and quantity of data on which risk estimate is based:	*Poor*

No epidemiological studies of malformations in the children of women treated with prazepam during pregnancy have been published.

In one study, the frequency of congenital anomalies was increased among the offspring of rats treated with prazepam during pregnancy in doses 1700-3300 times those used clinically, but such doses were toxic to the mothers (Kuriyama et al., 1978). The frequency of congenital anomalies was not increased in the offspring of pregnant rats treated with 40-400 times the usual human dose. Similarly, the frequency of malformations was not increased among the offspring of rabbits treated with 8-80 times the usual human dose of prazepam during pregnancy (Ota et al., 1979). The finding of an adverse fetal effect at very high maternally toxic doses in rats is unlikely to be relevant to therapeutic use of prazepam in human pregnancy.

Please see agent summary on diazepam for information on a closely related drug that has been more thoroughly studied.

Risk Related to Breast-feeding

Prazepam was not detected in the breast milk of five lactating mothers following oral administration of the compound; however, measurable amounts of one of the active metabolites of prazepam, N-descyclopropylmethylprazepam, were found in the breast milk (Brodie et al., 1981). On the basis of these data, the amount of N-descyclopropylmethylprazepam that the nursing infant would be expected to ingest is between 1.3-2.8% of the lowest dose that would be expected to have a therapeutic effect.*

The WHO Working Group on Drugs and Human Lactation (1988) regards low doses of prazepam to be safe to take while breast-feeding.

Key References

Brodie RR, Chasseaud LF, Taylor T: Concentrations of N-descyclopropylmethylprazepam in whole-blood plasma, and milk after administration of prazepam to humans. Biopharm Drug Dispos 2:59-68, 1981.

Kuriyama T, Nishigaki K, Ota T, et al.: [Safety studies of prazepam (K-373). VI. Teratological study in rats.] Oyo Yakuri (Pharmacometrics) 15:797-811, 1978.

Ota T, Okubo M, Kuriyama T, et al.: [Safety studies of prazepam (K-373). VIII. Teratological study in rabbits.] Oyo Yakuri (Pharmacometrics) 17:673-681, 1979.

WHO Working Group on Drugs and Human Lactation. In: Bennet PN (ed). *Drugs and Human Lactation*. Amsterdam: Elsevier, 1988, pp 369-370.

*This calculation is based on the following assumptions: maternal dose of prazepam: 60 mg/d; milk concentration of N-descyclopropylmethylprazepam: 0.04-0.09 mcg/mL; milk intake by the nursing infant: 150 mL/kg/d; estimated dose of N-descyclopropylmethylprazepam ingested by the nursing infant, assuming similar bioavailability, activity, and molecular weight: 0.006-0.01 mg/kg/d; lowest therapeutic dose of prazepam in adults: 0.47 mg/kg/d.

PRAZOSIN
(Minipress®)

Prazosin is an α_1-adrenergic blocking agent that is given orally to treat hypertension. The usual dose is 2-15 mg/d.

Teratogenic Risk

*Magnitude of teratogenic
risk to child born after
exposure during gestation:*   *Undetermined*

*Quality and quantity of data
on which risk estimate is based:*   *Poor*

No epidemiological studies of congenital anomalies among infants born to women treated with prazosin during pregnancy have been reported.

Studies in mice, rats, rabbits, and monkeys suggest that treatment of pregnant women with prazosin in usual therapeutic doses is unlikely to increase the children's risk of malformations greatly (Noguchi & Ohwaki, 1979; Mahalik & Hitner, 1992; USP DI, 1995).

Risk Related to Breast-feeding

Prazosin is excreted in breast milk in low concentrations (USP DI, 1995), although this has not been quantitated in published reports.

Key References

Mahalik MP, Hitner HW: Antagonism of cocaine-induced fetal anomalies by prazosin and diltiazem in mice. Reprod Toxicol 6:161-169, 1992.

Noguchi Y, Ohwaki Y: Reproductive and teratologic studies with prazosin hydrochloride in rats and rabbits. Oyo Yakuri 17:57-62, 1979.

USP DI: Prazosin. In: *USP DI (USP Dispensing Information), Volume 1. Drug Information for the Health Care Professional*, 15th ed. Rockville, Md.: The US Pharmacopeial Convention, 1995, p 2295.

PREDNISONE/PREDNISOLONE
(Deltasone®, Meticorten®, Orasone®)

Prednisone and prednisolone are synthetic glucocorticoids. Prednisone is biologically inert; it is converted to prednisolone, a biologically active compound, in the liver. Prednisone and prednisolone are used to treat a variety of allergic and inflammatory conditions. Prednisone is given orally but prednisolone may be given either orally or parenterally. The usual systemic dose of either agent is 5-60 mg/d, but doses up to 250 mg/d are sometimes used. Systemic absorption of prednisolone can occur from ophthalmic preparations, but the amount administered is usually small.

Teratogenic Risk

Magnitude of teratogenic
risk to child born after
exposure during gestation: *Unlikely*

Quality and quantity of data
on which risk estimate is based: *Poor to fair*

Therapeutic doses of prednisone and prednisolone are unlikely to pose a substantial teratogenic risk, but the data are insufficient to state that there is no risk.

The frequency of malformations was not increased among the children of 43 women who had been treated with prednisone during the first four lunar months of pregnancy in one epidemiological study (Heinonen et al., 1977). Malformations do not appear unusually frequent among the infants of women treated with prednisone during pregnancy in uncontrolled series of 20-40 livebirths (Nielsen et al., 1984; O'Donnell et al., 1985; Muirhead et al., 1992; Pollard et al., 1992; TambyRaja, 1993; Haugen et al., 1994).

Congenital immunodeficiency and lymphopenia have been reported in two infants born to women who had been treated with prednisone and azathioprine during pregnancy (Cote et al., 1974; DeWitte et al., 1984). It is uncertain whether or not the maternal immunosuppressive therapy played a role in development of this disease in the infants.

A high frequency of perinatal death has been observed in some series of women treated throughout gestation with prednisone or prednisolone (Walsh & Clark, 1967; Warrell & Taylor, 1968; Brown et al., 1991), but the perinatal death cannot be attributed to maternal steroid therapy because these women had serious illnesses requiring treatment, often with several drugs. Premature delivery and fetal growth retardation are also unsually frequent in some series of women treated during pregnancy with prednisone or prednisolone (Reinisch et al., 1978; Pirson et al., 1985; Petri et al., 1992; Rayburn, 1992; Silver et al., 1993), but the same confounding factors affect interpretation of the studies.

Fetal growth retardation occurs with increased frequency among the offspring of mice and rats treated in pregnancy with prednisone or prednisolone in doses within or above the human therapeutic range (Reinisch et al., 1978; Gandelman & Rosenthal, 1981; Gandelman & Guerriero, 1982; Neumann et al., 1986). Dose-dependent constriction of the ductus arteriosus was observed among the offspring of pregnant rats injected with prednisolone near term in doses 10-1000 times those used in humans (Momma et al., 1981).

Prednisolone, like other corticosteroids, causes an increased frequency of cleft palate in the offspring of pregnant mice treated with 1-40 times the human therapeutic dose (Pinsky & DiGeorge, 1965; Ballard et al., 1977). Increased frequencies of cleft palate are also observed among the offspring of pregnant rabbits and hamsters treated with prednisolone in doses respectively <1-2 and 80-240 times that used in humans (Walker, 1967; Shah & Kilistoff, 1976). An increase in the frequency of genital anomalies has been observed among the offspring of mice treated with 2-10 times the human therapeutic dose of prednisolone during pregnancy (Ballard et al., 1977; Gandelman & Rosenthal, 1981). Developmental and other behavioral alterations have been noted in mice born to mothers treated during pregnancy with prednisone or prednisolone in doses 1-4 times those used in humans (Reinisch et al., 1980; Gandelman & Rosenthal, 1981; Gandelman & Guerriero, 1982). The relevance, if any, of these observations to maternal treatment with prednisone or prednisolone in human pregnancy is unknown.

Risk Related to Breast-feeding

Prednisone and its active metabolite, prednisolone, are excreted in breast milk in low concentrations (Katz & Duncan, 1975; McKenzie et al., 1975; Ost et al., 1985; Greenberger et al., 1993). The amount of prednisone and prednisolone that the nursing infant would be expected to ingest is <1 and between <1-24% of the lowest therapeutic doses of prednisone and prednisolone, respectively, in children (Katz & Duncan, 1975; Ost et al., 1985).*

The American Academy of Pediatrics regards prednisone to be safe to use while breast-feeding (Committee on Drugs, American Academy of Pediatrics, 1994).

Key References

Ballard PD, Hearney EF, Smith MB: Comparative teratogenicity of selected glucocorticoids applied ocularly in mice. Teratology 16:175-180, 1977.

Brown JH, Maxwell AP, McGeown MG: Outcome of pregnancy following renal transplantation. Ir J Med Sci 160:255-256, 1991.

Committee on Drugs, American Academy of Pediatrics: The transfer of drugs and other chemicals into human milk. Pediatrics 93(1):137-150, 1994.

Cote CJ, Hilaire MD, Meuwissen JH, et al.: Effects on the neonate of prednisone and azathioprine administered to the mother during pregnancy. J Pediatr 85(3):324-328, 1974.

DeWitte DB, Buick MK, Cyran SE, et al.: Neonatal pancytopenia and severe combined immunodeficiency associated with antenatal administration of azathioprine and prednisone. J Pediatr 105(4):625-628, 1984.

Gandelman R, Guerriero LA: Brief prenatal exposure to prednisolone adversely affects behavioral development and body weight. Neurobehav Toxicol Teratol 4:289-292, 1982.

Gandelman R, Rosenthal C: Deleterious effects of prenatal prednisolone exposure upon morphological and behavioral development of mice. Teratology 24:293-301, 1981.

Greenberger PA, Odeh YK, Frederiksen MC, Atkinson AJ: Pharmacokinetics of prednisolone transfer into breast milk. Clin Pharmacol Ther 53:324-328, 1993.

Haugen G, Fauchald P, Sodal G, et al.: Pregnancy outcome in renal allograft recipients in Norway. Acta Obstet Gynecol Scand 73:541-546, 1994.

*This calculation is based on the following assumptions: maternal doses of prednisone and prednisolone: 10 mg and 10-80 mg, respectively; milk concentrations of prednisone and prednisolone: 0.03 mcg/mL and 0.002-0.32 mcg/mL, respectively; milk intake by the nursing infant: 150 mL/kg/d; estimated doses of prednisone and prednisolone ingested by the nursing infant: 0.0045 mg/kg/d and 0.0003-0.048 mg/kg/d, respectively; lowest therapeutic dose of prednisone and prednisolone: 2 mg/kg/d and 0.2 mg/kg/d, respectively.

Heinonen OP, Slone D, Shapiro S: *Birth Defects and Drugs in Pregnancy.* Littleton, Mass.: John Wright-PSG, 1977, pp 389, 391.

Katz FH, Duncan BR: Entry of prednisone into human milk. N Engl J Med 293:1154, 1975.

McKenzie SA, Selley JA, Agnew JE: Secretion of prednisolone into breast milk. Arch Dis Child 50:894-896, 1975.

Momma K, Nishihara S, Ota Y: Constriction of the fetal ductus arteriosus by glucocorticoid hormones. Pediatr Res 15:19-21, 1981.

Muirhead N, Sabharwal AR, Rieder MJ, et al.: The outcome of pregnancy following renal transplantation--The experience of a single center. Transplantation 54(3):429-432, 1992.

Neumann H-J, Garling H, Towe J: Zur wirkung von prednisolon-bisuccinat auf die pranatale entwicklung der Wistar ratte. Arzneimittelforsch 36:216-219, 1986.

Nielsen OH, Andreasson B, Bondesen S, et al.: Pregnancy in ulcerative colitis. Scand J Gastroenterol 19:724-732, 1984.

O'Donnell D, Sevitz H, Seggie JL, et al.: Pregnancy after renal transplantation. Aust NZ J Med 15:320-325, 1985.

Ost L, Wettrell G, Bjorkhem I, Rane A: Prednisolone excretion in human milk. J Pediatr 106:1008-1011, 1985.

Petri M, Howard D, Repke J, Goldman DW: The Hopkins Lupus Pregnancy Center: 1987-1991 update. Am J Reprod Immunol 28:188-191, 1992.

Pinsky L, DiGeorge AM: Cleft palate in the mouse: A teratogenic index of glucocorticoid potency. Science 147:402-403, 1965.

Pirson Y, van Lierde M, Ghysen J, et al.: Retardation of fetal growth in patients receiving immunosuppressive therapy. N Engl J Med 313:328, 1985.

Pollard JK, Scott JR, Branch DW: Outcome of children born to women treated during pregnancy for the antiphospholipid syndrome. Obstet Gynecol 80:365-368, 1992.

Rayburn WF: Glucocorticoid therapy for rheumatic diseases: Maternal, fetal, and breast-feeding considerations. Am J Reprod Immunol 28:138-140, 1992.

Reinisch JM, Simon NG, Gandelman R: Prenatal exposure to prednisone permanently alters fighting behavior of female mice. Pharmacol Biochem Behav 12:213-216, 1980.

Reinisch JM, Simon NG, Karow WG, Gandelman RG: Prenatal exposure to prednisone in humans and animals retards intrauterine growth. Science 202:436-438, 1978.

Shah RM, Kilistoff A: Cleft palate induction in hamster fetuses glucocorticoid hormones and their synthetic analogues. J Embryol Exp Morphol 36:101-108, 1976.

Silver RK, MacGregor SN, Sholl JS, et al.: Comparative trial of prednisone plus aspirin versus aspirin alone in the treatment of anticardiolipin antibody--positive obstetrics patients. Am J Obstet Gynecol 169:1411-1417, 1993.

TambyRaja RL: Fetal salvage in maternal systemic lupus erythematosus. Ann Acad Med Singapore 22:634-637, 1993.

Walker BE: Induction of cleft palate in rabbits by several glucocorticoids. Proc Soc Exp Biol Med 125:1281-1284, 1967.

Walsh SD, Clark FR: Pregnancy in patients on long-term corticosteroid therapy. Scott Med J 12:302-306, 1967.

Warrell DW, Taylor R: Outcome for the foetus of mothers receiving prednisolone during pregnancy. Lancet 1:117-118, 1968.

PRELESTONE® *See* Betamethasone

PRIMATENE MIST® *See* Epinephrine

PRINIVIL® *See* Lisinopril

PROCAINAMIDE
(Procan®, Pronestyl®, Rhythmin®)

Procainamide is used to treat cardiac arrhythmias. It is given orally or parenterally in a dose of 2000-6000 g/d.

Teratogenic Risk

Magnitude of teratogenic
risk to child born after
exposure during gestation: *Undetermined*

Quality and quantity of data
on which risk estimate is based: *None*

A small risk cannot be excluded, but there is no indication that the risk of congenital anomalies in the children of women treated with procainamide during pregnancy is likely to be great.

No epidemiological studies of congenital anomalies in the children of women treated with procainamide during pregnancy have been reported.

No animal teratology studies of procainamide have been published.

Procainamide has been used successfully in the treatment of fetal cardiac arrhythmias in the second and third trimesters of pregnancy (Hallak et al., 1991; Battiste et al., 1992; Kanzaki et al., 1993; Ito et al., 1994).

Risk Related to Breast-feeding

Procainamide and its active metabolite, N-acetylprocainamide, are excreted in the breast milk. The amount of procainamide and N-acetylprocainamide that the nursing infant would ingest is between 5-15% of the lowest weight-adjusted therapeutic dose, based on data from a single patient (Pittard & Glazier, 1983).*

The American Academy of Pediatrics (Committee on Drugs, American Academy of Pediatrics, 1994) regards procainamide to be safe to use while breast-feeding, but the WHO Working Group on Drugs and Human Lactation (1988), considers maternal use of procainamide to be incompatible with breast-feeding.

Key References

Battiste CE, Neff TW, Evans JF, Kline BW: In utero conversion of supraventricular tachycardia with digoxin and procainamide at 17 weeks' gestation. Am J Perinatol 9(4):302-303, 1992.

Committee on Drugs, American Academy of Pediatrics: The transfer of drugs and other chemicals into human milk. Pediatrics 93(1):137-150, 1994.

Hallack M, Neerhof MG, Perry R, et al.: Fetal supraventricular tachycardia and hydrops fetalis: Combined intensive, direct, and transplacental therapy. Obstet Gynecol 78:523-525, 1991.

Ito S, Magee L, Smallhorn J: Drug therapy for fetal arrhythmias. Clin Perinatol 21(3):543-572, 1994.

*This calculation is based on the following assumptions: maternal dose of procainamide: 1.5-2 g/d; milk concentrations of procainamide and N-acetylprocainamide: 2.6-10.2 mcg/mL and 2.2-5 mcg/mL, respectively; milk intake by the nursing infant: 150 mL/kg/d; estimated combined dose of procainamide and N-acetylprocainamide ingested by the nursing infant, assuming equivalent bioavailability, activity, and molecular weights: 0.73-2.3 mg/kg/d; lowest therapeutic dose of procainamide in adults: 15.6 mg/kg/d.

Kanzaki T, Murakami M, Kobayashi H, et al.: Hemodynamic changes during cardioversion in utero: A case report of supraventricular tachycardia and atrial flutter. Fetal Diagn Ther 8:37-44, 1993.

Pittard WB III, Glazier H: Procainamide excretion in human milk. J Pediatr 102:631-633, 1983.

WHO Working Group on Drugs and Human Lactation. In: Bennet PN (ed). *Drugs and Human Lactation.* Amsterdam: Elsevier, 1988, pp 106-107.

PROCAN® *See* Procainamide

PROCARDIA® *See* Nifedipine

PROCHLORPERAZINE
(Compazine®, Prorazin®, Stemetil®)

Prochlorperazine is a phenothiazine tranquilizer used in treatment of psychosis and as an antiemetic. Prochlorperazine is usually given orally in doses of 15-150 mg/d. The drug may also be administered rectally in doses of 30-50 mg/d or parenterally in doses as high as 200 mg/d.

Teratogenic Risk

Magnitude of teratogenic risk to child born after exposure during gestation:	*None*
Quality and quantity of data on which risk estimate is based:	*Good to excellent*

The frequencies of congenital anomalies in general, of major malformations, of minor anomalies, and of principle classes of anomalies were no greater than expected among the children of 877 women who took prochlorperazine during the first four lunar months of pregnancy in one epidemiological study (Heinonen et al., 1977). There was no increase in the frequency of congenital anomalies among the children of 2023 women who took prochlorperazine anytime during pregnancy in this study. The frequency of malformations was not increased among the children of 91, 433, and more than 50 women who took prochlorperazine during the first trimester of pregnancy in three other investigations (Kullander & Kallen, 1976; Milkovich & van den Berg, 1976; Jick et al., 1981).

An increased frequency of cleft palate was observed among the offspring of mice and rats treated during pregnancy with prochlorperazine in doses 17 or more and 3-23 times those used in humans (Roux, 1959; Szabo & Brent, 1974). The relevance of these observations to the therapeutic use of prochlorperazine in human pregnancy is unknown.

Risk Related to Breast-feeding

No information regarding the distribution of prochlorperazine in breast milk has been published.

Key References

Heinonen OP, Slone D, Shapiro S: *Birth Defects and Drugs in Pregnancy*. Littleton, Mass.: John Wright-PSG, 1977, pp 323-324, 437.

Jick H, Holmes LB, Hunter JR, et al.: First-trimester drug use and congenital disorders. JAMA 246:343-346, 1981.

Kullander S, Kallen B: A prospective study of drugs and pregnancy. II. Anti-emetic drugs. Acta Obstet Gynecol Scand 55:105-111, 1976.

Milkovich L, van den Berg BJ: An evaluation of the teratogenicity of certain antinauseant drugs. Am J Obstet Gynecol 125:244-248, 1976.

Roux CH: Teratogenic action of prochlorperazine. Arch Fr Pediatr 16:968-971, 1959.

Szabo KT, Brent RL: Species differences in experimental teratogenesis by tranquillising agents. Lancet 1:565, 1974.

PROCRIN® *See* Leuprolide

PROGESTASERT® *See* Progesterone

PROGESTERONE
(Femotrone®, Gesterol ®, Progestasert®)

Progesterone is a natural hormone secreted by the ovary and placenta. The functions of progesterone include maturation of the endometrium during the menstrual cycle, development of mammary tissue, and maintenance of pregnancy. Progesterone is given parenterally to treat amenorrhea and functional uterine bleeding. The usual dose is 50-100 mg as one injection or 5-10 mg/d for several days. Progesterone is also given in daily parenteral doses of 12.5 mg or daily rectal or vaginal doses of 50 mg early in pregnancy to treat corpus luteum insufficiency

This summary deals only with progesterone itself. Please see agent summaries on synthetic progestins and progesterone derivatives for information on these other agents. In assessing the teratogenic potential of progesterone, it is important to distinguish this natural hormone, the endogenous secretion of which is necessary for the maintenance of pregnancy, from synthetic progestins and progesterone derivatives (Wilson & Brent, 1981; Scialli, 1988). Unfortunately, this distinction has not always been made in the literature.

Teratogenic Risk

*Magnitude of teratogenic
risk to child born after
exposure during gestation:*
    Nongenital congenital anomalies: *Unlikely*
    Virilization of female fetus: *Unlikely*

*Quality and quantity of data
on which risk estimate is based:*
    Nongenital congenital anomalies: *Good*
    Virilization of female fetus: *Good*

Therapeutic doses of progesterone are unlikely to pose a substantial teratogenic risk, but the data are insufficient to state that there is no risk.

The frequencies of all malformations, of major malformations, and of minor congenital anomalies were no greater than expected among the children of 253 women treated with progesterone during the first four lunar months of pregnancy in one epidemiological study (Heinonen et al., 1977a). There was no increase in the frequency of cardiovascular malformations among these children (Heinonen et al, 1977b). The frequency of congenital anomalies among the children of 527 women treated with progesterone anytime in pregnancy in this study was a little less than expected (Heinonen et al., 1977a). The frequency of congenital anomalies was not increased in another study that included 186 infants born to women who had been given progesterone early in gestation (Michaelis et al., 1983). The frequency of malformations was not increased among the infants of 244 women who were treated with progesterone during pregnancy in one other study (Resseguie et al., 1985). Rates of congenital anomalies did not appear to be unusually high in clinical series that included 382 and 93 infants of women who had been treated with progesterone during the first trimester of pregnancy (Rock et al., 1985; Check et al., 1986).

Maternal treatment during pregnancy with synthetic progestins that have substantial androgen-like activity (e.g., ethisterone or norethindrone) can cause virilization of the external genitalia of female fetuses (Schardein, 1980, 1993). Hypospadias in male infants has also been observed in association with maternal use of various progestins during pregnancy, but this has been reported less often and less consistently (Schardein, 1993). Although cases of female virilization and male hypospadias have been reported among infants of women who were treated with progesterone early in pregnancy, such reports are uncommon. It seems likely that many of these occurrences are coincidental and that maternal progesterone treatment in usual doses during pregnancy rarely if ever causes genital abnormalities (Scialli, 1988; Schardein, 1993).

Studies in monkeys and rats suggest that treatment of pregnant women with progesterone in usual therapeutic doses is unlikely to increase the children's risk of malformations greatly (Lerner et al., 1962; Bartholomeusz & Bruce, 1976; Hendrickx et al., 1987).

Risk Related to Breast-feeding

Progesterone is excreted into breast milk (USP DI, 1995), although this has not been quantitated in published reports.

Key References

Bartholomeusz RK, Bruce NW: Effects of maternal progesterone supplementation on fetal, placental and corpus luteal weights in the rat. Biol Reprod 15:84-89, 1976.

Check JH, Rankin A, Teichman M: The risk of fetal anomalies as a result of progesterone therapy during pregnancy. Fertil Steril 45(4):575-577, 1986.

Heinonen OP, Slone D, Shapiro S: *Birth Defects and Drugs in Pregnancy.* Littleton, Mass.: John Wright-PSG, 1977a, p 389.

Heinonen OP, Slone D, Monson RR, et al.: Cardiovascular birth defects and antenatal exposure to female sex hormones. N Engl J Med 296:67-70, 1977b.

Hendrickx AG, Korte R, Leuschner F, et al.: Embryotoxicity of sex steroid hormone combinations in nonhuman primates: I. Norethisterone acetate + ethinyl estradiol and progesterone + estradiol benzoate (*Macaca mulatta, Macaca fasicularis,* and *Papio cynocephalus*). Teratology 35:119-127, 1987.

Lerner LJ, DePhillipo M, Yiacas E, et al.: Comparison of the acetophenone derivative of 16α, 17α-dihydroprogesterone with other progestational steroids for masculinization of the rat fetus. Endocrinology 71:448-451, 1962.

Michaelis J, Michaelis H, Gluck E, Koller S: Prospective study of suspected associations between certain drugs administered during early pregnancy and congenital malformations. Teratology 27:57-64, 1983.

Resseguie LJ, Hick JF, Bruen JA, et al.: Congenital malformations among offspring exposed in utero to progestins, Omstead County, Minnesota, 1936-1974. Fertil Steril 43:514-519, 1985.

Rock JA, Wentz AC, Cole KA et al.: Fetal malformations following progesterone therapy during pregnancy: A preliminary report. Fertil Steril 44(1):17-19, 1985.

Schardein JL: Congenital abnormalities and hormones during pregnancy: A clinical review. Teratology 22:251-270, 1980.

Schardein JL: *Chemically Induced Birth Defects,* 2nd ed. New York: Marcel Dekker, 1993, pp 291-292.

Scialli AR: Developmental effects of progesterone and its derivatives. Reprod Toxicol 2:3-11, 1988.

USP DI: Progestins: In: *USP DI (USP Dispensing Information), Volume 1. Drug Information for the Health Care Professional,* 15th ed. Rockville, Md.: The US Pharmacopeial Convention, 1995, p 2324.

Wilson JG, Brent RL: Are female sex hormones teratogenic? Am J Obstet Gynecol 141:567-580, 1981.

PROLOPRIM® *See* Trimethoprim

PROMETA® *See* Metaproterenol

PROMETHAZINE
(Histanil®, Phenergan®, Prorex®)

Promethazine is a phenothiazine that is used to treat allergic disorders, as a preoperative medication, and in the management of parkinsonian symptoms. Promethazine is given orally, parenterally, or rectally in doses of 25-150 mg/d.

Teratogenic Risk

*Magnitude of teratogenic
risk to child born after
exposure during gestation:*　　　　　*None*

*Quality and quantity of data
on which risk estimate is based:*　　　　　*Good to excellent*

This rating is for usual therapeutic doses of promethazine; the risk associated with toxic overdoses of this drug is unknown but may be greater.

The frequency of congenital anomalies was no greater than expected among the children of 63, 55, 114, and 529 women who were treated with promethazine during the first trimester of pregnancy in four epidemiological studies (Farkas & Farkas, 1971; Heinonen et al., 1977; Rumeau-Rouquette et al., 1977; Aselton et al., 1985). In one of these investigations, the frequency of congenital anomalies was no greater than expected among 746 children born to women who took promethazine anytime during pregnancy (Heinonen et al., 1977). No association with maternal use of promethazine during the first trimester of pregnancy was seen in studies of 175 and 836 children with congenital anomalies (Nelson & Forfar, 1971; Greenberg et al., 1977).

Among 19 pregnancies that were continued after the mother had taken a toxic overdose of promethazine, usually in combination with other drugs, there were two fetal deaths (one thought to be unrelated to the overdose), two children with mental retardation (who were siblings), and one child with borderline intellectual function (Czeizel et al., 1984, 1988). Three children had multiple naevi and one had strabismus; no malformations were noted. Most of the overdoses occurred in the second or third trimester; only two were in the first trimester of pregnancy. The relationship of the maternal overdose of promethazine to these outcomes is uncertain.

Studies in rats suggest that treatment of pregnant women with promethazine in usual therapeutic doses is unlikely to increase the children's risk of malformations greatly (King et al., 1965).

Maternal promethazine treatment during pregnancy has been used for Rh hemolytic disease (Gusdon, 1981). Altered immunological function has been demonstrated in the newborn infants of such treated women (Rubinstein et al., 1976; Eidelman et al., 1977), but the relationship of this problem to the maternal promethazine treatment is uncertain.

Abnormal in vitro tests of platelet function have been observed in infants born to women treated with promethazine during labor (Corby & Schulman, 1971). The clinical relevance of this observation is unknown.

Risk Related to Breast-feeding

No information regarding the distribution of promethazine in breast milk has been published.

Key References

Aselton P, Jick H, Milunsky A, et al.: First-trimester drug use and congenital disorders. Obstet Gynecol 65:451-455, 1985.

Corby DG, Schulman I: The effects of antenatal drug administration on aggregation of platelets of newborn infants. J Pediatr 79:307-313, 1971.

Czeizel A, Szentesi I, Szekeres I, et al.: A study of adverse effects on the progeny after intoxication during pregnancy. Arch Toxicol 62:1-7, 1988.

Czeizel A, Szentesi I, Szekeres I, et al.: Pregnancy outcome and health conditions of offspring of self-poisoned pregnant women. Acta Paediatr Hung 25(3):209-236, 1984.

Eidelman AI, Rubinstein A, Melamed J, et al.: More on the effect of maternal promethazine (P-HCl) on neonatal immunologic functions. J Pediatr 90(2):332-333, 1977.

Farkas VG, Farkas G Jr: Teratogenic action of hyperemesis in pregnancy and of medication used to treat it. Zentralbl Gynaekol 93:325-330, 1971.

Greenberg G, Inman WHW, Weatherall JAC, et al.: Maternal drug histories and congenital abnormalities. Br Med J 2:853-856, 1977.

Gusdon JP Jr: The treatment of erythroblastosis with promethazine hydrochloride. J Reprod Med 26(9):454-458, 1981.

Heinonen OP, Slone D, Shapiro S: *Birth Defects and Drugs in Pregnancy.* Littleton, Mass.: John Wright-PSG, 1977, pp 323, 437.

King CTG, Weaver SA, Narrod SA: Antihistamines and teratogenicity in the rat. J Pharmacol Exp Ther 147:391-398, 1965.

Nelson MM, Forfar JO: Associations between drugs administered during pregnancy and congenital abnormalities of the fetus. Br Med J 1:523-527, 1971.

Rubinstein A, Eidelman AI, Melamed J, et al.: Possible effect of maternal promethazine therapy on neonatal immunologic functions. J Pediatr 89(1):136-138, 1976.

Rumeau-Rouquette C, Goujard J, Huel G: Possible teratogenic effect of phenothiazines in human beings. Teratology 15:57-64, 1977.

PRONESTYL® *See* Procainamide

PROPOXYPHENE
(Darvon®, Doxaphene®, Novopropoxyn®)

Propoxyphene is a widely prescribed opioid analgesic that is given orally in the treatment of mild to moderate pain due to diseases such as arthritis, other musculoskeletal disorders, and cancer. The dose used is up to 390 mg/d (up to 600 mg/d of the napsylate salt).

Teratogenic Risk

Magnitude of teratogenic risk to child born after exposure during gestation:	*None*
Quality and quantity of data on which risk estimate is based:	*Good*

This assessment is for the use of propoxyphene in usual therapeutic doses.

The frequencies of congenital anomalies in general, major malformations, minor anomalies, and major classes of congenital anomalies were no greater than expected among the children of 686 women who took propoxyphene during the first four lunar months of pregnancy in a large epidemiological study (Heinonen et al., 1977). Similar findings were reported by Jick et al. (1981) in another study involving more than 100 pregnancies exposed to propoxyphene during the first trimester. The frequency of congenital anomalies was no greater than expected among the infants of 2914 women who took propoxyphene anytime during pregnancy (Heinonen et al., 1977). A few anecdotal cases of malformations in infants born after maternal exposure to propoxyphene during pregnancy have been reported (Boelter, 1980; Golden et al., 1982; Williams et al., 1983), but no recurrent pattern of anomalies is apparent and a causal relationship of the maternal exposure to the infants' malformations seems unlikely.

No teratogenic effect was observed in rats, rabbits, or hamsters after treatment during pregnancy with propoxyphene in doses as large as 10-40 times those used clinically (Emmerson et al., 1971; Geber & Schramm, 1975; Buttar & Moffatt, 1983). An increased frequency of malformations was observed among the offspring of pregnant hamsters treated with even larger doses of propoxyphene (Geber & Schramm, 1975). Long-lasting behavioral alterations have been noted among the offspring of rats treated during pregnancy with several times the human dose of propoxyphene (Vorhees et al., 1979; Saillenfait & Vannier, 1988). The clinical relevance of these observations is unknown.

Transient neonatal withdrawal symptoms occur in infants whose mothers took propoxyphene chronically during pregnancy (Tyson, 1974; Klein et al., 1975). Irritability, hyperactivity, tremors, and high-pitched cry are the usual clinical features.

Risk Related to Breast-feeding

Propoxyphene is excreted in breast milk in low concentrations. The amount of propoxyphene that the nursing infant would be expected to ingest is <1% of the lowest weight-adjusted therapeutic dose, based on data from six lactating women (Kunka et al., 1984).*

The American Academy of Pediatrics considers usual therapeutic amounts of propoxyphene to be safe to use during breast-feeding (Committee on Drugs, American Academy of Pediatrics, 1994).

Key References

Boelter W: Proposed fetal propoxyphene (Darvon®) syndrome. Clin Res 28:115A, 1980.

Committee on Drugs, American Academy of Pediatrics: The transfer of drugs and other chemicals into human milk. Pediatrics 93(1):137-150, 1994.

Buttar HS, Moffatt JH: Pre- and postnatal development of rats following concomitant intrauterine exposure to propoxyphene and chlordiazepoxide. Neurobehav Toxicol Teratol 5:549-556, 1983.

Emmerson JL, Owen NV, Koenig GR, et al.: Reproduction and teratology studies on propoxyphene napsylate. Toxicol Appl Pharmacol 19:471-479, 1971.

Geber WF, Schramm LC: Congenital malformations of the central nervous system produced by narcotic analgesics in the hamster. Am J Obstet Gynecol 123:705-713, 1975.

Golden NL, King KC, Sokol RJ: Propoxyphene and acetaminophen. Possible effects on the fetus. Clin Pediatr 21:752-754, 1982.

Heinonen OP, Slone D, Shapiro S: *Birth Defects and Drugs in Pregnancy*. Littleton, Mass.: John Wright-PSG, 1977, pp 287-288, 294, 434, 471, 484.

Jick H, Holmes LB, Hunter JR, et al.: First-trimester drug use and congenital disorders. JAMA 246:343-346, 1981.

Klein RB, Blatman S, Little GA: Probable neonatal propoxyphene withdrawal: A case report. Pediatrics 55:882-884, 1975.

Kunka RL, Venkataramanan R, Stern RM et al.: Excretion of propoxyphene and norpropoxyphene in breast milk. Clin Pharm Ther 35:675-680, 1984.

Saillenfait AM, Vannier B: Methodological proposal in behavioural teratogenicity testing: Assessment of propoxyphene, chlorpromazine, and vitamin A as positive controls. Teratology 37:185-199, 1988.

*This calculation is based on the following assumptions: maternal dose of propoxyphene: 390 mg/d; milk concentration of propoxyphene: 0.07-0.16 mcg/mL; milk intake by the nursing infant: 150 mL/kg/d; estimated dose of propoxyphene ingested by the nursing infant: 0.01-0.02 mg/kg/d; lowest therapeutic dose of propoxyphene in adults: 6.1 mg/kg/d.

Tyson HK: Neonatal withdrawal symptoms associated with maternal use of propoxyphene hydrochloride (Darvon®). J Pediatr 85:684-685, 1974.

Vorhees CV, Brunner RL, Butcher RE: Psychotropic drugs as behavioral teratogens. Science 205:1220-1225, 1979.

Williams DA, Weiss T, Wade E, Dignan P: Prune perineum syndrome: Report of a second case. Teratology 28:145-148, 1983.

PROPRANOLOL
(Detensol®, Inderal®)

Propranolol is a β-adrenergic receptor blocking agent. It is used in the treatment of hypertension, cardiac arrhythmias, hypertrophic subaortic stenosis, hyperthyroidism, and migraine headaches. Propranolol is given orally in doses of 30-640 mg/d or intravenously in smaller doses.

Teratogenic Risk

*Magnitude of teratogenic
risk to child born after
exposure during gestation:*   *Undetermined*

*Quality and quantity of data
on which risk estimate is based:*   *Poor*

A small risk cannot be excluded, but there is no indication that the risk of malformations in the children of women treated with propranolol during pregnancy is likely to be great.

Possible effects on fetal growth and perinatal adaptation are discussed below.

No significant association with maternal use of propranolol during the first three months of pregnancy was found in a study involving 726 infants with neural tube defects, 578 with cleft lip or palate, 1191 with hypospadias and 4470 with other congenital anomalies (Czeizel, 1989).

Chronic propranolol treatment of pregnant women in late pregnancy has been associated with fetal growth retardation (Eliahou et al., 1978; Lieberman et al., 1978; Oakley et al., 1979; Pruyn et al., 1979; Redmond, 1982). However, it is difficult in most studies to separate an action of the drug from an effect of the disease for which it has been given. Fetal weight appears to be most consistently affected;

head circumference may also be involved (Pruyn et al., 1979), but this measurement is not recorded in most studies. There are no data available in humans regarding whether or not the growth retardation associated with maternal propranolol use persists into childhood. The possibility that head (and presumably also brain) growth is deficient in children of mothers treated with propranolol during pregnancy is of concern, but no studies of neurological or intellectual function in these children have been reported.

The frequency of malformations was not increased among the offspring of rats or mice treated with propranolol during pregnancy in doses, respectively, 1-8 and 1 times those usually employed in humans (Fujii & Nishimura, 1974; Speiser et al., 1983; Kang & Manson, 1987). Treatment of pregnant rats with 4-12 times the maximum human dose of propranolol caused fetal growth retardation, but this effect was inconsistent or absent with lower doses (Schoenfeld et al., 1978; Harmon et al., 1986; Judlin et al., 1992; Erdtsieck-Ernste et al., 1993). Rats exposed prenatally to propranolol in doses similar to or slightly larger than those used in humans exhibited long-lasting alterations of behavior (Speiser et al., 1983, 1991).

Difficulties in perinatal adaptation including neonatal apnea, respiratory distress, bradycardia, and hypoglycemia have been associated with maternal treatment with propranolol, especially if the drug is given in a high dose and/or shortly before delivery (Rubin, 1981; Buechler & Palmer, 1982). Such effects are compatible with the known pharmacological actions of propranolol (Ayromlooi, 1983). The magnitude of these risks is uncertain.

Risk Related to Breast-feeding

Propranolol is excreted in the breast milk in low concentrations. The amount of propranolol that the nursing infant would be expected to ingest is between <1-2.8% of the lowest therapeutic dose in neonates, based on data from eight lactating women (Levitan & Manion, 1973; Karlberg et al., 1974; Bauer et al., 1979; Taylor & Turner, 1981; Smith et al., 1983).* No adverse effects on heart rate were observed in any of the breast-fed infants.

*This calculation is based on the following assumptions: maternal dose of propranolol: 20-160 mg/d; milk concentration of propranolol: 0.002-0.15 mcg/mL; milk intake by the nursing infant: 150 mL/kg/d; estimated dose of propranolol ingested by the nursing infant: 0.0003-0.022 mg/kg/d; lowest therapeutic dose of propranolol in neonates: 0.8 mg/kg/d.

Both the American Academy of Pediatrics (Committee on Drugs, American Academy of Pediatrics, 1994) and the WHO Working Group on Drugs and Human Lactation (1988) regard propranolol to be safe to use while breast-feeding. Although the risk of β-adrenergic blockade in nursing infants is small, infants whose mothers are taking propranolol while breast-feeding should be monitored for signs of bradycardia, hypotension, respiratory distress, and hypoglycemia.

Key References

Ayromlooi J: Effect of propranolol on the acid base balance and hemodynamics of 'chronically instrumented' pregnant sheep. Dev Pharmacol Ther 6:207-216, 1983.

Bauer JH, Pape B, Zajicek J, Groshong T: Propranolol in human plasma and breast milk. Am J Cardiol 43:860-862, 1979.

Buechler AA, Palmer SK: Intrapartum fetal death associated with propranolol; case report and review of physiology. Wis Med J 81:23-25, 1982.

Committee on Drugs, American Academy of Pediatrics: The transfer of drugs and other chemicals into human milk. Pediatrics 93(1):137-150, 1994.

Czeizel A: Teratogenicity of ergotamine. J Med Genet 26:69-70, 1989.

Eliahou HE, Silverberg DS, Reisin E, et al.: Propranolol for the treatment of hypertension in pregnancy. Br J Obstet Gynaecol 85:431-436, 1978.

Erdtsieck-Ernste EBHW, Feenstra MGP, Botterblom MHA, Boer GJ: Developmental changes in rat brain monoamine metabolism and β-adrenoceptor subtypes after chronic prenatal exposure to propranolol. Neurochem Int 22(6):589-598, 1993.

Fujii T, Nishimura H: Reduction in frequency of fetopathic effects of caffeine in mice by pretreatment with propranolol. Teratology 10:149-152, 1974.

Harmon JR, Delongchamp RR, Kimmel GL, Webb PJ: Effect of prenatal propranolol exposure on development of the postnatal rat heart. Teratogenesis Carcinog Mutagen 6:139-150, 1986.

Judlin PH, Boutroy MJ, Mallie JP: Rat neonates renal function after β-receptors and adrenoceptors blockade during pregnancy. Arch Int Physiol Biochim Biophys 100:355-359, 1992.

Kang YJ, Manson JM: Effect of prenatal propranolol-nitrofen exposure on pregnant rats. Teratology 35(2):58A, 1987.

Karlberg B, Lundberg D, Aberg H: Excretion of propranolol in human breast milk. Acta Pharmacol Toxicol 34:222-224, 1974.

Levitan AA, Manion JC: Propranolol therapy during pregnacy and lactation. Am J Cardiol 32:247, 1973.

Lieberman BA, Stirrat GM, Cohen SL, et al.: The possible adverse effect of propranolol on the fetus in pregnancies complicated by severe hypertension. Br J Obstet Gynaecol 85:678-683, 1978.

Oakley GDG, McGarry K, Limb DG, Oakley CM: Management of pregnancy in patients with hypertrophic cardiomyopathy. Br Med J 1:1749-1750, 1979.

Pruyn SC, Phelan JP, Buchanan GC: Long-term propranolol therapy in pregnancy: Maternal and fetal outcome. Am J Obstet Gynecol 135:485-489, 1979.

Redmond GP: Propranolol and fetal growth retardation. Semin Perinatol 6(2):142-147, 1982.

Rubin PC: β-blockers in pregnancy. N Engl J Med 305:1323-1326, 1981.

Schoenfeld N, Epstein O, Nemesh L, et al.: Effects of propranolol during pregnancy and development of rats. I. Adverse effects during pregnancy. Pediatr Res 12:747-750, 1978.

Smith MT, Livingstone I, Hooepr WD, et al.: Propranolol, propranolol glucuronide, and naphthoxylactic acid in breast milk and plasma. Ther Drug Monitor 5:87-93, 1983.

Speiser Z, Gordon I, Rehavi M, Gitter S: Behavioral and biochemical studies in rats following prenatal treatment with β-adrenoceptor antagonists. Eur J Pharmacol 195(1):75-83, 1991.

Speiser Z, Shved A, Gitter S: Effect of propranolol treatment in pregnant rats on motor activity and avoidance learning of the offspring. Psychopharmacology 79:148-154, 1983.

Taylor EA, Turner P: Anti-hypertensive therapy with propranolol during pregnancy and lactation. Postgrad Med J 57:427-430, 1981.

WHO Working Group on Drugs and Human Lactation. In: Bennet PN (ed). *Drugs and Human Lactation.* Amsterdam: Elsevier, 1988, pp 139-140.

PROPYCIL® *See Propylthiouracil*

PROPYLTHIOURACIL
(Propycil®, Propyl-Thyracil®)

Propylthiouracil is a thioamide derivative that is used to treat hyperthyroidism. Usual oral doses are 50-900 mg/d. Propylthiouracil may be given rectally in doses as high as 2400 mg/d to treat thyroid storm.

Teratogenic Risk

*Magnitude of teratogenic
risk to child born after
exposure during gestation:*
    Malformations: *None*
    Goiter: *Small to moderate*

*Quality and quantity of data
on which risk estimate is based:*
    Malformations: *Poor to fair*
    Goiter: *Good*

These ratings are for usual doses of propylthiouracil. The risk associated with maternal treatment with the very large doses used for thyroid storm is unknown but may be greater.

Propylthiouracil, when given to a pregnant woman, crosses the placenta and can cause suppression of fetal thyroid function. Since maternal thyroid hormones do not readily cross the placenta, fetal thyroid hyperplasia and goiter may develop as the fetus attempts to compensate for its hypothyroidism (Burrow, 1978; Solomon, 1981). It has been estimated that 1-5% of infants born to women treated with propylthiouracil during pregnancy develop significant transient neonatal hypothyroidism (Davis et al., 1989; Becks & Burrow, 1991), although clinically inapparent mild hypothyroxinemia is much more common (Cheron et al., 1981). Neonatal goiter is also seen in a few percent of infants born to women treated with propylthiouracil during pregnancy but is rarely large enough to cause respiratory compromise (Davis et al., 1989; Becks & Burrow, 1991). Large goiters are much more common in infants of women treated with both propylthiouracil and iodides during pregnancy (Mujtaba & Burrow, 1975).

Since either hypothyroidism or hyperthyroidism can occur among infants of women who have Graves' disease and are treated with propylthiouracil during pregnancy, thyroid function should be assessed in these children at the time of birth (Hayek & Brooks, 1975; Burrow, 1985). Both fetal goiter and hyperthyroidism have been diagnosed prenatally by ultrasonography in women with Graves' disease treated with propylthiouracil during pregnancy (Belfar et al., 1991; Soliman et al., 1994).

The frequency of malformations was not significantly increased among the children of 65 women with Graves' disease who were treated with propylthiouracil during pregnancy when compared to the children of untreated Graves' disease patients in one study (Momotani & Ito, 1991). Interpretation of this investigation is difficult because it appears to lack epidemiological rigor. The frequency of congenital anomalies not related to the thyroid gland does not appear unusual in clinical series of infants born to mothers treated with propylthiouracil during pregnancy (Burrow, 1965; Talbert et al., 1970; Goluboff et al., 1974; Wing et al., 1994).

No difference in intelligence test scores in comparison to unexposed siblings was found in 28 children in one study or 16 children in another study who were born to women treated with propylthiouracil during pregnancy (Burrow et al., 1978; Eisenstein et al., 1992).

Maternal treatment with propylthiouracil has been used to provide transplacental therapy to fetuses with hyperthyroidism (Bruinse et al., 1988; Hatjis, 1993).

Thyroid enlargement but no malformations were observed among the offspring of rabbits treated during pregnancy with propylthiouracil in a dose slightly greater than that used in humans (Krementz et al., 1957).

Risk Related to Breast-feeding

Propylthiouracil is excreted in low concentrations in the breast milk. The amount of propylthiouracil that the nursing infant would be expected to ingest is between 1.4-2% of the lowest therapeutic dose for infants, based on data from nine lactating women (Kampmann et al., 1980).*

No postnatal suppression of thyroid function was observed in 17 nursing infants whose mothers were treated with propylthiouracil (Kampmann et al., 1989; Momotani et al., 1989).

Both the American Academy of Pediatrics (Committee on Drugs, American Academy of Pediatrics, 1994) and the WHO Working Group on Drugs and Human Lactation (1988) regard propylthiouracil to be safe to use while breast-feeding. Although no adverse effects have been reported in nursing infants, it has been recommended that thyroid function of nursing infants whose mothers are taking high doses of propylthiouracil be monitored by measuring serum thyrotropin and thyroxine concentrations (USP DI, 1995).

Key References

Becks GP, Burrow GN: Thyroid disease and pregnancy. Med Clin North Am 75(1):121-150, 1991.

Belfar HL, Foley TP Jr, Hill LM, Kislak S: Sonographic findings in maternal hyperthroidism. Fetal hyperthyroidism/fetal goiter. J Ultrasound Med 10:281-284, 1991.

Bruinse HW, Vermeulen-Meiners C, Wit JM: Fetal treatment for thyrotoxicosis in non-thyrotoxic pregnant women. Fetal Ther 3:152-157, 1988.

Burrow GN: Hyperthyroidism during pregnancy. N Engl J Med 298(3):150-153, 1978.

Burrow GN: Neonatal goiter after maternal propylthiouracil therapy. J Clin Endocrinol Metab 25:403-408, 1965.

Burrow GN: The management of thyrotoxicosis in pregnancy. N Engl J Med 313(9):562-565, 1985.

Burrow GN, Klatskin EH, Genel M: Intellectual development in children whose mothers received propylthiouracil during pregnancy. Yale J Biol Med 51:151-156, 1978.

Cheron RG, Kaplan MM, Larsen PR, et al.: Neonatal thyroid function after propylthiouracil therapy for maternal Graves' disease. N Engl J Med 304(9):525-528, 1981.

---

*This calculation is based on the following assumptions: maternal dose of propylthiouracil: 400 mg/d; milk concentration of propylthiouracil: 0.5-0.7 mcg/mL; milk intake by the nursing infant: 150 mL/kg/d; estimated dose of propylthiouracil ingested by the nursing infant: 0.07-0.1 mg/kg/d; lowest therapeutic dose of propylthiouracil in infants: 5 mg/kg/d.

Committee on Drugs, American Academy of Pediatrics: The transfer of drugs and other chemicals into human milk. Pediatrics 93(1):137-150, 1994.

Davis LE, Lucas MJ, Hankins GDV, et al.: Thyrotoxicosis complicating pregnancy. Am J Obstet Gynecol 160(1):63-70, 1989.

Eisenstein Z, Weiss M, Katz Y, Bank H: Intellectual capacity of subjects exposed to methimazole or propylthiouracil in utero. Eur J Pediatr 151:558-559, 1992.

Goluboff LG, Sisson JC, Hamburger JI: Hyperthyroidism associated with pregnancy. Obstet Gynecol 44(1):107-116, 1974.

Hatjis CG: Diagnosis and successful treatment of fetal goitrous hyperthroidism caused by maternal Graves disease. Obstet Gynecol 81:837-839, 1993.

Hayek A, Brooks M: Neonatal hyperthyroidism following intrauterine hypothyroidism. J Pediatr 87(3):446-448, 1975.

Kampmann JP, Johansen K, Hansen JM, Helweg J: Propylthiouracil in human milk. Revision of a dogma. Lancet 1:736-737, 1980.

Krementz ET, Hooper RG, Kempson RL: The effect on the rabbit fetus of the maternal administration of propylthiouracil. Surgery 41(4):619-631, 1957.

Momotani N, Ito K: Treatment of pregnant patients with Basedow's disease. Exp Clin Endocrinol 97(2/3):268-274, 1991.

Momotani N, Yamashita R, Yoshimoto M, et al.: Recovery from foetal hypothyroidism: Evidence for the safety of breast-feeding while taking propylthiouracil. Clin Endocrinol 31:591-595, 1989.

Mujtaba Q, Burrow GN: Treatment of hyperthyroidism in pregnancy with propylthiouracil and methimazole. Obstet Gynecol 46:282-286, 1975.

Soliman S, McGrath F, Brennan B, Glazebrook K: Color doppler imaging of the thyroid gland in a fetus with congenital goiter: A case report. Am J Perinatol 11:21-23, 1994.

Solomon DH: Pregnancy and PTU. N Engl J Med 304(9):538-539, 1981.

Talbert LM, Thomas CG Jr, Holt WA, Rankin P: Hyperthyroidism during pregnancy. Obstet Gynecol 36(5):779-785, 1970.

USP DI: Antithyroid agents. In: *USP DI (USP Dispensing Information), Volume 1. Drug Information for the Health Care Professional*, 15th ed. Rockville, Md.: The US Pharmacopeial Convention, 1995, pp 375-376.

WHO Working Group on Drugs and Human Lactation. In: Bennet PN (ed). *Drugs and Human Lactation*. Amsterdam: Elsevier, 1988, pp 194-195.

Wing DA, Millar LK, Koonings PP, et al.: A comparison of propylthiouracil versus methimazole in the treatment of hyperthyroidism in pregnancy. Am J Obstet Gynecol 170:90-95, 1994.

PROPYL-THYRACIL® See Propylthiouracil

PRORAZIN® *See* Prochlorperazine

PROREX® *See* Promethazine

PROVATENE® *See* Beta-Carotene

PROVENTIL® *See* Albuterol

PROVERA® *See* Medroxyprogesterone

PROZAC® *See* Fluoxetine

PSEUDOEPHEDRINE
(Afrinol®, PediaCare®, Sudafed®)

Pseudoephedrine is a sympathomimetic agent that is used as a nasal and bronchial decongestant, often in combination with other drugs. The usual oral dose of pseudoephedrine is 240 mg/d.

Teratogenic Risk

Magnitude of teratogenic risk to child born after exposure during gestation:	*None to minimal*
Quality and quantity of data on which risk estimate is based:	*Fair*

The frequency of congenital anomalies was no higher than expected among the children of a total of 902 women who took pseudoephedrine during the first trimester of pregnancy in two cohorts of one epidemiological study (Jick et al., 1981; Aselton et al., 1985). The rate of congenital anomalies was not increased among children born to 39 women who took pseudoephedrine during the first four lunar months of pregnancy or the children of 194 women who took the drug anytime during pregnancy in another study (Heinonen et al., 1977). An association with maternal use of pseudoephedrine during the first trimester of pregnancy was observed in a study of 76 children with gastroschisis (Werler et al., 1992). No association was seen with such exposure in 416 infants with other congenital anomalies of possible vascular etiology. The authors concluded that the positive association of gastroschisis with maternal use of pseudoephedrine should be considered tentative until independent confirmation is obtained.

No animal teratology studies of pseudoephedrine have been published.

Risk Related to Breast-feeding

Pseudoephedrine is excreted in the breast milk in low concentrations. The amount of pseudoephedrine that the nursing infant would be expected to ingest is approximately 1% of the lowest weight-adjusted therapeutic dose, based on data from three lactating women (Findlay et al. 1984).*

Both the American Academy of Pediatrics (Committee on Drugs, American Academy of Pediatrics, 1994) and the WHO Working Group on Drugs and Human Lactation (1988) regard pseudoephedrine to be safe to use while breast-feeding.

Key References

Aselton P, Jick H, Milunsky A, et al.: First-trimester drug use and congenital disorders. Obstet Gynecol 65:451-455, 1985.

Committee on Drugs, American Academy of Pediatrics: The transfer of drugs and other chemicals into human milk. Pediatrics 93(1):137-150, 1994.

*This calculation is based on the following assumptions: maternal dose of pseudoephedrine: 60 mg; milk concentration of pseudoephedrine: 0.19-0.33 mcg/mL; milk intake by the nursing infant: 150 mL/kg/d; estimated dose of pseudoephedrine ingested by the nursing infant: 0.03-0.05 mg/kg/d; lowest therapeutic dose of pseudoephedrine in children: 4 mg/kg/d.

Findlay JWA, Butz RF, Sailstad JM, et al.: Pseudoephedrine and triprolidine in plasma and breast milk of nursing mothers. Br J Clin Pharmacol 18:901-906, 1984.

Heinonen OP, Slone D, Shapiro S: *Birth Defects and Drugs in Pregnancy.* Littleton, Mass.: John Wright-PSG, 1977, pp 346-347, 439.

Jick H, Holmes LB, Hunter JR, et al.: First-trimester drug use and congenital disorders. JAMA 246:343-346, 1981.

Werler MM, Mitchell AA, Shapiro S: First trimester maternal medication use in relation to gastroschisis. Teratology 45:361-367, 1992.

WHO Working Group on Drugs and Human Lactation. In: Bennet PN (ed). *Drugs and Human Lactation.* Amsterdam: Elsevier, 1988, p 413-414.

PSYLLIUM
(Fiberall®, Metamucil®, Serutan®)

Psyllium is a dietary fiber obtained from the husks of *Plantago* seeds. It is used as a bulk laxative. Psyllium is taken orally in doses of 1.7-18 g/d.

Teratogenic Risk

Magnitude of teratogenic risk to child born after exposure during gestation:	None
Quality and quantity of data on which risk estimate is based:	Poor to fair

The frequency of malformations was no greater than expected among the infants of more than 100 women who took psyllium during the first trimester of pregnancy in one epidemiological study (Jick et al., 1981).

No animal teratology studies of psyllium have been published.

Risk Related to Breast-feeding

No information regarding the distribution of psyllium in breast milk has been published.

Key References

Jick H, Holmes LB, Hunter JR, et al.: First-trimester drug use and congenital disorders. JAMA 246:343-346, 1981.

PURINOL *See* Allopurinol

PYRIDAMOLE® *See* Dipyridamole

PYRIDIUM® *See* Phenazopyridine

PYRIDOXINE
(Beesix®, Doxine®, Vitamin B₆)

Pyridoxine, vitamin B_6, is an essential nutrient that serves as an enzyme co-factor in intermediary metabolism. The dietary requirement for pyridoxine appears to be greater in pregnant women than in non-pregnant individuals (NRC, 1989; Driskell, 1994). The US Recommended Dietary Allowance (RDA) of pyridoxine in pregnancy is 2.2 mg/d. Deficiency states are treated with 25-600 mg/d of pyridoxine given orally or parenterally.

Teratogenic Risk

*Magnitude of teratogenic
risk to child born after
exposure during gestation:* None

*Quality and quantity of data
on which risk estimate is based:* Fair

This assessment refers to very high doses (hundreds of milligrams per day) of pyridoxine. Pyridoxine in small doses is a necessary dietary component.

No epidemiological studies of congenital anomalies among children born to women who used large ("megavitamin") doses of pyridoxine during pregnancy have been reported.

Studies in rats suggest that treatment of pregnant women with pyridoxine in usual "megavitamin" doses is unlikely to increase the children's risk of malformations greatly (Khera, 1975; Marathe & Thomas, 1986).

Risk Related to Breast-feeding

Pyridoxine is a normal constituent of breast milk. Maternal supplementation with pyridoxine during breast-feeding produces a dose-related increase in breast milk concentrations (Deodhar et al., 1964; Roepke & Kirksey, 1979; Thomas et al., 1979, 1980; Sneed et al., 1981; Andon et al., 1985; Styslinger & Kirksey, 1985; Kang-Yoon et al., 1992). However, this increase does not produce levels of pyridoxine in the nursing infant that exceed the RDA for infants.*

Key References

Andon MB, Howard MP, Moser PB, Reynolds RD: Nutritionally relevant supplementation of vitamin B6 in lactating women: Effect on plasma prolactin. Pediatrics 76:769-773, 1985.

Deodhar AD, Rajalakshmi R, Ramakrishnan CV: Studies on human lactation. Part III. Effect of dietary vitamin supplementation on vitamin contents of breast milk. Acta Paediatrica 53:42-48, 1964.

Driskell JA: Vitamin B-6 requirements of humans. Nutr Res 14(2):293-324, 1994.

Kang-Yoon SA, Kirksey A, Giacoia G, West K: Vitamin B-6 status of breast-fed neonates: Influence of pyridoxine supplementation on mothers and neonates. Am J Clin Nutr 56:548-558, 1992.

Khera KS: Teratogenicity study in rats given high doses of pyridoxine (vitamin B6) during organogenesis. Experientia 31:469-470, 1975.

Marathe MR, Thomas GP: Absence of teratogenicity of pyridoxine in Wistar rats. Indian J Physiol Pharmacol 30:264-266, 1986.

NRC (National Research Council): *Recommended Dietary Allowances, 10th ed. Report of the Subcommittee on the Tenth Edition of the RDAs, Food and Nutrition Board, Commission on Life Sciences.* Washington, DC: National Academy Press, 1989, p 262.

*The RDA of pyridoxine for infants under one year of age: 0.3-0.6 mg.

516

Roepke JLB, Kirksey A: Vitamin B_6 nutriture during pregnancy and lactation. I. Vitamin B_6 intake, levels of the vitamin in biological fluids, and condition of the infant at birth. Am J Clin Nutr 32:2249-2256, 1979.

Sneed SM, Zane C, Thomas MR: The effects of ascorbic acid, vitamin B_6, vitamin B_{12}, and folic acid supplementation on the breast milk and maternal nutritional status of low socioeconomic lactating women. Am J Clin Nutr 34:1338-1346, 1981.

Styslinger L, Kirksey A: Effects of different levels of vitamin B-6 supplementation on vitamin B-6 concentrations in human milk and vitamin B-6 intakes of breastfed infants. Am J Clin Nutr 41:21-31, 1985.

Thomas MR, Kawamoto J, Sneed SM, Eakin R: The effects of vitamin C, vitamin B_6, and vitamin B_{12} supplementation on the breast milk and maternal status of well-nourished women. Am J Clin Nutr 32:1679-1685, 1979.

Thomas MR, Sneed SM, Wei C, et al.: The effects of vitamin C, vitamin B_6, vitamin B_{12}, folic acid, riboflavin, and thiamin on the breast milk and maternal status of well-nourished women at 6 months postpartum. Am J Clin Nutr 33:2151-2156, 1980.

QUARZAN® *See* Clidinium Bromide

QUINALIN® *See* Quinidine

QUINIDINE
(Cardioquin®, Duraquin®, Quinalin®)

Quinidine is a drug used to prevent and treat cardiac arrhythmias. Quinidine is given orally in doses of 628-4000 mg/d or parenterally in doses of 500-5000 mg/d.

Teratogenic Risk

Magnitude of teratogenic
risk to child born after
exposure during gestation: *Undetermined*

Quality and quantity of data
on which risk estimate is based: *None*

No epidemiological studies of congenital anomalies in infants of women treated with quinidine during pregnancy have been reported.

No animal teratology studies of quinidine have been published.

Administration of quinidine to the mother has been used to treat fetal supraventricular tachycardia in the second and third trimesters of pregnancy (Spinnato et al., 1984; Guntheroth et al., 1985).

Risk Related to Breast-feeding

Quinidine is excreted in the breast milk in small quantities. The amount of quinidine that the nursing infant would be expected to ingest is between 3-4% of the lowest weight-adjusted therapeutic dose of quinidine, based on data from a single patient (Hill & Malkasian, 1979).*

The American Academy of Pediatrics regards quinidine to be safe to use while breast-feeding (Committee on Drugs, American Academy of Pediatrics, 1994).

Key References

Committee on Drugs, American Academy of Pediatrics: The transfer of drugs and other chemicals into human milk. Pediatrics 93(1):137-150, 1994.

Guntheroth WG, Cyr DR, Mack LA, et al.: Hydrops from reciprocating atrioventricular tachycardia in a 27-week fetus requiring quinidine for conversion. Obstet Gynecol 66:29S-33S, 1985.

Hill LM, Malkasian GD Jr: The use of quinidine sulfate throughout pregnancy. Obstet Gynecol 54:366-368, 1979.

Spinnato JA, Shaver DC, Flinn GS, et al.: Fetal supraventricular tachycardia: In utero therapy with digoxin and quinidine. Obstet Gynecol 64:730-735, 1984.

*This calculation is based on the following assumptions: maternal dose of quinidine: 1800 mg/d; milk concentration of quinidine: 6.4-8.2 mcg/mL; milk intake by the nursing infant: 150 mL/kg/d; estimated dose of quinidine ingested by the nursing infant: 1-1.2 mg/kg/d; lowest therapeutic dose of quinidine in children: 30 mg/kg/d.

RANITIDINE
(Zantac®)

Ranitidine is a histamine H_2-receptor antagonist used to reduce gastric acidity. It is given orally to treat or prevent gastric and duodenal ulcers, gastric hypersecretion, gastroesophageal reflux, and gastric mucosal damage associated with chronic use of nonsteroidal anti-inflammatory agents. Ranitidine is also used parenterally to prevent and treat stress-induced gastric mucosal damage and to prevent aspiration pneumonia associated with anesthesia. The usual dose is 150-300 mg/d, although doses up to 400 mg/d are sometimes used. Because most adverse effects are dose-related, occasional low-dose use is likely to be safer than chronic high-dose use.

Teratogenic Risk

Magnitude of teratogenic risk to child born after exposure during gestation:	*Undetermined*
Quality and quantity of data on which risk estimate is based:	*Poor*

There are no published epidemiological studies of congenital anomalies among children of women treated with ranitidine during pregnancy. One congenital anomaly (a large hemangioma) was observed among 12 infants born to women who had taken ranitidine during the first trimester of pregnancy in one series (Koren & Zemlickis, 1991). This anomaly may be unrelated to the mother's treatment.

Studies in rats and rabbits suggest that treatment of pregnant women with ranitidine in usual therapeutic doses is unlikely to increase the children's risk of malformations greatly (Higashida et al., 1983; Tamura et al., 1983).

Risk Related to Breast-feeding

Ranitidine is excreted into the breast milk. Based on data from a single patient, the amount of ranitidine that the nursing infant would be expected to ingest is between 2.5-10% of the lowest therapeutic dose on a weight-adjusted basis (Kearns et al., 1985)*

*This calculation is based on the following assumptions: maternal dose of ranitidine: 600 mg/d; milk concentration of ranitidine: 0.72-2.6 mcg/mL; milk intake by the nursing infant: 150 mL/kg/d; estimated dose of ranitidine ingested by the nursing infant: 0.1-0.4 mg/kg/d; lowest therapeutic dose of ranitidine in children: 4 mg/kg/d.

Key References

Higashida N, Kamada S, Sakanoue M, et al.: Teratogenicity study on ranitidine hydrochloride in rats. J Toxicol Sci 8(Suppl I):101-122, 1983.

Kearns GL, McConnell RF Jr, Trang JM, Kluza RB: Appearance of ranitidine in breast milk following multiple dosing. Clin Pharm 4:322-324, 1985.

Koren G, Zemlickis DM: Outcome of pregnancy after first trimester exposure to H₂ receptor antagonists. Am J Perinatol 8:37-38, 1991.

Tamura J, Sato N, Ezaki H, Yokoyama S: Teratological study on ranitidine hydrochloride in rabbits. J Toxicol Sci 8(Suppl I):141-150, 1983.

REACTINE® *See* Cetirizine

RESERPINE
(Sandril®, Serpalan®, Serpasil®)

Reserpine is a *Rauwolfia* alkaloid with central nervous system depressant action. It is given orally as an antihypertensive agent in a dose of 100-500 mcg/d, with much higher doses used in hypertensive emergencies.

Teratogenic Risk

Magnitude of teratogenic risk to child born after exposure during gestation:	*Unlikely*
Quality and quantity of data on which risk estimate is based:	*Fair*

Therapeutic doses of reserpine are unlikely to pose a substantial teratogenic risk, but the data are insufficient to state that there is no risk.

Transient neonatal respiratory distress may occur in infants born to women treated with reserpine late in pregnancy.

The frequency of congenital anomalies was not significantly greater than expected among the children of 48 women treated with reserpine or other *Rauwolfia* alkaloids during the first four lunar months of pregnancy or among 475 women treated with these agents anytime during pregnancy in one epidemiological investigation (Heinonen et al., 1977). The frequency of hydronephrosis and hydroureter appeared high among the children of women treated with reserpine or *Rauwolfia* alkaloids anytime in pregnancy, but studies such as this one that includes multiple comparisons between maternal drug exposures and various birth defect outcomes are expected to show occasional associations purely by chance.

The frequency of maternal reserpine use during pregnancy was no greater than expected among 6227 infants with various congenital anomalies in one large epidemiological study (Czeizel, 1988). There was no association with maternal use of reserpine during pregnancy among the infants in 11 malformation subgroups in this study. No information was provided regarding when in pregnancy the maternal exposures occurred, but it seems likely that most were late in gestation.

Maternal treatment with reserpine near term can produce transient nasal congestion, respiratory distress, and lethargy in newborn children (Budnick et al., 1955)

Increased frequencies of anophthalmia and other malformations were observed among the offspring of pregnant rats treated with reserpine in doses 80-200 times that used in humans (Goldman & Yakovac, 1965; Moriyama & Kanoh, 1978). Fetal or neonatal death often occurs when pregnant rats or guinea pigs are treated with 10 or more or with 0.5-10 times the human dose of reserpine, respectively (Deanesly, 1966; Towell & Hyman, 1966; Buelke-Sam et al., 1984; Harmon et al., 1987). Decreased brain and body weight occurred in rat offspring in association with maternal toxicity when the mothers were treated during pregnancy with 40 times the human dose of reserpine (Holson et al., 1994). Long-lasting behavioral alterations have been observed among the offspring of rats treated during pregnancy with 10 or more times the usual human dose of reserpine (Hoffeld et al., 1967, 1968; Buelke-Sam et al., 1989). The relevance of these findings to the clinical use of reserpine in human pregnancy is unknown.

Risk Related to Breast-feeding

Reserpine is excreted in breast milk (Anderson, 1977), although this has not been quantitated in published reports.

Key References

Anderson PO: Drugs and breast feeding - a review. Drug Intell Clin Pharm 11:208-223, 1977.

Budnick IS, Leikin S, Hoeck LE: Effect in the newborn infant of reserpine administered ante partum. Am J Dis Child 90:286-289, 1955.

Buelke-Sam J, Ali SF, Kimmel GL, et al.: Postnatal function following prenatal reserpine exposure in rats: Neurobehavioral toxicity. Neurotoxicol Teratol 11:515-522, 1989.

Buelke-Sam J, Kimmel GL, Webb PJ, et al.: Postnatal toxicity following prenatal reserpine exposure in rats: Effects of dose and dosing schedule. Fundam Appl Toxicol 4:983-991, 1984.

Czeizel A: Reserpine is not a human teratogen. J Med Genet 25:787, 1988.

Deanesly R: The effects of reserpine on ovulation and on the corpus luteum of the guinea-pig. J Reprod Fertil 11:429-438, 1966.

Goldman AS, Yakovac WC: Teratogenic action in rats of reserpine alone and in combination with salicylate and immobilization. Proc Soc Exp Biol Med 118:857-862, 1965.

Harmon JR, Kimmel GL, Webb PJ, Delongchamp RR: Effect of prenatal reserpine exposure on development of the postnatal rat heart. Teratogenesis Carcinog Mutagen 7:347-355, 1987.

Heinonen OP, Slone D, Shapiro S: *Birth Defects and Drugs in Pregnancy.* Littleton, Mass.: John Wright-PSG, 1977, pp 372-373, 441, 495.

Hoffeld DR, McNew J, Webster RL: Effect of tranquillizing drugs during pregnancy on activity of offspring. Nature 218:357-358, 1968.

Hoffeld DR, Webster RL, McNew J: Adverse effects on offspring of tranquillizing drugs during pregnancy. Nature 215:182-183, 1967.

Holson RR, Webb PJ, Grafton TF, Hansen DK: Prenatal neuroleptic exposure and growth stunting in the rat: An in vivo and in vitro examination of sensitive periods and possible mechanisms. Teratology 50:125-136, 1994.

Moriyama I, Kanoh S: Effect of reserpine on the pregnant rat. Acta Obstet Gynaecol Jpn 30(2):161-166, 1978.

Towell ME, Hyman AI: Catecholamine depletion in pregnancy. J Obstet Gynaecol Br Commonw 73:431-438, 1966.

RESTORIL® *See* Temazepam

RETIN-A® *See* Tretinoin

RETINOIC ACID *See* Tretinoin

RETINOL® *See* Vitamin A

RETOVIR® *See* Zidovudine

RHINALAR® *See* Flunisolide

RHYTHMIN® *See* Procainamide

RIBOFLAVIN
(Beflavin®, Flavitan®, Vitamin B$_2$)

Riboflavin (vitamin B$_2$) is a necessary dietary component. It functions as a coenzyme in intermediary metabolism. The US recommended dietary allowance (RDA) of riboflavin for pregnant and lactating women is 1.6 mg/d (NRC, 1989). Oral doses of 5-30 mg/d are usually given for the treatment of deficiency states.

Teratogenic Risk

*Magnitude of teratogenic
risk to child born after
exposure during gestation:*   *Undetermined*

*Quality and quantity of data
on which risk estimate is based:*   *Very poor*

A small risk cannot be excluded, but there is no indication that the risk of congenital anomalies in children of women who take large amounts of riboflavin during pregnancy is likely to be great.

No epidemiological studies of congenital anomalies in infants born to women who took unusually large amounts of riboflavin during pregnancy have been reported.

Studies in rats suggest that treatment of pregnant women with riboflavin in usual therapeutic doses is unlikely to increase the children's risk of malformations greatly (Chaube, 1973).

Risk Related to Breast-feeding

Riboflavin is a normal constituent of breast milk. Supplementation of both well-nourished and poorly-nourished breast-feeding mothers with riboflavin at levels up to six times the RDA increases breast milk concentrations but does not result in a riboflavin intake for the nursing infant that exceeds the infant RDA (Deodhar et al., 1964; Nail et al., 1980).*

The American Academy of Pediatrics regards riboflavin to be safe to take while breast-feeding (Committee on Drugs, American Academy of Pediatrics, 1994).

Key References

Chaube S: Protective effects of thymidine, 5-aminoimidazolecarboxamide, and riboflavin against fetal abnormalities produced in rats by 5-(3,3-dimethyl-1-triazeno)imidazole-4-carboxamide. Cancer Res 33:2231-2239, 1973.

Committee on Drug, American Academy of Pediatrics: The transfer of drugs and other chemicals into human milk. Pediatrics 93(1):137-150, 1994.

Deodhar AD, Rajalakshmi R, Ramakrishnan CV: Studies on human lactation. Part III. Effect of dietary vitamin supplementation on vitamin contents of breast milk. Acta Paediatr 53:42-48, 1964.

Nail PA, Thomas MR, Eakin R: The effect of thiamin and riboflavin supplementation on the level of those vitamins in human breast milk and urine. Am J Clin Nutr 33:198-204, 1980.

NRC (National Research Council): *Recommended Dietary Allowances, 10th ed. Report of the Subcommittee on the Tenth Edition of the RDAs, Food and Nutrition Board, Commission on Life Sciences.* Washington, DC: National Academy Press, 1989, p 262.

*RDA of riboflavin for infants less than one year: 0.4-0.5 mg.

RIFADIN® *See* Rifampin

RIFAMPIN
(Rifadin®, Rimactan®, Rofact®)

Rifampin is an antibiotic used in the treatment of tuberculosis. It is also used to treat leprosy and meningococcal carriers. Rifampin is given orally or parenterally in doses of 500-600 mg/d. It is also used in doses of 1200 mg/d for propylaxis of meningococcal carriers, as well as for some endocarditis.

Teratogenic Risk

*Magnitude of teratogenic
risk to child born after
exposure during gestation:*   *Unlikely*

*Quality and quantity of data
on which risk estimate is based:*   *Poor to fair*

Therapeutic doses of rifampin are unlikely to pose a substantial teratogenic risk, but the data are insufficient to state that there is no risk.

No controlled epidemiological studies of congenital anomalies among the infants of women treated with rifampin during pregnancy have been published. The frequency of malformations did not appear unusually high among the children of 442 women reported in various studies who were treated during pregnancy with rifampin, usually in combination with other antitubercular drugs (Snider et al., 1980). In 109 of these pregnancies, treatment with rifampin occurred during the first trimester.

The frequency of congenital anomalies was not increased among the offspring of mice or rats treated with 2.5-10 times the usual human dose of rifampin during pregnancy (Stratford, 1966), but an increased frequency of cleft palate was observed among the offspring of mice and an increased frequency of spina bifida among the offspring of rats treated with more than 15 times the human dose of rifampin (Anonymous, 1971; Steen & Stainton-Ellis, 1977). Congenital anomalies were not increased among the offspring of pregnant rabbits treated with similar doses (Stratford, 1966; Anonymous, 1971; Steen & Stainton-Ellis, 1977).

Risk Related to Breast-feeding

Rifampin is excreted in the breast milk. The amount of rifampin that a nursing infant would be expected to ingest is between 1.5-7% of the therapeutic dose of rifampin for infants (Lenzi & Santuari, 1969; Vorherr, 1974).*

The American Academy of Pediatrics regards rifampin to be safe to use while breast-feeding (Committee on Drugs, American Academy of Pediatrics, 1994).

Key References

Anonymous: Rifampicin: A review. Drugs 1:354-398, 1971.

Committee on Drugs, American Academy of Pediatrics: The transfer of drugs and other chemicals into human milk. Pediatrics 93(1):137-150, 1994.

Lenzi E, Santuari S: [Preliminary observations on the use of a new semi-synthetic rifamycin derivative in gynecology and obstetrics.] Atti Accad Lanisiana Roma 13(Suppl 1):87-94, 1969. Cited in Snider DE Jr, Powell KE: Should women taking antituberculosis drugs breast-feed? Arch Intern Med 144:589-590, 1984.

Snider DE Jr, Layde PM, Johnson MW, Lyle MA: Treatment of tuberculosis during pregnancy. Am Rev Respir Dis 122:65-79, 1980.

Steen JSM, Stainton-Ellis DM: Rifampicin in pregnancy. Lancet 2:604-605, 1977.

Stratford BF: Observations on laboratory rodents treated with "Rifamide" during pregnancy. Med J Aust 1:10-12, 1966.

Vorherr H: Drug excretion in breast milk. Postgrad Med 56(4):97-104, 1974.

*This calculation is based on the following assumptions: maternal dose of rifampin: 450-600 mg; milk concentration of rifampin: 1-5 mcg/mL; milk intake by the nursing infant: 150 mL/kg/d; estimated dose of rifampin ingested by the nursing infant: 0.15-0.75 mg/kg/d; lowest therapeutic dose of rifampin in infants: 10 mg/kg/d.

RIMACTAN® *See* Rifampin

RIVOTRIL® *See* Clonazepam

ROBITUSSIN® *See* Dextromethorphan

ROCALTROL® *See* Vitamin D

ROFACT® *See* Rifampin

RONASE® *See* Tolazamide

ROVAMYCINE® *See* Spiramycin

ROXANE® *See* Thiothixene

ROXANOL® *See* Morphine

ROXICODONE® *See* Oxycodone

RUBELLA VACCINE
(Meruvax®)

Rubella vaccine is a live attenuated virus vaccine used for the prevention of German measles.

Teratogenic Risk

*Magnitude of teratogenic
risk to child born after
exposure during gestation:*   *Unlikely*

*Quality and quantity of data
on which risk estimate is based:*   *Good*

Immunization with rubella vaccine is unlikely to pose a substantial teratogenic risk, but the data are insufficient to state that there is no risk.

No abnormalities characteristic of the congenital rubella syndrome were found among the infants of 230 susceptible women immunized with RA27/3 strain rubella vaccine, or among the infants of 94 susceptible women immunized with Cendehill or HPV-77 strain rubella vaccine in the three months immediately preceding or following conception (Preblud et al., 1981; Bart et al., 1985; Preblud, 1985; Anonymous, 1989; Best, 1991). No cases of congenital rubella syndrome were observed in two other studies among 144 or 42 infants born to mothers who were susceptible to rubella and had been immunized with rubella vaccine within three months before conception or during pregnancy (Enders, 1985; Sheppard et al., 1986; Best, 1991). On the basis of these data, the maximum risk for congenital rubella syndrome due to vaccination with RA27/3 strain vaccine during pregnancy was estimated to be 1.6% (Best, 1991). These studies included at least 122 women who were immunized from one week before to four weeks after conception, the period of presumed highest risk for fetal malformations (Anonymous, 1989). One case of cataract in a fetus with documented rubella vaccine virus infection has been observed after maternal immunization (Fleet et al., 1974).

All strains of rubella vaccine virus studied are capable of causing asymptomatic infection of the embryo or fetus after maternal immunization (Preblud, 1985; Anonymous, 1989; Best, 1991).

Fetal infection, but no increase in the frequency of malformations, was found among the offspring of rabbits injected with rubella vaccine virus during pregnancy (Cohen et al., 1971).

Risk Related to Breast-feeding

Rubella virus vaccine has been found to be excreted in the breast milk of some women following maternal vaccination (Losonsky et al., 1982a; Tingle et al., 1985). Virus shedding in breast milk generally lasts for two to three weeks when it occurs, but virus is not always found in the milk after maternal rubella immunization (Boue et al., 1969; Monif & Held, 1971; Grillner et al., 1973; Losonsky et al., 1982b).

Rubella virus or antigen has been recovered from the throat or nasopharynx of some breast-fed infants whose mothers were immunized with rubella vaccine, but none of these infants developed clinical manifestations of rubella infection (Buimovici-Klein et al., 1977; Losonsky et al., 1982b). Seroconversion occurred in four of 16 breast-fed infants of women who were immunized with rubella vaccine in one study (Losonsky et al., 1982b), but this immune response was transient and of low magnitude. None of these infants developed clinical manifestations of rubella. One case of rubella in a breast-fed infant attributed to maternal immunization has been reported (Landes et al., 1980), but the possibility of neonatal infection with natural rubella virus cannot be ruled out (Lerman, 1981).

Although there is a concern that breast-fed infants of vaccinated mothers may be sensitized to virus antigens, no conclusive evidence exists that these infants are at an increased risk of contracting rubella when exposed to the virus later in childhood (Losonsky et al., 1982a; Preblud et al., 1986).

The Advisory Committee on Immunization Practices considers live vaccines to be safe to administer to a mother during breast-feeding (ACIP, 1994).

Key References

ACIP: General recommendations on immunization. Recommendations of the Advisory Committee on Immunization Practices (ACIP). MMWR 43(RR-1):1-38, 1994.

Anonymous: Rubella vaccination during pregnancy--United States 1971-1988. MMWR 38(17):289-293, 1989.

Bart SW, Stetler HC, Preblud SR, et al.: Fetal risk associated with rubella vaccine: An update. Rev Infect Dis 7(Suppl 1):S95-S102, 1985.

Best JM: Rubella vaccines: Past, present and future. Epidemiol Infect 107:17-30, 1991.

Boue A, Papiernick-Berkhauer E, Levy-Thierry S: Attenuated rubella virus vaccine in women. Am J Dis Child 118:230-233, 1969.

Buimovici-Klein E, Hite RL, Byrne T, Cooper LZ: Isolation of rubella virus in milk after postpartum immunization. J Pediatr 91:939-941, 1977.

Cohen SM, Collins DN, Ward G, Deibel R: Transplacental transmission of rubella virus infection in rabbits. Appl Microbiol 21:76-78, 1971.

Enders G: Rubella antibody titers in vaccinated and nonvaccinated women and results of vaccination during pregnancy. Rev Infect Dis 7(Suppl 1):S103-S107, 1985.

Fleet WF Jr, Benz EW Jr, Karzon DT, et al.: Fetal consequences of maternal rubella immunization. JAMA 227:621-627, 1974.

Grillner L, Hedstrom C-E, Bergstrom H, et al.: Vaccination against rubella of newly delivered women. Scand J Infect Dis 5:237-241, 1973.

Landes RD, Bass JW, Millunchick EW, Oetgen WJ: Neonatal rubella following postpartum maternal immunization. J Pediatr 97:465-467, 1980.

Lerman SJ: Neonatal rubella following maternal immunization. J Pediatr 98:668-669, 1981.

Losonsky GA, Fishaut JM, Strussenberg J, Ogra PL: Effect of immunization against rubella on lactation products. I. Development and characterization of specific immunologic reactivity in breast milk. J Infect Dis 145(5):654-660, 1982a.

Losonsky GA, Fishaut JM, Strussenberg J, Ogra PL: Effect of immunization against rubella on lactation products. II. Maternal-neonatal interactions. J Infect Dis 145(5):661-666, 1982b.

Monif GRG, Held B: Noncontagiousness of the Cendehill vaccine strain of rubella virus from mother to newborn infant. J Pediatr 78:306-307, 1971.

Preblud SR: Some current issues relating to rubella vaccine. JAMA 254:253-256, 1985.

Preblud SR, Orenstein WA, Lopez C, et al.: Postpartum rubella immunization. J Infect Dis 154(2):367-368, 1986.

Preblud, SR, Stetler HC, Frank JA Jr, et al.: Fetal risk associated with rubella vaccine. JAMA 246:1413-1417, 1981.

Sheppard S, Smithells RW, Dickson A, Holzel H: Rubella vaccination and pregnancy: Preliminary report of a national survey. Br Med J 292:727, 1986.

Tingle AJ, Chantler JK, Pot KH, et al.: Postpartum rubella immunization: Association with development of prolonged arthritis, neurological sequelae, and chronic rubella viremia. J Infect Dis 152(3):606-612, 1985.

RUBION® *See* Cyanocobalamin

RYTHMODON® *See* Disopyramide

SALAGEN® *See* Pilocarpine

SALAZOPYRINE® *See* Sulfasalazine

SALICYLATES *See* Aspirin

SANDIMMUNE® *See* Cyclosporine

SANDRIL® *See* Reserpine

SCOPOLAMINE
(Transderm-Scop®, Transderm V®)

Scopolamine is an anticholinergic agent. It is used as a preoperative medication and in the treatment of motion sickness, mania, and delirium. Scopolamine is also used in ophthalmic preparations to produce mydriasis and cycloplegia. Scopolamine is usually given in oral doses of 1-80 mg/d. Individual parenteral doses range from 0.3-1 mg.

Teratogenic Risk

*Magnitude of teratogenic
risk to child born after
exposure during gestation:*   *Unlikely*

*Quality and quantity of data
on which risk estimate is based:*   *Poor to fair*

Therapeutic doses of scopolamine are unlikely to pose a substantial teratogenic risk, but the data are insufficient to state that there is no risk.

The frequency of congenital anomalies was no greater than expected among the children of 388 women treated with scopolamine during the first four lunar months of pregnancy or among the infants of 1053 women treated anytime during pregnancy in one epidemiological study (Heinonen et al., 1977).

No teratogenic effect was observed among the offspring of mice treated during pregnancy with 200-18,000 times the maximum human dose of scopolamine (George, 1987). An increased frequency of eye and skeletal anomalies was observed in a much smaller study in mice treated during pregnancy with 92-1180 times the maximum human dose of scopolamine (Yu et al., 1988). Studies in rats showed a teratogenic effect at 200 times the maximum human dose of scopolamine, but equivocal effects on fetal weight and anomalies were seen in association with maternal toxicity at higher doses (George et al., 1987). Eye anomalies were found in all 38 fetuses born to pregnant rabbits given scopolamine in doses several times the maximum used in humans in one study (McBride, 1983). Long-lasting alterations of behavior were observed among mice born to mothers treated with scopolamine during pregnancy in doses 50 times greater than those used in mice (Richardson et al., 1972). The relevance of these observations to the therapeutic use of scopolamine in human pregnancy is unknown.

When given to a pregnant woman just prior to delivery, scopolamine may alter fetal cardiac rate and activity (Ayromlooi et al., 1980). The clinical significance of this observation is unclear.

Risk Related to Breast-feeding

No information regarding the distribution of scopolamine in breast milk has been published. The American Academy of Pediatrics regards scopolamine to be safe to use while breast-feeding (Committee on Drugs, American Academy of Pediatrics, 1994).

Key References

Ayromlooi J, Tobias M, Berg P: The effects of scopolamine and ancillary analgesics upon the fetal heart rate recording. J Reprod Med 25:323-326, 1980.

Committee on Drugs, American Academy of Pediatrics: The transfer of drugs and other chemicals into human milk. Pediatrics 93(1):137-150, 1994.

George JD: Teratologic evaluation of scopolamine hydrobromide (CAS No. 114-49-8) administered to CD-1 mice on gestational days 6 through 15. NTIS (National Technical Information System) Report/PB87-209516, 1987.

George JD, Price CJ, Marr MC: Teratologic evaluation of scopolamine hydrobromide (CAS No. 114-49-8) administered to CD rats on gestational days 6 through 15. NTIS (National Technical Information Service) Report/PB87-235412, 1987.

Heinonen OP, Slone D, Shapiro S: *Birth Defects and Drugs in Pregnancy.* Littleton, Mass.: John Wright-PSG, 1977, pp 346, 439.

McBride WG: Note on the paper 'Effects of scopolamine hydrobromide on the development of the chick and rabbit embryo' by WG McBride, PH Vardy and J French. Aust J Biol Sci 36:171-172, 1983.

Richardson DL, Karczmar AG, Scudder CL: Effects of pre-natal cholinergic drug treatment on post-natal behavior and brain chemistry in mice. Fed Proc Fed Am Soc Exp Biol 31:596, 1972.

Yu J-F, Yang Y-S, Wang W-Y, et al.: Mutagenicity and teratogenicity of chlorpromazine and scopolamine. Chin Med J [Engl]
101(5):339-345, 1988.

SECOBARBITAL
(Novosecobarb®, Seconal®)

Secobarbital is a barbiturate that is used as a sedative and hypnotic.
Secobarbital is given orally in doses of 90-150 mg/d, but as much as
300 mg may be given in a single dose as an anesthetic.   Single
parenteral doses range from 50-250 mg.

Teratogenic Risk

*Magnitude of teratogenic
risk to child born after
exposure during gestation:*   *None*

*Quality and quantity of data
on which risk estimate is based:*   *Poor to fair*

*Neonatal withdrawal symptoms have been reported with chronic
use of secobarbital (see below).*

The frequencies of congenital anomalies in general, of major
malformations, of minor anomalies, and of principal classes of
malformations were no greater than expected among the children of
378 women who took secobarbital during the first four lunar months of
pregnancy in one epidemiological study (Heinonen et al., 1977).   The
frequency of congenital anomalies was not increased among the
children of 4248 women who took secobarbital anytime during
pregnancy in this study (Heinonen et al., 1977).

No animal teratology studies of secobarbital have been published.

Hyperirritability and seizures, thought to represent neonatal
withdrawal symptoms, have been reported in the infant of a woman
who took very large doses of secobarbital throughout pregnancy (Bleyer
& Marshall, 1972).

Risk Related to Breast-feeding

No information regarding the distribution of secobarbital in breast milk has been published. The American Academy of Pediatrics regards secobarbital to be safe to use while breast-feeding (Committee on Drugs, American Academy of Pediatrics, 1994).

Key References

Bleyer WA, Marshall RE: Barbiturate withdrawal syndrome in a passively addicted infant. JAMA 221:185-186, 1972.

Committee on Drugs, American Academy of Pediatrics: The transfer of drugs and other chemicals into human milk. Pediatrics 93(1):137-150, 1994.

Heinonen OP, Slone D, Shapiro S: *Birth Defects and Drugs in Pregnancy.* Littleton, Mass.: John Wright-PSG, 1977, pp 226-340, 344, 438, 476, 490.

SECONAL® *See* Secobarbital

SELDANE® *See* Terfenadine

SENNA
(Black Draught®, Fletcher's Castoria®, Senolax®)

Senna is an anthraquinone obtained from plants of the genus *Cassia*. It is usually taken by mouth as a laxative in doses of 320-1480 mg/d. Senna is not appreciably absorbed when taken in small doses.

Teratogenic Risk

Magnitude of teratogenic risk to child born after exposure during gestation:	*Undetermined*
Quality and quantity of data on which risk estimate is based:	*Very poor*

A small risk cannot be excluded, but a high risk of congenital anomalies in the children of women treated with senna during pregnancy is unlikely.

No epidemiological studies of congenital anomalies among infants born to women who took senna during pregnancy have been reported. Studies in rats and rabbits suggest that treatment of pregnant women with senna in usual therapeutic doses is unlikely to increase the children's risk of malformations greatly (Mengs, 1986).

Risk Related to Breast-feeding

The active sennoside metabolites of senna are excreted in breast milk in amounts that are either undetectable or far below those required to produce a laxative effect (Werthmann & Krees, 1973; Faber & Strenge-Hesse, 1988). No adverse effects of maternal use of senna have been observed in nursing infants (Baldwin, 1963; Werthmann & Krees, 1973; Anonymous, 1992).

Both the American Academy of Pediatrics (Committee on Drugs, American Academy of Pediatrics, 1994) and the WHO Working Group on Drugs and Human Lactation (1988) regard senna to be safe to use while breast-feeding.

Key References

Anonymous: Senna in the puerperium. Pharmacology 44(Suppl 1):23-25, 1992.

Baldwin WF: Clinical study of senna administration to nursing mothers: Assessment of effects on infant bowel habits. Can Med Assoc J 89:566-568, 1963.

Committee on Drugs, American Academy of Pediatrics: The transfer of drugs and other chemicals into human milk. Pediatrics 93(1):137-150, 1994.

Faber P, Strenge-Hesse A: Relevance of rhein excretion into breast milk. Pharmacology 36(Suppl 1):212-220, 1988.

Mengs U: Reproductive toxicological investigations with sennosides. Arzneimittelforsch 36:1355-1358, 1986.

Werthmann MW Jr, Krees SV: Quantitative excretion of Senokot® in human breast milk. Med Ann DC 42:4-5, 1973.

WHO Working Group on Drugs and Human Lactation. In: Bennet PN (ed). *Drugs and Human Lactation.* Amsterdam: Elsevier, 1988, pp 88-89.

SENOLAX® *See Senna*

SENSORCAINE® *See Bupivacaine*

SERPALAN® *See Reserpine*

SERPASIL® *See Reserpine*

SERTRALINE
(Zoloft®)

Sertraline is an inhibitor of presynaptic serotonin reuptake. It is administered orally in doses of 25-200 mg/d to treat depressive illnesses.

Teratogenic Risk

Magnitude of teratogenic risk to child born after exposure during gestation:	*Undetermined*
Quality and quantity of data on which risk estimate is based:	*Very poor*

No epidemiological studies of congenital anomalies among the children of women who were treated with sertraline during pregnancy have been reported.

No teratogenic effect is said to have occurred in unpublished studies among the offspring of pregnant rats or rabbits treated with 20 or 10 times the maximum daily human dose of sertraline; however, delayed ossification was observed in the offspring of animals exposed to 2.5-10 times the maximum daily human dose of sertraline (USP DI, 1995). The relevance of this observation to therapeutic use of sertraline in human pregnancy is unknown.

Risk Related to Breast-feeding

Sertraline is excreted in the breast milk in very low concentrations. Based on data from a single patient, the amount of sertraline that the nursing infant would be expected to ingest is <1% of the lowest therapeutic dose on a weight-adjusted basis (Altshuler et al., 1995).* Sertraline was not detected in the infant's serum and no apparent adverse effects of maternal treatment with sertraline were exhibited by the infant.

Key References

Altshuler LL, Burt VK, McMullen M, Hendrick V: Breastfeeding and sertraline: A 24-hour analysis. J Clin Psychiatry 56:243-245, 1995.

USP DI: Sertraline. In: *USP DI (USP Dispensing Information), Volume 1. Drug Information for the Health Care Professional,* 15th ed. Rockville, Md.: The US Pharmacopeial Convention, 1995, p 2451.

*This calculation is based on the following assumptions: maternal dose of sertraline: 100 mg/d; milk concentration of sertraline: 0.009-0.04 mcg/mL; milk intake by the nursing infant: 150 mL/kg/d; estimated dose of sertraline ingested by the nursing infant: 0.001-0.006 mg/kg/d; lowest therapeutic dose of sertraline in adults: 0.78 mg/kg/d.

SERUTAN® *See* Psyllium

SINEQUAN® *See* Doxepin

SINEX® *See* Phenylephrine

SLEEP-EZE D® *See* Diphenhydramine

SLOW-K *See* Potassium Chloride

SODIUM CROMOGLYCATE *See* Cromolyn

SOFARIN® *See* Warfarin

SOLATINE® *See* Beta-Carotene

SOLAZINE® *See* Trifluoperazine

SOLFOTON® *See* Phenobarbital

SOLGOL® *See* Nadolol

SOLUSTREP® *See* Streptomycin

SORIATANE® *See* Acitretin

SPASMOBAN® *See* Dicyclomine

SPIRAMYCIN
(Rovamycine®)

Spiramycin is a macrolide antibiotic that is used in the treatment of toxoplasmosis and other infections. Spiramycin is usually given orally but may also be administered intravenously or rectally. The usual dose is 2000-4000 mg/d.

Teratogenic Risk

Magnitude of teratogenic risk to child born after exposure during gestation:	*Undetermined*
Quality and quantity of data on which risk estimate is based:	*Very poor*

No epidemiological studies of congenital anomalies among the children of women treated with spiramycin during pregnancy have been reported. Spiramycin has been used for the treatment of pregnant women with acute *Toxoplasma gondii* infections without apparent adverse fetal effects (Desmonts & Couvreur et al., 1974; Couvreur et al., 1988; Stray-Pedersen, 1992).

No animal teratology studies of spiramycin have been published. The litter size and survival of offspring was not affected when pregnant mice were given spiramycin beginning in mid-gestation in a daily dose about 13 times the maximum used in humans (Nguyen & Stadtsbaeder, 1985).

Risk Related to Breast-feeding

Spiramycin is excreted in breast milk in high concentrations (USP DI, 1995). In one study, serum concentrations seven times the peak therapeutic serum level were found in nursing infants of mothers treated with spiramycin (Goisis & Cavalli, 1959).*

Key References

Couvreur J, Desmonts G, Thulliez Ph: Prophylaxis of congenital toxoplasmosis. Effects of spiramycin on placental infection. J Antimicrob Chemother 22(Suppl B):193-200, 1988.

Desmonts G, Couvreur J: Congenital toxoplasmosis. A prospective study of 378 pregnancies. N Engl J Med 290:1110-1116, 1974.

Goisis M, Cavalli P: Variations of the organoleptic properties of human milk under treatment with antibiotics. Minerva Ginac 11:794-804, 1959. Cited in: Onnis A, Grella P. *The Biochemical Effects of Drugs in Pregnancy*, Volume 2. Chichester: Ellis Horwood, Ltd, 1984, pp 340-341.

Nguyen BT, Stadtsbaeder S: Comparative effects of cotrimoxazole (trimethoprim-sulphamethoxazole) and spiramycin in pregnant mice infected with *Toxoplasma gondii* (Beverly strain). Br J Pharmacol 85:713-716, 1985.

Stray-Pedersen B: Treatment of toxoplasmosis in the pregnant mother and newborn child. Scand J Infect Dis (Suppl 84):23-31, 1992.

USP DI: Spiramycin. In: *USP DI (USP Dispensing Information), Volume 1. Drug Information for the Health Care Professional*, 15th ed. Rockville, Md.: The US Pharmacopeial Convention, 1995, p 2997.

*This calculation is based on the following assumptions: maternal dose of spiramycin: 1.5 g/d; serum concentration of spiramycin in infants: 20 mcg/mL; peak therapeutic serum level of spiramycin in adults: 3 mcg/mL.

SPIRONOLACTONE
(Aldactone®, Novospiroton®)

Spironolactone is a steroid that acts as a competitive inhibitor of aldosterone. Spironolactone is given orally in doses of 25-400 mg/d as a diuretic and antihypertensive agent.

Teratogenic Risk

Magnitude of teratogenic risk to child born after exposure during gestation:	*Undetermined*
Quality and quantity of data on which risk estimate is based:	*Very poor*

No epidemiological studies of congenital anomalies in the children of women treated with spironolactone during pregnancy have been reported.

No increase in the frequency of malformations was observed among the offspring of pregnant rats or mice treated with spironolactone in doses 2.5-10 times those used in humans (Miyakubo et al., 1977). Feminization of the external genitalia was seen in the male offspring of rats treated with spironolactone during late pregnancy in doses 5 times greater than those used in humans (Hecker et al., 1980). In another study, hypoprolactinemia and reduced weights of accessory sex organs were seen in adult male rats and increased ovarian and uterine weights in adult female rats born to dams that had been treated during pregnancy with spironolactone in doses 2.5 times those used in humans (Jaussan et al., 1985). The relevance of these observations to the therapeutic use of spironolactone in human pregnancy is unknown.

Risk Related to Breast-feeding

Unmetabolized spironolactone has not been detected in breast milk. However, canrenone, one of the active metabolites of spironolactone, was measured in the breast milk of one patient. On the basis of this data, the amount of canrenone that the nursing infant would be expected to ingest is equivalent to <1% of the lowest therapeutic dose of spironolactone, on a weight-adjusted basis.*

Both the American Academy of Pediatrics (Committee on Drugs, American Academy of Pediatrics, 1994) and the WHO Working Group on Drugs and Human Lactation (1988) regard spironolactone to be safe to use while breast-feeding.

Key References

Committee on Drugs, American Academy of Pediatrics: The transfer of drugs and other chemicals into human milk. Pediatrics 93(1):137-150, 1994.

Hecker A, Hasan SH, Neumann F: Disturbances in sexual differentiation of rat foetuses following spironolactone treatment. Acta Endocrinol 95:540-545, 1980.

Jaussan V, Lemarchand-Beraud T, Gomez F: Modifications of the gonadal function in the adult rat after fetal exposure to spironolactone. Biol Reprod 32:1051-1061, 1985.

Miyakubo H, Saito S, Tokunaga Y, et al.: [Toxicological studies of SC-14266. 5. Teratological study of SC-14266 in rats and mice.] Nichidai Igaku Zasshi 36:261-282, 1977.

WHO Working Group on Drugs and Human Lactation. In: Bennet PN (ed). *Drugs and Human Lactation.* Amsterdam: Elsevier, 1988, pp 133-134.

*This calculation is based on the following assumptions: maternal dose of spironolactone: 50 mg/d; milk concentration of canrenone: 0.05-0.1 mcg/mL; milk intake by the nursing infant: 150 mL/kg/d; estimated dose of canrenone ingested by the nursing infant, assuming 25% activity of spironolactone but similar bioavailability and molecular weight as spironolactone: 0.007-0.01 mg/kg/d; lowest therapeutic dose of spironolactone in children: 1.65 mg/kg/d.

STATEX® *See* Morphine

STAY-TRIM® *See* Phenylpropanolamine

STELAZINE® *See* Trifluoperazine

STEMETIL® *See* Prochlorperazine

STILBOESTROL® *See* Diethylstilbestrol

STOPASTHME® *See* Ephedrine

STREPTASE® *See* Streptokinase

STREPTOCOL® *See* Streptomycin

STREPTOKINASE
(Kabikinase®, Streptase®)

Streptokinase is a nonenzymatic protein produced by certain streptococcal bacteria that activates plasminogen in human plasma to plasmin, a fibrinolytic enzyme. Streptokinase is administered intravenously or intra-arterially to dissolve blood clots in conditions such as pulmonary thromboembolism, deep vein thrombosis, and coronary artery thrombosis. The usual dose is 250,000-1,500,00 units.

Teratogenic Risk

Magnitude of teratogenic risk to child born after exposure during gestation:	*Undetermined*
Quality and quantity of data on which risk estimate is based:	*None*

No epidemiological studies of congenital anomalies among infants born to women treated with streptokinase during pregnancy have been reported.

No animal teratology studies of streptokinase have been published.

Risk Related to Breast-feeding

No information regarding the distribution of streptokinase in breast milk has been published.

Key References

None available.

STREPTOMYCIN
(Novostrep®, Solustrep®, Streptocol®)

Streptomycin is an aminoglycoside antibiotic used in the treatment of tuberculosis and other bacterial infections. Streptomycin is given parenterally in doses of 1000-4000 mg/d.

Teratogenic Risk

Magnitude of teratogenic
risk to child born after
exposure during gestation:
Deafness:	*Small*
Malformations:	*None*

Quality and quantity of data
on which risk estimate is based:
Deafness:	*Fair to good*
Malformations:	*Fair to good*

The frequency of congenital anomalies was no greater than expected among the children of 135 women who took streptomycin in the first four lunar months of pregnancy or among the children of 335 women who took the drug anytime during pregnancy in one epidemiological study (Heinonen et al., 1977). Deafness was not included among the anomalies studied in this investigation.

A number of case reports of sensorineural deafness, sometimes with accompanying vestibular dysfunction, in children born to women treated with streptomycin during pregnancy have been published (Warkany, 1979; Snider et al., 1980; Donald & Sellars, 1981). No relationship to drug dosage or stage of pregnancy during which exposure occurred is apparent in these reports, but since auditory nerve damage is a well-known toxic effect of streptomycin in children and adults, it seems likely that similar toxicity could occur antenatally. Although asymptomatic abnormalities of auditory or vestibular function have been observed in up to 10% of children born to women treated with streptomycin during pregnancy, symptomatic disturbances appear to be much less common (Varpela et al., 1969; Warkany, 1979; Donald & Sellars, 1981).

No increase in the frequency of malformations was observed among the offspring of mice treated during pregnancy with streptomycin in doses 5-6 times those used in humans (Ericson-Strandvik & Gyllensten, 1963; Nomura et al., 1984). No abnormality of auditory response was observed in the offspring of pregnant rats and mice treated, respectively, with 2.5-7.5 and 2-10 times the usual human dose of streptomycin (Suzuki & Takeuchi, 1961), but histological evidence of inner ear damage was apparent among the offspring of pregnant mice treated with 3 times the human dose of streptomycin (Nakamoto et al., 1985). No functional or histological abnormality of the auditory or vestibular system was seen among the offspring of guinea pigs treated during pregnancy with streptomycin in doses similar to those used in humans (Riskaer et al., 1952).

Risk Related to Breast-feeding

Streptomycin is excreted in the breast milk in low concentrations. The amount of streptomycin that the nursing infant would be expected to receive is <1% of the lowest therapeutic weight-adjusted dose, based on data from eight lactating women (Snider & Powell, 1984).*

The American Academy of Pediatrics regards streptomycin to be safe to use while breast-feeding (Committee on Drugs, American Academy of Pediatrics, 1994).

Key References

Committee on Drugs, American Academy of Pediatrics: The transfer of drugs and other chemicals into human milk. Pediatrics 93(1):137-150, 1994.

Donald PR, Sellars SL: Streptomycin ototoxicity in the unborn child. S Afr Med J 60:316-318, 1981.

Ericson-Strandvik B, Gyllensten L: The central nervous system of foetal mice after administration of streptomycin. Acta Pathol Microbiol Scand 59:292-300, 1963.

Heinonen OP, Slone D, Shapiro S: *Birth Defects and Drugs in Pregnancy*. Littleton, Mass.: John Wright-PSG, 1977, pp 297, 435.

Nakamoto Y, Otani H, Tanaka O: Effects of aminoglycosides administered to pregnant mice on postnatal development of inner ear in their offspring. Teratology 32(3):34B, 1985.

*This calculation is based on the following assumptions: maternal dose of dihydros-treptomycin: 1g; milk concentration of streptomycin: 0.3-1.3 mcg/mL; milk intake by the nursing infant: 150 mL/kg/d; estimated dose of streptomycin ingested by the nursing infant: 0.004-0.19 mg/kg/d; lowest therapeutic dose of streptomycin in children: 20 mg/kg/d.

Nomura T, Kimura S, Kanzaki T, et al.: Induction of tumors and malformations in mice after prenatal treatment with some antibiotic drugs. Med J Osaka Univ 35(1-2):13-17, 1984.

Riskaer N, Christensen E, Hertz H: The toxic effects of streptomycin and dihydrosteptomycin in pregnancy, illustrated experimentally. Acta Tuber Pneumol Scand 27:211-216, 1952.

Snider DE, Layde PM, Johnson MW, Lyle MA: Treatment of tuberculosis during pregnancy. Am Rev Respir Dis 122:65-79, 1980.

Snider DE, Powell KE: Should women taking antituberculosis drugs breast-feed? Arch Intern Med 144:589-590, 1984.

Suzuki Y, Takeuchi S: [Experimental studies on effects of streptomycin on the auditory mechanism of the fetus after administration of various doses to the pregnant mother.] Keio J Med 10:31-41, 1961.

Varpela E, Hietalahti J, Aro MJT: Streptomycin and dihydrostreptomycin medication during pregnancy and their effect on the child's inner ear. Scand J Respir Dis 50:101-109, 1969.

Warkany J: Antituberculous drugs. Teratology 20:133-138, 1979.

SUDAFED® *See* Pseudoephedrine

SULFACETAMIDE
(Bleph-10®, Cetamide®, Sulfamide®)

Sulfacetamide is a sulfonamide that is used as an antibacterial agent in ophthalmic and vaginal preparations. Systemic absorption of locally administered sulfacetamide may occur.

Teratogenic Risk

Magnitude of teratogenic risk to child born after exposure during gestation:	*None*
Quality and quantity of data on which risk estimate is based:	*Poor to fair*

The frequency of congenital anomalies was no greater than expected among the children of 93 women who were treated with sulfacetamide during the first four lunar months of pregnancy in one epidemiological study (Heinonen et al., 1977).

No animal teratology studies of sulfacetamide have been published. *Please see agent summary on sulfamethoxazole for information on a related agent that has been more thoroughly studied.*

Risk Related to Breast-feeding

No information on the distribution of sulfacetamide in breast milk has been published.

Key References

Heinonen OP, Slone D, Shapiro S: *Birth Defects and Drugs in Pregnancy.* Littleton, Mass.: John Wright-PSG, 1977, pp 298, 301.

SULFADIAZINE
(Microsulfon®)

Sulfadiazine is a sulfonamide that is used to treat or to prevent bacterial and parasitic infections. It is given orally in a dose of 1000-8000 mg/d.

Teratogenic Risk

Magnitude of teratogenic risk to child born after exposure during gestation:	*Unlikely*
Quality and quantity of data on which risk estimate is based:	*Poor to fair*

Therapeutic doses of sulfadiazine are unlikely to pose a substantial teratogenic risk, but the data are insufficient to state that there is no risk.

The frequency of congenital anomalies was not increased among the children of 95 women treated with sulfadiazine during the first four lunar months of pregnancy or among the children of 293 women treated anytime in pregnancy in one epidemiological study (Heinonen et al., 1977).

Studies in rats, mice, and rabbits suggest that treatment of pregnant women with sulfadiazine in usual therapeutic doses is unlikely to increase the children's risk of malformations greatly (Loosli et al., 1964). Fetal death occurred in association with maternal toxicity when the pregnant animals were given several times the usual human dose of sulfadiazine (Loosli et al., 1964). The relevance of this observation to the therapeutic use of sulfadiazine in human pregnancy is unknown.

Please see agent summary on sulfisoxazole for information on a related drug that has been more thoroughly studied.

Risk Related to Breast-feeding

No information regarding the distribution of sulfadiazine in breast milk has been published.

Key References

Heinonen OP, Slone D, Shapiro S: *Birth Defects and Drugs in Pregnancy.* Littleton, Mass.: John Wright-PSG, 1977, pp 298, 301, 435.

Loosli R, Loustalot P, Schalch WR, et al.: Joint study in teratogenicity research. Preliminary communication. Proc Eur Soc Study Drug Toxic 4:214-217, 1964.

SULFAMETHAZINE

Sulfamethazine is a sulfonamide antibiotic that is given orally or parenterally. The usual dose is 6000 mg/d.

Teratogenic Risk

Magnitude of teratogenic risk to child born after exposure during gestation:	*Unlikely*
Quality and quantity of data on which risk estimate is based:	*Poor to fair*

Therapeutic doses of sulfamethazine during pregnancy are unlikely to pose a substantial teratogenic risk, but the data are insufficient to state that there is no risk.

The frequency of congenital anomalies was no greater than expected among the children of 47 women who were treated with sulfamethazine during the first four lunar months of pregnancy in one epidemiological study (Heinonen et al., 1977).

The frequencies of congenital anomalies (especially cleft palate, hydroureter, and hydronephrosis) were increased among the offspring of pregnant rats treated with 5.7-7.2 but not 4.5 times the human dose of sulfamethazine (Wolkowski-Tyl et al., 1982). This investigation has only been published as an abstract, and the relevance of its findings to therapeutic use of sulfamethazine in human pregnancy is unknown.

Please see agent summary on sulfisoxazole for information on a related agent that has been studied more thoroughly.

Risk Related to Breast-feeding

No information regarding the distribution of sulfamethazine in breast milk has been published.

Key References

Heinonen OP, Slone D, Shapiro S: *Birth Defects and Drugs in Pregnancy.* Littleton, Mass.: John Wright-PSG, 1977, pp 298, 301.

Wolkowski-Tyl R, Jones-Price C, Kimmel CA, et al.: Teratologic evaluation of sulfamethazine in CD rats. Teratology 25(2):81A-82A, 1982.

SULFAMETHOXAZOLE
(Gamazole®, Gantanol®, Methanoxanol®)

Sulfamethoxazole is a sulfonamide used primarily in the treatment of urinary tract infections. Sulfamethoxazole is given orally in doses of 2000-3000 mg/d.

Teratogenic Risk

Magnitude of teratogenic risk to child born after exposure during gestation:	*Unlikely*
Quality and quantity of data on which risk estimate is based:	*Poor to fair*

Therapeutic doses of sulfamethoxazole are unlikely to pose a substantial teratogenic risk, but the data are insufficient to state that there is no risk.

The frequency of congenital anomalies was no greater than expected among the children of 46 women treated with sulfamethoxazole in the first four lunar months of pregnancy or among the children of 210 women given this drug anytime during pregnancy in one epidemiological study (Heinonen et al., 1977). Congenital anomalies were no more frequent than expected among the children of 120 women treated with sulfamethoxazole and trimethoprim in a controlled trial of therapy for bacteriuria of pregnancy (Williams et al., 1969). Only ten of these women were treated with sulfamethoxazole during the first trimester.

An increased frequency of cleft palate was observed in the offspring of rats given 15 times the usual human dose of sulfamethoxazole during pregnancy (Udall, 1969). The relevance of this observation to the therapeutic use of sulfamethoxazole in human pregnancy is unknown.

Risk Related to Breast-feeding

Sulfamethoxazole is excreted in the breast milk (USP DI, 1995), although this has not been quantitated in published reports.

Key References

Heinonen OP, Slone D, Shapiro S: *Birth Defects and Drugs in Pregnancy.* Littleton, Mass.: John Wright-PSG, 1977, pp 298, 301, 435.

Udall V: Toxicology of sulphonamide-trimethoprim combinations. Postgrad Med J 45(Suppl 5):42-45, 1969.

USP DI: Sulfamethoxazole. In: *USPDI (USP Dispensing Information), Volume 1. Drug Information for the Health Care Professional,* 15th ed. Rockville, Md.: The US Pharmacopeial Convention, 1995, p 2528.

Williams JD, Condie AP, Brumfitt W, Reeves DS: The treatment of bacteriuria in pregnant women with sulphamethoxazole and trimethoprim. A microbiological, clinical and toxicological study. Postgrad Med J 45(Suppl 6):71-76, 1969.

SULFAMIDE® *See* Sulfacetamide

SULFASALAZINE
(Azaline®, Azulfidine®, Salazopyrine®)

Sulfasalazine is given orally or rectally in the treatment of inflammatory bowel disease. The usual dose of sulfasalazine is 1000-4000 mg/d. The drug is broken down in the intestine into its two components--sulfapyridine, a sulfonamide, and mesalazine, a salicylate.

Teratogenic Risk

Magnitude of teratogenic
risk to child born after
exposure during gestation: Unlikely

Quality and quantity of data
on which risk estimate is based: Fair

Therapeutic doses of sulfasalazine are unlikely to pose a substantial teratogenic risk, but the data are insufficient to state that there is no risk.

The frequency of congenital anomalies was no greater than expected among the children of women with inflammatory bowel disease treated during pregnancy with sulfasalazine with or without steroids in studies that included 60, 100, and 186 pregnancies, respectively (Willoughby & Truelove, 1980; Mogadam et al., 1981; Nielsen et al., 1983). Interpretation of these studies is confounded by the fact that the treatment occurred at various times and for various durations during the pregnancies and underascertainment of congenital anomalies appears to have occurred, at least in the largest study. Instances of congenital anomalies among infants born to women who had been treated with sulfasalazine during pregnancy have been reported (Craxi & Pagliarello, 1980; Haxton & Bell, 1983; Newman & Correy, 1983; Hoo et al., 1988), but no consistent pattern of malformations has been noted. A causal relationship between maternal sulfasalazine therapy during pregnancy and the congenital anomalies cannot be inferred from these anecdotal observations.

No animal teratology studies of sulfasalazine have been published.

The frequency of serious neonatal jaundice does not seem to be increased among the infants of women with inflammatory bowel disease treated with sulfasalazine during pregnancy (Willoughby & Truelove, 1980; Mogadam et al., 1981; Nielsen et al., 1983). Although there is a theoretical risk of kernicterus among infants of women treated with sulfonamides late in pregnancy because of displacement of bilirubin from albumin in the baby's blood, this problem appears to be of little practical concern (Jarnerot et al., 1981; Esbjorner et al., 1987).

Risk Related to Breast-feeding

Sulfasalazine and its active metabolite, sulfapyridine, are excreted in breast milk in low concentrations. The amount of sulfasalazine that the nursing infant would be expected to ingest is approximately <1.4% of the lowest therapeutic dose of sulfasalazine in infants (Azad Khan & Truelove, 1979; Esbjorner et al., 1987).[*] The amount of sulfapyridine that the nursing infant would be expected to receive is <1% of the therapeutic dose of sulfapyridine, on a weight-adjusted basis.[†]

Serum levels of sulfasalazine and sulfapyridine were respectively 0-10% and about 9% of those considered to be therapeutic in eight nursing infants of women treated with sulfasalazine in one study (Esbjorner et al., 1987).[‡]

Bloody diarrhea was described in one infant whose mother had been treated with sulfasalazine while breast-feeding (Branski et al., 1986). The symptoms resolved when the medication was discontinued. On the basis of this one case, the American Academy of Pediatrics recommends that sulfasalazine be used with caution in breast-feeding mothers (Committee on Drugs, American Academy of Pediatrics, 1994).

[*]This calculation is based on the following assumptions: maternal dose of sulfasalazine: 1-3 g/d; milk concentrations of sulfasalazine: 0.004-2.7 mcg/mL; milk intake by the nursing infant: 150 mL/kg/d; estimated dose of sulfasalazine ingested by the nursing infant: 0.0006-0.4 mg/kg/d; lowest therapeutic dose of sulfasalazine in infants: 30 mg/kg/d.

[†]This calculation is based on the following assumptions: milk concentration of sulfapyridine: 6-30 mcg/mL; estimated dose of sulfapyridine ingested by the nursing infant: 0.9-4.5 mg/kg/d; lowest therapeutic dose of sulfapyridine in adults: 1 g/d.

[‡]Infant serum levels of sulfasalazine and sulfapyridine: 0.001-0.002 mcg/mL and 0.001-0.005 mcg/mL, respectively; maternal serum levels of sulfasalazine and sulfapyridine: 0.002-0.018 mcg/mL and 0.013-0.06 mcg/mL, respectively.

Key References

Azad Khan AK, Truelove SC: Placental and mammary transfer of sulphasalazine. Br Med J 2:1553, 1979.

Branski D, Kerem E, Gross-Kieselstein E, et al.: Bloody diarrhea--a possible complication of sulfasalazine transferred through human breast milk. J Pediatr Gastroenterol Nutr 5:316-317, 1986.

Committee on Drugs, American Academy of Pediatrics: The transfer of drugs and other chemicals into human milk. Pediatrics 93(1):137-150, 1994.

Craxi A, Pagliarello F: Possible embryotoxicity of sulfasalazine. Arch Intern Med 140:1674, 1980.

Esbjorner E, Jarnerot G, Wranne L: Sulphasalazine and sulphapyridine serum levels in children to mothers treated with sulphasalazine during pregnancy and lactation. Acta Paediatr Scand 76:137-142, 1987.

Haxton MJ, Bell J: Fetal anatomical abnormalities and other associated factors in middle-trimester abortion and their relevance to patient counselling. Br J Obstet Gynaecol 90:501-506, 1983.

Hoo JJ, Hadro TA, von Behren P: Possible teratogenicity of sulfasalazine. N Engl J Med 318:1128, 1988.

Jarnerot G, Into-Malmberg M-B, Esbjorner E: Placental transfer of sulphasalazine and sulphapyridine and some of its metabolites. Scand J Gastroenterol 16:693-697, 1981.

Mogadam M, Dobbins WO III, Korelitz BI, Ahmed SW: Pregnancy in inflammatory bowel disease: Effect of sulfasalazine and corticosteroids on fetal outcome. Gastroenterology 80:72-76, 1981.

Newman NM, Correy JF: Possible teratogenicity of sulphasalazine. Med J Aust 1:528-529, 1983.

Nielsen OH, Andreasson B, Bondesen S, Jarnum S: Pregnancy in ulcerative colitis. Scand J Gastroenterol 18:735-742, 1983.

Willoughby CP, Truelove SC: Ulcerative colitis and pregnancy. Gut 21:469-474, 1980.

SULFISOXAZOLE
(Gantrisin®)

Sulfisoxazole is a sulfonamide used in the treatment of urinary tract and other infections. Sulfisoxazole is given orally in doses of 2-12 g/d. An ophthalmic preparation is also available.

Teratogenic Risk

*Magnitude of teratogenic
risk to child born after
exposure during gestation:*   *Unlikely*

*Quality and quantity of data
on which risk estimate is based:*   *Fair to good*

*Therapeutic doses of sulfisoxazole are unlikely to pose a
substantial teratogenic risk, but the data are insufficient to state that
there is no risk.*

The frequencies of congenital anomalies in general, of major
malformations, of minor anomalies, and of major classes of congenital
anomalies were no greater than expected among the children of 796
women who were treated with sulfisoxazole during the first four lunar
months of pregnancy in one epidemiological study (Heinonen et al.,
1977). The frequency of congenital anomalies was not increased
among the infants of 4287 women who were treated with this drug
anytime during pregnancy in this study. The frequency of congenital
anomalies was no greater than expected among the children of more
than 100 and 215 women, respectively, who had been treated with
sulfisoxazole during the first trimester of pregnancy in two separate
cohorts of another investigation (Jick et al., 1981; Aselton et al., 1985).

No teratogenic effect is said to have occurred in unpublished
studies among the offspring of pregnant rats and rabbits treated with 7
times the human therapeutic dose of sulfisoxazole (USP DI, 1995).
Increased frequencies of cleft palate and other facial malformations
have been observed among the offspring of mice and rats treated with 8
times the usual human dose of sulfisoxazole during pregnancy (Kato &
Kitagawa, 1973a, b; Lee & Chun, 1975). The relevance of this
observation to the therapeutic use of sulfisoxazole in human pregnancy
is unknown.

Risk Related to Breast-feeding

Sulfisoxazole and its active metabolite, N^4-acetyl sulfisoxazole, are
excreted in breast milk in low concentrations. Based on data from six
lactating women, the amount of sulfisoxazole and N^4-acetyl sulfisoxazole that the nursing infant would be expected to ingest is equivalent to

2% of the lowest therapeutic dose of sulfisoxazole in children (Kauffman et al., 1980).*

The American Academy of Pediatrics regards sulfisoxazole to be safe to use by breast-feeding mothers of nonhyperbilirubinemic or otherwise normal infants (Committee on Drugs, American Academy of Pediatrics, 1994).

Key References

Aselton P, Jick H, Milunsky A, et al.: First-trimester drug use and congenital disorders. Obstet Gynecol 65:451-455, 1985.

Committee on Drugs, American Academy of Pediatrics: The transfer of drugs and other chemicals into human milk. Pediatrics 93(1):137-150, 1994.

Heinonen OP, Slone D, Shapiro S: *Birth Defects and Drugs in Pregnancy.* Littleton, Mass.: John Wright-PSG, 1977, pp 306, 472, 485.

Jick H, Holmes LB, Hunter JR, et al.: First-trimester drug use and congenital disorders. JAMA 246:343-346, 1981.

Kato T, Kitagawa S: Production of congenital anomalies in fetuses of rats and mice with various sulfonamides. Congen Anom (Senten Ijo) 13:7-15, 1973b.

Kato T, Kitagawa S: Production of congenital skeletal anomalies in the fetuses of pregnant rats and mice treated with various sulfonamides. Congen Anom (Senten Ijo) 13:17-23, 1973a.

Kauffman RE, O'Brien C, Gilford P: Sulfisoxazole secretion into human milk. J Pediatr 97(5):839-841, 1980.

Lee KH, Chun KH: [Studies on the effects of sulfisoxazole on developing rat fetuses.] Ch'Oesin Uihak 18:295-300, 1975.

USP DI: Sulfisoxazole. In: *USP DI (USP Dispensing Information), Volume 1. Drug Information for the Health Care Professional,* 15th ed. Rockville, Md.: The US Pharmacopeial Convention, 1995, p 2543.

*This calculation is based on the following assumptions: estimated doses of sulfisoxazole and N^4-acetyl sulfisoxazole ingested by the nursing infant: 0.5 mg/kg/d and 1.73 mg/kg/d, respectively; total estimated dose of sulfisoxazole and N^4-acetyl sulfisoxazole ingested by the nursing infant, assuming similar bioavailability, activity, and molecular weights: 2.25 mg/kg/d; lowest therapeutic dose of sulfisoxazole in children: 100 mg/kg/d.

SULINDAC
(Arthrocine®, Clinoril®, Sulindal®)

Sulindac is a nonsteroidal anti-inflammatory agent with analgesic and antipyretic action. Sulindac is given orally in doses of 300-400 mg/d.

Teratogenic Risk

Magnitude of teratogenic risk to child born after exposure during gestation:	Undetermined
Quality and quantity of data on which risk estimate is based:	Very poor

No epidemiological studies of congenital anomalies in children born to women treated with sulindac during pregnancy have been reported. No therapy-related complications were observed among 18 infants of women who were treated with sulindac for preterm labor in one controlled trial (Carlan et al., 1992).

An increased frequency of cleft palate and other malformations was observed among the offspring of mice treated during pregnancy with sulindac in doses similar to those used in humans (Montenegro & Palomino, 1990). The relevance of this observation to the use of sulindac in human pregnancy is unknown.

In utero constriction or closure of the ductus arteriosus has been observed in rats given 1-100 times the usual human dose of sulindac late in pregnancy (Momma & Takeuchi, 1983a, b). Premature closure of the ductus arteriosus has been associated with maternal use of chemically related nonsteroidal anti-inflammatory agents in humans (Grella & Zanor, 1978).

Please see agent summary on indomethacin for information on a similar agent that has been more thoroughly studied.

Risk Related to Breast-feeding

No information regarding the distribution of sulindac in breast milk has been published.

Key References

Carlan SJ, O'Brien WF, O'Leary TD, Mastrogiannis D: Randomized comparative trial of indomethacin and sulindac for the treatment of refractory preterm labor. Obstet Gynecol 79:223-228, 1992.

Grella P, Zanor P: Premature labor and indomethacin. Prostaglandins 16:1007-1017, 1978.

Momma K, Takeuchi H: Constriction of fetal ductus arteriosus by nonsteroidal anti-inflammatory drugs. Adv Prostaglandin Thromboxane Leukotriene Res 12:499-503, 1983a.

Momma K, Takeuchi H: Constriction of fetal ductus arteriosus by non-steroidal anti-inflammatory drugs. Prostaglandins 26:631-643, 1983b.

Montenegro MA, Palomino H: Induction of cleft palate in mice by inhibitors of prostaglandin synthesis. J Craniofac Genet Dev Biol 10:83-94, 1990.

SULINDAL® *See* Sulindac

SUMATRIPTAN
(Imitrex®, Imigran®)

Sumatriptan is a serotonin receptor agonist used in the treatment of migraine headache. It is administered orally in doses of 100-300 mg/d or parenterally in doses of 6-12 mg/d.

Teratogenic Risk

Magnitude of teratogenic risk to child born after exposure during gestation:	*Undetermined*
Quality and quantity of data on which risk estimate is based:	*None*

No epidemiological studies of congenital anomalies among infants born to women treated with sumatriptan during pregnancy have been reported.

No animal teratology studies of sumatriptan have been published, although the manufacturer reports that they have been done in the rat and rabbit and were negative (Humphrey et al., 1991).

Risk Related to Breast-feeding

No information regarding the distribution of sumatriptan in breast milk has been published.

Key References

Humphrey PPA, Feniuk W, Marriott AS, et al.: Preclinical studies on the anti-migraine drug, sumatriptan. Eur Neurol 31:282-290, 1991.

SUPEUDOL® *See* Oxycodone

TAGAMET® *See* Cimetidine

TAMOFEN® *See* Tamoxifen

TAMOPLEX® *See* Tamoxifen

TAMOXIFEN
(Nolvadex®, Tamofen®, Tamoplex®)

Tamoxifen is a nonsteroidal antiestrogenic agent that also has some estrogenic activity. It is given orally to induce ovulation and to treat breast cancer. The usual dose is 20-40 mg/d.

Teratogenic Risk

Magnitude of teratogenic
risk to child born after
exposure during gestation: *Undetermined*

Quality and quantity of data
on which risk estimate is based: *Poor*

A small risk cannot be excluded, but a high risk of congenital anomalies in the children of women treated with tamoxifen during pregnancy is unlikely.

No congenital anomalies were observed among nine infants born to women whose pregnancies occurred after ovulation induction with tamoxifen in one series; five other pregnancies conceived after ovulation induction with tamoxifen in this study were spontaneously aborted (Ruiz-Velasco et al., 1979).

The frequency of malformations in the offspring was not altered but the frequency of embryonic loss or fetal death was increased after treatment of pregnant rabbits or rats with tamoxifen in doses similar to those used in humans (Furr et al., 1976, 1979; Esaki & Sakai, 1980; Furr & Jordan, 1984). Frequent miscarriage or failure of implantation was also observed in dogs treated early in pregnancy with tamoxifen in doses similar to those used in humans (Bowen et al., 1988). No fetal abnormalities were noted among the offspring of marmosets treated during pregnancy with tamoxifen in doses about 6 times greater than those used in humans (Furr et al., 1979; Furr & Jordan, 1984).

Risk Related to Breast-feeding

No information regarding the distribution of tamoxifen in breast milk has been published.

Key References

Bowen RA, Olson PN, Young S, Withrow SJ: Efficacy and toxicity of tamoxifen citrate for prevention and termination of pregnancy in bitches. Am J Vet Res 49:27-31, 1988.

Esaki K, Sakai Y: Influence of oral administration of tamoxifen on the rabbit fetus. Jitchuken Zenrinsho Kenkyuho 6:217-232, 1980.

Furr BJ, Patterson JS, Richardson DN, et al.: Tamoxifen. In: Goldberg ME (ed). *Pharmacological and Biochemical Properties of Drug Substances,* Volume 2. Washington, DC: American Pharmaceutical Association, 1979, pp 355-399.

Furr BJA, Jordan VC: The pharmacology and clinical uses of tamoxifen. Pharmacol Ther 25:127-205, 1984.

Furr BJA, Valcaccia B, Challis JRG: The effects of Nolvadex® (tamoxifen citrate; ICI 46,474) on pregnancy in rabbits. J Reprod Fertil 48:367-369, 1976.

Ruiz-Velasco V, Rosas-Arceo J, Matute MM: Chemical inducers of ovulation: Comparative results. Int J Fertil 24:61-64, 1979.

TAVIST® *See* Clemastine

TEGOPEN® *See* Cloxacillin

TEGRETOL® *See* Carbamazepine

TEMAZE® *See* Temazepam

TEMAZEPAM
(Restoril®, Temaze®)

Temazepam is a benzodiazepine that is used as a hypnotic. It is given orally in single doses of 7.5-30 mg.

Teratogenic Risk

Magnitude of teratogenic risk to child born after exposure during gestation:	*Undetermined*
Quality and quantity of data on which risk estimate is based:	*Very poor*

No epidemiological studies of congenital anomalies among the children of women treated with temazepam during pregnancy have been reported.

Increased fetal loss is said to have occurred in unpublished studies in which pregnant rats were treated with 100-400 times the human dose of temazepam (USP DI, 1995). Increased frequencies of skeletal variants are said to have been produced by treating pregnant rats or rabbits with temazepam in doses, respectively, 800 or 133 or more times those used in humans (USP DI, 1995). The relevance of these observations to therapeutic use of temazepam in human pregnancy is unknown.

Please see agent summary on diazepam for information on a chemically related agent which has been studied.

Risk Related to Breast-feeding

Temazepam is excreted in the breast milk in low concentrations. Based on data from 10 cases, the amount of temazepam that a nursing infant would be expected to ingest is approximately 0-3% of the lowest therapeutic dose on a weight-adjusted basis (Lebedevs et al., 1992).* No adverse effects of maternal temazepam treatment on the nursing infants were observed. Neither temazepam nor its metabolite, oxazepam, could be detected in serum sampled from two of these infants.

Because of its potential effects on the developing central nervous system, the American Academy of Pediatrics recommends that temazepam be used with caution in breast-feeding mothers (Committee on Drugs, American Academy of Pediatrics, 1994).

Key References

Committee on Drugs, American Academy of Pediatrics: The transfer of drugs and other chemicals into human milk. Pediatrics 93(1):137-150, 1994.
Lebedevs TH, Wojnar-Horton RE, Yapp P, et al.: Br J Clin Pharmacol 33:204-206, 1992.
USP DI: Benzodiazepines. In: *USP (USP Dispensing Information), Volume 1. Drug Information for the Health Care Professional,* 15th ed. Rockville, Md.: The US Pharmacopeial Convention, 1995, p 460.

*This calculation is based on the following assumptions: maternal dose of temazepam: 10-20 mg/d; milk concentration of temazepam: 0.026-0.028 mcg/mL; milk intake by the nursing infant: 150 mL/kg/d; estimated dose of temazepam ingested by the nursing infant: 0.004 mg/kg/d; lowest therapeutic dose of temazepam in adults: 0.12 mg/kg/d.

TENORMIN® *See* Atenolol

TERBUTALINE
(Brethaire®, Brethine®, Bricanyl®)

Terbutaline is a direct-acting sympathomimetic agent. It is used as a bronchodilator and to inhibit premature labor. Terbutaline may be administered orally, parenterally, or by aerosol. The oral dose is usually 7.5-15 mg/d; the dose by aerosol is 0.8-3.0 mg/d. Parenteral doses usually are less than 3 mg/d, although somewhat higher doses are sometimes used to arrest premature labor.

Teratogenic Risk

Magnitude of teratogenic risk to child born after exposure during gestation:	*Undetermined*
Quality and quantity of data on which risk estimate is based:	*Very poor*

No epidemiological studies of congenital anomalies in infants born to women who took terbutaline during early pregnancy have been reported.

No differences in growth or development in comparison to controls were found among 43 children studied for up to four years after delivery to women who had received terbutaline during pregnancy to inhibit premature labor (Laros et al., 1991). In another study, normal weight and development were observed in 21 18-month-old children born to women who had been treated with terbutaline for premature labor (Karlsson et al., 1980).

Fetal tachycardia and transient neonatal hypoglycemia have been observed following short-term maternal terbutaline therapy late in pregnancy (Sharif et al., 1990; Peterson et al., 1993). Neonatal myocardial dysfunction and necrosis have been reported in infants whose mothers were treated with terbutaline to inhibit premature labor (Fletcher et al., 1991; Thorkelsson & Loughead, 1991). A relationship to the maternal therapy was suggested but has been disputed (Bey et al., 1992; Kast & Hermer, 1993).

Maternal terbutaline therapy has been used to treat acute intrapartum fetal distress (Mendez-Bauer et al., 1987; Shekarloo et al., 1989).

Unpublished studies in rats, mice, and rabbits are said to provide no indication that maternal treatment with terbutaline in usual therapeutic doses is likely to increase the offspring's risk of malformations (USP DI, 1995). No adverse effect on fetal survival was seen after treatment of pregnant rats with 7-33 times the human dose of terbutaline late in pregnancy (Hou & Slotkin, 1989; Kudlacz et al., 1989, 1990). Decreased neonatal weight was observed in some of these studies at the higher dose, but the relevance of this observation to the use of terbutaline in therapeutic doses in human pregnancy is unknown.

Please see agent summary on metaproterenol for information on a similar agent that has been more thoroughly studied.

Risk Related to Breast-feeding

Terbutaline is excreted in the breast milk in low concentrations. Based on data from four nursing mothers, the amount of terbutaline that the nursing infant would be expected to ingest is <1% of the lowest therapeutic dose on a weight-adjusted basis (Lindberg et al., 1984).* No adverse effects of terbutaline on the nursing infants of these treated women were noted. No detectable levels of terbutaline were found in the serum of one of these infants studied.

The American Academy of Pediatrics regards terbutaline to be safe to use while breast-feeding (Committee on Drugs, American Academy of Pediatrics, 1994).

Key References

Bey M, Blanchard AC, Darnell J, Stephens K: Myocardial necrosis in a newborn after long-term maternal subcutaneous terbutaline for suppression of premature labor. Am J Obstet Gynecol 167:292-293, 1992.

Committee on Drugs, American Academy of Pediatrics: The transfer of drugs and other chemicals into human milk. Pediatrics 93(1):137-150, 1994.

Fletcher SE, Fyfe DA, Case CL, et al.: Myocardial necrosis in a newborn after long-term maternal subcutaneous terbutaline infusion for suppression of preterm labor. Am J Obstet Gynecol 165:1401-1404, 1991.

Hou Q-C, Slotkin TA: Effects of prenatal dexamethasone or terbutaline exposure on development of neural and intrinsic control of heart rate. Pediatr Res 26(6):554-557, 1989.

Karlsson K, Krantz M, Hamberger L: Comparison of various betamimetics on preterm labor, survival and development of the child. J Perinat Med 8:19-26, 1980.

Kast A, Hermer M: β-adrenoceptor tocolysis and effects on the heart of fetus and neonate. A review. J Perinat Med 21:97-106, 1993.

*This calculation is based on the following assumptions: maternal dose of terbutaline: 7.5-15 mg/d; milk concentration of terbutaline: 0.002-0.005 mcg/mL; milk intake by the nursing infant: 150 mL/kg/d; estimated dose of terbutaline ingested by the nursing infant: 0.0003-0.0007 mg/kg/d; lowest therapeutic dose of terbutaline in adults: 0.12 mg/kg/d.

Kudlacz EM, Navarro HA, Eylers JP, et al.: Effects of prenatal terbutaline exposure on cellular development in lung and liver of neonatal rat: Ornithine decarboxylase activity and macromolecules. Pediatr Res 25(6):617-622, 1989.

Kudlacz EM, Navarro HA, Slotkin TA: Regulation of β-adrenergic receptor-mediated processes in fetal rat lung: Selective desensitization caused by chronic terbutaline exposure. J Dev Physiol 14:103-108, 1990.

Laros RK Jr, Kitterman JA, Heilbron DC, et al.: Outcome of very-low-birth-weight infants exposed to β-sympathomimetics in utero. Am J Obstet Gynecol 164:1657-1665, 1991.

Lindberg C, Boreus LO, de Chateau P, et al.: Transfer of terbutaline into breast milk. Eur J Respir Dis 65(Suppl 134):87-91, 1984.

Mendez-Bauer C, Shekarloo A, Cook V, Freese U: Treatment of acute intrapartum fetal distress by β₂-sympathomimetics. Am J Obstet Gynecol 156:638-642, 1987.

Peterson A, Peterson K, Tongen S, et al.: Glucose intolerance as a consequence of oral terbutaline treatment for preterm labor. J Fam Pract 36:25-31, 1993.

Sharif DS, Huhta JC, Moise KJ Jr, et al.: Changes in fetal hemodynamics with terbutaline treatment and premature labor. J Clin Ultrasound 18:85-89, 1990.

Shekarloo A, Mendez-Bauer C, Cook V, Freese U: Terbutaline (intravenous bolus) for the treatment of acute intrapartum fetal distress. Am J Obstet Gynecol 160:615-618, 1989.

Thorkelsson T, Loughead JL: Long-term subcutaneous terbutaline tocolysis: Report of possible neonatal toxicity. J Perinatol 11(3):235-238, 1991.

USP DI: Terbutaline. In: *USP DI (USP Dispensing Information), Volume 1. Drug Information for the Health Care Professional,* 15th ed. Rockville, Md.: The US Pharmacopeial Convention, 1995, p 536.

TERFENADINE
(Seldane®)

Terfenadine is an antihistamine used to relieve seasonal allergic reactions such as sneezing, rhinorrhea, pruritis, and lacrimation. Terfenadine is given orally; the usual dose is 120 mg/d.

Teratogenic Risk

Magnitude of teratogenic
risk to child born after
exposure during gestation: *Undetermined*

Quality and quantity of data
on which risk estimate is based: *Poor*

A small risk cannot be excluded, but a high risk of congenital anomalies in the children of women treated with terfenadine during pregnancy is unlikely.

The frequency of congenital anomalies was no greater than expected among 105 infants of women who had taken terfenadine during the first or early second trimester of pregnancy in one study (Schick et al., 1994).

Studies in rats and rabbits suggest that treatment of pregnant women with terfenadine in usual therapeutic doses is unlikely to increase the children's risk of malformations greatly (Gibson et al., 1982).

Risk Related to Breast-feeding

Terfenadine was not detected in the milk of four mothers who were treated while breast-feeding, but small amounts of terfenadine carboxylic acid, an active metabolite, were found (Lucas et al., 1995). Based on these data, the amount of terfenadine carboxylic acid that the nursing infant would be expected to ingest is <1% of the lowest therapeutic dose on a weight-adjusted basis.*

Key References

Gibson JP, Huffman KW, Newborne JW: Preclinical safety studies with terfenadine. Arzneimittelforsch 22:1179-1184, 1982.

*This calculation is based on the following assumptions: maternal dose of terfenadine: 120 mg/d; milk concentration of terfenadine carboxylic acid: 0.02-0.06 mcg/mL; milk intake by the nursing infant: 150 mL/kg/d; estimated dose of terfenadine carboxylic acid ingested by the nursing infant: 0.003-0.009 mg/kg/d; lowest therapeutic dose of terfenadine in adults: 1.87 mg/kg/d.

Lucas BD Jr, Purdy CY, Scarim SK, et al.: Terfenadine pharmacokinetics in breast milk in lactating women. Clin Pharmacol Ther 57:398-402, 1995.

Schick B, Hom M, Librizzi R, et al.: Terfenadine (Seldane®) exposure in early pregnancy. Teratology 49(5):417, 1994.

TERFLUZINE® *See* Trifluoperazine

TESOPREL® *See* Bromperidol

TESSALON® *See* Benzonatate

TETANUS TOXOID

Tetanus toxoid is inactivated *Clostridium tetani* toxin. Tetanus toxoid is administered intramuscularly or subcutaneously to induce active immunity to tetanus.

Teratogenic Risk

Magnitude of teratogenic risk to child born after exposure during gestation:	*Unlikely*
Quality and quantity of data on which risk estimate is based:	*Poor to fair*

Administration of tetanus toxoid in usual doses is unlikely to pose a substantial teratogenic risk, but the data are insufficient to state that there is no risk.

Jaundice in newborn infants due to ABO incompatibility may be more frequent than expected after maternal immunization with tetanus toxoid late in pregnancy (see below).

The frequencies of major congenital anomalies, of minor anomalies, and of major classes of malformations were not significantly increased among the children of 337 women who received immunization with tetanus toxoid during the first four lunar months of pregnancy in one epidemiological study (Heinonen et al., 1977). The frequency of congenital anomalies was no greater than expected among the children of 853 women immunized with tetanus toxoid anytime during pregnancy in this investigation.

The frequency of neonatal jaundice associated with ABO incompatibility was increased among infants of type O women who received immunization with tetanus toxoid during the third trimester of pregnancy in one study (Gupte & Bhatia, 1980). This effect may be due to the nonspecific elevation of anti-A and anti-B titers that normally occurs in response to immunization.

Studies in rats suggest that immunization of pregnant women with tetanus toxoid is unlikely to increase the children's risk of malformations greatly (Sethi et al., 1991).

Risk Related to Breast-feeding

No information regarding the distribution of tetanus toxoid in breast milk has been published. The Advisory Committee on Immunization Practices considers inactivated vaccines to be safe to administer to a mother during breast-feeding (ACIP, 1994).

Key References

ACIP: General recommendations on immunization. Recommendations of the Advisory Committee on Immunization Practices (ACIP). MMWR 43(RR-1):1-38, 1994.

Gupte SC, Bhatia HM: Increased incidence of haemolytic disease of the new-born caused by ABO-incompatibility when tetanus toxoid is given during pregnancy. Vox Sang 38:22-28, 1980.

Heinonen OP, Slone D, Shapiro S: *Birth Defects and Drugs in Pregnancy.* Littleton, Mass.: John Wright-PSG, 1977, pp 314-320, 436, 474, 488.

Sethi N, Srivastava RK, Singh RK: Teratological evaluation of a new potent tetanus vaccine (250 Lf) in Charles Foster rats. Pharmacol Toxicol 68:226-227, 1991.

TETRACYCLINE
(Achromycin®, Cyclospar®, Panmycin®)

Tetracycline is a broad-spectrum antibiotic. It is frequently used in treatment of respiratory tract infections, acne, and other infections. The drug is usually administered orally in a dose of 1000-2000 mg/d.

Teratogenic Risk

Magnitude of teratogenic
risk to child born after
exposure during gestation:
  Dental staining: High
  Malformations: None to minimal

Quality and quantity of data
on which risk estimate is based:
  Dental staining: Excellent
  Malformations: Fair

Tetracycline causes staining of the primary dentition in fetuses exposed during the second or third trimesters of pregnancy (Toaff & Ravid, 1966; Cohlan, 1977).

The frequencies of congenital anomalies in general, of major malformations, and of minor anomalies were no greater than expected among the children of 341 women treated with tetracycline during the first four lunar months of pregnancy in a large epidemiological study (Heinonen et al., 1977). The frequency of congenital anomalies was not increased among the children of 1336 women treated with this medicine anytime during pregnancy. No increase in malformations was found among more than 274 infants of women who took tetracycline during the first trimester of pregnancy in another epidemiological investigation (Jick et al., 1981; Aselton et al., 1985). An association with maternal use of tetracycline during pregnancy was seen among 46 infants with transposition of the great arteries in one study (Zierler & Rothman, 1985), but this finding requires independent confirmation.

The dental staining caused by in utero exposure to tetracycline appears to be only of cosmetic significance, not affecting development of the enamel or the likelihood of forming caries (Genot et al., 1970; Rebich et al., 1985). Similar staining has been found in the bones and lenses of fetuses whose mothers were treated with tetracycline during gestation (Cohlan et al., 1963; Totterman & Saxen, 1969; Krejci & Brettschneider, 1983). Tetracycline administration has been associated with decreased rates of bone growth in premature infants (Cohlan et al., 1963). Tetracycline exposure during the first trimester of gestation was reported for four babies with congenital or infantile cataracts (Farrar & Mackie, 1964; Harley et al., 1964). These observations were not made in controlled studies, and no definite conclusion can be drawn regarding a possible association between maternal tetracycline exposure and development of cataracts.

Most studies in rats and rabbits suggest that treatment of pregnant women with tetracycline in usual therapeutic doses is unlikely to increase the children's risk of malformations greatly (Mennie, 1962; Hurley et al., 1963; Brown et al., 1968).

Risk Related to Breast-feeding

Tetracycline is excreted into breast milk in low concentrations. Based on data from six lactating women, the amount of tetracycline that a nursing infant would be expected to ingest is approximately 1% of the lowest therapeutic dose on a weight-adjusted basis (Posner et al., 1955).* No tetracycline was detected in the infants' sera and no adverse effect of the maternal treatment on the infants was observed.

Both the American Academy of Pediatrics (Committee on Drugs, American Academy of Pediatrics, 1994) and the WHO Working Group on Drugs and Human Lactation (1988) regard maternal tetracycline treatment to be safe for the nursing infant.

Key References

Aselton P, Jick H, Milunsky A, et al.: First-trimester drug use and congenital disorders. Obstet Gynecol 65:451-455, 1985.

Brown DM, Harper KH, Palmer AK, Tesh SA: Effect of antibiotics upon pregnancy in the rabbit. Toxicol Appl Pharmacol 12:295, 1968.

Cohlan SQ: Tetracycline staining of teeth. Teratology 15:127-130, 1977.

Cohlan SQ, Bevelander G, Tiamsic T: Growth inhibition of prematures receiving tetracycline. Am J Dis Child 105:453-461, 1963.

Committee on Drugs, American Academy of Pediatrics: The transfer of drugs and other chemicals into human milk. Pediatrics 93(1):137-150, 1994.

Farrar JF, Mackie IJ: Survey of possible causes of congenital malformation. Med J Aust 2:702-704, 1964.

Genot MT, Golan HP, Porter PJ, Kass EH: Effect of administration of tetracycline in pregnancy on the primary dentition of the offspring. J Oral Med 25:75-79, 1970.

*This calculation is based on the following assumptions: maternal dose of tetracycline: 2 g/d; milk concentration of tetracycline: 0.43-2.58 mcg/mL; milk intake by the nursing infant: 150 mL/kg/d; estimated dose of tetracycline ingested by the nursing infant: 0.06-0.4 mg/kg/d; lowest therapeutic dose of tetracycline in children: 25 mg/kg/d.

Harley JD, Farrar JF, Gray JB, Dunlop IC: Aromatic drugs and congenital cataracts. Lancet 1:472-473, 1964.

Heinonen O, Slone D, Shapiro S: *Birth Defects and Drugs in Pregnancy*. Littleton, Mass.: John Wright-PSG, 1977, pp 296-313.

Hurley LS, Tuchmann-Duplessis H: Influence of tetracycline on the pre- and postnatal development of the rat. C R Acad Sci (Paris) 257:302-304, 1963.

Jick H, Holmes LB, Hunter JR, et al.: First trimester drug use and congenital disorders. JAMA 246:343-346, 1981.

Krejci L, Brettschneider I: Congenital cataract due to tetracycline. Animal experiments and clinical observation. Ophthalmic Paediatr Genet 3(1):59-60, 1983.

Mennie AT: Tetracycline and congenital limb abnormalities. Br Med J 2:480, 1962.

Posner AC, Prigot A, Konicoff NG: Further observations on the use of tetracycline hydrochloride in prophylaxis and treatment of obstetric infections. In: *Antibiotics Annual 1954-1955*. New York: Medical Encyclopedia, 1955, pp 594-598.

Rebich T, Kumar J, Brustman B: Dental caries and tetracycline-stained dentition in an American Indian population. J Dent Res 64(3):462-464, 1985.

Toaff R, Ravid R: Tetracyclines and the teeth. Lancet 2:281-282, 1966.

Totterman LE, Saxen L: Incorporation of tetracycline into human foetal bones after maternal drug administration. Acta Obstet Gynecol Scand 48:542-549, 1969.

WHO Working Group on Drugs and Human Lactation: In: Bennet PN (ed): *Drugs and Human Lactation*. Amsterdam: Elsevier, 1988, pp 219-220.

Zierler S, Rothman KJ: Congenital heart disease in relation to maternal use of Bendectin and other drugs in early pregnancy. N Engl J Med 313:347-352, 1985.

THALIDOMIDE

Thalidomide, the best known human teratogen, is a sedative and hypnotic agent that also has immunosuppressive activity. Thalidomide is used in the treatment of oropharyngeal and esophageal ulcers in patients with AIDS and in the therapy of various other immunologically-mediated diseases including dicoid lupus erythematosis, Behcet's syndrome, graft-versus-host disease, and leprosy. Thalidomide is given orally; the usual dose is 25-400 mg/d, although doses as great as 1600 mg/d are sometimes used in graft-versus-host disease.

Teratogenic Risk

Magnitude of teratogenic risk to child born after exposure during gestation: High

Quality and quantity of data on which risk estimate is based: Excellent

Thalidomide embryopathy was recognized as a very unusual and characteristic pattern of congenital anomalies that occurs in most children born to women who were treated with thalidomide during the susceptible period of pregnancy (Smithells, 1973; McBride, 1977; Newman, 1985, 1986; Smithells & Newman, 1992). This susceptible period is thought to last from about 34 to 50 days after the beginning of the mother's last menstrual period (Lenz & Knapp, 1962; Kreipe, 1967; Kajii et al., 1973). The characteristic limb malformations of thalidomide embryopathy are reduction defects (Smithells, 1973; Newman, 1985; Smithells & Newman, 1992). In the upper limb the malformations are usually rather symmetrical and involve the components in a remarkably consistent order. The thumb is most often affected, then the radius, the humerus, the ulna, and the ulnar digits. The lower limbs are less frequently involved than the upper limbs, and the long bones are most likely to be deficient or absent in the lower limbs. Club feet and supernumerary toes are common. Most individuals with thalidomide embryopathy have abnormalities of the ears, eyes, facial or external ocular muscles, and/or tear glands (Smithells & Newman, 1992; Stromland & Miller, 1993). Congenital heart disease, ranging from complex conotruncal defects to simple ventricular or atrial septal defects, is frequent and may cause death in early childhood (Smithells & Newman, 1992). Poor linear growth, mental retardation, autism, orofacial clefts, and malformations of the urogenital or gastrointestinal systems or of the spine may occur (McFie & Robertson, 1973; Brook et al., 1977; Smithells & Newman, 1992; Stromland et al., 1994).

Although no formal epidemiological studies of malformations among children of women who took thalidomide during early pregnancy have been published, a striking temporal association between the sales of thalidomide in Germany and the occurrence of malformations characteristic of thalidomide embryopathy has been observed (Eskes, 1984).

Thalidomide embryopathy has been diagnosed by ultrasound examination at 17 weeks gestation (Gollop et al., 1987).

Limb and other malformations typical of thalidomide embryopathy occur in the offspring of pregnant baboons, macaques, and green monkeys treated during critical times of embryogenesis with thalidomide in doses similar to those used in humans (Hendrickx et al., 1966; Hendrickx & Sawyer, 1978; Newman & Hendrickx, 1981, 1985). Increased frequencies of fetal death, growth retardation, and malformations of the limbs, heart, gastrointestinal system, kidneys, and eyes occur among the offspring of pregnant rabbits treated with 1.5-14 times the maximum human dose of thalidomide (Fabro & Smith, 1966; Pearn & Vickers, 1966; Vickers, 1967; Schumacher et al., 1968; Lehmann & Niggeschulze, 1971; Sterz et al., 1987). Teratogenic effects of thalidomide have also been demonstrated among the offspring of pregnant cats, hamsters, rats, and mice given thalidomide in large doses (Homburger et al., 1965; Jonsson, 1972; Khera, 1975; Scott et al., 1977; Parkhie & Webb, 1983; Bila & Kren, 1994).

Risk Related to Breast-feeding

No information regarding the distribution of thalidomide in breast milk has been published.

Key References

Bila V, Kren V: Evidence for teratogenicity of thalidomide using congenic and recombinant inbred rat strains. Folia Biol (Praha) 40:161-171, 1994.

Brook CGD, Jarvis SN, Newman CGH: Linear growth of children with limb deformities following exposure to thalidomide in utero. Acta Paediatr Scand 66:673-675, 1977.

Eskes TKAB: Classic illustration. Eur J Obstet Gynecol Reprod Biol 16:365, 1984.

Fabro S, Smith RL: The teratogenic activity of thalidomide in the rabbit. J Pathol Bacteriol 91:511-519, 1966.

Gollop TR, Eigier A: Prenatal diagnosis of thalidomide syndrome. Prenat Diagn 7:295-298, 1987.

Hendrickx AG, Axelrod LR, Clayborn LD: "Thalidomide" syndrome in baboons. Nature 210:958-959, 1966.

Hendrickx AG, Sawyer RH: Developmental staging and thalidomide teratogenicity in the green monkey (*Cercopithecus aethiops*). Teratology 18:393-404, 1978.

Homburger F, Chaube S, Eppenberger M, et al.: Susceptibility of certain inbred strains of hamsters to teratogenic effects of thalidomide. Toxicol Appl Pharmacol 7:686-693, 1965.

Jonsson BG: Teratological studies on thalidomide in rats. Acta Pharmacol Toxicol 31:11-16, 1972.

Kajii T, Kida M, Takahashi K: The effect of thalidomide intake during 113 human pregnancies. Teratology 8:163-166, 1973.

Khera KS: Fetal cardiovascular and other defects induced by thalidomide in cats. Teratology 11:65-72, 1975.

Kreipe U: [Miszbildungen innerer organe bei thalidomidembryonpathie.] Arch Kinderheilkunde 176:33-61, 1967.

Lehmann H, Niggeschulze A: The teratologic effects of thalidomide in Himalayan rabbits. Toxicol Appl Pharmacol 18:208-219, 1971.

Lenz W, Knapp K: [Die thalidomid-embryopathie.] Dtsch Med Wochenschr 87:1232-1242, 1962.

McBride WG: Thalidomide embryopathy. Teratology 16:79-82, 1977.

McFie J, Robertson J: Psychological test results of children with thalidomide deformities. Dev Med Child Neurol 15:719-727, 1973.

Newman CGH: Teratogen Update: Clinical aspects of thalidomide embryopathy--A continuing preoccupation. Teratology 32:133-144, 1985.

Newman CGH: The thalidomide syndrome: Risks of exposure and spectrum of malformations. Clin Perinatol 13(3):555-573, 1986.

Newman LH, Hendrickx AG: Fetal ear malformations induced by maternal ingestion of thalidomide in the bonnet monkey (*Macaca radiata*). Teratology 23:351-364, 1981.

Newman LH, Hendrickx AG: Temporomandibular malformations in the bonnet monkey (*Macaca radiata*) fetus following maternal ingestion of thalidomide. J Craniofac Genet Dev Biol 5:147-157, 1985.

Parkhie M, Webb M: Embryotoxicity and teratogenicity of thalidomide in rats. Teratology 27:327-332, 1983.

Pearn JH, Vickers TH: The rabbit thalidomide embryopathy. Br J Exp Pathol 47:186-192, 1966.

Schumacher H, Blake DA, Gurian JM, Gillette JR: A comparison of the teratogenic activity of thalidomide in rabbits and rats. J Pharmacol Exp Ther 160:189-200, 1968.

Scott WJ, Fradkin R, Wilson JG: Non-confirmation of thalidomide induced teratogenesis in rats and mice. Teratology 16:333-336, 1977.

Smithells RW: Defects and disabilities of thalidomide children. Br Med J 1:269-272, 1973.

Smithells RW, Newman CGH: Recognition of thalidomide defects. J Med Genet 29:716-723, 1992.

Sterz H, Nothdurft H, Lexa P, Ockenfels H: Teratologic studies on the Himalayan rabbit: New aspects of thalidomide-induced teratogenesis. Arch Toxicol 60:376-381, 1987.

Stromland K, Miller MT: Thalidomide embryopathy: Revisited 27 years later. Acta Ophthalmol 71(2):238-245, 1993.

Stromland K, Nordin V, Miller M, et al.: Autism in thalidomide embryopathy: A population study. Dev Med Child Neurol 36:351-356, 1994.

Vickers TH: The thalidomide embryopathy in hybrid rabbits. Br J Exp Pathol 48:107-117, 1967.

THEOPHYL® *See* Theophylline

THEOPHYLLINE
(Aerolate®, Bronkodyl®, Theophyl®)

Theophylline is a xanthine derivative with strong diuretic action. It is used as a bronchodilator and as a stimulant of myocardial and respiratory function. Theophylline is found in many teas. Aminophylline is the ethylenediamine salt of theophylline; aminophylline releases free theophylline in the body. Dosages of both aminophylline and theophylline are calculated as the equivalent of anydrous theophylline: The usual oral or parenteral dose is 150-900 mg/d. Theophylline serum levels of 10-20 mcg/mL are considered to be therapeutic.

Teratogenic Risk

*Magnitude of teratogenic
risk to child born after
exposure during gestation:*   *Unlikely*

*Quality and quantity of data
on which risk estimate is based:*   *Poor to fair*

573

Therapeutic doses of theophylline are unlikely to pose a substantial teratogenic risk, but the data are insufficient to state that there is no risk.

The frequency of congenital anomalies was no greater than expected among the children of 193 women who took medications containing theophylline during the first four lunar months of pregnancy or among the children of 653 women who took such medicines anytime during pregnancy in one epidemiological study (Heinonen et al., 1977). The frequency of stillbirth was not increased among the pregnancies of 253 asthmatic women treated with theophylline in this study (Neff & Leviton, 1990). Three infants with various severe cardiovascular malformations who were born to asthmatic women treated with theophylline throughout pregnancy have been reported (Park et al., 1990), but no cause and effect relationship can be inferred from these anecdotal observations.

An increased frequency of congenital anomalies was observed among the offspring of pregnant mice and rats treated with theophylline in doses 6-25 times those used therapeutically in humans (Tucci & Skalko, 1978; Lindstrom et al., 1990). Cleft palate and skeletal anomalies were most frequently observed. The relevance of these observations to the therapeutic use of theophylline in human pregnancy is unknown.

Transient theophylline toxicity characterized by jitteriness and tachycardia has been observed in infants born shortly after maternal ingestion of theophylline (Turner et al., 1980; Spector, 1984).

Risk Related to Breast-feeding

Theophylline is excreted in breast milk. Based on data from eight lactating women, the amount of theophylline that a nursing infant would be expected to ingest is between 16-90% of the lowest therapeutic dose of theophylline in neonates (Yurchak & Jusko, 1976; Stec et al., 1980).* No adverse effects of theophylline treatment were observed in these nursing infants.

*This calculation is based on the following assumptions: maternal dose of theophylline: 200 mg aminophylline (orally) or 3.2-5.3 mg/kg (intravenously); milk concentration of theophylline: 2.2-12 mcg/mL; milk intake by the nursing infant: 150 mL/kg/d; estimated dose of theophylline ingested by the nursing infant: 0.33-1.8 mg/kg/d; lowest therapeutic dose of theophylline in neonates: 2 mg/kg/d.

The American Academy of Pediatrics regards theophylline to be safe to use while breast-feeding (Committee on Drugs, American Academy of Pediatrics, 1994).

Key References

Committee on Drugs, American Academy of Pediatrics: The transfer of drugs and other chemicals into human milk. Pediatrics 93(1):137-150, 1994.

Heinonen OP, Slone D, Shapiro S: *Birth Defects and Drugs in Pregnancy.* Littleton, Mass.: John Wright-PSG, 1977, pp 366-370.

Lindstrom P, Morrissey RE, George JD, et al.: The developmental toxicity of orally administered theophylline in rats and mice. Fundam Appl Toxicol 14:167-178, 1990.

Neff RK, Leviton A: Maternal theophylline consumption and the risk of stillbirth. Chest 97:1266-1267, 1990.

Park JM, Schmer V, Myers TL: Cardiovascular anomalies associated with prenatal exposure to theophylline. South Med J 83(12):1487-1488, 1990.

Spector SL: Reciprocal relationship between pregnancy and pulmonary disease. State of the art. Chest 86(Suppl):1S-5S, 1984.

Stec GP, Greenberger P, Ruo TI, et al.: Kinetics of theophylline transfer to breast milk. Clin Pharmacol Ther 28:404-408, 1980.

Tucci SM, Skalko RG: The teratogenic effects of theophylline in mice. Toxicol Lett 1:337-341, 1978.

Turner ES, Greenberger PA, Patterson R: Management of the pregnant asthmatic patient. Ann Intern Med 6:905-918, 1980.

Yurchak AM, Jusko WJ: Theophylline secretion into breast milk. Pediatrics 57(4):518-525, 1976.

THERAZID® *See* Aminosalicylic Acid

THIAMINE
(Betaxin®, Biamine®, Vitamin B₁)

Thiamine (vitamin B₁) is an essential dietary component that is used as a coenzyme in intermediary metabolism. The US recommended dietary allowance (RDA) of thiamine in pregnancy is 1.5 mg/d (NRC, 1989). Doses 15-40 mg/d are ofen used orally to treat deficiency states. Doses as large as 300 mg/d are sometimes given parenterally.

Teratogenic Risk

*Magnitude of teratogenic
risk to child born after
exposure during gestation:*   Undetermined

*Quality and quantity of data
on which risk estimate is based:*   Very poor

A small risk cannot be excluded, but there is no indication that the risk of congenital anomalies in the children of women who take large amounts of thiamine during pregnancy is likely to be great.

No epidemiological studies of congenital anomalies in infants born to women who took very large amounts of thiamine during pregnancy have been reported.

Survival and weight gain of newborn rats were not affected by treatment of the mother with thiamine during pregnancy in doses about 130 times the human RDA (Schumacher et al., 1965) or about 50 times the rat daily requirement (Morrison & Sarett, 1959).

Risk Related to Breast-feeding

Thiamine is a normal constituent of breast milk (DeBuse, 1992).* Supplementation of well-nourished breast-feeding mothers with a multi-vitamin containing thiamine at levels above the RDA has not been found to significantly increase breast milk concentrations of thiamine (Nail et al., 1980; Thomas et al., 1980). On the other hand, progressive supplementation with thiamine up to 20 mg/d in poorly-nourished breast-feeding women increased the breast milk concentrations of thiamine above those of women not receiving supplementation (Deodhar et al., 1964); however, the amount of thiamine ingested by their nursing infants did not exceed the RDA for infants[†].

*Average concentration of thiamine in breast milk: 0.142 mcg/mL.
[†]RDA of thiamine for infants: 0.075 mg/kg.

Thiamine deficiency may develop in infants exclusively breast-fed by mothers who consume a diet inadequate in thiamine (Rao & Subrahmanyam, 1964; Higginbottom et al., 1978; DeBuse, 1992). A case of *Shoshin beriberi* (cardiac failure accompanied by vasoconstriction, hypotension, and metabolic acidosis) in the infant of a breast-feeding mother deficient in thiamine was reported by DeBuse (1992). Recovery occurred when 50 mg of thiamine was administered intravenously to the infant.

Key References

DeBuse PJ: Shoshin beriberi in an infant of a thiamine-deficient mother. Acta Paediatr 81:723-724, 1992.

Deodhar AD, Rajalakshmi R, Ramakrishnan CV: Studies on human lactation. Part III. Effect of dietary vitamin supplementation on vitamin contents of breast milk. Acta Paediatr 53:42-48, 1964.

Higginbottom MC, Sweetman L, Nyan WL: A syndrome of methylmalonic aciduria, homocystinuria, megaloblastic anemia and neurologic abnormalities in vitamin B_{12} deficient breast fed infant of a strict vegetarian. N Engl J Med 299:317, 1978.

Morrison AB, Sarett HP: Effects of excess thiamine and pyridoxine on growth and reproduction in rats. J Nutr 69:111-116, 1959.

Nail PA, Thomas MR, Eakin R: The effect of thiamin and riboflavin supplementation on the level of those vitamins in human breast milk and urine. Am J Clin Nutr 33:198-204, 1980.

NRC (National Research Council): *Recommended Dietary Allowances, 10th ed. Report of the Subcommittee on the Tenth Edition of the RDAs, Food and Nutrition Board, Commission on Life Sciences.* Washington, DC: National Academy Press, 1989, p 262.

Rao RR, Subrahmanyam I: An investigation on the thiamine content of mother's milk in relation to infantile convulsions. Ind J Med Res 52(11):1198-1201, 1964.

Schumacher MF, Williams MA, Lyman RL: Effect of high intakes of thiamine, riboflavin and pyridoxine on reproduction in rats and vitamin requirements of the offspring. J Nutr 86:343-349, 1965.

Thomas MR, Sneed SM, Wei C, et al.: The effects of vitamin C, vitamin B_6, vitamin B_{12}, folic acid, riboflavin, and thiamin on the breast milk and maternal status of well-nourished women at 6 months postpartum. Am J Clin Nutr 33:2151-2156, 1980.

THIORIDAZINE
(Mellaril®, Millazine®)

Thioridazine is a phenothiazine tranquilizer that is used in the treatment of psychoses, moderate and severe emotional disorders, and severe behavioral problems. Thioridazine is given orally in doses of 20-800 mg/d.

Teratogenic Risk

Magnitude of teratogenic
risk to child born after
exposure during gestation: *Undetermined*

Quality and quantity of data
on which risk estimate is based: *Poor*

Although a small risk cannot be excluded, a high risk of congenital anomalies in the children of women treated with thioridazine during pregnancy is unlikely.

No congenital anomalies were found in a series of 23 infants born to women treated with thioridazine during the first trimester of pregnancy (Scanlan, 1972).

Increased frequencies of cleft palate were observed among the offspring of rats and mice treated, respectively, with 50 times and more than 12 times the usual human dose of thioridazine during pregnancy (Szabo & Brent, 1974), but the effect appeared to be attributable largely to a drug-induced reduction of maternal feeding (Szabo & Brent, 1975). No alteration of litter size, neonatal mortality, or neonatal weight gain was noted among the offspring of rats treated during pregnancy with thioridazine in doses equivalent to those used in humans (Murphree et al., 1962). The relevance of these observations to the therapeutic use of thioridazine in human pregnancy is unknown.

Please see agent summary on chlorpromazine for information on a related agent that has been more thoroughly studied.

Risk Related to Breast-feeding

No information regarding the distribution of thioridazine in breast milk has been published.

Key References

Murphree OD, Monroe BL, Seager LD: Survival of offspring of rats administered phenothiazines during pregnancy. J Neuropsychiatry 3:295-297, 1962.

Scanlan FJ: The use of thioridazine (Mellaril®) during the first trimester. Med J Aust 1:1271-1272, 1972.

Szabo KT, Brent RL: Reduction of drug-induced cleft palate in mice. Lancet 1:1296-1297, 1975.

Szabo KT, Brent RL: Species differences in experimental teratogenesis by tranquillising agents. Lancet 1:565, 1974.

THIOTHIXENE
(Navane®, Roxane®)

Thiothixene is a thioxanthine tranquilizer that is used to treat psychosis. Thiothixene is given orally in doses of 6-60 mg/d or intramuscularly in doses of 8-30 mg/d.

Teratogenic Risk

Magnitude of teratogenic risk to child born after exposure during gestation:	*Undetermined*
Quality and quantity of data on which risk estimate is based:	*Very poor*

No epidemiological studies of congenital anomalies in infants born to women treated with thiothixene during pregnancy have been reported.

Studies in mice and rabbits suggest that treatment of pregnant women with thiothixene in usual therapeutic doses is unlikely to increase the children's risk of malformations greatly (Owaki et al., 1969a, b).

Please see agent summary on chlorpromazine for information on a related drug that has been more thoroughly studied.

Risk Related to Breast-feeding

No information regarding the distribution of thiothixene in breast milk has been published.

Key References

Owaki Y, Momiyama H, Yokoi Y: [Teratological studies on thiothixene (Navane®) in mice.] Oyo Yakuri 3:315-320, 1969a.
Owaki Y, Momiyama H, Yokoi Y: [Teratological studies on thiothixene (Navane®) in rabbits.] Oyo Yakuri 3:321-324, 1969b.

THORAZINE® *See* Chlorpromazine

THOR-PROM® *See* Chlorpromazine

TIMOLOL
(Blocadren®, Timoptic®)

Timolol is a β-adrenergic receptor blocking agent. It is used for treating hypertension, vascular headaches, myocardial infarction, and glaucoma. When given orally, the dosage is usually 20-60 mg/d. Although systemic absorption may occur when timolol drops are used in the eye, the dosage is very much smaller.

Teratogenic Risk

Magnitude of teratogenic risk to child born after exposure during gestation:	*Undetermined*
Quality and quantity of data on which risk estimate is based:	*Very poor*

No epidemiological studies of congenital anomalies among infants born to women treated with timolol during pregnancy have been reported.

The frequency of malformations is said not to have been increased in unpublished studies in mice and rabbits in which the mother was treated with up to 50 times the maximum human dose of timolol during pregnancy (USP DI, 1995). Increased fetal death was seen in pregnant mice and rabbits given 1000 and 100 times the maximum human dose, respectively (USP DI, 1995). Fetal bradycardia and blockage of the fetal response to hypoxia were observed in pregnant sheep given timolol during the third trimester of pregnancy in doses less than those used clinically (Cottle et al., 1983). The relevance of these observations for the use of timolol in therapeutic doses in human pregnancy is unknown.

Please see agent summary on propranolol for information on a related agent that has been more thoroughly studied.

Risk Related to Breast-feeding

Timolol is excreted in the breast milk. Based on data from 14 lactating women, the amount of timolol that the nursing infant would be expected to ingest is <1-8.4% of the lowest therapeutic dose of timolol, on a weight-adjusted basis (Fidler et al., 1983; Lustgarten & Podos, 1983).*

Both the American Academy of Pediatrics (Committee on Drugs, American Academy of Pediatrics, 1994) and the WHO Working Group on Drugs and Human Lactation (1988) regard timolol to be safe to use while breast-feeding.

Key References

Committee on Drugs, American Academy of Pediatrics: The transfer of drugs and other chemicals into human milk. Pediatrics 93(1):137-150, 1994.

Cottle MKW, Van Petten GR, van Muyden P: Maternal and fetal cardiovascular indices during fetal hypoxia due to cord compression in chronically cannulated sheep. I. Responses to timolol. Am J Obstet Gynecol 146:678-685, 1983.

Fidler J, Smith V, De Swiet M: Excretion of oxprenolol and timolol in breast milk. Br J Obstet Gynecol 90:961-965, 1983.

Lustgarten JS, Podos SM: Topical timolol and the nursing mother. Arch Ophthalmol 101:1381-1382, 1983.

*This calculation is based on the following assumptions: maternal doses of timolol: 15-30 mg/d (orally) in 13 mothers, 0.5% timolol in ophthalmic drops in 1 mother; milk concentration of timolol: 0.002-0.09 mcg/mL; milk intake by the nursing infant: 150 mL/kg/d; estimated dose of timolol ingested by the nursing infant: 0.0003-0.013 mg/kg/d; lowest therapeutic dose of timolol in adults: 0.16 mg/kg/d.

USP DI: Beta-adrenergic blocking agents. In: *USP DI (USP Dispensing Information), Volume 1. Drug Information for the Health Care Professional*, 15th ed. Rockville, Md.: The US Pharmacopeial Convention, 1995, p 494.

WHO Working Group on Drugs and Human Lactation. In: Bennet PN (ed). *Drugs and Human Lactation*. Amsterdam: Elsevier, 1988, p 141-142.

TIMOPTIC® *See* Timolol

TIPRAMINE® *See* Imipramine

TOBACCO *See* Cigarette Smoking

TOCOPHERCAPS® *See* Vitamin E

TOFRANIL® *See* Imipramine

TOLAZAMIDE
(Ronase®, Tolinase®)

Tolazamide is a sulfonylurea compound that is used as an oral hypoglycemic agent. The usual dose is 100-1000 mg/d.

Teratogenic Risk

Magnitude of teratogenic risk to child born after exposure during gestation:	*Undetermined*
Quality and quantity of data on which risk estimate is based:	*None*

No epidemiological studies of congenital anomalies in infants born to women who were treated with tolazamide during pregnancy have been reported.

No experimental animal teratology studies of tolazamide have been published.

Risk Related to Breast-feeding

No information regarding the distribution of tolazamide in breast milk has been published.

Key References

None available.

TOLBUTAMIDE
(Novobutamide®, Oramide®, Orinase®)

Tolbutamide is a sulfonylurea compound that is used as an oral hypoglycemic agent. The usual dose is 250-3000 mg/d.

Teratogenic Risk

*Magnitude of teratogenic
risk to child born after
exposure during gestation:*   *Unlikely*

*Quality and quantity of data
on which risk estimate is based:*   *Poor to fair*

Therapeutic doses of tolbutamide are unlikely to pose a substantial teratogenic risk, but the data are insufficient to state that there is no risk.

The frequency of congenital anomalies was no greater than expected among the children of 42 women who had been treated with tolbutamide during pregnancy in one epidemiological study; only 13 of these women were treated during the first trimester (Heinonen et al., 1977). Results of clinical series suggest that malformations among infants born to women treated with tolbutamide during pregnancy do not occur substantially more often than expected among infants of diabetic mothers (Dolger et al., 1969; Notelovitz, 1971; Coetzee & Jackson, 1984).

The frequency of malformations was no greater than expected among the offspring of mice, rats, or rabbits treated with tolbutamide during pregnancy in doses 5-20 times those used in humans, although

583

increased rates of fetal death and delayed skeletal maturation were seen in some studies (Lazarus & Volk, 1963; McColl et al., 1965, 1967; Belisle & Long, 1976). Fetal malformations including exencephaly were induced by maternal treatment with tolbutamide in one study in mice, but the dose used, about 50 times the human therapeutic dose, often killed the mothers (Smithberg & Runner, 1963). The relevance of these observations to the therapeutic use of tolbutamide in human pregnancy is unknown.

Risk Related to Breast-feeding

Tolbutamide is excreted in the breast milk. Based on data from two lactating women, the amount of tolbutamide that the nursing infant would be expected to ingest is between 8-77% of the lowest therapeutic dose of tolbutamide, on a weight-adjusted basis (Moiel & Ryan, 1967).* This amount of tolbutamide causes concern because of its hypoglycemic properties; however, the American Academy of Pediatrics regards tolbutamide to be safe to use while breast-feeding (Committee on Drugs, American Academy of Pediatrics, 1994).

Key References

Belisle RJ, Long SY: Tolbutamide treatment of pregnant mice: Repeated administration reduces fetal lethality. Teratology 13:65-70, 1976.

Coetzee EJ, Jackson WPU: Oral hypoglycaemics in the first trimester and fetal outcome. S Afr Med J 65:635-637, 1984.

Committee on Drugs, American Academy of Pediatrics: The transfer of drugs and other chemicals into human milk. Pediatrics 93(1):137-150, 1994.

Dolger H, Bookman JJ, Nechemias C: Tolbutamide in pregnancy and diabetes. J Mt Sinai Hosp 36:471-474, 1969.

Heinonen OP, Slone D, Shapiro S: *Birth Defects and Drugs in Pregnancy.* Littleton, Mass.: John Wright-PSG, 1977, p 443.

Lazarus SS, Volk BW: Absence of teratogenic effect of tolbutamide in rabbits. J Clin Endocrinol Metab 23:597-599, 1963.

*This calculation is based on the following assumptions: maternal dose of tolbutamide: 1 g/d; milk concentration of tolbutamide: 2-20 mcg/mL; milk intake by the nursing infant: 150 mL/kg/d; estimated dose of tolbutamide ingested by the nursing infant: 0.3-3 mg/kg/d; lowest therapeutic dose of tolbutamide in adults: 3.9 mg/kg/d.

McColl JD, Globus M, Robinson S: Effect of some therapeutic agents on the developing rat fetus. Toxicol Appl Pharmacol 7:409-417, 1965.

McColl JD, Robinson S, Globus M: Effect of some therapeutic agents on the rabbit fetus. Toxicol Appl Pharmacol 10:244-252, 1967.

Moiel RH, Ryan JR: Tolbutamide orinase in human breast milk. Clin Pediatr 6(8):480, 1967.

Notelovitz M: Sulphonylurea therapy in the treatment of the pregnant diabetic. S Afr Med J 45:226-229, 1971.

Smithberg M, Runner MN: Teratogenic effects of hypoglycemic treatments in inbred strains of mice. Am J Anat 113:479-489, 1963.

TOLECTIN® *See* Tolbutamide

TOLINASE® *See* Tolazamide

TOLMETIN
(Tolectin®)

Tolmetin is a nonsteroidal anti-inflammatory agent with analgesic and antipyretic action. Tolmetin is given orally in doses of 600-2000 mg/d to treat rheumatic and musculoskeletal disorders.

Teratogenic Risk

*Magnitude of teratogenic
risk to child born after
exposure during gestation:*   *Undetermined*

*Quality and quantity of data
on which risk estimate is based:*   *Very poor*

Maternal treatment with tolmetin late in pregnancy may be associated with premature closure of the fetal ductus arteriosus (see below).

No epidemiological studies of congenital anomalies among children of women treated with tolmetin during pregnancy have been published.

The frequency of malformations was not increased among the offspring of pregnant rabbits treated with tolmetin in doses 1-4 times those used in humans (Nishimura et al., 1977). Increased fetal mortality occurred at the high dose levels, but such doses were also toxic to the mothers.

Alterations of perinatal cardiopulmonary adaptation have been reported in infants born to women who took pharmacologically-related nonsteroidal anti-inflammatory agents shortly before delivery (Manchester et al., 1976; Levin et al., 1978; Itskovitz et al., 1980). Premature closure of the ductus arteriosus was seen among the offspring of rats treated just prior to delivery with tolmetin in doses 1-4 times those used in humans (Momma & Takeuchi, 1983; Nishimura et al., 1984). It seems likely that tolmetin can produce premature ductus closure in humans as well.

Please see agent summary on indomethacin for information on a related agent that has been more thoroughly studied.

Risk Related to Breast-feeding

Tolmetin is excreted in the breast milk in low concentrations. Based on data from a single patient, the amount of tolmetin that the nursing infant would be expected to receive is <1% of the lowest therapeutic dose, on a weight-adjusted basis (Sagraves et al., 1985).*

The American Academy of Pediatrics regards tolmetin to be safe to use while breast-feeding (Committee on Drugs, American Academy of Pediatrics, 1994).

Key References

Committee on Drugs, American Academy of Pediatrics: The transfer of drugs and other chemicals into human milk. Pediatrics 93(1):137-150, 1994.

Itskovitz J, Abramovici H, Brandes JM: Oligohydramnion, meconium and perinatal death concurrent with indomethacin treatment in human pregnancy. J Reprod Med 24:137-140, 1980.

Levin DL, Fixler DE, Morriss FC, Tyson J: Morphologic analysis of the pulmonary vascular bed in infants exposed in utero to prostaglandin synthetase inhibitors. J Pediatr 92:478-483, 1978.

*This calculation is based on the following assumptions: maternal dose of tolmetin: 400 mg; milk concentration of tolmetin: <0.03-0.18 mcg/mL; milk intake by the nursing infant: 150 mL/kg/d; estimated dose of tolmetin ingested by the nursing infant: <0.01-0.03 mg/kg/d; lowest therapeutic dose of tolmetin in children: 15 mg/kg/d.

Manchester D, Margolis HS, Sheldon RE: Possible association between maternal indomethacin therapy and primary pulmonary hypertension of the newborn. Am J Obstet Gynecol 126:467-469, 1976.

Momma K, Takeuchi H: Constriction of fetal ductus arteriosus by non-steroidal anti-inflammatory drugs. Prostaglandins 26(4):631-643, 1983.

Nishimura K, Fukagawa S, Shigematsu K, et al.: Teratogenicity study of 1-methyl-5-p-toluoylpyrrole-2-acetate sodium dihydrate (tolmetin sodium) in rabbits. Iyakuhin Kenkyu 8:158-164, 1977.

Nishimura K, Sato K, Nanto T, Yoshida K: Constriction of fetal ductus arteriosus by anti-inflammatory agents in rats. Teratology 30:35A, 1984.

Sagraves R, Waller ES, Goehrs HR: Tolmetin in breast milk. Drug Intell Clin Pharm 19:55-56, 1985.

TOLUENE
(Toluol)

Toluene is an organic solvent that is widely used, especially in the paint, printing, and adhesive industries. Toluene is also abused by inhalation. Maternal exposure can be monitored by measuring toluene in the blood or its major metabolite, hippuric acid, in the urine (Low et al., 1988). The threshold limit value (TLV) for occupational exposure to toluene in air is 50 ppm (375 mg/cu m) as an 8-hour time-weighted average. The odor threshold is 2.14 ppm (8 mg/cu m) (HSDB, 1995).

Teratogenic Risk

Magnitude of teratogenic
risk to child born after
exposure during gestation:
    For usual occupational exposure: *Unlikely*
    For abuse: *Moderate to high*

Quality and quantity of data
on which risk estimate is based:
    For usual occupational exposure: *Poor to fair*
    For abuse: *Fair*

Occupational exposure to toluene at less than the threshold limit value is unlikely to pose a substantial teratogenic risk, but the data are insufficient to state that there is no risk.

Commercial solvents that have toluene as an ingredient ordinarily contain a mixture of volatile hydrocarbons. The teratogenic effects attributed to toluene could be due to concomitant exposure to other volatile hydrocarbons alone or in combination with toluene.

"Occupational exposure" is used here to mean chronic exposure to toluene in amounts less than the TLV that do not cause symptoms in the mother.

More than 30 children whose mothers regularly abused toluene during pregnancy have been reported with a similar pattern of congenital anomalies (Hersh et al., 1985; Goodwin, 1988; Hersh, 1989; Lindemann, 1991; Wilkins-Haug & Gabow, 1991; Arnold et al., 1994; Pearson et al., 1994). The children exhibit central nervous system dysfunction, developmental delay, attention deficit disorder, microcephaly, growth deficiency, short palpebral fissures, deep-set eyes, microagnathia, abnormal auricles, and small fingernails. The features appear to constitute a "toluene embryopathy" that resembles the fetal alcohol syndrome. Among 35 pregnancies in women who chronically abused toluene in one series (Wilkins-Haug & Gabow, 1991; Arnold et al., 1994), there were three perinatal deaths. Many of the infants were born prematurely and had fetal growth retardation and neonatal hyertonia. Growth retardation for height, weight, and head circumference persisted at least through the first year of life, and developmental delay was common (Wilkins-Haug & Gabow, 1991; Arnold et al., 1994).

An increased frequency of occupational exposure to aromatic solvents was found in one epidemiological study of mothers of 301 infants with major congenital anomalies; the excess exposure was attributable almost entirely to toluene (McDonald et al., 1987). The malformations in the infants of mothers who had aromatic solvent exposure in this study were quite heterogeneous, and the exposures reported by the women were low level. Studies such as this one that include multiple comparisons between maternal occupational exposures and birth defect outcomes are expected to show occasional associations with nominal statistical significance purely by chance.

Toluene exposure during pregnancy was no more frequent than expected in a study of 38 women who had miscarriages while working in pharmaceutical factories (Taskinen et al., 1986). The frequency of miscarriage was no greater than expected among 166 pregnancies of women who were exposed to toluene while working in university laboratories (Axelsson et al., 1984). In a study of women with occupational exposure to high levels of toluene (50-150 ppm), an increased rate of spontaneous abortion was observed (Ng et al., 1992). However, the rate of miscarriage among the exposed group in this study is similar to what would be expected in the general population (12.4%), while the rates in the comparison groups were inexplicably low.

The frequency of malformations was not increased among the offspring of rats, mice, or rabbits treated by toluene inhalation in chronic doses equivalent to 1-50, 1-10, or <1-10 times the human occupational TLV (Shigeta et al., 1982; Ungvary et al., 1983; Anonymous, 1984, 1985; Ungvary & Tatrai, 1985; Courtney et al., 1986; Klimisch et al., 1992; Roberts et al., 1993). Fetal growth and developmental retardation and fetal death were sometimes seen at the higher doses, often in association with signs of maternal toxicity. Behavioral alterations have been observed among the offspring of pregnant rats and hamsters exposed to toluene vapors at a dose about twice the human occupational TLV (Da-Silva et al., 1990).

Transient neonatal hyperchloremic acidosis has been observed in infants of women who chronically abused toluene during pregnancy (Goodwin, 1988; Lindmann, 1991). Renal tubular dysfunction with consequent hyperchloremic acidosis is a frequent manifestation of chronic toluene toxicity in pregnant women as well (Wilkins-Haug & Gabow, 1991).

Risk Related to Breast-feeding

No information regarding the distribution of toluene in breast milk has been published.

Key References

Anonymous: Two generation inhalation reproduction/fertility study on a petroleum-derived hydrocarbon with toluene with submittal letter dated 082085. EPA/OTS; Doc #FYI-AX-0885-0294, 1985.

Anonymous: Two generation inhalation study on a petroleum-derived hydrocarbon with cover letter dated 021384 and EPA acknowledgment dated 031984. EPA/OTS; Doc #FYI-AX-0284-0294 Initial Sequence A, 1984.

Arnold GL, Kirby RS, Langendoerfer S, Wilkins-Haug L: Toluene embryopathy: Clinical delineation and developmental follow-up. Pediatrics 93:216-220, 1994.

Axelsson G, Lutz C, Rylander R: Exposure to solvents and outcome of pregnancy in university laboratory employees. Br J Ind Med 41:305-312, 1984.

Courtney KD, Andrews JE, Springer J, et al.: A perinatal study of toluene in CD-1 mice. Fundam Appl Toxicol 6:145-154, 1986.

Da-Silva VA, Malheiros LR, Bueno FMR: Effects of toluene exposure during gestation on neurobehavioral development of rats and hamsters. Braz J Med Biol Res 23:533-538, 1990.

Goodwin TM: Toluene abuse and renal tubular acidosis in pregnancy. Obstet Gynecol 71(5):715-718, 1988.

Hersh JH: Toluene embryopathy: Two new cases. J Med Genet 26(5):333-337, 1989.

Hersh JH, Podruch PE, Rogers G, Weisskopf B: Toluene embryopathy. J Pediatr 106:922-927, 1985.

HSDB [database online]. Bethesda, Md.: National Library of Medicine; 1985- [updated 1995 September 15]. Available from: National Library of Medicine; BRS Information Technologies, McLean, Va.

Klimisch H-J, Hellwig J, Hofmann A: Studies on the prenatal toxicity of toluene in rabbits following inhalation exposure and proposal of a pregnancy guidance value. Arch Toxicol 66:373-381, 1992.

Lindemann R: Congenital renal tubular dysfunction associated with maternal sniffing of organic solvents. Acta Paediatr Scand 80:882-884, 1991.

Low LK, Meeks JR, Mackerer CR: Health effects of the alkylbenzenes. I. Toluene. Toxicol Ind Health 4:49-76, 1988.

McDonald JC, Lavoie J, Cote R, McDonald AD: Chemical exposures at work in early pregnancy and congenital defect: A case-referent study. Br J Ind Med 44:527-533, 1987.

Ng TP, Foo SC, Yoong T: Risk of spontaneous abortion in workers exposed to toluene. Br J Ind Med 49:804-808, 1992.

Pearson MA, Hoyme HE, Seaver LH, Rimsza ME: Toluene embryopathy: Delineation of phenotype and comparison with fetal alcohol syndrome. Pediatrics 93:211-215, 1994.

Roberts L, Vernot E, Bevan C, et al.: Developmental toxicity of toluene in the rat. Teratology 47:434, 1993.

Shigeta S, Aikawa H, Misawa T: Effects of maternal exposure to toluene during pregnancy on mouse embryos and fetuses. Tokai J Exp Clin Med 7:265-270, 1982.

Taskinen H, Lindbohm M-L, Hemminki K: Spontaneous abortions among women working in the pharmaceutical industry. Br J Ind Med 43:199-205, 1986.

Ungvary G, Tatrai E: On the embryotoxic effects of benzene and its alkyl derivatives in mice, rats and rabbits. Arch Toxicol (Suppl 8):425-430, 1985.

Ungvary G, Tatrai E, Lorincz M, Barcza G: Combined embryotoxic action of toluene, a widely used industrial chemical, and acetylsalicylic acid (Aspirin). Teratology 27:261-269, 1983.

Wilkins-Haug L, Gabow PA: Toluene abuse during pregnancy: Obstetric complications and perinatal outcomes. Obstet Gynecol 77:504-509, 1991.

TOLUOL® *See* Toluene

TOPICORT® *See* Desoximetasone

TRANSDERM-SCOP® *See* Scopolamine

TRANSDERM V® *See* Scopolamine

TRANXENE® *See* Chlorazepate

TRAZODONE
(Desyrel®, Trazon®, Trialodine®)

Trazodone is an antidepressant with sedative action. Trazodone is given orally in doses of 50-600 mg/d.

Teratogenic Risk

*Magnitude of teratogenic
risk to child born after
exposure during gestation:*   *Undetermined*

*Quality and quantity of data
on which risk estimate is based:*   *Very poor*

591

No epidemiological studies of congenital anomalies in the children of women who were treated with trazodone during pregnancy have been reported.

The frequency of malformations was not significantly increased among the offspring of pregnant rats and rabbits treated with trazodone in doses 2.5-38 times those used in humans (Barcellona, 1970; Rivett & Barcellona, 1974; Suzuki, 1974; Ono et al., 1989). Fetal death and growth retardation were seen in association with maternal toxicity at the higher doses.

Risk Related to Breast-feeding

Trazodone is excreted in the breast milk in low concentrations. Based on data from six lactating women, the amount of trazodone that the nursing infant would be expected to ingest is between 0.07-1% of the lowest therapeutic dose of trazodone, on a weight-adjusted basis (Verbeeck et al., 1986).*

The American Academy of Pediatrics recommends that trazodone be used with caution in breast-feeding mothers because of its potential to alter central nervous system development in nursing infants (Committee on Drugs, American Academy of Pediatrics, 1994).

Key References

Barcellona PS: Investigations on the possible teratogenic effects of trazodone in rats and rabbits. Boll Chim Farm 109:323-332, 1970.

Committee on Drugs, American Academy of Pediatrics: The transfer of drugs and other chemicals into human milk. Pediatrics 93(1):137-150, 1994.

Ono C, Kiwaki S, Furuko T, et al.: [Reproduction study in rats of trazodone hydrochloride (KB-831) orally administered during the period of fetal organogenesis.] Yakuri To Chiryo 17(Suppl 5):51-67, 1989.

Rivett KF, Barcellona PS: Toxicology of trazodone. Mod Probl Pharmacopsychiatry 9:76-86, 1974.

Suzuki Y: Teratogenicity and placental transfer of trazodone. Mod Probl Pharmacopsychiatry 9:87-94, 1974.

*This calculation is based on the following assumptions: maternal dose of trazodone: 50 mg; milk concentration of trazodone: 0.01-0.1 mcg/mL; milk intake by the nursing infant: 150 mL/kg/d; estimated dose of trazodone ingested by the nursing infant: 0.001-0.015 mg/kg/d; lowest therapeutic dose of trazodone in children: 1.5 mg/kg/d.

Verbeeck RK, Ross SG, McKenna EA: Excretion of trazodone in breast milk. Br J Clin Pharmacol 22:367-370, 1986.

TRAZON® *See* Trazodone

TRETINOIN
(Retin-A®, Retinoic Acid)

Tretinoin (all-trans-retinoic acid) is a vitamin A congener used topically in the treatment of acne and other dermatologic diseases. Tretinoin is poorly absorbed through the skin (De Wals et al., 1991; Kalivas, 1992).

Teratogenic Risk

*Magnitude of teratogenic
risk to child born after
exposure during gestation:* Unlikely

*Quality and quantity of data
on which risk estimate is based:* Fair

Topical treatment with tretinoin is unlikely to pose a substantial teratogenic risk, but the data are insufficient to state that there is no risk.

The frequency of major congenital anomalies was not increased among 212 infants of women who had become pregnant within four months of receiving a prescription for topical tretinoin or who obtained such a prescription during the first three months of pregnancy in one epidemiological study (Jick et al., 1993). Three infants with holoprosencephaly whose mothers used tretinoin topically during pregnancy have been reported to the US Food and Drug Administration, but no history of tretinoin use during pregnancy was found among the mothers of 16 infants with holoprosencephaly in a study designed to look for such an association (De Wals et al., 1991).

A child with low birth weight and a dysplastic auricle who was born to a mother who used tretinoin cream throughout the first 11 weeks of pregnancy has been reported (Camera & Pregliasco, 1992). In another case report, a child with supraumbilical exomphalos, anterior diaphragmatic hernia, pericardial defect, and a severe upper limb defect was born to a woman who used an alcohol-based liquid tretinoin preparation during the first five weeks of pregnancy (Lipson et al., 1993). No causal relationship can be established on the basis of these anecdotal observations.

Teratogenic effects similar to those demonstrated with other retinoids have been observed among the offspring of pregnant monkeys, rabbits, mice, rats, and hamsters treated systemically with tretinoin in doses of 2-10 mg/kg/d or greater (Kochhar et al., 1984; Alles & Sulik, 1990; Granstom & Kullaa-Mikkonen, 1990; Hendrickx & Hummler, 1992). Genetically predisposed animals may exhibit teratogenic effects after maternal treatment with single systemic doses as low as 0.3 mg/kg (Sulik et al., 1993). Malformations observed among affected fetuses include those of the ear, face, palate, limb, central nervous system, and heart. Fetal death is frequent.

Studies have also been done of the teratogenicity of topical tretinoin preparations applied to the skin of experimental animals. It is difficult to compare the dosages used in these studies to those used in humans because the experimental investigations involve relatively large areas of application and conditions that promote absorption of the drug. It seems likely that the absorbed dose of tretinoin in all of these studies is substantially greater than that usually encountered therapeutically in humans.

Increased rates of fetal death have been observed among pregnant rabbits treated topically with tretinoin (Zbinden, 1975). Skeletal malformations were seen with increased frequency among the offspring of rats treated topically with large amounts of tretinoin in some studies but not others (Zbinden, 1975; Chahoud et al., 1989, 1991; Seegmiller et al., 1990). Cleft palate was seen with increased frequency among the offspring of mice treated topically with tretinoin during pregnancy (Caldwell & Seegmiller, 1991). The relevance of these observations to use of topical tretinoin preparations in human pregnancy is uncertain.

Risk Related to Breast-feeding

No information regarding the distribution of tretinoin in breast milk has been published.

Key References

Alles AJ, Sulik KK: Retinoic acid-induced spina bifida: Evidence for a pathogenetic mechanism. Development 108:73-81, 1990.

Caldwell AP, Seegmiller RE: Evaluation of the teratogenic potential of topically applied all-trans retinoic acid (RA) in mice. Teratology 43(5):443, 1991.

Camera G, Pregliasco P: Ear malformation in baby born to mother using tretinoin cream. Lancet 339:687, 1992.

Chahoud I, Lofberg B, Mittmann B, Nau H: Teratogenicity and pharmacokinetics of vitamin A acid (tretinoin, all-trans retinoic acid) after dermal application in the rat. Naunyn Schmiedebergs Arch Pharmacol 339(Suppl):R30, 1989.

Chahoud I, Nau H, Tzimas G, et al.: Teratogenicity und pharmacokinetics of tretinoin after topical and oral application in the rat. Teratology 44(3):15A, 1991.

De Wals P, Bloch D, Calabro A, et al.: Association between holoprosencephaly and exposure to topical retinoids: Results of the EUROCAT survey. Paediatr Perinat Epidemiol 5:445-447, 1991.

Granstrom G, Kullaa-Mikkonen A: Experimental craniofacial malformations induced by retinoids and resembling branchial arch syndromes. Scand J Plast Reconstr Hand Surg 24:3-12, 1990.

Hendrickx AG, Hummler H: Teratogenicity of all-trans retinoic acid during early embryonic development in the cynomolgus monkey (Macaca fascicularis). Teratology 45:65-74, 1992.

Jick SS, Terris BZ, Jick H: First trimester topical tretinoin and congenital disorders. Lancet 341:1181-1182, 1993.

Kalivas J: Retinoids: Uses and abuses. Compr Ther 18(4):2-5, 1992.

Kochhar DM, Penner JD, Tellone CI: Comparative teratogenic activities of two retinoids: Effects on palate and limb development. Teratogenesis Carcinog Mutagen 4:377-387, 1984.

Lipson AH, Collins F, Webster WS: Multiple congenital defects associated with maternal use of topical tretinoin. Lancet 341:1352-1353, 1993.

Seegmiller RE, Carter MW, Ford WH, White RD: Induction of maternal toxicity in the rat by dermal application of retinoic acid and its effect on fetal outcome. Reprod Toxicol 4(4):277-281, 1990.

Sulik KK, Dehart D, Rogers JM, Chernoff N: Teratogenicity of low doses of all-trans retinoic acid. Teratology 47(5):383, 1993.

Zbinden G: Investigations on the toxicity of tretinoin administered systemically to animals. Acta Derm Venereol Suppl 74:36-40, 1975.

TRIADIPIN® *See* Doxepin

TRIALODINE® *See* Trazodone

TRIAMCINOLONE
(Aristocort®, Kenacort®, Ledercort®)

Triamcinolone is a synthetic glucocorticoid used to treat allergic and inflammatory conditions. It is employed in oral, parenteral, and aerosol forms as well as in local injectable and topical preparations, from which substantial absorption may occur. Dosages vary widely from <1 mg/d in many topical preparations to as much as 60 mg/d orally.

Teratogenic Risk

Magnitude of teratogenic risk to child born after exposure during gestation:	*Undetermined*
Quality and quantity of data on which risk estimate is based:	*Poor*

Chronic use of triamcinolone at high doses may be associated with fetal growth retardation.

No epidemiological studies of congenital anomalies in children of women treated with triamcinolone during pregnancy have been reported. Severe fetal growth retardation has been observed in the infant of a woman who was treated chronically with large amounts of topical triamcinolone during pregnancy (Katz et al., 1990). This anecdotal report is of concern because similar findings have been observed in nonhuman primates (see below).

An increased frequency of malformations was found among the offspring of three species of nonhuman primates treated during pregnancy with triamcinolone in doses <1-20 times those used clinically (Bacher & Michejda, 1988; Jerome & Hendrickx, 1988; Tarara et al., 1988; Hendrickx & Tarara, 1990). Neural tube defects and other central nervous system abnormalities, craniofacial malformations, and skeletal anomalies were seen most often; fetal growth retardation and fetal or neonatal death also occurred commonly.

Cleft palate occurs with increased frequency among the offspring of mice, rats, and hamsters treated during pregnancy with triamcinolone in doses within the human therapeutic range or greater (Melnick et al., 1981; Rowland & Hendrickx, 1983; Marazita et al., 1988; Wise et al., 1991; Zhou & Walker, 1993). The relevance of these findings to the risk of malformations in children of women treated with triamcinolone during pregnancy is unknown. *Please see agent summary on prednisone/prednisolone for information on a related agent.*

Risk Related to Breast-feeding

No information regarding the distribution of triamcinolone in breast milk has been published.

Key References

Bacher JD, Michejda M: Allogeneic fetal bone cranioplasty in *Macaca mulatta*. Fetal Ther 3:108-117, 1988.

Hendrickx AG, Tarara RP: Triamcinolone acetonide-induced meningocele and meningoencephalocele in rhesus monkeys. Am J Pathol 136(3):725-727, 1990.

Jerome CP, Hendrickx AG: Comparative teratogenicity of triamcinolone acetonide and dexamethasone in the rhesus monkey *(Macaca mulatta)*. J Med Primatol 17:195-203, 1988.

Katz VL, Thorp JM Jr, Bowes WA Jr: Severe symmetric intrauterine growth retardation associated with the topical use of triamcinolone. Am J Obstet Gynecol 162(2):396-397, 1990.

Marazita ML, Jaskoll T, Melnick M: Corticosteroid-induced cleft palate in short-ear mice. J Craniofac Genet Dev Biol 8:47-51, 1988.

Melnick M, Jaskoll T, Slavkin HC: Corticosteroid-induced cleft palate in mice and H-2 Haplotype: Maternal and embryonic effects. Immunogenetics 13:443-450, 1981.

Rowland JM, Hendrickx AG: Teratogenicity of triamcinolone acetonide in rats. Teratology 27:13-18, 1983.

Tarara RP, Wheeldon EB, Hendrickx AG: Central nervous system malformations induced by triamcinolone acetonide in nonhuman primates: Pathogenesis. Teratology 38:259-270, 1988.

Wise LD, Vetter CM, Anderson CA, et al.: Reversible effects of triamcinolone and lack of effects with aspirin or L-656,224 on external genitalia of male Sprague-Dawley rats exposed in utero. Teratology 44:507-520, 1991.

Zhou M, Walker BE: Potentiation of triamcinolone-induced cleft palate in mice by maternal high dietary fat. Teratology 48:53-57, 1993.

TRIAMTERENE
(Dyrenium®)

Triamterene is a mild diuretic with potassium-sparing effects. It is administered orally, usually in association with a diuretic of another kind, in the treatment of edema and hypertension. The usual dose is 100-300 mg/d.

Teratogenic Risk

Magnitude of teratogenic risk to child born after exposure during gestation:	*Undetermined*
Quality and quantity of data on which risk estimate is based:	*Very poor*

The frequency of congenital anomalies was no greater than expected among the children of 271 women treated with triamterene during pregnancy in a large epidemiological study (Heinonen et al., 1977). Only five of these women were treated during the first four lunar months of gestation.

Studies in rats suggest that treatment of pregnant women with triamterene in usual therapeutic doses is unlikely to increase the children's risk of malformations greatly (Ellison & Maren, 1972; Posner, 1972).

Risk Related to Breast-feeding

No information regarding the distribution of triamterene in breast milk has been published.

Key References

Ellison AC, Maren TH: The effect of potassium metabolism on acetazolamide-induced teratogenesis. Johns Hopkins Med J 130:105-115, 1972.

Heinonen OP, Slone D, Shapiro S: *Birth Defects and Drugs in Pregnancy.* Littleton, Mass.: John Wright-PSG, 1977, pp 372, 341.

Posner HS: Significance of cleft palate induced by chemicals in the rat and mouse. Food Cosmet Toxicol 10:839-855, 1972.

TRIAZOLAM
(Halcion®)

Triazolam is a benzodiazepine derivative used as a hypnotic. Triazolam is given orally, usually in a single dose of 125-250 mcg.

Teratogenic Risk

Magnitude of teratogenic risk to child born after exposure during gestation:	*Unlikely*
Quality and quantity of data on which risk estimate is based:	*Very poor*

Therapeutic doses of triazolam are unlikely to pose a substantial teratogenic risk, but the data are insufficient to state that there is no risk.

No epidemiological studies of congenital anomalies in infants born to women who took triazolam during pregnancy have been reported.

Studies in rats and rabbits suggest that treatment of pregnant women with triazolam in usual therapeutic doses is unlikely to increase the children's risk of malformations greatly (Matsuo et al., 1979).

Please see agent summary on diazepam for information on a related agent that has been more thoroughly studied.

Risk Related to Breast-feeding

No information regarding the distribution of triazolam in breast milk has been published.

Key References

Matsuo A, Kast A, Tsunenari Y: Reproduction studies of triazolam in rats and rabbits. Iyakuhin Kenkyu 10:52-67, 1979.

TRICODEINE® *See* Codeine

TRIFLUOPERAZINE
(Salazine®, Stelazine®, Terfluzine®)

Trifluoperazine is a phenothiazine used to treat psychoses and other psychiatric illnesses. Trifluoperazine is given orally in doses of 1-100 mg/d or parenterally in doses of 4-10 mg/d.

Teratogenic Risk

*Magnitude of teratogenic
risk to child born after
exposure during gestation:*   *Unlikely*

*Quality and quantity of data
on which risk estimate is based:*   *Fair*

Therapeutic doses of trifluoperazine are unlikely to pose a substantial teratogenic risk, but the data are insufficient to state that there is no risk.

The frequency of congenital anomalies was no higher than expected among the children of 42 women who took trifluoperazine during the first four lunar months of pregnancy in one epidemiological study (Heinonen et al., 1977). The frequency of congenital anomalies was not increased among the infants of 59 women treated with trifluoperazine during the first trimester of pregnancy in another study (General Practitioner Research Group, 1963). The incidence of malformations did not appear to be increased in a survey regarding the infants of 480 pregnant women treated with trifluoperazine (Moriarty & Nance, 1963).

The frequency of malformations was no higher than expected among the offspring of rabbits and mice treated during pregnancy with 20-80 and 290-1150 times those used clinically (Khan & Azam, 1969). A reduction of fetal weight occurred among the rabbits and an increased frequency of fetal loss occurred among the mice in this study. Szabo & Brent (1974) reported an increased frequency of cleft palate in the offspring of mice treated with 70-300 times the usual human dose of trifluoperazine during pregnancy. The relevance of these observations to the therapeutic use of trifluoperazine in human pregnancy in unknown.

Risk Related to Breast-feeding

No information regarding the distribution of trifluoperazine in breast milk has been published.

Key References

General Practitioner Research Group: Drugs in pregnancy survey. Practitioner 191:775-780, 1963.

Heinonen OP, Slone D, Shapiro S: *Birth Defects and Drugs in Pregnancy.* Littleton, Mass.: John Wright-PSG, 1977, pp 323-325.

Khan I, Azam A: Study of teratogenic activity of trifluoperazine, amitriptyline, ethionamide and thalidomide in pregnant rabbits and mice. Proc Eur Soc Study Drug Toxic 10:235-242, 1969.

Moriarty AJ, Nance MR: Trifluoperazine and pregnancy. Can Med Assoc J 88:375-376, 1963.

Szabo KT, Brent RL: Species differences in experimental teratogenesis by tranquillising agents. Lancet 1:565, 1974.

TRIMETHOPRIM
(Proloprim®, Trimpex®)

Trimethoprim is a competitive inhibitor of dihydrofolate reductase with specificity for microbial rather than mammalian systems (Mandell & Sande, 1990). It is used as an oral antimicrobial agent, often in combination with a sulfonamide. The usual dose of trimethoprim is 200 mg/d, but doses greater than 600 mg/d are often employed in the treatment of *Pneumocystis carnii* pneumonia.

Teratogenic Risk

*Magnitude of teratogenic
risk to child born after
exposure during gestation:*   Unlikely

*Quality and quantity of data
on which risk estimate is based:*   Poor to fair

Therapeutic doses of trimethoprim are unlikely to pose a substantial teratogenic risk, but the data are insufficient to state that there is no risk.

This risk estimate is for treatment of pregnant women with trimethoprim in conventional doses. The risk related to treatment with the very high doses often used for Pneumocystis carnii pneumonia is undetermined.

The frequency of congenital anomalies was no greater than expected among the infants of 89 women treated with trimethoprim in combination with sulfamethoxazole during the first trimester of pregnancy or of 211 treated with this agent anytime during pregnancy in one epidemiological study (Colley et al., 1982). No congenital anomalies were observed among the infants of 42 women treated with trimethoprim in combination with sulfamethoxazole in a clinical trial of treatment for bacteriuria in the first trimester of pregnancy (Bailey, 1984). In another trial, the frequency of congenital anomalies was no higher than expected among the infants of 120 women treated with trimethoprim and sulfamethoxazole, but only ten of these women were treated during the first trimester (Williams et al., 1969).

An association with maternal use of trimethoprim-sulfamethoxazole during pregnancy was observed in a study of 6228 infants with congenital anomalies (Czeizel, 1990). The association was seen with treatment at all gestational ages including the first trimester and involved a variety of congenital anomalies. No characteristic pattern was observed among exposed cases that had multiple congenital anomalies. The author concluded that the association between maternal exposure to trimethoprim-sulfamethoxazole and congenital anomalies was probably due to the underlying maternal disorder and not to the drugs per se.

No teratogenic effect was observed among the offspring of rats treated during pregnancy with trimethoprim in doses less than 10 times greater than those conventionally used in humans, but treatment with doses 16-117 times conventional human doses produced increased frequencies of embryonic malformations and death as well as maternal toxicity (Udall, 1969; Kreutz, 1981). The anomalies seen primarily affected the skeleton and were similar to those that occur with folate antagonists such as aminopterin and methotrexate. The relevance of these observations to the use of trimethoprim in conventional therapeutic doses in human pregnancy is uncertain. Neither the rate of embryonic death nor the rate of exencephaly was increased among the offspring of pregnant mice given trimethoprim in a dose 12.5 times those used conventionally in humans (Elmazar & Nau, 1993).

Risk Related to Breast-feeding

Trimethoprim is excreted in the breast milk. Based on data from 70 lactating women, the amount of trimethoprim that the nursing infant would be expected to ingest is between 3-14% of the lowest therapeutic dose of trimethoprim, on a weight-adjusted basis (Arnauld et al., 1972; Miller & Salter, 1974).*

The American Academy of Pediatrics regards trimethoprim to be safe to use while breast-feeding (Committee on Drugs, American Academy of Pediatrics, 1994).

Key References

Arnauld R, Soutoul JH, Gallier J, et al.: [A study of the passage of trimethoprim into the maternal milk.] Quest Med 25:959-964, 1972.

Bailey RR: Single-dose antibacterial treatment for bacteriuria in pregnancy. Drugs 27:183-186, 1984.

Colley DP, Kay J, Gibson GT: Study of the use in pregnancy of co-trimoxazole sulfamethizole. Aust J Pharm 63:570-575, 1982.

Committee on Drugs, American Academy of Pediatrics: The transfer of drugs and other chemicals into human milk. Pediatrics 93(1):137-150, 1994.

Czeizel A: A case-control analysis of the teratogenic effects of co-trimoxazole. Reprod Toxicol 4(4):305-313, 1990.

Elmazar MMA, Nau H: Trimethoprim potentiates valproic acid-induced neural tube defects (NTDs) in mice. Reprod Toxicol 7:249-254, 1993.

Kreutz VR: Investigation on the influence of trimethoprim at the intrauterine development in the rat. Anat Anz 149:151-159, 1981.

Mandell GL, Sande MA: Antimicrobial agents (continued). Sulfonamides, trimethoprim-sulfamethoxazole, quinolones, and agents for urinary tract infections. In: Gilman AG, Rall TW, Nies AS, Taylor P (eds). *Goodman and Gilman's The Pharmacological Basis of Therapeutics*, 8th ed. New York: Pergamon Press, 1990, pp 1047-1064.

*This calculation is based on the following assumptions: maternal dose of trimethoprim: 320-480 mg/d; milk concentration of trimethoprim: 1.2-5.5 mcg/mL; milk intake by the nursing infant: 150 mL/kg/d; estimated dose of trimethoprim ingested by the nursing infant: 0.18-0.82 mg/kg/d; lowest therapeutic dose of trimethoprim in children: 6 mg/kg/d.

Miller RD, Salter AJ: The passage of trimethoprim/sulphamethoxazole into breast milk and its significance. In: Daikos GK (ed). *Progress in Chemotherapy, Proceedings of the Eighth International, Congress of Chemotherapy*, Athens, 1973. Athens: Hellenic Society for Chemotherapy, 1974, pp 687-691.

Udall V: Toxicology of sulphonamide-trimethoprim combinations. Postgrad Med J 45:42-45, 1969.

Williams JD, Brumfitt W, Condie AP, Reeves DS: The treatment of bacteriuria in pregnant women with sulphamethoxazole and trimethoprim: A microbiological, clinical and toxicological study. Postgrad Med J 45(Suppl):71-76, 1969.

TRIMPEX® *See* Trimethoprim

TRINALIN REPETABS® *See* Azatadine

TUBASOL® *See* Aminosalicylic Acid

TUMS® *See* Calcium Salts

TYLENOL® *See* Acetaminophen

ULTRACEF® *See* Cefadroxil

UNISOM® *See* Doxylamine

UROPAN® *See* Nalidixic Acid

VALIUM® *See* Diazepam

VALPROIC ACID
(Depakene®, Depakote®, Epival®)

Valproic acid is a commonly used oral anticonvulsant. It is also employed to treat manic-depressive illness. Divalproex (Depakote®, Epival®)

is a compound composed of equal parts of valproic acid and sodium valproate. Divalproex breaks down in the stomach to form two valproate molecules, so equivalent oral doses of divalproex and valproic acid produce similar blood levels of valproate. Doses range from 5-60 mg/kg/d. Therapeutic serum levels for most patients are 50-100 mcg/mL.

Teratogenic Risk

Magnitude of teratogenic risk to child born after exposure during gestation:	
Neural tube defects:	*Small to moderate*
Other congenital anomalies:	*Small to moderate*
Quality and quantity of data on which risk estimate is based:	
Neural tube defects:	*Good*
Other congenital anomalies:	*Poor to fair*
These risks are additive.	

Epidemiological studies of malformations in infants born to women who took valproic acid during pregnancy can be difficult to interpret because assessment of the effects of anticonvulsant treatment is confounded by many other factors (Dansky & Finnell, 1991; Kaneko, 1991; Yerby, 1994). Among these confounders are the facts that most women with seizures are treated with some anticonvulsant drug, that many women are treated with more than one anticonvulsant at a time, that women who are not treated or are treated with a single agent probably have milder disease, and that valproic acid treatment is uncommon in women without seizures.

Many epidemiological studies and clinical series support the existence of an association between maternal use of valproic acid in pregnancy and the occurrence of spina bifida in infants (Anonymous, 1983; Mastroiacovo et al., 1983; Robert et al., 1983; Bertollini et al., 1985; Lammer et al., 1987; Robert, 1988; Kallen et al., 1989; Martinez-Frias, 1990; Rosa, 1991; Battino et al., 1992; Dravet et al., 1992; Kaneko et al., 1992, 1993; Lindhout et al., 1992a, b; Omtzigt et al., 1992a; Guibaud et al., 1993; Laegreid et al., 1993; Kallen, 1994). The defect observed is usually lumbar or sacral spina bifida; it is often associated with hydrocephalus (Lindhout et al., 1992b). Anencephaly is rarely seen. The best available estimate of the risk of spina bifida among the children of women treated with valproic acid during the first trimester of pregnancy is about 2% in populations in which the background rate of spina bifida is about 1/1000. The risk may be greater in populations with a higher background rate.

Spina bifida can be detected prenatally by high-resolution ultrasonography and measurement of amniotic fluid acetylcholinesterase and α-fetoprotein concentration (Omtzigt et al., 1992b; Guibaud et al., 1993). Maternal serum α-fetoprotein measurements appear to be less sensitive for detection of fetal neural tube defects in cases associated with maternal valproic acid therapy than in other circumstances. Women of childbearing age who are being treated with valproic acid should take folic acid supplements to reduce the risk of neural tube defects among children who are subsequently conceived (Oakeshott & Hunt, 1994).

A distinctive pattern of minor anomalies of the face and digits, i.e., a "fetal valproate syndrome," occurs in some infants born to women treated with valproic acid during pregnancy (DiLiberti et al., 1984; Winter et al., 1987; Ardinger et al., 1988; Christianson et al., 1994). Features include growth retardation, microcephaly, developmental delay, midface hypoplasia, epicanthal folds, short nose, broad nasal bridge, thin upper lip, thick lower lip, and micrognathia. In one series, nine (53%) of 17 infants born to epileptic women who had been treated with valproate during pregnancy had features of fetal valproate syndrome (Thisted & Ebbesen, 1993).

An epidemiological study of 12,506 children with congenital anomalies other than spina bifida found maternal use of valproic acid during pregnancy more frequently than expected (Martinez-Frias et al., 1989). Congenital anomalies were observed more often than expected among 79 infants born to women who were treated with valproic acid for seizure disorders during pregnancy (Dravet et al., 1992). A variety of malformations including cleft palate, congenital heart disease, hypospadias, club feet, and defects of the radius and related digital rays have been observed in children born to women who were treated with valproic acid for seizure disorders during pregnancy (Lammer et al., 1987; Sharony et al., 1993; Langer et al., 1994; Ylagan & Budorick, 1994).

Experimental studies demonstrate the teratogenic potential of valproic acid in other mammalian species. Treatment of pregnant rhesus monkeys with valproic acid in doses that produce blood levels similar to or greater than those considered to be therapeutic in humans produces craniofacial and skeletal anomalies in the offspring (Mast et al., 1986; Hendrickx et al., 1988). Exposure of pregnant mice, rats, or hamsters to valproic acid in doses that are associated with blood levels above the human therapeutic range causes skeletal, cardiac, and other malformations including neural tube defects in the offspring (Nau & Scott, 1986; Finnell & Dansky, 1991; Nau et al., 1991). Behavioral alterations occur among the offspring of rats treated with valproic acid during pregnancy in doses equivalent to those used in humans (Sobrian & Nandedkar, 1986; Vorhees, 1987).

Perinatal distress and unusual neonatal behavior have been noted in infants born to women treated with valproic acid or a variety of other anticonvulsants during pregnancy (Koch et al., 1985; Jager-Roman et al., 1986, 1987; Thisted & Ebbesen, 1993). There are also anecdotal reports of afibrinogenemia and hepatic failure in infants born to women who were treated with valproic acid during pregnancy (Legius et al., 1987; Majer & Green, 1987). Similar complications have been reported in children and adults on such therapy.

Risk Related to Breast-feeding

Valproic acid is excreted in breast milk in low concentrations. Based on data from 31 lactating women, the amount of valproic acid that the nursing infant would be expected to ingest is between <1-7% of the lowest therapeutic dose of valproic acid, on a weight-adjusted basis (Espir et al., 1976; Alexander, 1979; Dickinson et al., 1979; Nau et al., 1981; Bardy et al., 1982; von Unruh et al., 1984).*

Serum levels of valproic acid in seven of the infants from which samples were taken fall within the therapeutic range of valproic acid for adults (Alexander, 1979; Bardy et al., 1982; von Unruh et al., 1984).[†]

Both the American Academy of Pediatrics (Committee on Drugs, American Academy of Pediatrics, 1994) and the WHO Working Group on Drugs and Human Lactation (1988) regard valproic acid to be safe to use while breast-feeding.

Key References

Alexander FW: Sodium valproate and pregnancy. Arch Dis Child 54:240, 1979.

Anonymous: Valproate: A new cause of birth defects - Report from Italy and follow-up from France. CDC Morbid Mortal Week Rep 32:438-439, 1983.

*This calculation is based on the following assumptions: maternal dose of valproic acid: 4.1-32.7 mg/kg/d; milk concentration of valproic acid: 0.17-7.2 mcg/mL; milk intake by the nursing infant: 150 mL/kg/d; estimated dose of valproic acid ingested by the nursing infant: 0.026-1.1 mg/kg/d; lowest therapeutic dose in children: 15 mg/kg/d.

[†]Infant serum levels of valproic acid: <0.43-64.9 mcg/mL; range of therapeutic serum levels of valproic acid in adults: 30-100 mcg/mL.

Ardinger HH, Atkin JF, Blackston RD, et al.: Verification of the fetal valproate syndrome phenotype. Am J Med Genet 29:171-185, 1988.

Bardy AH, Granstrom M-L, Hiilesmaa VK: Valproic acid and breast-feeding. In: Janz D, Bossi L, Dam M, Richens A, Schmidt D (eds). *Epilepsy, Pregnancy, and the Child.* New York: Raven Press, 1982, pp 359-360.

Battino D, Binelli S, Caccamo ML, et al.: Malformations in off-spring of 305 epileptic women: A prospective study. Acta Neurol Scand 85:204-207, 1992.

Bertollini R, Mastroiacovo P, Segni G: Maternal epilepsy and birth defects: A case-control study in the Italian Multicentric Registry of Birth Defects (IPIMC). Eur J Epidemiol 1:67-72, 1985.

Christianson AL, Chesler N, Kromberg JGR: Fetal valproate syndrome: Clinical and neurodevelopmental features in two sibling pairs. Dev Med Child Neurol 36:361-369, 1994.

Committee on Drugs, American Academy of Pediatrics: The transfer of drugs and other chemicals into human milk. Pediatrics 93(1):137-150, 1994.

Dansky LV, Finnell RH: Parental epilepsy, anticonvulsant drugs, and reproductive outcome: Epidemiologic and experimental findings spanning three decades; 2: Human studies. Reprod Toxicol 5(4):301-335, 1991.

Dickinson RG, Harland RC, Lynn RK, et al.: Transmission of valproic acid (Depakene®) across the placenta: Half-life of the drug in mother and baby. J Pediatr 94:832-835, 1979.

DiLiberti JH, Farndon PA, Dennis NR, Curry CJR: The fetal valproate syndrome. Am J Med Genet 19:473-481, 1984.

Dravet C, Julian C, Legras C, et al.: Epilepsy, antiepileptic drugs, and malformations in children of women with epilepsy: A French prospective cohort study. Neurology 42(Suppl 5):75-82, 1992.

Espir MLE, Benton P, Will E, et al.: Sodium valproate (Epilim)--some clinical and pharmacological aspects. In: Legg (ed). *Clinical and Pharmacological Aspects of Sodium Valproate (Epilim) in the Treatment of Epilepsy.* Tunbridge Wells: MCS Consultants, 1976, pp 145-151.

Finnell RH, Dansky LV: Parental epilepsy, anticonvulsant drugs, and reproductive outcome: Epidemiologic and experimental findings spanning three decades; 1: Animal studies. Reprod Toxicol 5(4):281-299, 1991.

Guibaud S, Robert E, Simplot A, et al.: Prenatal diagnosis of spina bifida aperta after first-trimester valproate exposure. Prenat Diagn 13:772-773, 1993.

Hendrickx AG, Nau H, Binkerd P, et al.: Valproic acid developmental toxicity and pharmacokinetics in the rhesus monkey: An interspecies comparison. Teratology 38:329-345, 1988.

Jager-Roman E, Deichl A, Jakob S, et al.: Fetal growth, major malformations, and minor anomalies in infants born to women receiving valproic acid. J Pediatr 108:997-1004, 1986.

Jager-Roman E, Koch S, Helge H: Gentamicin pharmacokinetics in cystic fibrosis. J Pediatr 111:309-310, 1987.

Kallen AJB: Maternal carbamazepine and infant spina bifida. Reprod Toxicol 8(3):203-205, 1994.

Kallen B, Robert E, Mastroiacovo P, et al.: Anticonvulsant drugs and malformations: Is there a drug specificity? Eur J Epidemiol 5(1):31-36, 1989.

Kaneko S: Antiepileptic drug therapy and reproductive consequences: Functional and morphologic effects. Reprod Toxicol 5(3):179-198, 1991.

Kaneko S, Otani K, Kondo T, et al.: Malformation in infants of mothers with epilepsy receiving antiepileptic drugs. Neurology 42(Suppl 5):68-74, 1992.

Kaneko S, Otani K, Kondo T, et al.: Teratogenicity of antiepileptic drugs and drug specific malformations. Jpn J Psychol Neurol 47(2):306-308, 1993.

Koch S, Gopfert-Geyer I, Hauser I, et al: Neonatal behavior disturbances in infants of epileptic women treated during pregnancy. Prog Clin Biol Res 163B:453-461, 1985.

Laegreid L, Kyllerman M Hedner T, et al.: Benzodiazepine amplification of valproate teratogenic effects in children of mothers with absence epilepsy. Neuropediatrics 24:88-92, 1993.

Lammer EJ, Sever LE, Oakley GP Jr: Teratogen update: Valproic acid. Teratology 35:465-473, 1987.

Langer B, Haddad J, Gasser B, et al.: Isolated fetal bilateral ray reduction associated with valproic acid usage. Fetal Diagn Ther 9:155-158, 1994.

Legius E, Jaeken J, Eggermont E: Sodium valproate, pregnancy, and infantile fatal liver failure. Lancet 2:1518-1519, 1987.

Lindhout D, Meinardi H, Meijer JWA, Nau H: Antiepileptic drugs and teratogenesis in two consecutive cohorts: Changes in prescription policy paralleled by changes in pattern of malformations. Neurology 42(Suppl 5):94-110, 1992a.

Lindhout D, Omtzigt JGC, Cornel MC: Spectrum of neural-tube defects in 34 infants prenatally exposed to antiepileptic drugs. Neurology 42(Suppl 5):111-118, 1992b.

Majer RV, Green PJ: Neonatal afibrinogenaemia due to sodium valproate. Lancet 2:740-741, 1987.

Martinez-Frias ML: Clinical manifestation of prenatal exposure to valproic acid using case reports and epidemiologic information. Am J Med Genet 37:277-282, 1990.

Martinez-Frias ML, Rodriguez-Pinilla E, Salvador J: Valproate and spina bifida. Lancet 1:611-612, 1989.

Mast TJ, Cukierski MA, Nau H, Hendrickx AG: Predicting the human teratogenic potential of the anticonvulsant, valproic acid, from a non-human primate model. Toxicology 39:111-119, 1986.

Mastroiacovo P, Bertollini R, Morandini S, Segni G: Maternal epilepsy, valproate exposure, and birth defects. Lancet 2:1499, 1983.

Nau H, Hauck R-S, Ehlers K: Valproic acid-induced neural tube defects in mouse and human: Aspects of chirality, alternative drug development, pharmacokinetics and possible mechanisms. Pharmacol Toxicol 69:310-321, 1991.

Nau H, Rating D, Koch S, et al.: Valproic acid and its metabolites: Placental transfer, neonatal pharmacokinetics, transfer via mother's milk and clinical status in neonates of epileptic mothers. J Pharmacol Exp Ther 219(3):768-776, 1981.

Nau H, Scott WJ Jr: Weak acids may act as teratogens by accumulating in the basic milieu of the early mammalian embryo. Nature 323:276-278, 1986.

Oakeshott P, Hunt G: Prevention of neural tube defects. Lancet 343:123, 1994.

Omtzigt JGC, Los FJ, Grobbee DE, et al.: The risk of spina bifida aperta after first-trimester exposure to valproate in a prenatal cohort. Neurology 42(Suppl 5):119-125, 1992a.

Omtzigt JGC, Nau H, Los FJ, et al.: The disposition of valproate and its metabolites in the late first trimester and early second trimester of pregnancy in maternal serum, urine, and amniotic fluid: Effect of dose, co-medication, and the presence of spina bifida. Eur J Clin Pharmacol 43:381-388, 1992b.

Robert E: Valproic acid as a human teratogen. Congen Anom 28(Suppl):S71-S80, 1988.

Robert E, Robert JM, Lapras C: [Is valproic acid teratogenic?] Rev Neurol 139:445-447, 1983.

Rosa FW: Spina Bifida in infants of women treated with carbamazepine during pregnancy. N Engl J Med 324(10):674-677, 1991.

Sharony R, Garber A, Viskochil D, et al.: Preaxial ray reduction defects as part of valproic acid embryofetopathy. Prenat Diagn 13:909-918, 1993.

Sobrian SK, Nandedkar AKN: Prenatal antiepileptic drug exposure alters seizure susceptibility in rats. Pharmacol Biochem Behav 24:1383-1391, 1986.

Thisted E, Ebbesen F: Malformations, withdrawal manifestations, and hypoglycaemia after exposure to valproate in utero. Arch Dis Child 69:288-291, 1993.

von Unruh GE, Froescher W, Hoffmann F, Niesen M: Valproic acid in breast milk: How much is really there? Ther Drug Monit 6:272-276, 1984.

Vorhees CV: Teratogenicity and developmental toxicity of valproic acid in rats. Teratology 35:195-202, 1987.

WHO Working Group on Drugs and Human Lactation. In: Bennet PN (ed). *Drugs and Human Lactation.* Amsterdam: Elsevier, 1988, p 341-342.

Winter RM, Donnai D, Burn J, Tucker SM: Fetal valproate syndrome: Is there a recognisable phenotype? J Med Genet 24:692-695, 1987.

Yerby MS: Pregnancy, teratogenesis and epilepsy. Neurol Clin 12(40):749-771, 1994.

Ylagan LR, Budorick NE: Radial ray aplasia in utero: A prenatal finding associated with valproic acid exposure. J Ultrasound Med 13:408-411, 1994.

VANCERASE® *See* Beclomethasone

VARICELLA-RIT® *See* Varicella-Zoster Vaccine

VARICELLA-ZOSTER IMMUNE GLOBULIN
(VZIG)

Varicella-zoster immune globulin is human immunoglobulin (largely IgG) obtained from individuals with high antibody titers to varicella-zoster virus. Varicella-zoster immune globulin is administered intramuscularly to confer passive immunity against chickenpox.

Teratogenic Risk

*Magnitude of teratogenic
risk to child born after
exposure during gestation:*   Undetermined

*Quality and quantity of data
on which risk estimate is based:*   None

A small risk cannot be excluded, but a greatly increased risk of congenital anomalies among the children of women treated with varicella-zoster immune globulin during pregnancy is unlikely.

No epidemiological studies of congenital anomalies in children of women who were given varicella-zoster immune globulin during pregnancy have been reported.

No animal teratology studies of varicella-zoster immune globulin have been published.

Risk Related to Breast-feeding

No information regarding the distribution of varicella-zoster immune globulin in breast milk has been published.

Key References

None available.

VARICELLA-ZOSTER VACCINE
(Varicella-RIT®, Varivax®)

Varicella-zoster vaccine is an attenuated live virus vaccine that is injected subcutaneously to produce active immunity to chickenpox (Feldman & Moffitt, 1990; Gershon, 1995).

Teratogenic Risk

*Magnitude of teratogenic
risk to child born after
exposure during gestation:*   Undetermined

No epidemiological studies of congenital anomalies in children born to women who were immunized with varicella-zoster vaccine during pregnancy have been reported. No adverse fetal effects are said to have occurred in a small number of women who became pregnant within a few weeks of being immunized with varicella-zoster vaccine in investigative trials (Clements & Katz, 1993). A detailed description of this experience has not been published.

No animal teratology studies of varicella-zoster vaccine have been reported.

Risk Related to Breast-feeding

No information regarding the distribution of varicella-zoster vaccine in breast milk has been published. The Advisory Committee on Immunization Practices considers live vaccinations to be safe to administer while the mother is breast-feeding (ACIP, 1994).

Key References

ACIP: General recommendations on immunization. Recommendations of the Advisory Committee on Immunization Practices (ACIP). MMWR 43(RR-1):1-38, 1994.

Clements DA, Katz SL: Varicella in a susceptible pregnant woman. Curr Clin Top Infect Dis 13:123-130, 1993.

Feldman S, Moffitt JE: Varicella vaccine. Pediatr Ann 19:721-726, 1990.

Gershon AA: Varicella-zoster virus: Prospects for control. Adv Pediatr Infect Dis 10:93-124, 1995.

VARIVAX® *See* Varicella-Zoster Vaccine

VASOTEC® *See* Enalapril

VELOSULIN® *See* Insulin

VENTOLIN® *See* Albuterol

VERAPAMIL
(Calan®, Isoptin®, Verelan®)

Verapamil is a calcium channel blocking agent that is used as an antihypertensive and to treat cardiac arrhythmias and angina pectoris. Verapamil is given orally or parenterally; the dose is usually 180-480 mg/d.

Teratogenic Risk

*Magnitude of teratogenic
risk to child born after
exposure during gestation:*   None to Minimal

*Quality and quantity of data
on which risk estimate is based:*   Poor

The frequency of congenital anomalies was not significantly increased among 57 infants of women who had been treated with verapamil or another calcium channel blocking agent during the first trimester of pregnancy in one study (Magee et al., 1994). No adverse drug-related effects were observed among the infants of 90 or 47 hypertensive women treated with verapamil in late pregnancy in two therapeutic trials (Orlandi et al., 1986; Marlettini et al., 1990).

Decreased litter size and reduced fetal weight were observed among pregnant rats treated parenterally with verapamil in doses similar to those used in humans (Spatz et al., 1986). This treatment also produced maternal toxicity in the rats. The relevance of these observations to the therapeutic use of verapamil in human pregnancy is unknown.

Verapamil has been employed in combination with other tocolytic agents in the therapy of premature labor in women (Gummerus, 1977; Carstensen et al., 1983). Verapamil has also been used to treat fetal cardiac arrhythmias during the second and third trimesters of pregnancy (Wladimiroff et al., 1989; Ito et al., 1994). Unexplained fetal death has occurred after successful therapy of fetal supraventricular tachycardia with verapamil (Owen et al., 1988).

Risk Related to Breast-feeding

Verapamil and its active metabolite, norverapamil, are excreted in the breast milk in very low concentrations. Based on data from four lactating women, the amount of verapamil that the nursing infant would be expected to ingest is between 0.02-1% of the lowest therapeutic dose of verapamil in infants (Inoue et al., 1984; Miller et al., 1986; Anderson et al., 1987).*

Norverapamil concentrations were measured in the breast milk of two lactating women (Miller et al., 1986; Anderson et al., 1987). The maximum amount of norverapamil that the nursing infant would be expected to receive is equivalent to <1% of the lowest therapeutic dose of verapamil in infants.[†]

The serum level of verapamil in one of three infants from whom samples were taken was 2.5% of the lowest therapeutic serum level in adults; no verapamil was detected in the serum of the other two infants (Anderson, 1983; Miller et al., 1986; Anderson et al., 1987).[‡] Also, norverapamil was not detected in the infants' serum.

Both the American Academy of Pediatrics (Committee on Drugs, American Academy of Pediatrics, 1994) and the WHO Working Group on Drugs and Human Lactation (1988) regard verapamil to be safe to use while breast-feeding.

Key References

Anderson HJ: Excretion of verapamil in human milk. Eur J Clin Pharmacol 25:279-280, 1983.

Anderson HJ, Bondesson U, Mattiasson I, Johansson BW: Verapamil and norverapamil in plasma and breast milk during breast feeding. Eur J Clin Pharmacol 31:623-627, 1987.

Carstensen MH, Bahnsen J, Sterzing E: [Tocolysis with β-sympathicomimetics alone or combined with the calcium antagonist verapamil.] Geburtshilfe Frauenheilkd 43:431-437, 1983.

*This calculation is based on the following assumptions: maternal dose of verapamil: 240-360 mg/d; milk concentration of verapamil: 0.01-0.3 mcg/mL; milk intake by the nursing infant: 150 mL/kg/d; estimated dose of verapamil: 0.001-0.04 mg/kg/d; lowest therapeutic dose of verapamil in infants: 4 mg/kg/d.

†This calculation is based on the following assumptions: milk concentration of norverapamil: 0.006-0.065 mcg/mL; estimated dose of norverapamil: 0.45-9.7 mcg/kg/d; equivalent dose of verapamil, assuming 12% activity of norverapamil: 0.06-1.2 mcg/kg/d.

‡Infant serum level of verapamil: 0.002 mcg/mL; lowest therapeutic serum level of verapamil in adults: 0.08 mcg/mL.

Committee on Drug, American Academy of Pediatrics: The transfer of drugs and other chemicals into human milk. Pediatrics 93(1):137-150, 1994.

Gummerus M: [Treatment of premature labour and antagonization of the side effects of tocolytic therapy with verapamil.] Z Geburtshife Perinatol 181:334-340, 1977.

Inoue H, Unno N, Ou M-C, et al.: Level of verapamil in human milk. Eur J Clin Pharmacol 26:657-658, 1984.

Ito S, Magee L, Smallhorn J: Drug therapy for fetal arrhythmias. Clin Perinatol 21(3):543-572, 1994.

Magee LA, Conover B, Schick B, et al.: Exposure to calcium channel blockers in human pregnancy. A prospective, controlled, multicentre cohort study. Teratology 49(5):372, 1994.

Marlettini MG, Crippa S, Morselli-Labate AM, et al.: Randomized comparison of calcium antagonists and β-blockers in the treatment of pregnancy-induced hypertension. Curr Ther Res 48(4):684-692, 1990.

Miller MR, Withers R, Bhamra R, Holt DW: Verapamil and breast-feeding. Eur J Clin Pharmacol 30:125-126, 1986.

Orlandi C, Marlettini MG, Cassani A, et al.: Treatment of hypertension during pregnancy with the calcium antagonist verapamil. Curr Ther Res 39(6):884-893, 1986.

Owen J, Colvin EV, Davis RO: Fetal death after successful conversion of fetal supraventricular tachycardia with digoxin and verapamil. Am J Obstet Gynecol 158:1169-1170, 1988.

Spatz RJ, Pillalamari ED, Diab GM, et al: Verapamil effect on fetus in rat. Proc West Pharmacol Soc 29:319-322, 1986.

WHO Working Group on Drugs and Human Lactation. In: Bennet PN (ed). *Drugs and Human Lactation*. Amsterdam: Elsevier, 1988, pp 122-123.

Wladimiroff JW, Stewart PA, Reuss A: Medical treatment of the fetus. In: Rodeck CH (ed). *Fetal Medicine*. Oxford: Blackwell, 1989, pp 154-176.

VERELAN® *See* Verapamil

VIBRAMYCIN® *See* Doxycycline

VITAMIN A (RETINOIDS)
(Aquasol A®, Retinol)

Vitamin A, a fat-soluble nutrient, is essential for normal vision. Retinoids, including retinol, retinaldehyde, and retinoic acid, possess vitamin A activity directly; carotenoids such as beta-carotene can be metabolized to form vitamin A. *This summary deals only with retinoids. Please see agent summary on beta-carotene for information on carotenoids.*

The current US recommended dietary allowance (RDA) for vitamin A in pregnant women is the equivalent of 800 mcg (2667 IU) of retinol per day (0.3 mcg of all-trans retinol is equivalent to one international unit [IU] of vitamin A). In lactating women, the RDA is increased to 1200-1300 mcg (4000-4300 IU). Vitamin A has a long biological half-life and accumulates in the body (Hathcock et al., 1990).

Doses of vitamin A as large as 7500-15,000 mcg of retinol per day are used to treat deficiency states and certain skin diseases. Vitamin A has also been taken in even larger amounts by some individuals for various other purported health benefits, but this use is not generally accepted. Vitamin A is usually taken orally, but it may also be given parenterally.

Teratogenic Risk

Magnitude of teratogenic
risk to child born after
exposure during gestation:
    Low dose (<10,000 IU):   *None*
    High dose (>25,000 IU):   *Undetermined*

Quality and quantity of data
on which risk estimate is based:
    Low dose (<10,000 IU):   *Good*
    High dose (>25,000 IU):   *Poor*

Although the teratogenicity of retinol has not been established in humans, there is reason to suspect that the risk of congenital anomalies may be increased among children of women who take very large amounts of this substance early in pregnancy. Very high doses of retinol or retinoic acid are teratogenic in many species of experimental animals, and isotretinoin, a closely related compound, is a recognized human teratogen. Teratogenic dosages of retinol in experimental animals are hundreds to thousands of times greater than the human RDA (Anonymous, 1987; Pinnock & Alderman, 1992); such doses are rarely if ever encountered among pregnant women, even those who take "megadose" vitamins.

Large amounts of retinol may be found in some food sources (e.g., liver) (Nelson, 1990; Sanders, 1990).

The frequency of congenital anomalies was no greater than expected among 1203 children of women who took 6000 IU of vitamin A daily throughout the first trimester of pregnancy in a randomized trial of vitamin supplementation (Dudas & Czeizel, 1992). No significant association was observed with maternal use of 10,000 IU or more per day of vitamin A in an epidemiological study that included 11,293 children with minor and major congenital anomalies (Martinez-Frias & Salvador, 1988, 1990). Neither of these studies specified whether the vitamin A preparations used contained retinoids or carotenoids.

An association of marginal statistical significance was seen with maternal use of retinoid supplements during the first lunar month of pregnancy in a study of 2658 infants with congenital anomalies involving structures derived at least in part from the neural crest, an embryonic cell type thought to be involved in retinoid embryopathy in experimental animals (Werler et al., 1990). The dose of the supplements used by these women was unknown. None of the mothers of 172 infants in this study who had a pattern of malformations consistent with isotretinoin embryopathy had taken retinoid supplements in the first trimester of pregnancy.

Several instances of congenital anomalies in infants born to mothers who took large amounts of vitamin A during pregnancy have been reported (Rosa et al., 1986; Evans & Hickey-Dwyer, 1991; Rosa, 1991), but no consistent pattern of anomalies has been observed. Although such cases are of concern, the number reported is far less than would be expected to occur by chance even if "megadoses" of retinoids were not teratogenic in humans (Rosa, 1987). No congenital anomalies were observed in 14 pregnancies with first-trimester exposures to high doses (25,000 IU or greater) of vitamin A in one series, although three other similarly-exposed pregnancies resulted in spontaneous abortion (Zuber et al., 1987). In another series, no malformations were observed among seven infants born to women who took more than 25,000 IU of vitamin A daily at various times during pregnancy (Bonati et al., 1995).

Increased frequencies of fetal death and congenital anomalies have consistently been observed among the offspring of rats, mice, and hamsters treated during pregnancy with 750 to many thousands of times the human RDA of retinol or retinoic acid (Cohlan, 1954; Kalter & Warkany, 1961; Marin-Padilla & Ferm, 1965; Kochhar, 1967; Willhite, 1984; Eckhoff et al., 1989). Many different malformations are seen in affected offspring, but craniofacial, central nervous system, and skeletal anomalies are most frequent. Cardiac and eye anomalies have been reported in the offspring of pigs and cleft palate in the offspring of dogs treated during pregnancy with very large doses of vitamin A (Palludan, 1966; Wiersig & Swenson, 1967). Malformations have been produced in the offspring of pregnant rabbits treated with retinol in doses about 300 times greater than the human RDA (Kamm, 1982).

Please see agent summary on isotretinoin for more information on this closely related compound. Please see agent summary on beta-carotene for information on this vitamin A precursor.

Risk Related to Breast-feeding

Vitamin A is a normal constitutent in milk (Wallingford & Underwood, 1986; Newman, 1993). Maternal supplementation with vitamin A late in pregnancy and during breast-feeding has been associated with higher milk concentrations of vitamin A (Kon & Mawson, 1950; Venkatachalam et al., 1962; Prentice et al., 1980; Wallingford & Underwood, 1986; Newman, 1993; Stolzfus et al., 1993).

High dose supplementation immediately following delivery has been recommended for vitamin-deficient nursing mothers (Underwood, 1994). Single boluses of 200,000-300,000 IU of vitamin A have not produced adverse effects in nursing infants (Wallingford & Underwood, 1986; Newman, 1993).

Key References

Anonymous: Teratology Society Position Paper: Recommendations for vitamin A use during pregnancy. Teratology 35:269-275, 1987.

Bonati M, Nannini S, Addis A: Vitamin A supplementation during pregnancy in developed countries. Lancet 345:736-737, 1995.

Cohlan SQ: Congenital anomalies in the rat produced by excessive intake of vitamin A during pregnancy. Pediatrics 13:556-569, 1954.

Dudas I, Czeizel AE: Use of 6,000 IU Vitamin A during early pregnancy without teratogenic effect. Teratology 45:335-336, 1992.

Eckhoff CH, Lofberg B, Chahoud I, et al.: Transplacental pharmacokinetics and teratogenicity of a single dose of retinol (vitamin A) during organogenesis in the mouse. Toxicol Lett 48:171-184, 1989.

Evans K, Hickey-Dwyer MU: Cleft anterior segment with maternal hypervitaminosis A. Br J Ophthalmol 75:691-692, 1991.

Hathcock JN, Hattan DG, Jenkins MY, et al.: Evaluation of vitamin A toxicity. Am J Clin Nutr 52:183-202, 1990.

Kalter H, Warkany J: Experimental production of congenital malformations in strains of inbred mice by maternal treatment with hypervitaminosis A. Am J Pathol 38:1-21, 1961.

Kamm JJ: Toxicology, carcinogenicity, and teratogenicity of some orally administered retinoids. J Am Acad Dermatol 6(4):652-659, 1982.

Kochhar DM: Teratogenic activity of retinoic acid. Acta Pathol Microbiol Scand 70:398-404, 1967.

Kon SK, Mawson EH: *Human milk: Wartime Studies of Certain Vitamins and Other Constituents. Medical Research Council Special Report Series*, No. 269. London: HMSO, 1950. Cited in: Bates CJ: Vitamin A in pregnancy and lactation. Proc Nutr Soc 42:65-79, 1983.

Marin-Padilla M, Ferm VH: Somite necrosis and developmental malformations induced by vitamin A in the golden hamster. J Embryol Exp Morphol 13:1-8, 1965.

Martinez-Frias ML, Salvador J: Epidemiological aspects of prenatal exposure to high doses of vitamin A in Spain. Eur J Epidemiol 6(2):118-123, 1990.

Martinez-Frias ML, Salvador J: Megadose vitamin A and teratogenicity. Lancet 1:236, 1988.

Nelson M: Vitamin A, liver consumption, and risk of birth defects. BMJ 301:1176, 1990.

Newman V: *Vitamin A and breastfeeding: A Comparison of Data From Developed and Developing Countries.* San Diego, Calif.: Wellstart International, 1993.

Palludan B: Swine in teratological studies. In: Bustad LK, McClellan RO (eds). *Swine in Biomedical Research.* Columbus, Oh.: Battelle Memorial Institute, 1966, pp 51-78.

Pinnock CB, Alderman CP: The potential for teratogenicity of vitamin A and its congeners. Med J Aust 157:804-809, 1992.

Prentice AM, Whitehead RG, Roberts SB, et al.: Dietary supplementation of Gambian nursing mothers and lactational performance. Lancet 2:886-887, 1980.

Rosa F: Detecting human retinoid embryopathy. Teratology 43(5):419, 1991.

Rosa FW: Difficulties with vitamin A human teratology. Teratology 35(3):28A, 1987.

Rosa FW, Wilk AL, Kelsey FO: Teratogen update: Vitamin A congeners. Teratology 33:355-364, 1986.

Sanders TAB: Vitamin A and pregnancy. Lancet 336:1375, 1990.

Stolzfus RJ, Hakimi M, Miller KW, et al.: High dose vitamin A supplementation of breast-feeding Indonesian mothers: Effects on the vitamin A status of mother and infant. J Nutr 123:666-675, 1993.

Underwood BA: Maternal vitamin A status and its importance in infancy and early childhood. Am J Clin Nutr 59(Suppl):517S-524S, 1994.

Venkatachalam PS, Belavady B, Gopalan C: Studies on vitamin A nutritional status of mothers and infants in poor communities of India. Trop Pediatr 61:262, 1962.

Wallingford JC, Underwood BA: Vitamin A deficiency in pregnancy, lactation, and the nursing child. In: Bauernfeind JC (ed). *Vitamin A Deficiency and Its Control*. New York: Academic Press, 1986, pp 101-152.

Werler MM, Lammer EJ, Rosenberg L, Mitchell AA: Maternal vitamin A supplementation in relation to selected birth defects. Teratology 42:497-503, 1990.

Wiersig DO, Swenson MJ: Teratogenicity of vitamin A in the canine. Fed Proc 26:486, 1967.

Willhite CC: Dose-response relationships of retinol in production of the Arnold-Chiari malformation. Toxicol Lett 20:257-262, 1984.

Zuber C, Librizzi RJ, Vogt BL: Outcomes of pregnancies exposed to high doses vitamin A. Teratology 35(2):42A,1987.

VITAMIN B_1 *See* Thiamine

VITAMIN B_2 *See* Riboflavin

VITAMIN B_3 *See* Niacin

VITAMIN B_6 *See* Pyridoxine

VITAMIN C *See* Ascorbic Acid

VITAMIN D
(Calcifediol®, Deltalin®, Rocaltrol®)

Vitamin D includes a series of compounds that are able to prevent and cure rickets. Vitamin D synthesis occurs in the skin in the presence of sunlight. Many foods also contain this fat-soluble vitamin. The current US recommended dietary allowance (RDA) of vitamin D in pregnancy and lactation is 10 mcg (400 units) per day (NRC, 1989). Larger doses are given orally or parenterally to treat deficiency states; these doses vary greatly depending on the particular form of vitamin D being used.

Teratogenic Risk

Magnitude of teratogenic risk to child born after exposure during gestation:	*Unlikely*
Quality and quantity of data on which risk estimate is based:	*Poor*

This assessment refers to risks associated with very high doses of vitamin D. Vitamin D in small doses is a necessary dietary component.

High doses of vitamin D are unlikely to pose a substantial teratogenic risk, although the data are insufficient to state that there is no risk.

In one clinical series, no malformations were observed among 15 children born to hypoparathyroid women who took an average of more than 200 times the RDA of vitamin D throughout pregnancy (Goodenday & Gordon, 1971). In another series, no malformations were seen among 19 infants with elevated vitamin D levels whose mothers had drank milk containing excessive vitamin D supplements (100-600 times the RDA) during pregnancy (O'Brien et al., 1993).

Maternal vitamin D deficiency during pregnancy can produce rachitic skeletal anomalies in newborns (Ford et al., 1973; Moncrieff & Fadahunsi, 1974).

Administration of vitamin D to pregnant rabbits and rats in doses hundreds to thousands of times greater than the human RDA produces cardiovascular and craniofacial anomalies in the offspring similar to those seen in the human Williams syndrome (supravalvular aortic stenosis, unusual facies, and infantile hypercalcemia) (Friedman & Roberts, 1966; Friedman & Mills, 1969; Chan et al., 1979). Although it was suggested that the Williams syndrome in humans may be related to maternal ingestion of large amounts of vitamin D (Friedman, 1968), Williams syndrome is now known to be due to a contiguous gene deletion (Ewart et al., 1993).

Risk Related to Breast-feeding

Vitamin D is a normal constituent of breast milk. Breast milk concentrations of vitamin D are influenced by the maternal vitamin D status. Maternal doses of 500-40,000 IU/d were associated with increases in the vitamin D content of breast milk (Polskin et al., 1945; Hollis et al., 1982; Ala-Houhala, 1985). Nevertheless, the amount of vitamin D that the nursing infant would be expected to ingest is below the RDA of vitamin D for infants.*

A massive maternal dose of 100,400 IU of vitamin D per day for 25 days postpartum resulted in significantly increased breast milk concentrations (Greer et al., 1984). Although the estimated amount of vitamin D that the nursing infant ingested was 14 times the RDA, no clinical symptoms of vitamin D toxicity or hypercalcemia were observed in the infant.

Nursing infants whose mothers were supplemented with 500 or 1000 IU of vitamin D per day for six weeks had significantly higher serum concentrations of 25-hydroxyvitamin D than nursing infants whose mothers were not supplemented (Rothberg et al., 1982). No adverse effects were observed in the infants.

The American Academy of Pediatrics regards vitamin D to be safe to take while breast-feeding (Committee on Drugs, American Academy of Pediatrics, 1994).

Key References

Ala-Houhala M: 25-hydroxyvitamin D levels during breast-feeding with or without maternal or infantile supplementation of vitamin D. J Pediatr Gastroenterol Nutr 4:220-226, 1985.

Chan GM, Buchino JJ, Mehlhorn D, et al.: Effect of vitamin D on pregnant rabbits and their offspring. Pediatr Res 13:121-126, 1979.

*RDA for infants six months or younger: 75 IU/kg.

Committee on Drugs, American Academy of Pediatrics: The transfer of drugs and other chemicals into human milk. Pediatrics 93(1):137-150, 1994.

Ewart AK, Morris CA, Atkinson D, et al.: Hemizygosity at the elastin locus in a developmental disorder, Williams syndrome. Nature Genet 5:11-16, 1993.

Ford JA, Davidson DC, McIntosh WB, et al.: Neonatal rickets in Asian immigrant population. Br Med J 3:211-212, 1973.

Friedman WF: Vitamin D and the supravalvular aortic stenosis syndrome. Adv Teratol 3:85-96, 1968.

Friedman WF, Mills LF: The relationship between vitamin D and the craniofacial and dental anomalies of the supravalvular aortic stenosis syndrome. Pediatrics 43:12-18, 1969.

Friedman WF, Roberts WC: Vitamin D and the supravalvar aortic stenosis syndrome. The transplacental effects of vitamin D on the aorta of the rabbit. Circulation 34:77-86, 1966.

Goodenday LS, Gordon GS: No risk from vitamin D in pregnancy. Ann Intern Med 75:807-808, 1971.

Greer FR, Hollis BW, Napoli JL: High concentrations of vitamin D_2 in human milk associated with pharmacologic doses of vitamin D_2. J Pediatr 105(1):61-64, 1984.

Hollis BW, Breer FR, Tsang RC: The effects of oral vitamin D supplementation and ultraviolet phototherapy on the antirachitic sterol content of human milk. Calcif Tissue Int Suppl 34:552, 1982.

Moncrieff M, Fadahunsi TO: Congenital rickets due to maternal vitamin D deficiency. Arch Dis Child 49:810-811, 1974.

NRC (National Research Council): *Recommended Dietary Allowances, 10th ed. Report of the Subcommittee on the Tenth Edition of the RDAs, Food and Nutrition Board, Commission on Life Sciences.* Washington, DC: National Academy Press, 1989, p 262.

O'Brien J, Rosenwasser S, Feingold M, Lin A: Prenatal exposure to milk with excessive vitamin D supplements. Teratology 47(5):387, 1993.

Polskin LJ, Kramer B, Sobel AE: Secretion of vitamin D in milk of women fed fish liver oil. J Nutr 30:451, 1945.

Rothberg AD, Pettifor JM, Cohen DF, et al.: Maternal-infant vitamin D relationships during breast-feeding. J Pediatr 101(4):500-503, 1982.

VITAMIN E
(Aquasol E®, TocopherCaps®, Vita-Plus E®)

Vitamin E is an essential nutrient. This fat-soluble vitamin has been used in large doses as an antioxidant. The US recommended dietary allowance (RDA) of vitamin E in pregnancy is 16.7 units (10 mg)/d (NRC, 1989). Oral doses of 60-75 units/d are used to treat deficiency states.

Teratogenic Risk

Magnitude of teratogenic risk to child born after exposure during gestation:	*Undetermined*
Quality and quantity of data on which risk estimate is based:	*Poor*

No epidemiological studies of congenital anomalies in infants born to women who took large doses of vitamin E during pregnancy have been reported.

In most studies, the frequency of malformations was no greater than expected among the offspring of rats or mice treated with vitamin E during pregnancy in doses hundreds to thousands of times the human RDA (Sato et al., 1973; Hook et al., 1974; Krasavage & Terhaar, 1977; Hurley et al., 1983; Kappus & Diplock, 1992). An increased frequency of cleft palate was observed in the offspring of mice given 750-1500 times the human RDA of vitamin E in one investigation (Momose et al., 1972). The relevance of this observation to the use of vitamin E in conventional doses in human pregnancy is unknown.

Risk Related to Breast-feeding

Vitamin E is a normal constituent of breast milk. Levels of vitamin E are highest in colostrum, and by four to six days postpartum infant serum levels reach those found in adult serum (Marx, 1985; Ostrea et al., 1986; Zheng et al., 1993).

Topical application of vitamin E to sore nipples each time after nursing for 2.5 days induced a significant increase in serum levels of the infants compared to those of infants whose mothers used no topical treatment (Marx et al., 1985). It is not known if the elevated serum levels were the result of higher breast milk concentrations of vitamin E or direct ingestion by the nursing infant. Nevertheless, the serum levels measured in the exposed infants were still within the normal range of vitamin E for infants. No adverse effects were observed in any of the nursed infants.

Key References

Hook EB, Healy KM, Niles AM, Skalko RG: Vitamin E: Teratogen or anti-teratogen? Lancet 1:809, 1974.

Hurley LS, Dungan DD, Keen CL, Lonnerdal B: The effects of vitamin E on zinc deficiency teratogenesis in rats. J Nutr 113:1875-1877, 1983.

Kappus H, Diplock AT: Tolerance and safety of vitamin E: A toxicological position report. Free Radic Biol Med 13(1):55-74, 1992.

Krasavage WJ, Terhaar CJ: d-α-Tocopheryl poly(ethylene glycol) 1000 succinate. Acute toxicity, subchronic feeding, reproduction, and teratologic studies in the rat. J Agric Food Chem 25:273-278, 1977.

Marx CM, Izquierdo A, Driscoll JW, et al.: Vitamin E concentrations in serum of newborn infants after topical use of vitamin E by nursing mothers. Am J Obstet Gynecol 152:668-670, 1985.

Momose Y, Akiyoshi S, Mori K, et al.: On teratogenicity of vitamin E. Mie Kenritsu Daigakubu Igakubu Kaibogaku Kyoshitsu Gyosekishu 20:27-35, 1972.

NRC (National Research Council): *Recommended Dietary Allowances, 10th ed. Report of the Subcommittee on the Tenth Edition of the RDAs, Food and Nutrition Board, Commission on Life Sciences.* Washington, DC: National Academy Press, 1989 p 262.

Ostrea EM, Balun JE, Winkler R, Porter T: Influence of breastfeeding on the restoration of the low serum concentration of vitamin E and beta-carotene in the newborn infant. Am J Obstet Gynecol 154:1014-1017, 1986.

Sato Y: [Study of developmental pharmacology on vitamin E.] Folia Pharmacol Jpn 69:293-298, 1973.

Zheng M-C, Zhou LS, Zhang GF: α-tocopherol content of breast milk in China. J Nutr Sci Vitaminol 39:517-520, 1993.

VITAPLUS E® *See Vitamin E*

VIVARIN® *See Caffeine*

VOLMAX® *See* Albuterol

VZIG *See* Varicella-Zoster Immune Globulin

WARFARIN
(Coumadin®, Panwarfin®, Sofarin®)

Warfarin is an anticoagulant that depresses synthesis of vitamin K-dependent clotting factors. Warfarin is given orally or parenterally in doses of 2-15 mg/d to treat thromboembolic disorders. Warfarin is also employed as a rodenticide.

Teratogenic Risk

*Magnitude of teratogenic
risk to child born after
exposure during gestation:*   *Small to moderate*

*Quality and quantity of data
on which risk estimate is based:*   *Good*

Available data deal with chronic use of warfarin in therapeutic doses.

A very uncommon but strikingly similar pattern of congenital anomalies has been observed in more than 50 children born to women treated with warfarin during pregnancy (Warkany, 1976; Hall et al., 1980; Stevenson et al., 1980; Stein et al., 1984; Zakzouk, 1986; Khera, 1987; Wong et al., 1993). Frequent features of this pattern of anomalies, which is called the "warfarin embryopathy" or "fetal warfarin syndrome," include nasal hypoplasia, stippled epiphyses on radiographs, and growth retardation.

The greatest period of susceptibility to the skeletal features of fetal warfarin syndrome is in the latter half of the first trimester of pregnancy. On the basis of published experience with warfarin use in pregnancy (an obviously biased sample), it has been estimated that about 10% of infants born alive to mothers who take warfarin during pregnancy have warfarin embryopathy (Hall et al., 1980). In one series of 38 children who had been born to women treated with warfarin throughout pregnancy and in whom physical examinations were performed to look for features of warfarin embryopathy, one child (3%) had typical features of warfarin embryopathy and two others (5%) had mild manifestations of this condition (Salazar et al., 1984). In another series of 37 infants born to women who were treated with "coumarin-like" drugs throughout the first and second trimesters of pregnancy, three (8%) had typical features of warfarin embryopathy (Born et al., 1992). In contrast, none of 20 children born to women treated with a strictly controlled low (5 mg/d or less) dose of warfarin throughout pregnancy had warfarin embryopathy on thorough evaluation (Cotrufo et al., 1991). No infants with warfarin embryopathy were seen among 36 born to women who took warfarin throughout pregnancy in another series (Sbarouni & Oakley, 1994).

Central nervous system (CNS) and eye anomalies have been observed unusually often among the children of mothers who were treated with warfarin during pregnancy (Ville et al., 1993; Wong et al., 1993; Pati & Helmbrecht, 1994). These abnormalities may occur in association with other features of warfarin embryopathy or in otherwise unaffected infants whose mothers took warfarin during gestation. These CNS and eye anomalies may occur with maternal use of warfarin after the first trimester. On the basis of published experience, the frequency of CNS structural anomalies among liveborn infants whose mothers took warfarin during pregnancy has been estimated to be about 3% (Hall et al., 1980).

Two infants with fatal diaphragmatic hernia who were born to women treated with warfarin throughout pregnancy have been described (O'Donnell et al., 1985; Normann & Stray-Pedersen, 1989). Neither child was noted to have features of warfarin embryopathy, but the clinical description is quite limited in both reports. It is not clear whether diaphragmatic hernia is an occasional feature of warfarin embryopathy.

The frequency of stillbirth appears to be substantially increased in warfarin-exposed pregnancies, and spontaneous abortion is also more common than expected (Hall et al., 1980; Sheikhzadeh et al., 1983; Vitali et al., 1986; Sareli et al., 1989; Sbarouni & Oakley, 1994). In a series of 128 pregnancies in women who were treated throughout gestation with warfarin because of cardiac valve replacement, the rate of stillbirth was 7% and the rate of miscarriage was 28% (Salazar et al., 1984).

Maternal warfarin use late in pregnancy has been associated with fetal, placental, and neonatal hemorrhage (Stevenson et al., 1980; Salazar et al., 1984; Vitali et al., 1986; Sareli et al., 1989). Such hemorrhage may result from the pharmacologic action of warfarin.

An increased frequency of fetal death has been reported among the offspring of mice treated during pregnancy with warfarin in doses 1-4 times those used in humans (Kronick et al., 1974). An increased frequency of minor skeletal anomalies was also observed in this study. No increase in the frequency of major malformations was observed among the offspring of pregnant rabbits treated with 10-100 times the usual human dose of warfarin (Grote & Weinmann, 1973). Increased frequencies of fetal death and of hemorrhages of the brain, face, eyes, ears, and occasionally limbs were seen among the offspring of rats treated during pregnancy with warfarin in doses 15-500 times those used in humans (Howe & Webster, 1990). Skeletal anomalies were not seen in the affected fetuses in this study, but similar treatment of the pups postnatally produced marked maxillonasal hypoplasia (Howe & Webster, 1992). Much of the skeletal maturation that occurs prenatally in humans does not occur until after birth in rats.

Risk Related to Breast-feeding

Warfarin was undetectable in the breast milk of 13 lactating women who were treated with warfarin (Orme et al., 1977). No warfarin was detected in the serum of the seven infants which were nursed. All infants had normal prothrombin times (de Swiet & Lewis, 1977).

The American Academy of Pediatrics regards warfarin to be safe to use while breast-feeding (Committee on Drugs, American Academy of Pediatrics, 1994).

Key References

Born D, Martinez EE, Almeida PAM, et al.: Pregnancy in patients with prosthetic heart valves: The effects of anticoagulation on mother, fetus, and neonate. Am Heart J 124:413-417, 1992.

Committee on Drugs, American Academy of Pediatarics: The transfer of drugs and other chemicals into human milk. Pediatrics 93(1):137-150, 1994.

Cotrufo M, de Luca TSL, Calabro R, et al.: Coumarin anticoagulation during pregnancy in patients with mechanical valve prostheses. Eur J Cardiothorac Surg 5:300-305, 1991.

de Swiet M, Lewis PJ: Excretion of anticoagulants in human milk. N Engl J Med 297:1471, 1977.

Grote VW, Weinmann I: [Examination of the active substances coumarin and rutin in a teratogenic trial with rabbits.] Arzneimittelforsch 23:1319-1320, 1973.

Hall JG, Pauli RM, Wilson KM: Maternal and fetal sequelae of anticoagulation during pregnancy. Am J Med 68:122-140, 1980.

Howe AM, Webster WS: Exposure of the pregnant rat to warfarin and vitamin K1: An animal model of intraventricular hemorrhage in the fetus. Teratology 42:413-420, 1990.

Howe AM, Webster WS: The warfarin embryopathy: A rat model showing maxillonasal hypoplasia and other skeletal disturbances. Teratology 46:379-390, 1992.

Khera KS: Maternal toxicity of drugs and metabolic disorders - A possible etiologic factor in the intrauterine death and congenital malformation: A critique on human data. CRC Crit Rev Toxicol 17:345-375, 1987.

Kronick J, Phelps NE, McCallion DJ, Hirsh J: Effects of sodium warfarin administered during pregnancy in mice. Am J Obstet Gynecol 118:819-823, 1974.

Normann EK, Stray-Pedersen B: Warfarin-induced fetal diaphragmatic hernia. Case report. Br J Obstet Gynaecol 96:729-730, 1989.

O'Donnell D, Meyers AM, Sevitz H, et al.: Pregnancy after renal transplantation. Aust NZ J Med 15:320-325, 1985.

Orme M, Lewis PJ, de Swiet M, et al.: May mothers given warfarin breast-feed their infants? Br Med J 1:1564-1565, 1977.

Pati S, Helmbrecht GD: Congenital schizencephaly associated with in utero warfarin exposure. Reprod Toxicol 8(2):115-120, 1994.

Salazar E, Zajarias A, Gutierrez N, Iturbe I: The problem of cardiac valve prostheses, anticoagulants, and pregnancy. Circulation 70(Suppl I):I169-I177, 1984.

Sareli P, England JM, Berk MR, et al.: Maternal and fetal sequelae of anticoagulation during pregnancy in patients with mechanical heart valve prostheses. Am J Cardiol 63:1462-1465, 1989.

Sbarouni E, Oakley CM: Outcome of pregnancy in women with valve prostheses. Br Heart J 71:196-201, 1994.

Sheikhzadeh A, Ghabusi P, Hakim SH, et al.: Congestive heart failure in valvular heart disease in pregnancies with and without valvular prostheses and anticoagulant therapy. Clin Cardiol 6:465-470, 1983.

Stevenson RE, Burton M, Ferlauto GJ, Taylor HA: Hazards of oral anticoagulants during pregnancy. JAMA 243:1549-1551, 1980.

Stein Z, Kline J, Kharrazi M: What is a teratogen? Epidemiological criteria. Issues Rev Teratol 2:23-66, 1984.

Ville Y, Jenkins E, Shearer MJ, et al.: Fetal intraventricular haemorrhage and maternal warfarin. Lancet 341:1211, 1993.

Vitali E, Donatelli F, Quaini E, et al.: Pregnancy in patients with mechanical prosthetic heart valves. J Cardiovasc Surg 27:221-227, 1986.

Warkany J: Warfarin embryopathy. Teratology 14:205-210, 1976.

Wong V, Cheng CH, Chan KC: Fetal and neonatal outcome of exposure to anticoagulants during pregnancy. Am J Med Genet 45:17-21, 1993.

Zakzouk MS: The congenital warfarin syndrome. J Laryngol Otol 100:215-219, 1986.

WYMOX® *See* Amoxicillin

XANAX® *See* Alprazolam

ZANTAC® *See* Ranitidine

ZARONTIN® *See* Ethosuximide

ZIDOVUDINE
(AZT®, Retovir®)

Zidovudine (AZT) is a thymidine analog that is given orally to treat AIDS or AIDS-related complex and to prevent the transmission during pregnancy of human immunodeficiency virus (HIV) from mother to child. The usual oral dose of zidovudine is 600 mg/d. Zidovudine may also be given parenterally in doses of 6-12 mg/kg of body weight (300-600 mg for a 110 pound woman) per day.

Teratogenic Risk

*Magnitude of teratogenic
risk to child born after
exposure during gestation:*   *Unlikely*

*Quality and quantity of data
on which risk estimate is based:*   *Poor to fair*

Therapeutic doses of zidovudine are unlikely to pose a substantial teratogenic risk, but the data are insufficient to state that there is no risk.

No congenital anomalies attributable to zidovudine were noted among 45 infants born to pregnant women treated with this medication for HIV infection in one series (Sperling et al., 1992). Twelve of these pregnancies were treated in the first trimester. No serious or persistent adverse effect of maternal zidovudine treatment during the second and third trimester of pregnancy was found among 180 infants born to treated women in a randomized controlled trial (ACTG, 1994) or in small series of children born to women with HIV infection and followed to one to two years of age (Ferrazin et al., 1993; O'Sullivan et al., 1993).

Macrocytic anemia, which is usually mild and transient, is often observed among the infants of women who have been treated with zidovudine during pregnancy (Watts et al., 1991; Sperling et al., 1992; Ferrazin et al., 1993; O'Sullivan et al., 1993; ACTG, 1994). Anemia is a common side effect of zidovudine treatment in adults.

Fetal or neonatal death and hematological alterations often occurred among the offspring of macaques treated during pregnancy with up to 2.5 times the human dose of zidovudine (Tarantal et al., 1993). Increased rates of embryonic death were observed among pregnant mice given zidovudine in doses that were greater than those used in humans but which produced blood levels below those encountered with human therapeutic doses (Toltzis et al., 1991; Gogu et al., 1992). No increase in malformations was observed among the offspring of pregnant mice, rats, or rabbits treated, respectively, with <1-12.5, 5-25 or 5-21 times the human dose of zidovudine (Ayers, 1988; Stahlmann et al., 1989; Sieh et al., 1992). A high rate of postnatal death was observed among the pups of rats treated with high doses in one study (Stahlmann et al., 1989). The relevance of these observations to the therapeutic use of zidovudine in human pregnancy is unknown.

Risk Related to Breast-feeding

No information regarding the distribution of zidovudine in breast milk has been published. Because of the possibility that HIV may be transmitted from the mother to the nursing infant, the USP DI (1995) recommends that women taking zidovudine for treatment of HIV refrain from breast-feeding.

Key References

ACTG (AIDS Clinical Trials Group): Clinical alert: Important therapeutic information on the benefit of zidovudine (AZT) for the prevention of the transmission of HIV from mother to infant. Study conducted by the Pediatric ACTG of the National Institute of Allergy & Infectious Diseases in collaboration with the National Institute of Child Health and Human Development and Institut National de la Sante et de la Recherche Medicale and Agence Nationale de Recheres sur le SIDA. Cited by: National Library of Medicine; BRS Information Technologies, MacLean VA, 1994.

Ayers K: Preclinical toxicology of zidovudine. Am J Med 85(Suppl 2A):186-188, 1988.

Ferrazin A, De Maria A, Gotta C, et al.: Zidovudine therapy of HIV-1 infection during pregnancy: Assessment of the effect on the newborns. J Acquir Immune Defic Syndr 6:376-379, 1993.

Gogu SR, Beckman BS, Agrawal KC: Amelioration of zidovudine-induced fetal toxicity in pregnant mice. Antimicrob Agents Chemother 36(11):2370-2374, 1992.

O'Sullivan MJ, Boyer PJJ, Scott GB, et al.: The pharmacokinetics and safety of zidovudine in the third trimester of pregnancy for women infected with human immunodeficiency virus and their infants: Phase I Acquired Immunodeficiency Syndrome Clinical Trials Group study (protocol 082). Am J Obstet Gynecol 168:1510-1516, 1993.

Sieh E, Coluzzi ML, Cusella de Angelis MG, et al.: The effects of AZT and DDI on pre- and postimplantation mammalian embryos: An in vivo and in vitro study. AIDS Res Hum Retroviruses 8(5):639-649, 1992.

Sperling RS, Stratton P, O'Sullivan MJ, et al.: A survey of zidovudine use in pregnant women with human immunodeficiency virus infection. N Engl J Med 326(13):857-861, 1992.

Stahlmann R, Rahn U, Baumann-Wilschke I, Thiel R: Pharmacokinetics, prenatal toxicity and hematotoxicity of zidovudine in rats. Nauyn-Schmiedebergs Arch Pharmacol 339(Suppl):R30, 1989.

Tarantal AF, Spanggord RJ, Hendrickx AG: Prenatal treatment of the macaque fetus (*M. mulatta*) with AZT in utero. Teratology 47(5):437, 1993.

Toltzis P, Marx CM, Kleinman N, et al.: Zidovudine-associated embryonic toxicity in mice. J Infect Dis 163:1212-1218, 1991.

Watts DH, Brown ZA, Tartaglione T, et al.: Pharmacokinetic disposition of zidovudine during pregnancy. J Infect Dis 163:226-232, 1991.

USP DI: Zidovudine. In: *USP DI (USP Dispensing Information), Volume 1. Drug Information for the Health Care Professional,* 15th ed. Rockville, Md.: The US Pharmacopeial Convention, 1995, p 2823.

ZIDOVUDINE IN PREGNANCY REGISTRY

A registry on the inadvertent use of zidovudine during pregnancy has been established by Burroughs Wellcome with collaboration of the Centers for Disease Control and the American Social Health Association. The registry attempts to prospectively follow such pregnancy to ascertain exposure information and the pregnancy outcome. A report summarizing the progress and findings of the registry is prepared periodically, and is available to health professionals from the address below.

Health professionals are encouraged to report all cases of zidovudine use during pregnancy to Dr. Elizabeth B. Andrews at the address below, or by telephone: (800) 722-9292, ext. 8465.

Elizabeth B. Andrews, Ph.D.
Head, Epidemiology Section
Epidemiology, Surveillance & Pharmacoeconomics Division
Burroughs Wellcome Co.
3030 Cornwallis Rd.
Research Triangle Park, NC 27709

ZINACEF® *See* Cefuroxime

ZIRTEK® *See* Cetirizine

ZOLOFT® *See* Sertraline

ZOVIRAX® *See* Acyclovir

ZYLOPRIM® *See* Allopurinol

APPENDIX 1

List of Agents Available in TERIS

Note: Numbers following the agent names are TERIS reference numbers

1,1,2,2-Tetrachloroethane	1940	Aminosalicylic Acid	1569
1,1,2-Trichloroethane	5912	Amiodarone	5337
Acebutolol	1510	Amitriptyline	1088
Acetaldehyde	1207	Ammonium Lactate	5191
Acetaminophen	1017	Amobarbital	5340
Acetic Acid	3000	Amoxapine	1375
Acetohexamide	3001	Amoxicillin	1374
Acetohydroxamic Acid	1512	Amphotericin B	1450
Acetyl Tributyl Citrate	5176	Ampicillin	1019
Acetylcysteine	3002	Amrinone	1265
Acetyldigitoxin	1264	Amsacrine	5343
Acitretin	3201	Amyl Nitrite	5192
Actodigin	3069	Amylase	5193
Acyclovir	1079	Amylocaine	1289
Aflatoxins	1568	Anisotropine	5195
Alanine	5177	Anthralin	5196
Albumin	5178	Anti-Inhibitor Coagulant	5198
Albuterol	1073	Antihemophilic Factor	5117
Alclometasone Dipropionate	5179	Antipyrine	1360
Alcohol	1127	Antivenin (Crotalidae)	5199
Aldicarb	1782	Antivenin (Micrurus Fulvius)	2830
Alfentanil	3003	Aprobarbital	3006
Aliflurane	1244	Aptocaine	1290
Allantoin	3004	Arginine	1263
Allopurinol	1063	Articaine	1296
Aloe	2835	Ascorbic Acid	1183
Alpha Interferon	4032	Asparaginase	3007
Alpha-1-Proteinase Inhibitor	5180	Aspartame	1102
Alpha-Ketoglutaric Acid	5181	Aspirin	1010
Alphaxalone/Alphadolone	1224	Astemizole	1508
Alprazolam	1048	Atenolol	1033
Alprenolol	1884	Atracurium	3008
Alprostadil	2546	Atropine	1081
Alteplase	5182	Auranofin	1341
Aluminum Hydroxide	1338	Aurothioglucose	1342
Amantadine	1522	Aurothioglycanide	1343
Ambruticin	1266	Azacitidine	5355
Amcinonide	5184	Azaconazole	1424
Amdinocillin/Pivamdinocillin	5185	Azatadine	1352
Amikacin	1526	Azathioprine	1204
Amiloride	1075	Azlocillin	5200
Aminacrine	3005	Bacampicillin	5360
Aminobenzoate	5020	Bacitracin	1091
Aminocaproic Acid	2836	Barium	1337
Aminoglutethimide	2837	BCG Vaccine	5201
Aminohippurate	6050	Beclomethasone	1152
Aminopterin	1011	Belladonna	1335

Bendectin	1007	Capsaicin	2643
Bendroflumethiazide	3009	Captan	1482
Benomyl	1483	Captopril	1103
Benoxinate	1308	Caramiphen	1319
Benzalkonium Salts	1840	Carbamazepine	1118
Benzamine	1291	Carbazeran	1080
Benzene	1032	Carbenicillin	1700
Benzocaine	1292	Carbidopa	1129
Benzonatate	3010	Carbinoxamine	1162
Benzoyl Peroxide	5037	Carboxymethylcellulose	2874
Benzphetamine	3011	Carbutamide	1487
Benzthiazide	3012	Carisoprodol	3020
Benztropine	1125	Carmustine	1399
Benzyl Benzoate	1334	Cascara Sagrada	4110
Beta-Carotene	1909	Cefaclor	1053
Beta-Interferon	1696	Cefadroxil	1149
Betamethasone	1101	Cefazolin	2880
Betaxolol	1631	Cefotaxime	1384
Bethanechol	3013	Cefuroxime	1706
Bifonazole	1464	Cellulose, Microcrystalline	1364
Biphenamine	1316	Cephalexin	1027
Bisacodyl	3014	Cephalothin	2068
Bismuth Subgallate	1336	Cephradine	3021
Bisoprolol	1634	Cetirizine	1507
Bleomycin	4026	Cetyl Alcohol	2849
Borate	5085	Cetylpyridinium	1929
Bromocriptine	5377	Charcoal, Activated	3022
Bromodiphenhydramine	2845	Chloral Hydrate	1356
Bromperidol	1116	Chloramphenicol	1215
Brompheniramine	1089	Chlordane	1029
Buclizine	1876	Chlordantoin	1467
Bufexamac	4073	Chlordiazepoxide	1114
Bumetanide	3015	Chlormezanone	1370
Bupivacaine	1267	Chloroform	1031
Bupropion	3148	Chloroprocaine	1269
Buspirone	3016	Chloroquine	1216
Butabarbital	5086	Chlorothiazide	1158
Butacaine	1293	Chloroxine	3023
Butalbital	1061	Chloroxylenol	3024
Butamben	1295	Chlorpheniramine	1085
Butanilicaine	1294	Chlorpromazine	1164
Butethamine	1268	Chlorpropamide	1028
Butoconazole	1425	Chlorpyrifos	1956
Butopamine	1261	Chlortetracycline	1951
Caffeine	1128	Chlorthalidone	1062
Calamine	3017	Chlorzoxazone	1117
Calcitonin	1640	Cholera Vaccine	3026
Calcium Salts	1362	Chorionic Gonadotropin	2187
Camphor	3018	Chromium Salts	3027
Cantharidin	3019	Ciclopirox	1468
Capreomycin	2754	Cigarette Smoking	1166

Cilastatin	5025	Denofungin	1427
Cimetidine	1024	Deslanoside	1406
Cinoxacin	1966	Desmopressin	3039
Ciprofloxacin	5005	Desonide	3040
Citrate	1134	Desoximetasone	1163
Clarithromycin	2857	Dexamethasone	1643
Clemastine	3028	Dexivacaine	1252
Clidinium Bromide	1115	Dexpanthenol	3041
Clindamycin	1972	Dextranomer	5164
Clioquinol	3029	Dextroamphetamine	4001
Clofazimine	4002	Dextromethorphan	1187
Clomiphene	1977	Dextrothyroxine	5089
Clomipramine	4003	Diamocaine	1270
Clonazepam	1387	Diazepam	1003
Clonidine	1060	Diazoxide	3043
Clorazepate	1052	Dibromochloropropane	5490
Clotrimazole	1100	Dibucaine	1271
Cloxacillin	1711	Diclofenac	5501
Coal Tar	3031	Dicloxacillin	1713
Coal Tar Naphtha	2395	Dicumarol	2051
Cocaine	1005	Dicyclomine	1021
Codeine	1023	Diethylpropion	1333
Colchicine	1982	Diethylstilbestrol	1220
Colistimethate	3032	Difenoxin	2895
Copper Deficiency	3068	Diflorasone	2057
Copper Iud's	1339	Diflunisal	1113
Cortisone	1094	Digoxin	1013
Coumarin	2772	Dihydroergotamine	1321
Cromolyn	3033	Dihydroxyacetone	2854
Crotamiton	2866	Diloxanide	2762
Cuprimyxin	1426	Diltiazem	1076
Cyanocobalamin	5470	Dimenhydrinate	2063
Cyclacillin	3034	Dimercaprol	1390
Cyclobenzaprine	1097	Dimethisoquin	1298
Cyclomethycaine	1297	Dimethyl Sulfoxide (DMSO)	2071
Cyclopropane	1226	Dinitrophenol	1490
Cycloserine	2755	Dinoseb	2076
Cyclosporine	1377	Dioxybenzone	2900
Cyprex	1779	Diperodon	1299
Cyproheptadine	1320	Diphenhydramine	1050
Cytarabine	5473	Diphenidol	3044
Cytomegalovirus	1184	Diphenoxylate	1112
Dacarbazine	3035	Diphenylpyraline	3045
Danazol	2017	Diphtheria Antitoxin	3046
Danthron	4101	Dipotassium Phosphate	3047
Dapsone	2746	Dipyridamole	1057
Daunorubicin	2019	Dipyrithione	1428
Deferoxamine	3036	Dipyrone	5528
Dehydrocholic Acid	3037	Disodium Phosphate	3048
Demecarium	3038	Disopyramide	1135
Demeclocycline	6087	Disulfiram	1391

Divalproex	3049	Etoposide	5558
Dobutamine	1407	Etoxadrol	1253
Doconazole	1452	Etretinate	2137
Docusate	3050	Euprocin	1301
Doxepin	1090	Factor IX Complex	5116
Doxorubicin	2901	Famotidine	2139
Doxycycline	1148	Felbamate	2960
Doxylamine	1020	Fenoprofen	1105
Drocode	1131	Fenticonazole	1429
Droperidol	3051	Filgrastim	3090
Dyclonine	1300	Filipin	1430
Echothiophate	3052	Flavoxate	4025
Econazole	1469	Flecainide	3065
Edrophonium	3053	Floxuridine	3066
Electrical Shock	4117	Fluconazole	1181
Electroconvulsive Therapy	1379	Flucytosine	1454
Emetine	2763	Flunarizine	5568
Emotional Stress	1180	Flunisolide	4024
Enalapril	2103	Fluocinolone	2954
Encainide	3056	Fluocinonide	1140
Enflurane	1227	Fluoride	5060
Enilconazole	1453	Fluorouracil	4023
Enoximone	1416	Fluoxetine	5993
Ephedrine	1369	Fluoxymesterone	4022
Epinephrine	1210	Flurandrenolide	4021
Epoetin Alfa	2728	Flurazepam	1045
Epstein-Barr Virus	1202	Flurbiprofen	1710
Ergoloid Mesylates	1157	Fluroxene	1245
Ergotamin	5541	Folic Acid	1612
Erythrityl Tetranitrate	3058	Fomocaine	1302
Erythromycin	1038	Formaldehyde	2159
Ethacrynic Acid	3057	Framycetin	2957
Ethambutol	2115	Fungimycin	1431
Ethaverine	2956	Furazolidone	4051
Ethchlorvynol	3059	Furosemide	1009
Ether	1228	Gabapentin	2729
Ethinamate	3060	Gasoline	1199
Ethinyl Estradiol	1258	Gemeprost	3136
Ethionamide	2118	Gemfibrozil	4016
Ethoheptazine	2081	Gentamicin	5026
Ethosuximide	1388	Gentian Violet	4020
Ethotoin	1394	Glipizide	4017
Ethyl Chloride	1229	Glutethimide	2180
Ethylene	5070	Glyburide	3070
Ethylene Oxide	5172	Glycerin	4018
Ethylnorepinephrine	3061	Gold Sodium Thiomalate	1344
Ethynodiol Diacetate	2133	Gold-198	3256
Etidocaine	1272	Gonadorelin	3071
Etidronate	3062	Gramicidin	1092
Etomidate	1230	Griseofulvin	1455

Guaifenesin	1119	Influenza Vaccine	1485
Guanabenz	2189	Inositol	4031
Guanadrel	3072	Insulin	1211
Guanethidine	2190	Iodinated Glycerol	2923
Guanfacine	2191	Iodoquinol	4034
Halazepam	3073	Iohexol	4035
Halcinonide	3074	Ipecac	1353
Halofantrine	5009	Iron	1190
Haloperidol	1077	Isobucaine	1274
Haloprogin	3075	Isobutamben	1317
Halothane	1223	Isoetharine	4036
Hamycin	1456	Isoflurane	1231
Heparin	2202	Isomazole	1417
Hepatitis B Immune Globulin	5118	Isometheptene	2929
Hepatitis B Vaccine	2752	Isoniazid	2260
Heptachlor	1380	Isopropamide	1354
Heroin	1109	Isopropyl Myristate	2930
Herpes Simplex Virus	1108	Isoproterenol	2262
Hesperidin	3076	Isosorbide Dinitrate	1054
Hetastarch	3077	Isotretinoin	1041
Hexachlorophene	2208	Isoxsuprine	4028
Hexocyclium Methylsulfate	3078	Kalafungin	1432
Hexothiocaine	1303	Kanamycin	2272
Hexylcaine	1273	Kaolin	4037
Homatropin	1361	Ketamine	1232
Human Immunodeficiency		Ketoconazole	1457
Virus	1126	Ketorolac	2902
Hyaluronidase	3079	Labetalol	2279
Hydralazine	1120	Lactic Acid (Lactate)	4038
Hydrochlorothiazide	1014	Lactulose	1401
Hydrocodone	1322	Lanatoside C	1409
Hydrocortisone	1093	Lanolin	4039
Hydroflumethiazide	3080	Lecithins	4040
Hydrogen Peroxide	5029	Leucinocaine	1304
Hydromorphone	4008	Leuprolide	3085
Hydroquinone	4009	Levodopa	1130
Hydroxocobalamin	4010	Levonordefrin	4041
Hydroxyamphetamine	4011	Levorphanol	4043
Hydroxychloroquine	2765	Levothyroxine	1035
Hydroxydione	1257	Levoxadrol	1275
Hydroxyethyl Cellulose	4019	Lidocaine	1276
Hydroxypropyl Cellulose	4029	Lindane	1154
Hydroxyurea	2223	Lisinopril	6112
Hydroxyzine	1098	Lithium	1200
Hyoscyamine	1082	Lobeline	5204
Ibuprofen	1016	Lomofungin	1433
Ichthammol	4030	Lomustine	1400
Idoxuridine	4000	Loperamide	1355
Imipenem	2750	Loratadine	2659
Imipramine	1110	Lorazepam	1037
Indomethacin	1040	Lovastatin	2367

Lydimycin	1434	Metaraminol	4060
Lyme Disease	4098	Metaxalone	4061
Lymphocytic		Methacrylates	2323
Choriomeningitis		Methacycline	4062
Virus (LCMV)	5688	Methadone	2324
Lynestrenol	1260	Methamphetamine	1167
Lysergide	1170	Metharbital	4063
Mafenide	2305	Methazolamide	4064
Magaldrate	4044	Methdilazine	4065
Magnesium Hydroxide	4168	Methenamine	2331
Magnesium Sulfate	1616	Methimazole	2333
Malathion	1030	Methionine	2334
Manganese	5693	Methixene	1221
Mannitol	4045	Methocarbamol	4068
Maprotiline	1159	Methohexital	1233
Marijuana	1068	Methoserpidine	1600
Mazindol	4046	Methotrexate	1012
Measles Vaccine, Live	5122	Methoxamine	4069
Mebendazole	2312	Methoxsalen	4070
Mecamylamine	4047	Methoxyflurane	1234
Mechlorethamine	4048	Methsuximide	4072
Meclizine	1099	Methyclothiazide	1137
Meclocycline	4049	Methyl Mercaptan	1422
Meclofenamate	1144	Methylbenzethonium	4074
Medroxyprogesterone	2246	Methyldopa	1026
Mefenamic Acid	4052	Methylene Blue	2347
Mefloquine	3135	Methylergonovine	4075
Megestrol	4053	Methylparaben	6001
Melphalan	4054	Methylphenidate	2357
Menadiol	4055	Methylprednisolone	1147
Meningococcal		Methyltestosterone	2359
Polysaccharide Vaccine	4056	Methyprylon	4076
Menthol	4057	Methysergide	1222
Mepartricin	1471	Metoclopramide	1106
Mepenzolate	4058	Metocurine	4077
Meperidine	1383	Metolazone	1156
Mephenesin	1376	Metoprolol	1034
Mephenytoin	1395	Metronidazole	1002
Mephobarbital	1389	Metyrapone	4078
Mepivacaine	1277	Metyrosine	4079
Meprobamate	1372	Mexiletine	2368
Meprylcaine	1278	Mezlocillin	1716
Mercaptopurine	4059	Miconazole	1051
Mercury (Elemental)	1348	Midazolam	1250
Mesalamine	5187	Mifepristone (RU-486)	5174
Mescaline	1171	Milrinone	1410
Mesoridazine	2319	Minaxolone	1254
Mestranol	1262	Mineral Oil	4080
Metabutethamine	1279	Minocycline	1136
Metabutoxycaine	1305	Minoxidil	2374
Metaproterenol	1069	Mitomycin	1367

Mitotane	4081	Nystatin	1123
Molindone	4082	Octanoic Acid	1472
Molybdenum	2382	Octocrylene	2940
Mometasone Furoate	4083	Octodrine	1280
Monensin	1458	Octyl Methoxycinnamate	5002
Monobenzone	4084	Olsalazine	5052
Morphine	2387	Omega-3 Polyunsaturates	5003
Morrhuate	4085	Omega-6 Polyunsaturates	5051
Moxalactam	1392	Opium	5004
Mumps Skin Test Antigen	4086	Orconazole	1437
Mumps Virus	5021	Organic Mercury	1347
Mumps Virus Vaccine	4087	Orphenadrine	1323
Mupirocin	2937	Orthocaine	1306
Muromonab-CD3	4088	Ouabain	1411
Nabilone	2391	Ox Bile Extract	5006
Nadolol	1056	Oxacillin	1718
Nafcillin	1385	Oxamniquine	2768
Naftifine	1459	Oxandrolone	5007
Nalbuphine	1382	Oxazepam	1138
Nalidixic Acid	5173	Oxethazaine	1307
Naloxone	4089	Oxidized Cellulose	5008
Naltrexone	2393	Oxifungin	1438
Nandrolone	4090	Oxybenzone	5010
Naphazoline	4091	Oxybutynin	5011
Naproxen	1039	Oxychlorosene	5092
Narcobarbital	1256	Oxycodone	1074
Neomycin	1095	Oxymetazoline	5012
Neostigmine	1393	Oxymetholone	5013
Netilmicin	2402	Oxymorphone	5014
Niacin	1192	Oxyquinoline	5015
Niacinamide	4093	Oxytetracycline	2445
Niclosamide	2767	Oxytocin	1203
Nifedipine	1047	Padimate O	5001
Nifuratel	1460	Pamabrom	1357
Nifurmerone	1435	Pancuronium	5017
Nikethamide	4099	Pantothenate	1609
Nitralamine	1436	Papain	5018
Nitrofurantoin	1104	Papaverine	2455
Nitrofurazone	4095	Paraldehyde	1396
Nitroglycerin	1067	Parconazole	1439
Nitromersol	1174	Pargyline	5023
Nitrous Oxide	1235	Paromomycin	2769
Nizatidine	2938	Paroxetine	1768
Nonoxynols	1189	Partricin	1440
Norethindrone	2245	Parvovirus B19	4097
Norethynodrel	2244	Pectin	2942
Norfloxacin	2431	Pelrinone	1418
Norflurane	1246	Pemoline	5024
Norgestrel	2247	Pempidine	5121
Nortriptyline	4027	Penicillamine	5027
Nylidrin	5000	Penicillin	1066

Pentachlorophenol	2468	Polythiazide	5053
Pentaerythritol Tetranitrate	2471	Potassium Chloride	1043
Pentagastrin	5028	Povidone	1363
Pentamidine	2770	Pramoxine	1311
Pentazocine	1206	Prazepam	1139
Pentobarbital	5093	Praziquantel	2773
Pentoxifylline	2472	Prazosin	1049
Pepsin	5033	Prednisone/Prednisolone	1155
Permethrin	2771	Prilocaine	1281
Perphenazine	1324	Primidolol	1213
Peruvian Balsam	1491	Primidone	1214
Petrolatum	5030	Probenecid	4004
Phenacaine	1309	Probucol	2535
Phenacetin	2475	Procainamide	1133
Phenazopyridine	1151	Procaine	1282
Phencyclidine	1168	Prochlorperazine	1145
Phendimetrazine	5034	Proclonol	1441
Phenelzine	2477	Procyclidine	5055
Phenindamine	5035	Progestrone	1107
Pheniramine	1368	Proguanil	1936
Phenmetrazine	2479	Promethazine	1141
Phenobarbital	1083	Propanidid	1236
Phenol	2480	Propanocaine	1312
Phenolphthalein	1365	Proparacaine	1313
Phensuximide	1398	Propionate	5095
Phentermine	1325	Propofol	1251
Phenylbutazone	1326	Propoxycaine	1283
Phenylephrine	1086	Propoxyphene	1025
Phenylpropanolamine	1087	Propranolol	1006
Phenyltoloxamine	1327	Propylparaben	6002
Phenytoin	1022	Propylthiouracil	2544
Pilocarpine	1165	Proscillaridin	1412
Pimozide	2506	Protirelin	5864
Pindolol	5040	Protriptyline	5059
Piperacillin	1719	Pseudoephedrine	1161
Piperazine	5019	Psilocybine	1176
Piperocaine	1310	Psyllium	1193
Piperonyl Butoxide	2511	Pyrantel	2775
Piroxicam	1044	Pyrazinamide	2757
Piroximone	1419	Pyrethrins	2776
Pitcher Plant Distillate	5041	Pyridostigmine	1397
Plague Vaccine	5042	Pyridoxine	1018
Plasma Protein Fraction	5043	Pyrilamine	1358
Plicamycin	5044	Pyrimethamine	1217
Pneumococcal Vaccine	5045	Pyrithione	1473
Podophyllum	2524	Pyrrocaine	1284
Poliovirus Vaccine,	5047	Pyrrolnitrin	1474
Poliovirus Vaccine, Live	5048	Quazepam	1587
Polyestradiol Phosphate	5049	Quazinone	1415
Polyethylene Glycol	5050	Quazodine	1413
Polymyxin B	1096	Quinacrine	2557

Quinestrol	2558	Somatrem	5099
Quinethazone	5061	Somatropin	5098
Quinidine	1153	Sorbitol	1371
Quinine	1218	Spectinomycin	2751
Rabies Antiserum	5062	Spiramycin	3260
Rabies Immune Globulin	5063	Spironolactone	1122
Radon	4096	Stanozolol	5101
Ranitidine	1055	Staphylococcus Vaccine	2608
Rescinnamine	5066	Streptokinase	5102
Reserpine	1328	Streptomycin	1212
Resorcinol	5067	Sucralfate	5104
Rho(D) Immune Globulin	5071	Sulbactam	2616
Rhus Extracts	5046	Sulconazole	1445
Ribavirin	2574	Sulfabenzamide	5106
Riboflavin	1197	Sulfacetamide	1330
Ricinoleic Acid	5072	Sulfadiazine	6015
Rifampin	2758	Sulfadoxine	5107
Risocaine	1285	Sulfamethazine	1578
Rodocaine	1286	Sulfamethoxazole	1071
Roflurane	1247	Sulfapyridine	1495
Rubella Vaccine	1178	Sulfasalazine	1493
Rubella Virus	1177	Sulfathiazole	5108
Rutamycin	1442	Sulfinpyrazone	1402
Saccharin	1179	Sulfisoxazole	1331
Salicyl Alcohol	1287	Sulfurated Lime	5111
Salicylamide	1373	Sulindac	1058
Salmeterol	6166	Sumatriptan	5022
Salsalate	5075	Sutilains	5113
Scopafungin	1443	Talbutal	5124
Scopolamine	1084	Tamoxifen	2638
Sebacic Acid	2898	Tazolol	1414
Secobarbital	1690	Teflurane	1249
Selenium Sulfide	5076	Temazepam	1059
Senna	5077	Terazosin	5125
Sertraline	2720	Terbutaline	1111
Sevoflurane	1248	Terconazole	1462
Shark Liver Oil	5078	Terfenadine	4007
Simethicone	5079	Terpin Hydrate	1366
Sinefungin	1444	Testolactone	5126
Skin Test Antigens	5080	Testosterone	2646
Sodium Bicarbonate	5083	Tetanus Immune Globulin	5120
Sodium Chloride	1670	Tetanus Toxoid	3257
Sodium Citrate	1329	Tetracaine	1288
Sodium Lauryl Sulfate	1737	Tetrachloroethylene	2649
Sodium Oxybate	1237	Tetracycline	1004
Sodium Phosphates	1677	Tetrahydrozoline	5128
Sodium Polystyrene Sulfonate	1693	Thalidomide	2653
Sodium Salicylate	1502	Theophylline	1036
Sodium Sulfate	1679	Thiabendazole	2657
Sodium Tetradecyl Sulfate	1741	Thialbarbitone	1239
Sodium Thiosulfate	1642	Thiamine	1196

Thiamphenicol	1205	Trimethoprim	1072
Thiamylal	1238	Trimipramine	4071
Thiethylperazine	5129	Triprolidine	1332
Thimerosal	1349	Trolamine	5144
Thiopental	1240	Tryptophan	1381
Thioridazine	1065	Tubocurarine	2701
Thiothixene	1160	Ubiquinone	2705
Thiram	1476	Undecylenic Acid	1480
Ticarcillin	5136	Urethane	1142
Ticlatone	1477	Urofollitropin	5156
Tilactase	2932	Urokinase	2711
Tiletamine	1255	Valproic Acid	1008
Timolol	1046	Vancomycin	2753
Tin, Inorganic	1350	Varicella-Zoster Immune	
Tioconazole	1463	Globulin	3258
Tobramycin	2675	Varicella-Zoster Vaccine	3259
Tocainide	5137	Varicella-Zoster Virus	1201
Tolazamide	1064	Vecuronium	5158
Tolazoline	5139	Verapamil	1150
Tolbutamide	1143	Vidarabine	1386
Tolciclate	1478	Video Display Units	1175
Tolindate	1446	Vinblastine	5130
Tolmetin	1121	Vincristine	2724
Tolnaftate	5140	Vinyl Ether	1243
Toluene	1198	Viridofulvin	1448
Tolycaine	1314	Vitamin A	1182
Toxoplasmosis	1185	Vitamin D	1194
Tramazoline	1601	Vitamin E	1195
Tranylcypromine	2681	Warfarin	1078
Trazodone	1132	Xylometazoline	2739
Tretinoin	1572	Yeast Cell Derivative	5165
Triacetin	1479	Yellow Fever Vaccine	5166
Triafungin	1447	Yohimbine	5168
Triamcinolone	1124	Zalcitabine	2798
Triamterene	1015	Zidovudine	5169
Triazolam	1070	Zinc Oxide	2251
Tribromoethanol	1241	Zinc Salts	1351
Trichlormethiazide	5141	Zinc Undecylenate	1481
Trichloroethylene	1242	Zinoconazole	1449
Tridihexethyl	5142	Zolamine	1318
Trientine	2692	Zolpidem	2461
Trifluoperazine	1146		
Trifluridine	5145		
Trimecaine	1315		
Trimethadione/			
Paramethadione	1001		
Trimethobenzamide	1492		

APPENDIX 2

Resources for Information on
Pregnancy Exposures

Books

Barlow SM, Sullivan FM: *Reproductive Hazards of Industrial Chemicals*. London: Academic Press, 1982.

This book reviews the available clinical and animal data on the reproductive toxicity of approximately 50 industrial chemicals. Information regarding the teratogenic, mutagenic, and carcinogenic effects of each chemical is included.

Briggs GG, Freeman RK, Yaffe SJ: *Drugs in Pregnancy and Lactation, 4th ed*. Baltimore, Md.: Williams & Wilkins, 1994.

This reference contains over 700 monographs on fetal risks associated with prenatal exposure to drugs. The monographs also provide information regarding risks associated with the use of these drugs during lactation. Most of the information is based on human studies, although animal studies are included for a few of the monographs.

Folb PI, Graham Dukes MN (eds). *Drug Safety in Pregnancy*. Amsterdam: Elsevier Science Publishers BV, 1990.

This book provides a comprehensive review of the clinical literature pertaining to the safety of drugs for the fetus and pregnant woman. Animal and pharmacological data are included when relevant to the understanding of fetal toxicity. Material is presented according to categories of drugs.

Friedman JM, Polifka JE: *Teratogenic Effects of Drugs: A Resource for Clinicians (TERIS)*. Baltimore, Md.: The Johns Hopkins University Press, 1994.

This book was designed to assist physicians and other health care professionals in counseling pregnant women who have concerns about the possible effects of drugs and other agents on their developing babies. Risk assessments based on a consensus of ratings by the authors and five internationally-recognized authorities in clinical teratology are provided for each agent in the book.

Gilstrap LC, Little BB: *Drugs and Pregnancy*. New York: Elsevier, 1992.

This book provides clinicians with useful guidelines for clinical evaluation and patient counseling as well as information regarding the reproductive effects of commonly-used medications, occupational agents, and substances of abuse.

Koren G (ed). *Maternal-Fetal Toxicology. A Clinician's Guide*, 2nd ed. New York: Marcel Dekker, 1994

This book provides practical information for health care practitioners who counsel pregnant women regarding pregnancy exposures. In addition to briefly summarizing the relevant data on the teratogenic effects of various environmental and physical agents, the book includes a list of teratogen information programs. The editor's approach to counseling pregnant women regarding teratogenic risks is also described.

Paul M: *Occupational and Environmental Reproductive Hazards: A Guide for Clinicians*. Baltimore: Williams & Wilkins, 1993.

This is a general review of the principles of reproductive and developmental toxicology, the research methods used to assess the reproductive toxicity of common occupational and environmental agents, and the clinical management of patients faced with such agents. In addition, information on the reproductive toxicity of commonly-encountered agents, such as organic solvents, video display terminals, and household chemicals is included.

Schardein JL: *Chemically Induced Birth Defects, 2nd ed.* New York: Marcel Dekker, 1993.

This comprehensive reference book reviews available animal and human studies on the teratogenic effects of drugs and chemicals. Emphasis is placed on studies in which exposures took place during the period of organogenesis.

Scialli AR, Lione A, Boyle Padgett GK: *Reproductive Effects of Chemical, Physical, and Biologic Agents*. Baltimore, Md.: The Johns Hopkins University Press, 1995.

This book contains information on the reproductive toxicology of over 2800 physical and chemical agents. The summaries include information on the effects of these agents on male and female fertility and the infants of breast-feeding mothers as well as on embryonic and fetal development.

Shepard TH: *Catalog of Teratogenic Agents, 8th ed.* Baltimore, Md.: The Johns Hopkins University Press, 1995.

Shepard's Catalog provides a comprehensive compilation of animal and human research on the teratogenicity of chemical and environmental agents. The Catalog contains information on over 2500 agents and includes many references from the Japanese as well as the American and European literature.

Computerized Databases

REPROTEXT: Reproductive Hazard Reference by Betty Dabney.
Available on CD-ROM as part of the REPRORISK system (see below).

This database includes reviews of the reproductive, carcinogenic, and genetic effects of acute and chronic exposures to over 600 commonly-encountered industrial chemicals. The reviews include a numerical scale that ranks the general toxicity and a "grade-card" scale that suggests the level of reproductive hazard associated with each chemical.

REPROTOX: Reproductive Hazard Information by Anthony R. Scialli.
Available online, in a disk-based version for MS-DOS personal computers, and CD-ROM format from the Reproductive Toxicology Center, Columbia Hospital for Women Medical Center, Washington, DC. The database is also available on CD-ROM as part of the REPRORISK system (see below).

This is a frequently-updated version of the book by Dr. Scialli and his associates described above.

SHEPARD'S CATALOG OF TERATOGENIC AGENTS by Thomas H. Shepard.
Available online from the Department of Pediatrics, Box 356320 University of Washington, Seattle, WA 98195. The database is also available online and in a disk-based version for MS-DOS personal computers in conjunction with the TERIS database and on CD-ROM as part of the REPRORISK system (see both below).

This is a frequently-updated version of the Shepard's Catalog described above.

TERIS: Teratogen Information System by J.M. Friedman and Janine E. Polifka.

Available online and in a disk-based version for MS-DOS personal computers from Janine E. Polifka, TERIS Box 357920, University of Washington, Seattle, WA 98195-7920 and as part of the REPRORISK system (see below).

This is a frequently-updated version of the book by Friedman and Polifka described above. The electronic version includes an extensive list of alternate agent names that can be used to access the summaries.

REPRORISK system

This is a commercially-available CD-ROM that contains electronic versions of Reprotext, REPROTOX, Shepard's Catalog, and TERIS. The system is available from MICROMEDEX, Inc., 6200 S. Syracuse Way, Suite 300, Englewood , CO 80111-4740.

Drug Compendiums and Indexes

The following reference books include general pharmacology and prescribing information on drugs. Such information is essential when a physician is deciding whether or not to treat a pregnant or lacating woman with a particular medication. Some of these references provide pregnancy risk information; however, this is usually in the form of a legal disclaimer that does little to help the clinician assess pregnancy risks associated with use of a particular drug. We strongly discourage quoting pregnancy risks from these books to patients. Doing so frequently provokes unnecessary anxiety and usually does not provide a balanced view of the risk from the patient's perspective.

Drug Facts and Comparisons® St. Louis, Mo.: Fact and Comparisons, 1995.

Gilman AG, Rall TW, Nies AS, Taylor P (eds). *Goodman and Gilman's The Pharmacological Basis of Therapeutics*, 9th ed. New York: Pergamon Press, 1996.

Physician's Desk Reference, 49th ed. Montvale, NJ: Medical Economics Data, 1995.

Reynolds JEF, Parfitt K, Parsons AV, Sweetman SC (eds). *Martindale: The Extra Pharmacopeia*, 30th ed. London: Pharmaceutical Press, 1993.

USP DI (USP Dispensing Information), Volume 1. Drug Information for the Health Care Professional, 15th ed. Rockville, Md.: The US Pharmacopeial Convention, 1995.